PEDIATRIC GAST
APH
321-841-3339

Pediatric Gastroenterology   THE REQUISITES IN PEDIATRICS

SERIES EDITOR **Louis M. Bell,** MD
Patrick S. Pasquariello, Jr. Chair in General Pediatrics
Professor of Pediatrics
University of Pennsylvania School of Medicine
Chief, Division of General Pediatrics
Attending Physician, General Pediatrics and Infectious Diseases
The Children's Hospital of Philadelphia
Philadelphia, Pennsylvania

OTHER VOLUMES IN
THE REQUISITES IN PEDIATRICS SERIES

Orthopaedics and Sports Medicine

Endocrinology

Nephrology and Urology

Pulmonology

Cardiology

Otolaryngology

COMING SOON IN
THE REQUISITES IN PEDIATRICS SERIES

Adolescent Medicine

Infectious Diseases

Hematology and Oncology

Pediatric Gastroenterology

THE REQUISITES IN PEDIATRICS

Chris A. Liacouras, MD
Co-Director of Pediatric Endoscopy and Attending
  Gastroenterologist
The Children's Hospital of Philadelphia
Professor of Pediatrics
University of Pennsylvania School of Medicine
Philadelphia, Pennsylvania

David A. Piccoli, MD
Chief, Division of Gastroenterology and Nutrition
Co-Director, Biesecker Center for Pediatric Liver
  Disease
The Children's Hospital of Philadelphia
Professor of Pediatrics
University of Pennsylvania School of Medicine
Philadelphia, Pennsylvania

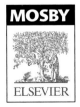

1600 John F. Kennedy Blvd.
Ste 1800
Philadelphia, PA 19103-2899

PEDIATRIC GASTROENTEROLOGY: THE REQUISITES IN PEDIATRICS   ISBN: 978-0-323-03280-3

THE REQUISITES is a proprietary trademark of Mosby, Inc.

Copyright © 2008 by Mosby, Inc., an affiliate of Elsevier Inc.

All rights reserved. No part of this publication may be reproduced or transmitted in any form or by any means, electronic or mechanical, including photocopying, recording, or any information storage and retrieval system, without permission in writing from the publisher.

Permissions may be sought directly from Elsevier's Rights Department: phone: (+1) 215 239 3804 (US) or (+44) 1865 843830 (UK), fax: (+44) 1865 853333; e-mail: healthpermissions@elsevier.com. You may also complete your request on-line via the Elsevier website at http://www.elsevier.com/permissions.

Notice

Knowledge and best practice in this field are constantly changing. As new research and experience broaden our knowledge, changes in practice, treatment, and drug therapy may become necessary or appropriate. Readers are advised to check the most current information provided (i) on procedures featured or (ii) by the manufacturer of each product to be administered, to verify the recommended dose or formula, the method and duration of administration, and contraindications. It is the responsibility of the practitioner, relying on his or her experience and knowledge of the patient, to make diagnoses, to determine dosages and the best treatment for each individual patient, and to take all appropriate safety precautions. To the fullest extent of the law, neither the Publisher nor the Editors assume any liability for any injury and/or damage to persons or property arising out of or related to any use of the material contained in this book.

The Publisher

Library of Congress Cataloging-in-Publication Data

Pediatric gastroenterology / [edited by] Chris Liacouras, David Piccoli. — 1st ed.
    p. ; cm. — (The requisites in pediatrics)
  Includes bibliographical references and index.
  ISBN 978-0-323-03280-3
  1. Pediatric gastroenterology. 2. Children—Diseases. I. Liacouras, Christopher A. II. Piccoli, David A. III. Series.
   [DLNM: 1. Gastrointestinal Diseases. 2. Child. 3. Liver Diseases. 4. Pancreatic Diseases. WS 310 P37123 2008]
   RJ446.P34 2008   618.92'33—dc22   2007007902

Acquisitions Editor: Judith Fletcher
Developmental Editor: Colleen McGonigal
Publishing Services Manager: Frank Polizzano
Project Manager: Jeff Gunning
Design Direction: Lou Forgione

Printed in the United States of America

Working together to grow libraries in developing countries
www.elsevier.com | www.bookaid.org | www.sabre.org
ELSEVIER   BOOK AID International   Sabre Foundation

Last digit is the print number: 9 8 7 6 5 4 3 2 1

This book is dedicated to the hard-working, conscientious medical staff of The Children's Hospital of Philadelphia. These professionals include the physicians, nurses, fellows, residents, and medical secretaries who have devoted their lives to the care of ill children. Although the primary doctor typically receives praise from the patient and his or her family when an illness is correctly diagnosed and treated, many times proper medical care would not be possible without the effort and selflessness put forth by the other members of the health care team.

Contributors

Robert Baldassano, MD
Director, Inflammatory Bowel Disease Center, The Children's Hospital of Philadelphia; Professor of Pediatrics, University of Pennsylvania School of Medicine, Philadelphia, Pennsylvania

Dorsey Bass, MD
Associate Professor of Pediatrics, Division of Pediatric Gastroenterology, Stanford University School of Medicine, Stanford, California

Vincent Biank, MD
Assistant Professor of Pediatrics, Department of Pediatrics, Division of Gastroenterology and Nutrition, Medical College of Wisconsin; Attending Physician, Children's Hospital of Wisconsin, Milwaukee, Wisconsin

Dana Boctor, MSC, MD, FRCPC
Clinical Assistant Professor, University of Calgary Faculty of Medicine; Gastroenterologist, Division of Gastroenterology and Nutrition, Alberta Children's Hospital, Calgary, Alberta, Canada

Joseph M. Croffie, MD, MPH
Associate Professor of Clinical Pediatrics, Indiana University School of Medicine; Director, Pediatric GI Motility Laboratory, James Whitcomb Riley Hospital for Children, Indianapolis, Indiana

Vera De Matos, MD
Fellow in Gastroenterology, Hepatology, and Nutrition, University of Pennsylvania School of Medicine/The Children's Hospital of Philadelphia, Philadelphia, Pennsylvania

Patricia A. DeRusso, MD, MS
Assistant Professor of Pediatrics, Division of Pediatric Gastroenterology and Nutrition, Johns Hopkins University School of Medicine, Baltimore, Maryland

Edwin deZoeten, MD
Attending Gastroenterologist, The Children's Hospital of Philadelphia; Assistant Professor of Pediatrics, University of Pennsylvania School of Medicine, Philadelphia, Pennsylvania

Rosalyn Diaz, MD
Instructor, Department of Pediatrics, University of Pennsylvania School of Medicine; Attending Physician, Department of Gastroenterology, Hepatology, and Nutrition, The Children's Hospital of Philadelphia, Philadelphia, Pennsylvania

Udeme Ekong, MBBS, MRCP(UK)
Assistant Professor of Pediatrics, Northwestern University Feinberg School of Medicine; Attending Physician, Pediatric Gastroenterology, Hepatology, and Nutrition Division, Children's Memorial Hospital, Chicago, Illinois

Karan M. Emerick, MD
Attending Physician, Pediatric Digestive Diseases, Connecticut Children's Medical Center, Hartford, Connecticut

Joseph F. Fitzgerald, MD
Professor of Pediatrics, Indiana University School of Medicine; Director Emeritus, Section of Pediatric Gastroenterology, Hepatology, and Nutrition, James Whitcomb Riley Hospital for Children, Indianapolis, Indiana

Jonathan Flick, MD
Clinical Associate Professor of Pediatrics, University of Pennsylvania School of Medicine; Attending Physician, The Children's Hospital of Philadelphia, Philadelphia, Pennsylvania

Alejandro Flores, MD
Professor of Pediatrics, Tufts University School of Medicine; Chief, Division of Pediatric Gastroenterology and Nutrition, Floating Hospital for Children, Boston, Massachusetts

James P. Franciosi, MD, MS
Fellow-Physician, Division of Gastroenterology, Hepatology, and Nutrition, The Children's Hospital of Philadelphia, Philadelphia, Pennsylvania

Joshua R. Friedman, MD
Attending Gastroeneterologist, The Children's Hospital of Philadelphia; Professor of Pediatrics, University of Pennsylvania School of Medicine, Philadelphia, Pennsylvania

Benjamin D. Gold, MD
Professor of Pediatrics and Microbiology and Marcus Professor and Director, Division of Pediatric Gastroenterology, Hepatology and Nutrition, Department of Pediatrics, Emory Children's Center, Emory University School of Medicine; Chief, Gastroenterology Service, and Medical Director, Gastroenterology Endoscopy and Diagnostic Laboratory, Children's Healthcare of Atlanta, Egleston Children's Hospital Campus, Atlanta, Georgia

Andrew B. Grossman, MD
Instructor, University of Pennsylvania School of Medicine; Fellow, Division of Gastroenterology, Hepatology, and Nutrition, The Children's Hospital of Philadelphia, Philadelphia, Pennsylvania

Barbara A. Haber, MD
Associate Professor of Pediatrics, University of Pennsylvania School of Medicine; Attending Physician, Division of Gastroenterology, Hepatology, and Nutrition, The Children's Hospital of Philadelphia, Philadelphia, Pennsylvania

Analice S. Hoffenberg, MD
Clinical Instructor, University of Colorado School of Medicine, Denver, Colorado

Edward J. Hoffenberg, MD
Associate Professor of Pediatrics, University of Colorado School of Medicine; Attending Physician, The Children's Hospital, Denver, Colorado

Douglas Jacobstein, MD
Attending Physician, Division of Pediatric Gastroenterology and Nutrition, The Herman and Walter Samuelson Children's Hospital at Sinai, The Sinai Hospital of Baltimore, Baltimore, Maryland

Muralidhar Jatla, MD
Instructor, Department of Pediatrics, University of Pennsylvania School of Medicine; Fellow, Division of Gastroenterology, Hepatology, and Nutrition, The Children's Hospital of Philadelphia, Philadelphia, Pennsylvania

Binita M. Kamath, MBBC
Assistant Professor of Pediatrics, University of Pennsylvania School of Medicine; Attending Physician, Division of Gastroenterology, Hepatology, and Nutrition, The Children's Hospital of Philadelphia, Philadelphia, Pennsylvania

Marsha Kay, MD
Staff Physician, Department of Pediatric Gastroenterology and Nutrition, The Children's Hospital, Cleveland Clinic, Cleveland, Ohio

Janice A. Kelly, MD
Clinical Assistant Professor, Department of Pediatrics, University of Pennsylvania School of Medicine; Attending Physician, The Children's Hospital of Philadelphia, Philadelphia, Pennsylvania

Phillip P. Le, MD, PhD
Resident, Doheny Eye Institute, Los Angeles, California

Chris A. Liacouras, MD
Co-Director of Pediatric Endoscopy and Attending Gastroenterologist, The Children's Hospital of Philadelphia; Professor of Pediatrics, University of Pennsylvania School of Medicine, Philadelphia, Pennsylvania

Kathleen M. Loomes, MD
Assistant Professor of Pediatrics, University of Pennsylvania School of Medicine; Attending Physician, The Children's Hospital of Philadelphia, Philadelphia, Pennsylvania

David Mack, MD
Professor, Department of Pediatrics and Biochemistry, Microbiology, and Immunology, University of Ottawa Faculty of Medicine; Head, Pediatric Gastroenterology, Hepatology and Nutrition, Children's Hospital of Eastern Ontario, Ottawa, Ontario, Canada

Petar Mamula, MD
Assistant Professor of Pediatrics, University of Pennsylvania School of Medicine; Director, Pediatric Endoscopy, The Children's Hospital of Philadelphia, Philadelphia, Pennsylvania

Asim Maqbool, MD
Assistant Professor of Pediatrics, University of Pennsylvania School of Medicine; Attending Physician, Division of Gastroenterology, Hepatology, and Nutrition, The Children's Hospital of Philadelphia, Philadelphia, Pennsylvania

Jonathan E. Markowitz, MD
Attending Physician, Center for Digestive Health, Greenville Children's Hospital, Greenville, South Carolina

Maria Mascarenhas, MBBS
Associate Professor of Pediatrics, University of Pennsylvania School of Medicine; Section Chief, Nutrition, Division of Gastroenterology, Hepatology, and Nutrition, The Children's Hospital of Philadelphia, Philadelphia, Pennsylvania

Peter Mattei, MD
Assistant Professor of Surgery, University of Pennsylvania School of Medicine; Attending Physician, Division of General, Thoracic, and Fetal Surgery, The Children's Hospital of Philadelphia, Philadelphia, Pennsylvania

Randolph P. Matthews, MD, PhD
Assistant Professor of Pediatrics, University of Pennsylvania School of Medicine; Attending Physician, Division of Gastroenterology, Hepatology, and Nutrition, The Children's Hospital of Philadelphia, Philadelphia, Pennsylvania

Michael L. Nance, MD
Associate Professor of Surgery, University of Pennsylvania School of Medicine; Attending Surgeon and John and Josephine Templeton Endowed Chair in Pediatric Trauma, The Children's Hospital of Philadelphia, Philadelphia, Pennsylvania

Peter F. Nichol, MD, PhD
Assistant Professor, University of Utah Department of Surgery; Pediatric Surgeon, Primary Children's Medical Center, Salt Lake City, Utah

Gilberto Pereira, MD
Professor of Pediatrics, University of Pennsylvania School of Medicine; Neonatologist, The Children's Hospital of Philadelphia, Philadelphia, Pennsylvania

David A. Piccoli, MD
Professor of Pediatrics, University of Pennsylvania School of Medicine; Chief, Division of Gastroenterology, Hepatology, and Nutrition, The Children's Hospital of Philadelphia, Philadelphia, Pennsylvania

Michael Posencheg, MD
Assistant Professor of Clinical Pediatrics, University of Pennsylvania School of Medicine; Associate Medical Director, Intensive Care Nursery, Hospital of the University of Pennsylvania, Philadelphia, Pennsylvania

Elizabeth Rand, MD
Director, Pediatric Liver Transplant Program and Attending Gastroenterologist, The Children's Hospital of Philadelphia; Associate Professor of Pediatrics, University of Pennsylvania School of Medicine, Philadelphia, Pennsylvania

Matthew R. Riley, MD
Pediatric Gastroenterologist, Legacy Emanuel Children's Hospital and Providence St. Vincent's Medical Center, Portland, Oregon

Leonel Rodriguez, MD, MS
Instructor in Pediatrics, Harvard Medical School; Director, Pediatric Gastrointestinal Motility Program, and Medical Director, Pediatric Intestinal Rehabilitation Program, Massachusetts General Hospital, Boston, Massachusetts

Colin D. Rudolph, MD, PhD
Professor of Pediatrics, Medical College of Wisconsin; Chief, Division of Pediatric Gastroenterology and Nutrition, Children's Hospital of Wisconsin, Milwaukee, Wisconsin

Anil Rustgi, MD
T. Grier Miller Professor of Medicine and Genetics and Director, Center for Molecular Studies in Digestive and Liver Disease, University of Pennsylvania School of Medicine; Chief, Gastroenterology Division, Hospital of the University of Pennsylvania, Philadelphia, Pennsylvania

Matthew J. Ryan, MD
Assistant Professor of Pediatrics, University of Pennsylvania School of Medicine; Attending Physician, Division of Gastroenterology, Hepatology, and Nutrition, The Children's Hospital of Philadelphia, Philadelphia, Pennsylvania

Edisio Semeao, MD
Attending Gastroenterologist, The Children's Hospital of Philadelphia; Clinical Assistant Professor of Pediatrics, University of Pennsylvania School of Medicine, Philadelphia, Pennsylvania

Timothy A.S. Sentongo, MD
Assistant Professor, Department of Pediatrics, University of Chicago Pritzker School of Medicine; Director, Pediatric Nutrition Support, University of Chicago Comer Children's Hospital, Chicago, Illinois

Manu R. Sood, MBBS, MD(UK), FRCPCH
Associate Professor of Pediatrics, Medical College of Wisconsin; Director of Motility, Children's Hospital of Wisconsin, Milwaukee, Wisconsin

Raman Sreedharan, MD, DCH, MRCPCH
Attending Physician, Division of Gastroenterology, Hepatology, and Nutrition, The Children's Hospital of Philadelphia, Philadelphia, Pennsylvania

Michael C. Stephens, MD
Assistant Professor of Pediatrics, Department of Pediatrics, Section of GI and Nutrition, Medical College of Wisconsin; Attending Physician, Children's Hospital of Wisconsin, Milwaukee, Wisconsin

Gregorz Telega, MD
Assistant Professor of Pediatrics, Medical College of Wisconsin; Consulting Physician, Children's Hospital of Wisconsin, Milwaukee, Wisconsin

John Tung, MD
Pediatric Gastroenterologist, South Jersey Pediatric GI, LLC, Mays Landing, New Jersey

Elizabeth Utterson, MD
Children's Gastroenterology of St. Louis, St. Luke's Hospital, Chesterfield, Missouri

Ritu Verma, MD
Attending Gastroenterologist, The Children's Hospital of Philadelphia; Clinical Associate Professor of Pediatrics, University of Pennsylvania School of Medicine, Philadelphia, Pennsylvania

Mei-Lun Wang, MD
Assistant Professor, Department of Pediatrics, University of Pennsylvania School of Medicine; Attending Physician, Division of Gastroenterology, Hepatology, and Nutrition, The Children's Hospital of Philadelphia, Philadelphia, Pennsylvania

Robert Willie, MD
Chair, Division of Pediatrics, and Physician-in-Chief, Children's Hospital; Calabrese Chair of Pediatrics, Cleveland Clinic, Cleveland, Ohio

Tracie Wong, MD
Fellow in Pediatric Gastroenterology, Hepatology, and Nutrition, The Children's Hospital of Philadelphia, Philadelphia, Pennsylvania

Foreword

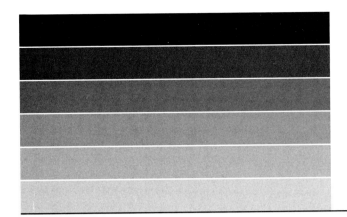

As a review of the table of contents will show, *Pediatric Gastroenterology: The Requisites in Pediatrics* has "something for everyone." Today's primary care pediatricians and other practitioners and students of pediatrics can expect to be involved in treating virtually all of the diseases described in this book. Included are chapters on disorders that often are managed primarily by general pediatricians, such as constipation, failure to thrive, and gastroesophageal reflux. This book also includes topics of interest typically found in other subspecialty textbooks, such as pediatric infectious diseases (infectious diarrhea and parasitic infections, for example), pediatric surgery (for intussusception, malrotation, volvulus, or Hirschsprung's disease), pediatric emergency medicine (foreign bodies, gastrointestinal bleed), pulmonology (cystic fibrosis), and neonatology (necrotizing entercolitis). The diversity of information, all from a gastroenterology perspective, makes this book a wonderful addition to the **Requisites in Pediatrics** series.

Dr. Liacouras' and Dr. Piccoli's expert editing adhered to the goals of this **Requisites** series. The editors and authors were asked to consider and discuss the common pediatric conditions within their specialty and to include practical information that would guide primary care providers, resident physicians, nurse practitioners, and students in the care of patients and their families.

The volume is divided into three parts. Part 1, Gastrointestinal Disorders, includes 25 chapters, each on a common gastrointestinal disease or condition. Part 2 focuses on hepatic disorders, with 11 chapters of interest, and Part 3 reviews pancreatic disorders. Information is presented in a well-organized, clinically relevant format: Each chapter begins with a case presentation that anchors the subsequent sections on epidemiology, pathophysiology, differential diagnosis, testing, and treatment. A section describing the outcome of the example case follows; for convenience, a summary of chapter content is provided as well.

I thoroughly enjoyed reading *Pediatric Gastroenterology*. The information included here is easily accessible and quite relevant for primary care pediatricians and pediatric hospitalists alike. I congratulate Dr. Liacouras, Dr. Piccoli, and the authors for their expert and insightful contributions in this seventh volume of **The Requisites in Pediatrics** series. The book should prove to be a useful and informative resource for anyone involved in the care of children with gastroenterologic diseases.

Louis M. Bell, MD
Patrick S. Pasquariello, Jr. Chair in General Pediatrics
Professor of Pediatrics
University of Pennsylvania School of Medicine
Chief, Division of General Pediatrics
Attending Physician, General Pediatrics and Infectious Diseases
The Children's Hospital of Philadelphia
Philadelphia, Pennsylvania

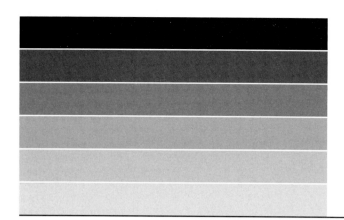

Preface

Gastroenterology, hepatology, and nutrition are among the newest of the pediatric medical specialties. Three decades ago, only a handful of relatively new gastroenterologic/gastrointestinal training programs were in existence; these were destined to produce the first group of leaders in the field. At that time, the diagnostic technology was extraordinarily limited. The mainstay of diagnosis was the radiologic examination performed with conventional techniques, augmented by the advent of computed tomography, which also was in its infancy. Flexible endoscopy was achieving considerable success in adult gastroenterology, but the lack of appropriate-sized instrumentation and the limited availability of this technology made its use in pediatrics extremely rare. Pediatric endoscopic therapy relied on either suction biopsy, using instruments that could be deployed only a limited distance from an orifice, or use of a rudimentary capsule attached to a cable that could retrieve small bowel specimens blindly. The next decade, however, saw spectacular advances in the miniaturization of fiberoptic endoscopic equipment. Even more profound success was achieved for pediatric patients with the advent of digital endoscopic imaging. Likewise, technology developed for adult gastroenterology was applied to pediatrics in the fields of motility, pH measurement, and wireless capsule endoscopy. These technical advances led directly to an increased ability to diagnose peptic, allergic, and inflammatory diseases and to ascertain their pathogenesis. At the same time, a concerted effort was directed at elucidation of pharmacokinetics and the development of medication preparations tailored for use in infants and young children. These advances were paralleled by an increase in laboratory, clinical, and translational research. Taken together, these factors have resulted in rapid, dramatic improvement in the understanding of and therapy for pediatric enteric diseases.

Two decades ago, the field of pediatric nutrition was being developed at several centers in North America. The primary area of focus was the undernutrition of macro- and micronutrients and the consequences of these deficits in children with chronic disease, not limited to the gastrointestinal tract. More recently, however, pediatric nutrition specialists have focused on the extraordinary problem of childhood obesity, which is now a major cause for morbidity and early mortality in the United States. The shortage of pediatric nutrition experts remains significant, and it is incumbent on the pediatrician to understand these problems and to intervene at an early age, when therapy is likely to be of optimal benefit.

The field of pediatric hepatology is the newest of the gastrointestinal subspecialty areas. Over the past decade, a virtual explosion occurred in the understanding of the mechanisms of pediatric liver diseases. This was made possible by advances in molecular and cellular biology that have given the hepatologist specific tools to diagnose and treat the nearly 200 pediatric liver diseases that affect children. Specific training programs in pediatric hepatology have emerged, and pediatric liver transplantation is now a highly successful therapy for children with liver disease.

Contents

Color Plates follow page xvi.

PART 1
GASTROINTESTINAL DISORDERS 1

1 Abdominal Mass 3
Michael L. Nance and Peter F. Nichol

2 Achalasia 13
Manu R. Sood and Colin D. Rudolph

3 Caustic Ingestions 19
Jonathan Flick

4 Celiac Disease 24
Edward J. Hoffenberg, Elizabeth Utterson, and Analice S. Hoffenberg

5 Constipation and Irritable Bowel Syndrome 30
Joseph M. Croffie and Joseph F. Fitzgerald

6 Eosinophilic Esophagitis 42
Edwin deZoeten and Jonathan E. Markowitz

7 Failure to Thrive 48
Asim Maqbool

8 Foreign Bodies and Bezoars 64
Marsha Kay and Robert Wyllie

9 Gastroesophageal Reflux 74
Andrew B. Grossman and Chris A. Liacouras

10 Gastrointestinal Bleeding 87
Binita M. Kamath and Petar Mamula

11 *Helicobacter pylori* Infection 98
Benjamin D. Gold

12 Hirschsprung's Disease 114
Peter Mattei

13 Infectious Diarrhea 123
Matthew R. Riley and Dorsey Bass

14 Inflammatory Bowel Disease 131
Douglas Jacobstein and Robert Baldassano

15 Intussusception 142
Janice A. Kelly

16 Lactose Intolerance 146
Raman Sreedharan and John Tung

17 Malrotation and Volvulus 152
Vincent Biank and Michael C. Stephens

18 Meckel's Diverticulum 158
Edisio Semeao

19 Necrotizing Enterocolitis 163
Michael Posencheg and Gilberto Pereira

20 Parasitic Infections 170
Rosalyn Diaz and Asim Maqbool

21 Perianal Anomalies 187
Gregorz Telega

22 Polyps and Polyposis Syndromes 192
Mei-Lun Wang and Anil Rustgi

23 Chronic Intestinal Pseudo-Obstruction 200
Leonel Rodriguez and Alejandro Flores

24 Short Bowel Syndrome 211
Maria Mascarenhas and Matthew J. Ryan

25 Small Bowel Bacterial Overgrowth 217
Timothy A.S. Sentongo

PART 2
HEPATIC DISORDERS 225

26 Alagille Syndrome 227
Binita M. Kamath and David A. Piccoli

27 Alpha$_1$-Antitrypsin Deficiency 233
Phillip P. Le and Joshua R. Friedman

28 Autoimmune Hepatitis 237
Udeme Ekong and Karan M. Emerick

29 Cholelithiasis 243
Dana Boctor

30 Congenital Hepatic Fibrosis 253
Kathleen M. Loomes and Matthew J. Ryan

31 Hemochromatosis 261
Patricia A. DeRusso

32 Metabolic Liver Disease: Tyrosinemia, Galactosemia, and Hereditary Fructose Intolerance 267
Randolph P. Matthews

33 Jaundice 276
Muralidhar Jatla and Barbara A. Haber

34 Primary Sclerosing Cholangitis 285
Elizabeth Rand and Matthew J. Ryan

35 **Viral Hepatitis** 289
Barbara A. Haber

36 **Wilson Disease** 298
James P. Franciosi and Kathleen M. Loomes

PART 3
PANCREATIC DISORDERS **305**

37 **Congenital Anomalies** 307
Raman Sreedharan and Petar Mamula

38 **Cystic Fibrosis** 314
Vera De Matos and Maria Mascarenhas

39 **Pancreatitis** 322
Ritu Verma and Tracie Wong

40 **Shwachman-Diamond Syndrome** 329
David Mack

Index 335

Color Plates

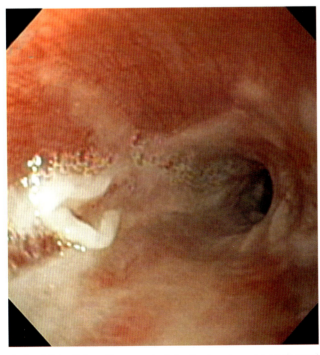

Color Plate 3-1 Upper gastrointestinal endoscopy performed approximately 8 hours after ingestion of liquid drain cleaner reveals focal areas of mid-esophageal mucosal ulceration and intraluminal exudate.

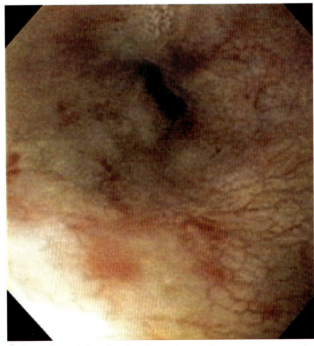

Color Plate 3-2 The distal esophagus demonstrates coagulation necrosis and areas of scattered hemorrhage.

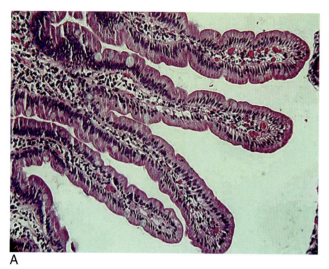

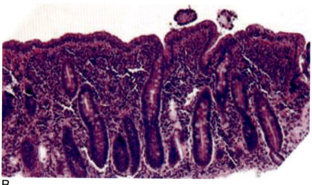

Color Plate 4-2 Hematoxylin and eosin stain of duodenal biopsy obtained by grasp forceps during esophagogastroduodenoscopy. **A,** Normal, long slender villi (200×). **B,** Villous atrophy with increased numbers of intraepithelial lymphocytes, characteristic of celiac disease (100×).

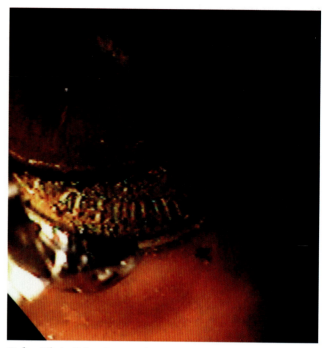

Color Plate 8-1 Retained gastric quarter and a penny in a 4-year-old with autism. Note the eroded appearance of the penny. The coins were believed to be in place for 6 weeks. The coins adhered to each other at the time of endoscopy, which may have contributed to their nonpassage but were easily removed endoscopically using alligator forceps.

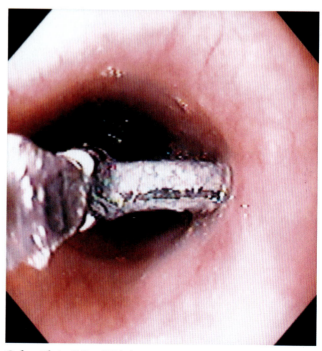

Color Plate 8-2 Withdrawal of a swallowed key using alligator forceps. Note the key is withdrawn parallel to the axis of the esophagus.

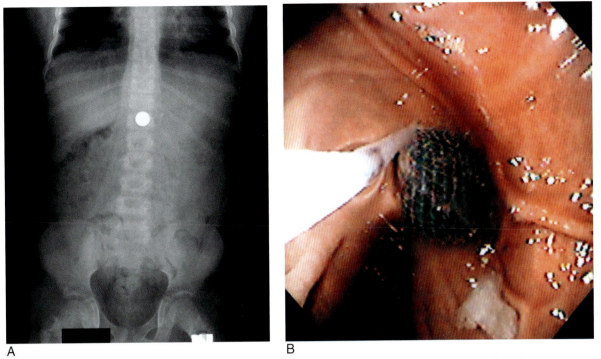

Color Plate 8-3 **A** and **B,** Magnetic marble demonstrated on KUB and in the stomach at the time of endoscopic retrieval using the Roth Net. The marble was part of a toy game and weighed 12 g.

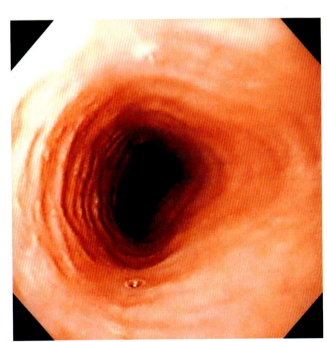

Color Plate 8-4 Ringed esophagus in a teenager with a meat impaction. Note that the mucosal appearance of the esophagus resembles that of the trachea. The patient had eosinophilic esophagitis on endoscopic biopsy.

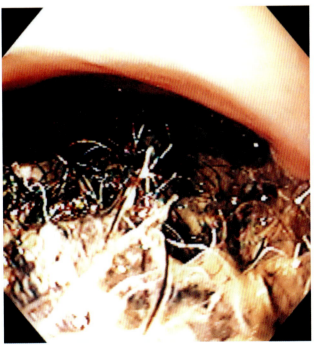

Color Plate 8-5 Endoscopic images of a massive trichobezoar in a 3-year-old patient who presented with acute abdominal pain and a palpable abdominal mass. The patient also had anorexia and significant iron deficiency anemia. The bezoar was composed of hair and a variety of fibers and required surgical removal because of its size and extension into the small intestine. Image courtesy of Vera Hupertz, M.D. and Franziska Mohr, M.D.

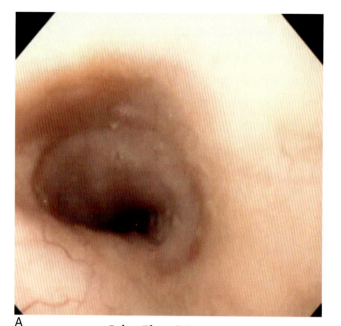 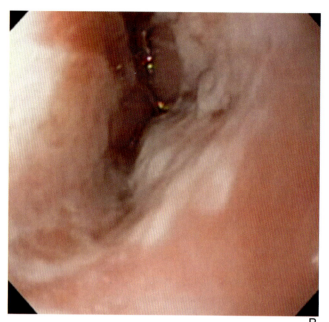

Color Plate 9-1 **A,** Smooth endoscopic appearance of normal esophageal mucosa. **B,** Erythematous, inflamed, irregular appearance of distal esophageal mucosa from patient with gastroesophageal reflux disease (GERD). No discrete ulcers are noted.

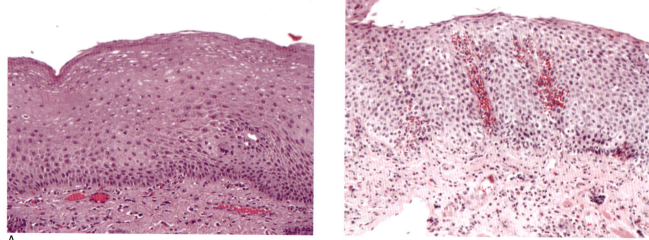

Color Plate 9-2 **A,** Normal esophageal mucosa. **B,** Reflux esophagitis as shown by expanded basal cell layer and scattered inflammatory cells. (**A** and **B** × 100). (**A** and **B** courtesy E. Ruchelli, MD, Division of Pathology, Children's Hospital of Philadelphia and the University of Pennsylvania School of Medicine.)

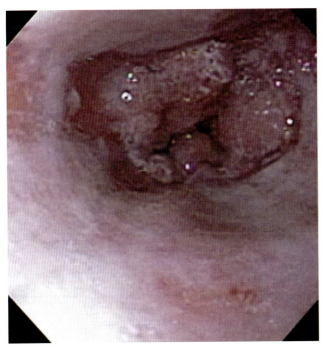

Color Plate 10-2 Erosive esophagitis.

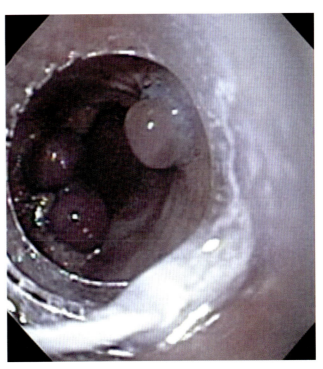

Color Plate 10-4 Postligation appearance of banded esophageal varices.

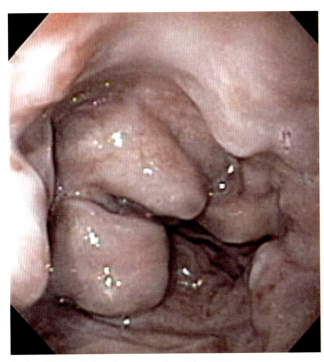

Color Plate 10-3 Large esophageal varices.

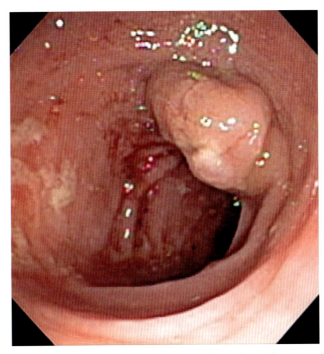

Color Plate 10-5 Large polyp in the descending colon.

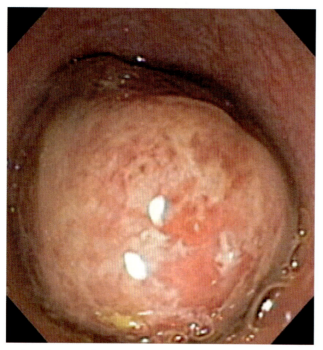

Color Plate 10-6 Postpolypectomy appearance of a juvenile polyp.

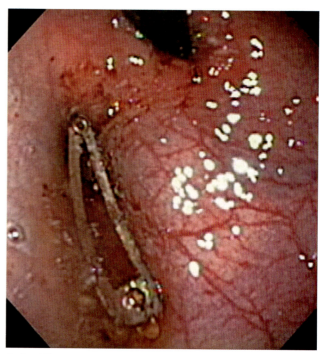

Color Plate 10-8 Foreign body (hairpin) in the stomach.

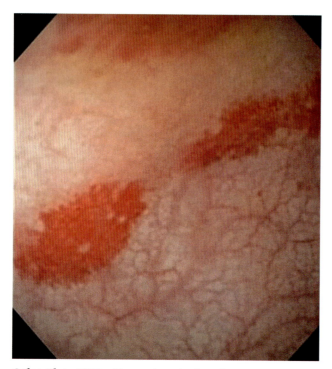

Color Plate 10-7 Hemangioma in the colon.

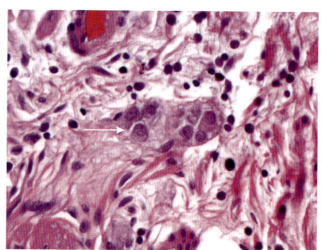

Color Plate 12-1 Ganglion cells within the myenteric plexus of the rectum *(arrow)*. (Hematoxylin and eosin stain, × 400.)

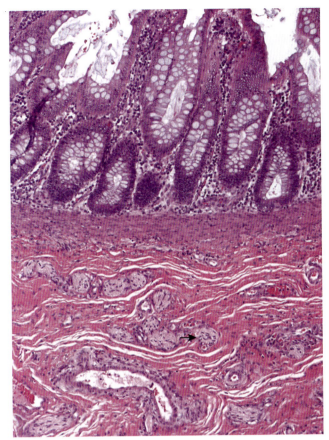

Color Plate 12-4 Rectal biopsy of a patient with Hirschsprung's disease. There are no ganglion cells to be found within the myenteric plexus. There are hypertrophied nerves *(arrow)*, however, which serves to confirm the diagnosis of Hirschsprung's disease. (Hematoxylin and eosin stain, × 400.)

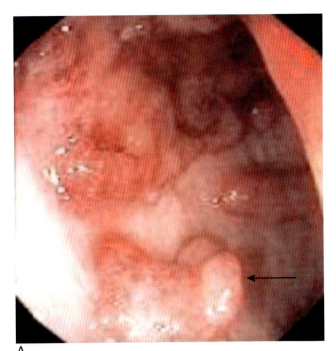

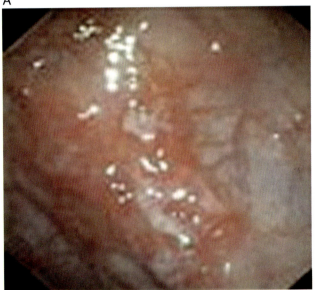

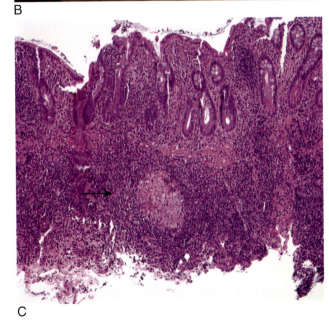

Color Plate 14-1 Macroscopic and microscopic findings of Crohn's disease. **A,** Characteristic pseudopolyps demonstrating chronic inflammation *(arrow)* within the terminal ileum. **B,** Aphthous ulcers and erythema surrounded by normal mucosa. **C,** Noncaseating granuloma of the intestine.

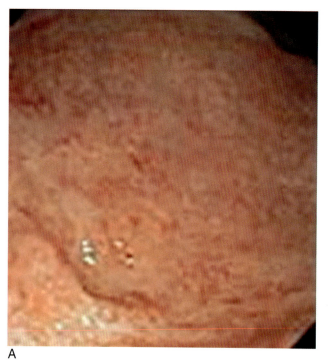

A

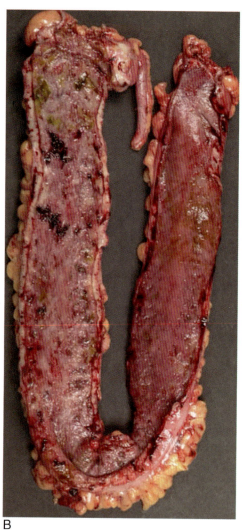

B

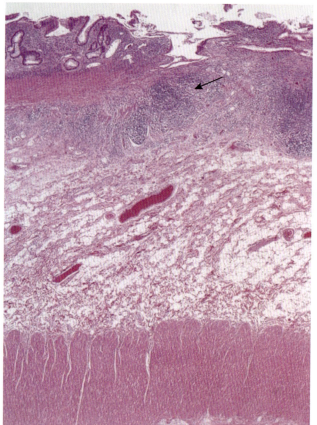

C

Color Plate 14-2 Ulcerative colitis. **A,** Characteristic macroscopic appearance of ulcerative colitis with erythema, continuous irritation, and ulceration. **B,** Colectomy specimen from a patient with ulcerative colitis. **C,** Microscopically there is inflammation located only within the luminal surface.

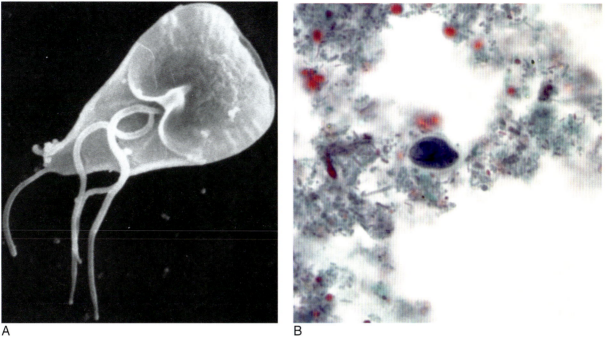

Color Plate 20-1 **A,** Scanning electron microscopy of *Giardia lamblia* showing its flagella. **B,** Trichrome stain revealing cystic form of *Giardia* (in blue in center). (**A,** From the Public Health Image Library from the Centers for Disease Control and Prevention [CDC] website, http://phil.cdc.gov [provider CDC/Janice Carr]; **B,** from the Public Health Image Library from the CDC website, http://phil.cdc.gov [provider CDC/DPDx /Melanie Moser].)

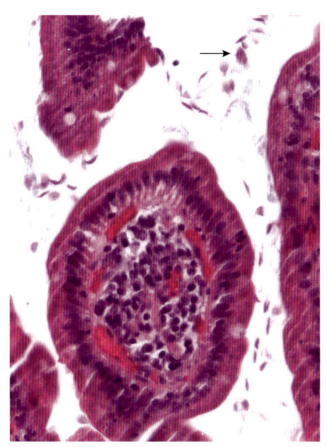

Color Plate 20-2 Light microscopy of *Giardia (arrow)* in a duodenal biopsy.

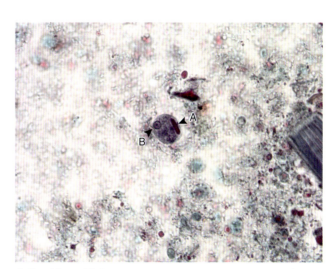

Color Plate 20-3 *Entamoeba histolytica.* Notice in this trichrome stain the cystic form of *Entamoeba* with a body *(A)* and well-demarcated nucleus *(B)*. (From the Public Health Image Library from the Centers for Disease Control and Prevention (CDC) website, http://phil.cdc.gov [provider CDC/DPDx /Melanie Moser].)

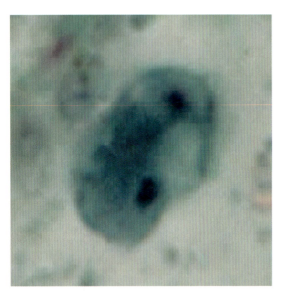

Color Plate 20-4 *Dientamoeba fragilis*. Trichrome stain of a binucleated trophozoite. (From the Public Health Image Library from the Centers for Disease Control and Prevention [CDC] website, http://phil.cdc.gov [provider CDC].)

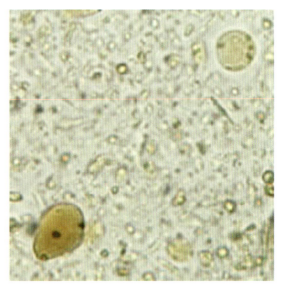

Color Plate 20-5 *Blastocystis hominis*. Iodine stain of the cyst-like form of *Blastocystis*. (From the Public Health Image Library from the Centers for Disease Control and Prevention [CDC] website, http://phil.cdc.gov [provider CDC].)

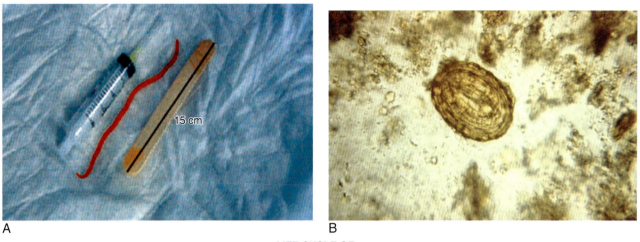
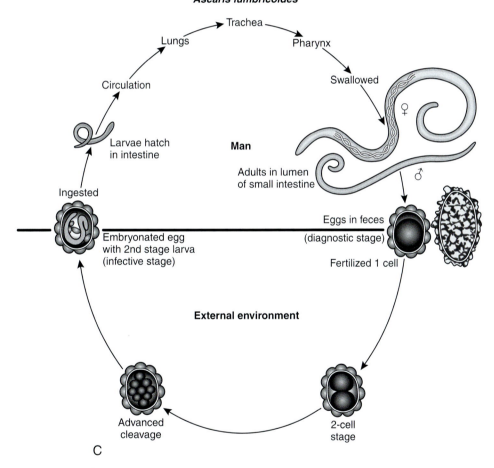

Color Plate 20-6 **A,** Adult ascaris male. **B,** Fertilized ascaris egg. **C,** Life cycle of ascaris. (**A,** From Batyraliev T: Pulmonary edema associated with *Ascaris lumbricoides* in a patient with mild mitral stenosis: A case report. Eur J Gen Med I:43-45, 2004; **B,** from the Public Health Image Library from the Centers for Disease Control and Prevention [CDC] website, http://phil.cdc.gov [provider CDC]; **C,** from Public Health Image Library from the CDC website, http://phil.cdc.gov [provider CDC].)

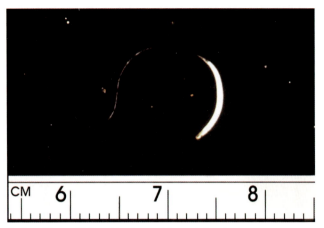

Color Plate 20-7 *Trichuris.* This adult whipworm measures approximately 4 cm in length. (From the Public Health Image Library from the Centers for Disease Control and Prevention [CDC] website, http://phil.cdc.gov [provider CDC/Dr. Mae Melvin].)

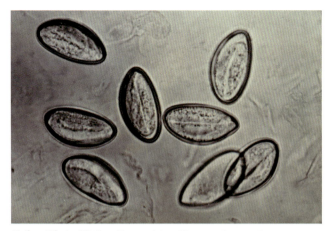

Color Plate 20-8 *Enterobius.* Picture shows pinworm eggs caught on cellulose tape. (From the Public Health Image Library from the Centers for Disease Control and Prevention [CDC] website, http://phil.cdc.gov [provider CDC].)

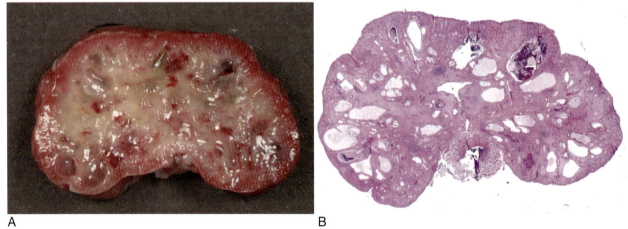

Color Plate 22-1 **A,** Cut surface of a typical juvenile (hamartomatous) polyp. **B,** Hematoxylin and eosin–stained hamartomatous polyp with dilated mucin-filled cystic glands and inflammatory infiltrate. (Courtesy Eduardo D. Ruchelli, MD, Children's Hospital of Philadelphia.)

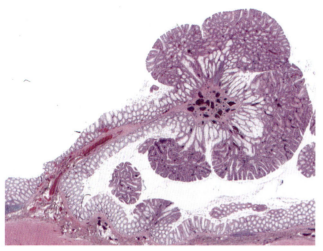

Color Plate 22-2 Hematoxylin and eosin–stained adenoma, with a multilobulated surface (×100). (Courtesy Eduardo D. Ruchelli, MD, Children's Hospital of Philadelphia.)

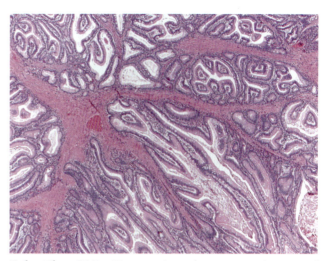

Color Plate 22-5 Hematoxylin and eosin–stained section of Peutz-Jeghers polyp. Note the appearance of "arborizing" smooth muscle within the polyp, which distinguishes these polyps from typical hamartomatous polyps. (Courtesy Eduardo D. Ruchelli, MD, Children's Hospital of Philadelphia.)

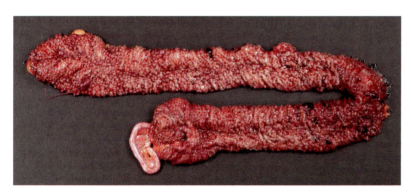

Color Plate 22-7 Familial adenomatous polyposis coli. Cut surface of resected specimen demonstrates the presence of polyps throughout the colon. (Courtesy Eduardo D. Ruchelli, MD, Children's Hospital of Philadelphia.)

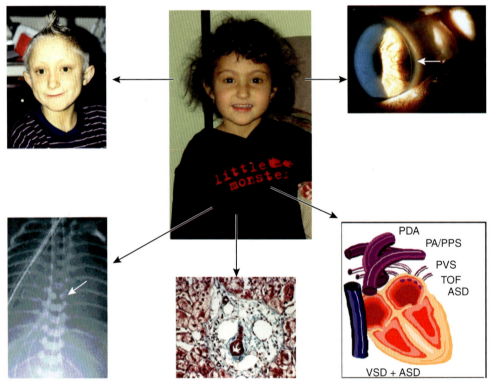

Color Plate 26-1 Clinical manifestations of Alagille syndrome. Clockwise upper right and central panels: facial features; posterior embryotoxon; common cardiac anomalies; liver biopsy showing bile duct paucity; butterfly vertebrae on thoracic x-ray. ASD, atrial septal defect; PA/PPS, pulmonary atresia/peripheral pulmonary stenosis; PVS, pulmonary valve stenosis; TOF, tetralogy of Fallot; VSD, ventricular septal defect.

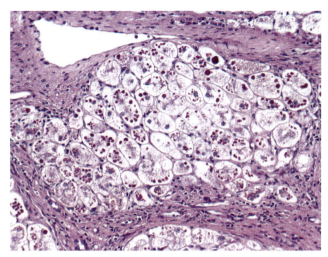

Color Plate 27-1 Explant liver section from a patient with α_1-AT deficiency and cirrhosis stained with periodic acid–Schiff (PAS). The hepatocytes within the cirrhotic nodule are slightly swollen and contain numerous PAS-positive globules. (Magnification ×200) (Courtesy Eduardo Ruchelli, MD, Children's Hospital of Philadelphia.)

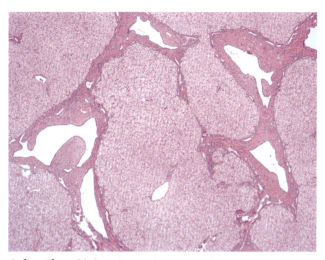

Color Plate 30-3 Typical features of ductal plate malformation include persistence of embryonic ductal structures surrounding the periphery of the portal tracts, dilated cystic ducts and increased fibroconnective tissue. (H&E staining, 100×)

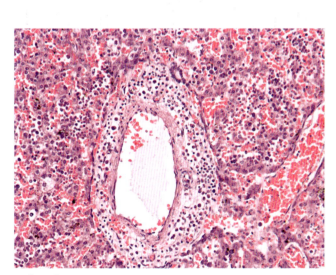

Color Plate 30-1 Normal ductal plate in a human fetal liver at 22 weeks' gestation. (H&E staining, 400×)

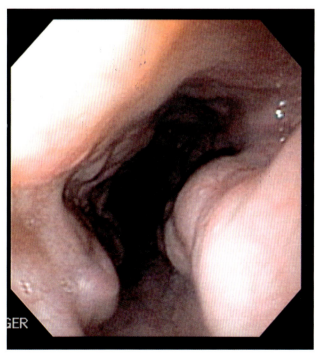

Color Plate 30-4 Esophageal varices.

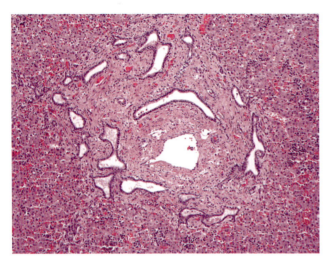

Color Plate 30-5 Needle biopsy, congenital hepatic fibrosis (CHF) (cytokeratin stain). Wide bands of bridging fibrosis are seen encircling nodules of normal liver parenchyma. Portal tracts are expanded with proliferation of abnormal dilated bile ducts. (H&E staining, 100×)

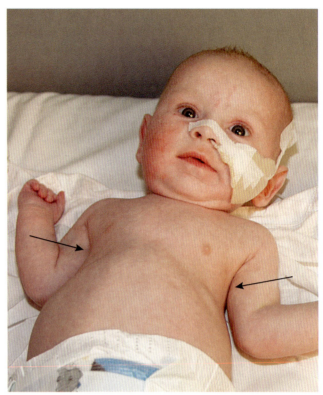

Color Plate 40-2 Thoracic dystrophy *(arrows)* can be noted. The patient also had a fine scaly rash over the entire body.

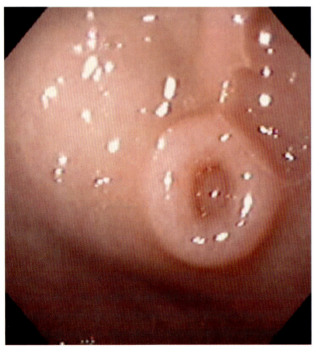

Color Plate 37-3 Endoscopic appearance of heterotopic pancreas (pancreatic rest) in the antrum of stomach.

GASTROINTESTINAL DISORDERS

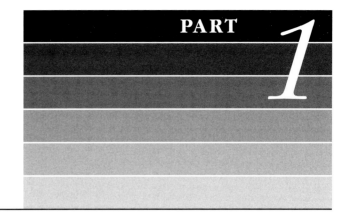

PART 1

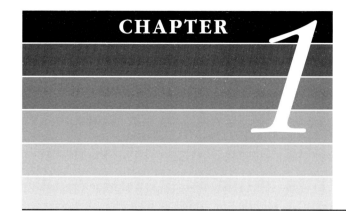

CHAPTER 1

Abdominal Mass

MICHAEL L. NANCE
PETER F. NICHOL

Disease Description
Case Presentation
Differential Diagnosis
Diagnostic Testing
   History and Physical Examination
   Laboratory Studies
   Imaging Studies
Congenital and Acquired Masses
   Choledochal Cyst
   Duplication Cyst
   Pyloric Stenosis
   Incarcerated Umbilical Hernia
   Incarcerated Inguinal Hernia
Infectious and Inflammatory Masses
   Abdominal Wall Abscesses
   Appendicitis
   Crohn's Phlegmon
   Intussusception
   Urachal Remnant
   Tubo-Ovarian Abscess
   Pancreatic Pseudocysts
Neoplastic Origin
   Hepatic Neoplasm
   Lymphoma
   Sarcoma
   Neuroblastoma
   Pancreatic Neoplasm
   Sacrococcygeal Teratoma
   Renal Neoplasms
   Ovarian Neoplasms
   Other Abdominal Masses
Approach to the Case
Summary
Major Points

DISEASE DESCRIPTION

Abdominal masses are relatively common in the pediatric age-group. Because of the considerable volume available for growth afforded by the peritoneal cavity, many masses will grow quite large before detection. Masses come to medical attention once they have achieved a size sufficient to palpate or observe externally, due to mass effect on adjacent structures, or from associated symptoms such as pain. One of the critical steps in assessment of the patient with an abdominal mass is distinguishing the patient with a process in need of urgent or emergent intervention. Regardless of presentation, a systematic approach is desirable in the management of the child with an abdominal mass.

CASE PRESENTATION

A 30-month-old previously well female was noted by her mother to have fullness in her abdomen. She was brought to the pediatrician for examination, at which time a large, palpable mass was noted in the left side of the abdomen. For several days before this evaluation, she had a low-grade fever (<100° F) and a decrease in oral intake. She also was noted to be somewhat less active than her usual baseline. There was no history of weight loss, change in bowel or bladder habits, or extra-abdominal complaints. Her medical history was unremarkable, she had not undergone any surgeries, and she had no recent trauma. The family history was noncontributory; she was on no medications and had no known allergies to medications. On examination, the child was lethargic with a fever of 99.5° F. The abdominal examination revealed a very large, firm fixed mass occupying the left side of the abdomen. The mass and the remainder of the abdomen were nontender. The nonabdominal portion of the physical examination was unrevealing. A neoplastic process was strongly suspected and the patient was referred to the oncology service for further assessment. Initial laboratory values at the time of her oncologic evaluation demonstrated a hemoglobin of 10.1 g/dL, with a normal white blood cell count and differential. The serum lactate dehydrogenase (LDH) was elevated at 3996 units/L (normal, 500 to 920 units/L). The electrolytes, calcium, phosphorus, magnesium, urea nitrogen, and creatinine levels were normal. The urine was of insufficient concentration to analyze for tumor markers (vanillylmandelic acid [VMA], metanephrine). An abdominal x-ray demonstrated a nonspecific bowel gas pattern.

DIFFERENTIAL DIAGNOSIS

Abdominal masses can be categorized based on the etiology (e.g., neoplasm, congenital anomaly; Table 1-1). A differential diagnosis list also can be created by considering the age of the patient at presentation (Table 1-2). Whereas some lesions can be diagnosed throughout the pediatric age range (e.g., choledochal cyst), others occur at characteristic times (e.g., pyloric stenosis or mesoblastic nephroma in the infant age range, or Crohn's phlegmon in older children). The location of the lesion on examination or imaging may also provide insight as to the diagnosis (Table 1-3). Based on these considerations, a differential diagnosis list can be formulated to help establish a management plan. The remainder of this chapter discusses the more common abdominal masses encountered in the pediatric population.

DIAGNOSTIC TESTING

History and Physical Examination

As with any disease process, evaluation of the patient should begin with a thorough history and physical examination, which in most instances will be sufficient to make an initial determination regarding the need for urgent operative intervention and help guide the choice of the most appropriate imaging or laboratory studies (Fig. 1-1). In the history, the physician should determine the precise nature and duration of symptoms, and whether onset was acute or insidious, persistent or intermittent. Pain, if present, should be characterized (e.g., sharp vs. dull, diffuse vs. focal, radiating vs. localized) as best as possible based on patient age. Gastrointestinal symptoms such as nausea, emesis, satiety, or a change in bowel habits should be documented. The presence of other constitutional symptoms such as fever, night sweats, or weight loss also should be elicited.

With the substantial improvement in the resolution of ultrasound, masses are more frequently detected in the prenatal period. Such data should be sought when applicable. The past medical history may reveal associated or predisposing conditions. A past surgical history may be relevant, particularly if abdominal surgeries were

Table 1-1 Etiology of Abdominal Masses

Congenital/Acquired Anatomic Abnormality	Neoplastic	Inflammatory/Infectious	Other
Choledochal cyst	Neuroblastoma	Appendicitis (phlegmon)	Pregnancy
Meckel's diverticulum	Wilms' tumor	Crohn's disease (phlegmon)	Neurogenic bladder
Hernia (umbilical/inguinal)	Mesoblastic nephroma	Infected urachal remnant	Hydrometrocolpos
Enteric duplication cyst	Multicystic dysplastic kidney	Tubo-ovarian abscess	Hematocolpos
Retroperitoneal hemorrhage	Gastrointestinal stromal tumors	Pancreatic pseudocyst	Renal vein thrombosis
Omphalocele/gastroschisis	Sarcoma	Intussusception	Fecal impaction
Hydronephrosis	Lymphangioma		
Posterior urethral valves	Mesenteric cyst		
Pyloric stenosis	Ovarian cyst		
	Ovarian teratoma		
	Liver tumors		
	Cavernous hemangioma		
	Hamartoma		
	Hepatoblastoma		
	Hemangioendothelioma		
	Lymphoma		
	Sacrococcygeal teratoma		
	Pancreatoblastoma		

Table 1-2 Abdominal Masses by Age at Presentation			
Newborn (<1 month)	**Infant (<1 year)**	**Child (1-12 years)**	**Teen (>12 years)**
Adrenal hemorrhage	Anterior meningomyelocele	Appendiceal phlegmon	Appendiceal phlegmon
Anterior meningomyelocele	Cavernous hemangioma	Choledochal cyst	Choledochal cyst
Cavernous hemangioma	Choledochal cyst	Constipation	Constipation
Choledochal cyst	Constipation	Crohn's phlegmon	Crohn's phlegmon
Enteric duplication cyst	Enteric duplication cyst	Enteric duplication cyst	Enteric duplication cyst
Hamartoma	Hamartoma	Mesenteric cyst	Ovarian cyst
Hemangioendothelioma	Hemangioendothelioma	Ovarian cyst	Ovarian teratoma
Hepatoblastoma	Hepatoblastoma	Ovarian teratoma	Ovarian torsion
Hydrometrocolpos	Intussusception	Ovarian torsion	Pregnancy
Hydronephrosis	Mesenteric cyst	Tubo-ovarian abscess	Retroperitoneal hematoma
Meconium ileus	Mesoblastic nephroma	Wilms' tumor	Tubo-ovarian abscess
Mesenteric cyst	Ovarian cyst	Fecal impaction	Fecal impaction
Mesoblastic nephroma	Ovarian torsion		
Multicystic dysplastic kidney	Sacrococcygeal teratoma		
Neurogenic bladder	Wilms' tumor		
Ovarian cyst	Fecal impaction		
Ovarian torsion			
Polycystic kidney			
Posterior urethral valves			
Pyloric stenosis			
Renal vein thrombosis			
Sacrococcygeal teratoma			
Fecal impaction			

performed. A family history may reveal prior inheritable malignancies, inflammatory bowel disease, or genetic abnormalities. A history of trauma is also important.

Anatomically, the abdomen is defined externally as the area of the body that is inferior to the costal margin, anterior to the midaxillary lines laterally, and stretching inferiorly and medially from the anterior superior iliac spines to the femoral regions bilaterally. Internally, it includes all viscera within the peritoneal cavity inferior to the diaphragm and extending down to the floor of the true pelvis. On physical examination the clinician should begin with inspection of the abdomen to determine if the mass is visible. The presence or absence of external findings (e.g., abdominal wall induration or erythema) should be noted. Second, the abdomen should be palpated. If palpable, the location of the mass is helpful in establishing a differential. The size, shape, and mobility of the mass are also important features. Tenderness, if present, should be characterized as focal or diffuse. Guarding and/or rebound tenderness should be assessed.

Laboratory Studies

The history and physical examination is the first step in establishing a list of possible diagnoses. Accordingly, the need for additional testing will be determined. Laboratory studies may provide necessary information in the evaluation of a pediatric patient with an abdominal mass. For patients with acute symptomatology, a white blood cell count (± differential), and, at times, C-reactive protein, may provide insight regarding the infectious or inflammatory nature of a lesion. If the patient is likely to require operative intervention, a hemoglobin (or hematocrit), type, and screen (and in the adolescent female a pregnancy test) should be obtained. Coagulation parameters also may be indicated if extensive surgery is anticipated. Chemistry values such as a basic metabolic panel, amylase, lipase, and liver function studies should be ordered as indicated. For suspected neoplasms, tumor markers should be obtained (e.g., alpha-fetoprotein [AFP], beta-human chorionic gonadotropin [β-hCG]). Urine may be sent for microscopic analysis and, in the case of suspected neuroblastoma, for VMA and metanephrine.

Imaging Studies

Imaging studies are frequently a vital component of the evaluation of an abdominal mass. The choice of imaging modality is critical and should be based on the differential diagnoses established by the history and physical examination. Communication with the radiologist is key to determine the most reliable means to assess the individual patient and optimize the study. The plain film of the abdomen may demonstrate calcifications (e.g., neuroblastoma, meconium peritonitis), mass effect, or abnormal bowel gas pattern. Ultrasound is

Table 1-3 Abdominal Masses by Location of Mass					
RUQ	**LUQ**	**Epigastrium**	**Suprapubic**	**RLQ**	**LLQ**
Gastrointestinal stromal tumor	Gastrointestinal stromal tumor	Gastrointestinal stromal tumor	Ovarian mass	Gastrointestinal stromal tumor	Gastrointestinal stromal tumor
Neuroblastoma	Neuroblastoma	Neuroblastoma	Ovarian cyst	Neuroblastoma	Neuroblastoma
Duplication cyst	Duplication cyst	Duplication cyst	Ovarian teratoma	Duplication cyst	Duplication cyst
Sarcoma	Sarcoma	Sarcoma	Tubo-ovarian abscess	Sarcoma	Sarcoma
Lymphoma	Lymphoma	Lymphoma	Ovarian torsion	Lymphoma	Lymphoma
Mesenteric cyst	Mesenteric cyst	Mesenteric cyst	Urinary retention	Mesenteric cyst	Mesenteric cyst
Choledochal cyst	Intussusception	Pancreatic mass	Sacrococcygeal teratoma	Intussusception	Ovarian mass
Renal mass	Renal mass	Pancreatic pseudocyst	Anterior meningomyelocele	Ovarian mass	Ovarian cyst
Wilms' tumor	Wilms' tumor	Pancreaticoblastoma	Hydrometrocolpos	Ovarian cyst	Ovarian teratoma
Mesoblastic nephroma	Mesoblastic nephroma	Pyloric stenosis	Urachal remnant	Tubo-ovarian abscess	Tubo-ovarian abscess
Hydronephrosis	Hydronephrosis	Umbilical hernia	Pregnancy	Ovarian teratoma	Ovarian torsion
Polycystic kidney	Polycystic kidney	Pregnancy	Sarcoma	Ovarian torsion	Renal mass
Multicystic dysplastic kidney	Multicystic dysplastic kidney	Crohn's phlegmon	Crohn's phlegmon	Renal mass	Wilms' tumor
Posterior urethral valves	Posterior urethral valves	Fecal impaction	Fecal impaction	Wilms' tumor	Mesoblastic nephroma
Renal vein thrombosis	Renal vein thrombosis			Mesoblastic nephroma	Hydronephrosis
Liver mass	Adrenal hemorrhage			Hydronephrosis	Polycystic kidney
Cavernous hemangioma	Splenic cyst			Polycystic kidney	Multicystic dysplastic kidney
Hamartoma	Crohn's phlegmon			Multicystic dysplastic kidney	Posterior urethral valves
Hepatoblastoma	Fecal impaction			Posterior urethral valves	Renal vein thrombosis
Hemangioendothelioma				Renal vein thrombosis	Sacrococcygeal teratoma
Adrenal hemorrhage				Sacrococcygeal teratoma	Inguinal hernia
Crohn's phlegmon				Inguinal hernia	Crohn's phlegmon
Fecal impaction				Appendiceal phlegmon	Fecal impaction
				Crohn's phlegmon	
				Fecal impaction	

LLQ, left lower quadrant; LUQ, left upper quadrant; RLQ, right lower quadrant; RUQ, right upper quadrant.

particularly useful in evaluating the hepatobiliary system, pancreas, and pelvic structures in the female. In assessment of the ovaries, ultrasound can be used to determine adequacy of blood flow if there is concern for torsion. Ultrasound is the imaging modality of choice for select radiologists to evaluate the patient with suspected appendicitis. Ultrasound is appealing because of its lack of radiation exposure and there is no need for sedation.

Cross-sectional imaging, such as computed tomography (CT) or magnetic resonance imaging (MRI), may provide detailed information about the origin and extent of the mass as well as its relation to other intra-abdominal structures. CT offers rapid scan acquisition times and is widely available. MRI has proved quite versatile and is being used more frequently. Magnetic resonance cholangiopancreatography (MRCP) provides a detailed anatomic assessment of the pancreatobiliary structures and is particularly useful in the younger child in whom more traditional endoscopic techniques might not be possible.

Fluoroscopic studies such as an upper gastrointestinal (UGI) or contrast enema will provide anatomic details about the bowel. Such information may help distinguish extrinsic compression on the bowel from an intrinsic lesion. Nuclear medicine studies may be useful in select patients. A tagged white blood cell scan (gallium scan) may be useful in identifying sites of infection. A hepatobiliary nuclear medicine scan provides anatomic and functional information about the hepatobiliary tree. Angiography may on occasion be necessary to evaluate blood flow to lesions. Studies are often complementary, providing different information. For instance, a CT scan may be performed to evaluate the

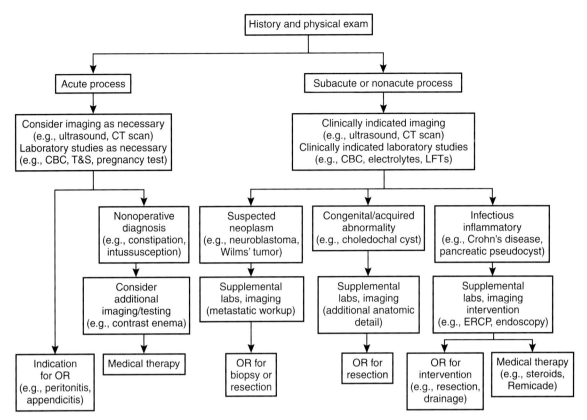

Figure 1-1 Management algorithm for the patient with an abdominal mass. CBC, complete blood count; CT, computed tomography; ERCP, endoscopic retrograde cholangiopancreatography; LFTs, liver function tests; T&S, type and screen; OR, operating room.

extent of a suspected renal neoplasm, and an ultrasound may be performed to evaluate flow through the vena cava and exclude the possibility of an associated thrombosis; a bone scan can evaluate for osseous metastases.

CONGENITAL AND ACQUIRED MASSES

Choledochal Cyst

The etiology of a choledochal cyst is poorly understood, although a leading theory postulates that the chronic reflux of pancreatic enzymes into the common bile duct results in damage and dilation. Choledochal cysts are increasingly being detected on prenatal screening ultrasounds. Beyond the newborn period, patients present with vague right upper quadrant pain and at times abnormalities in liver function. Five distinct anatomic variants have been described, ranging from involvement of a discrete area of the common bile duct to more extensive involvement of the intra- and extrahepatic biliary system. Because ultrasound is the preferred method for routine imaging of the biliary tract, it is often the first test to demonstrate the abnormality. MRCP or endoscopic retrograde cholangiopancreatography (ERCP) also may be useful to clarify the anatomy. Surgery is indicated in all cases because of the risk of cholangitis or malignant degeneration (as high as 15%) of the cyst mucosa over time. Resection of the cyst and reconnection of the biliary tract with the bowel are necessary.

Duplication Cyst

Duplications of the gastrointestinal tract can occur anywhere from the upper esophagus to the anus. Presentation is variable and can include obstructive symptoms from impingement of the cyst on adjacent bowel to bleeding or pain. The cysts can be tubular or spherical; typically they have a mucosal lining and contain fluid. The cysts are located on the mesenteric border and may or may not have a communication with the bowel. The cyst may result in symptoms leading to imaging studies such as a CT scan or UGI. Others are detected incidentally on imaging studies or as painless masses on examination. Management involves resection of the cyst. Depending on the location of the cyst, adjacent bowel may also require removal.

Pyloric Stenosis

An infant with pyloric stenosis typically presents with nonbilious emesis. The emesis is often described as projectile and increases in frequency over time. On examination, a palpable mass is often present in the epigastrium. Given the appropriate clinical setting and examination, no diagnostic imaging is necessary. If uncertain, an ultrasound or UGI can be obtained to confirm the diagnosis. Treatment is surgical once the electrolytes are confirmed to be normal or are corrected. Surgery involves splitting the hypertrophied muscle to relieve the obstruction and can be performed by a traditional open technique or by an increasingly popular laparoscopic approach.

Incarcerated Umbilical Hernia

Umbilical hernias are typically noted at birth. In most, the fascial defect closes by 4 to 5 years of age. On occasion, omentum or bowel can incarcerate through the defect. In such cases, the patient will usually present with a painful mass on the abdominal wall. If the bowel is incarcerated, the patient may also demonstrate obstructive symptoms. Emergent repair of the defect and assessment of the incarcerated bowel are necessary.

Incarcerated Inguinal Hernia

Inguinal hernias are present in as many as 3% to 5% of newborn males. Incarceration is a risk at any age and manifests most commonly with a painful mass in the inguinal region. Incarceration may result in strangulation and compromise of the bowel. Like umbilical incarceration, emergent repair and attention to the bowel are indicated.

INFECTIOUS AND INFLAMMATORY MASSES

Abdominal Wall Abscesses

Abdominal wall abscesses tend to occur in the inguinal regions and often manifest with a rim of cellulitis. They also can be seen in the anterior labial region in girls. Diagnosis is made by examination and on occasion, ultrasound. Drainage is the mainstay of therapy, with the addition of antibiotics if clinically indicated.

Appendicitis

Appendicitis is the most frequent diagnosis necessitating emergent surgical intervention in the pediatric population, yet it often is one of the most challenging diagnoses to make. The peak incidence is in the second decade of life; however, it can occur at any age. The majority of children present with some combination of fever, abdominal pain, and right-sided tenderness of 12 to 24 hours' duration. Younger children are at greater risk for perforation because of the difficulty in interpreting signs and symptoms and the associated delay in definitive treatment. One sequela of perforated appendicitis is an abscess or phlegmon. Children with an abscess typically have a prolonged history of fever and abdominal complaints. The diagnosis may be suggested by history and examination (including presence of a right lower quadrant mass) and frequently is supported by imaging. The imaging of choice is of considerable debate: Ultrasound has traditionally been a useful tool given its ease of use and accuracy, but more recently, imaging protocols based on CT scan have been effective. Children with appendicitis require operative intervention (either open or laparoscopic) to remove the appendix and wash out any contamination. Most surgeons advocate an extended course of antibiotics (either PO or IV) in the setting of perforation. On occasion, a child presents with a delay in diagnosis, and a well-formed abscess or phlegmon is noted on imaging. In select cases, treatment with IV antibiotics to "cool down" the infectious process with delayed appendectomy (at 4 to 6 weeks) may be indicated.

Crohn's Phlegmon

Crohn's disease can manifest in many different ways. The most common segment of the gastrointestinal tract affected by Crohn's disease is the terminal ileum. Transmural bowel wall involvement, the hallmark of Crohn's disease, can result in a localized abscess or inflammatory mass (i.e., phlegmon). These patients typically present with fever, abdominal pain, and a palpable mass in the right lower quadrant. In the patient with a known history of Crohn's disease, the diagnosis would be suspected based on the history and examination. In a patient with an initial presentation of Crohn's disease, the diagnosis can be quite difficult and is often mistaken for a perforated appendicitis. A CT scan of the abdomen is the most useful initial imaging study. In suspected Crohn's disease, an upper GI series is obtained to evaluate the extent of small bowel disease. Treatment is multidisciplinary, but resection with primary anastomosis is required when obstruction, abscess, failure of medical therapy, or failure to thrive occurs.

Intussusception

Intussusception, the telescoping of proximal bowel into distal bowel (classically the terminal ileum into the colon), can manifest with an abdominal mass. The peak incidence is between 3 months and 3 years of age. The cause of the intussusception is most commonly idiopathic in young children, with the risk of a pathologic lead point increasing with age. History is often suggestive, with symptoms such as fever, intermittent colicky abdominal pain, and vomiting. Between episodes of pain, the patient is often well appearing. Examination may reveal a mass in the right lower quadrant, the result of bowel within bowel. A suggestive history and/or physical examination mandate imaging. The study of choice varies by radiologist, but the more common methods include ultrasound or contrast enema. The majority of intussusceptions can be corrected with hydrostatic reduction by the radiologist. Failure to reduce or a child with a late diagnosis and septic shock warrant surgical reduction and possible bowel resection in the fluoroscopy suite. The recurrence rate is between 2% and 20%, and a recurrence is less likely following operative reduction.

Urachal Remnant

The urachus usually obliterates before birth. Incomplete obliteration of the structure could lead to formation of a cyst, which can grow large and present as an abdominal mass. In other cases, the urachal remnant can be infected and present as a tender mass. This presentation will often be confused with appendicitis. An ultrasound or CT scan help in the diagnosis. Resection of the urachal remnant is indicated with a course of antibiotics if infected.

Tubo-Ovarian Abscess

A sequela of pelvic inflammatory disease, a tuboovarian abscess, presents with fever, pain, and, if large enough, an abdominal mass. The findings at presentation may be difficult to distinguish from appendicitis or complicated Crohn's disease. The diagnosis should be considered in the adolescent female and is usually confirmed by imaging such as ultrasound or CT scan. Treatment requires broad-spectrum antibiotics and, in exceptional cases, drainage.

Pancreatic Pseudocysts

In the pediatric population, a pancreatic pseudocyst occurs as a sequela of either pancreatitis or pancreatic trauma. Pancreatitis can cause destruction of the gland with leak of caustic enzymes from the ducts. The intense inflammatory response will often wall off the process, resulting in a pseudocyst. Similarly, in trauma, an injury to a duct results in a leak of pancreatic enzymes and subsequent pseudocyst formation. A pseudocyst may evolve soon after the inciting event or in a much delayed fashion. Often a palpable mass is present in the epigastrium. Management is based on the symptomatology of the patient and the underlying cause. Percutaneous drainage or cyst enterostomy has been used to treat the cyst.

NEOPLASTIC ORIGIN

Hepatic Neoplasm

Liver tumors are uncommon and account for less than 2% of all pediatric neoplasms. The most common liver tumor is hepatoblastoma, representing 79% of all hepatic malignancies. Hepatocellular carcinoma is the second most common and portends a particularly poor prognosis. A variety of vascular neoplasms arise in the liver. The most common is the infantile hemangioendothelioma. This vascular lesion can grow quite large, resulting in high-output cardiac failure, respiratory compromise, and/or failure to thrive. The mass is often detected on a well-baby exam. Other hepatic neoplasms include malignant angiosarcoma and embryonal sarcoma, as well as the benign hamartoma. Evaluation relies heavily on imaging such as CT scanning or MRI to fully define the anatomy. Of critical importance is the relation of the mass to the surrounding ductal and vascular structures. Surgery is generally required for a tissue diagnosis (i.e., biopsy) or definitive resection.

Lymphoma

Lymphoma involving the gastrointestinal tract can manifest as a palpable mass or may develop obstructive symptoms due either to infiltration and growth into the bowel or extrinsic compression. Based on the symptoms at presentation, workup may begin with a UGI if obstructive symptoms predominate or a CT scan if evaluating a mass. Treatment is largely medical; however, a biopsy to confirm the diagnosis is often needed.

Sarcoma

Sarcomas can occur anywhere in the soft tissues. This includes the abdominal wall, small and large bowel, stomach, liver, uterus, bladder, and prostate. When on the abdominal wall or retroperitoneum, these masses tend to be fixed. Cross-sectional imaging is necessary to define the anatomy and localize the origin, and biopsy is required for definitive diagnosis. The goal of surgical therapy is complete excision, and adjuvant therapy is usually required.

Neuroblastoma

Neuroblastoma is the most common extracranial malignancy in the young child. These tumors arise from cells derived from the neural crest and can be found anywhere such cells are present. The adrenal gland is a common location as is the sympathetic chain. These tumors often grow quite large before detection and can spread to regional lymph nodes, often encasing central abdominal vasculature. Evaluation of these lesions may begin with an abdominal radiograph. Small calcifications are often noted on plain films. A CT scan demonstrates the mass and its relation to surrounding structures. In cases of suspected neuroblastoma, urine analyses for metanephrine and VMA should be obtained to determine if the lesion is biologically active. If amenable, primary resection is desirable. A tissue diagnosis is necessary to determine treatment. For large, unresectable tumors, chemotherapy is used with delayed resection.

Pancreatic Neoplasm

Pancreatic tumors are extremely rare in children. Symptoms are typically of vague abdominal pain. Diagnosis is usually made by CT scan. Hormonally active tumors include insulinoma (the most common islet cell tumor), gastrinoma, and vasoactive intestinal polypeptide-secreting tumor (VIPoma). Insulinoma should be suspected in a child with persistent hypoglycemia and is confirmed by imaging and a high insulin level in the face of a low serum glucose. Cystadenoma, cystadenocarcinomas, and carcinomas in children are rare. More commonly, papillary-cystic epithelial neoplasms are seen. They are more common in girls and young women and are hormonally inactive. They have a good prognosis, but have malignant potential, with metastasis being reported in 5% of cases. Surgery plays a primary role in the management of these lesions.

Sacrococcygeal Teratoma

Sacrococcygeal teratomas originate from the coccyx. These lesions typically present at birth as perineal masses. In a smaller subset, the lesion is predominantly intrapelvic, with little if any perineal component. Tumors with no perineal component can grow until palpable on abdominal exam. Malignancy in the newborn period is less than 10%, but without resection (as a result of pelvic location and delay in diagnosis) increases to 75% by 2 years. The optimal imaging study for these patients is MRI. Resection may require a perineal as well as an abdominal approach. It is critical the coccyx be resected in these cases, otherwise the recurrence rate exceeds 50%.

Renal Neoplasms

A large palpable abdominal mass is the most common presenting complaint for renal tumors in the pediatric age range. Ultrasound is a good initial imaging study to distinguish cystic abnormalities from solid lesions. Most patients will require baseline laboratory studies such as a complete blood count (CBC), blood urea nitrogen (BUN), and creatinine as well as a urinalysis. Mesoblastic nephroma is the most common renal mass in the newborn. Often quite large, it is usually first detected by palpation of the abdomen. Nephrectomy alone is typically adequate therapy, with chemotherapy reserved for the occasional unresectable tumor or if there is extension into adjacent structures. Wilms' tumor is the most frequent renal tumor in infants and children. The association of Wilms' tumor and seral syndromes (e.g., Denys-Drash, Beckwith-Wiedemann) suggests a genetic predisposition. The treatment of Wilms' tumor depends on surgical staging and the histologic characteristics. Surgery is indicated for definitive resection when possible or biopsy for a tissue diagnosis. Treatment is multimodal including chemotherapy and, for higher-stage lesions, radiation therapy. For most children, survival now exceeds 90%.

Ovarian Neoplasms

Benign cystic and solid tumors of the ovary are relatively common. In addition, several malignant tumors of the ovary present in the pediatric age group. Ovarian cysts in children are uniformly benign and can originate from either the ovary or the tube. Simple cysts most commonly present with cyclical pain or pain from rupture or torsion. Ultrasound and CT are useful in the diagnosis. Simple cysts should be treated if they exceed 4 cm in size or if they present with torsion. Ovarian desmoid tumors typically present as large, painless abdominal masses in prepubertal and teenage girls. These tumors can contain elements of ectoderm, endoderm, and/or mesoderm. The history is typically of a slow increase in abdominal girth. The examiner will find a large, firm mobile mass that resides in the lower abdomen. CT scan and ultrasound will demonstrate calcifications within a heterogeneous mass. Along with imaging, a serum β-hCG and AFP should be obtained. These are benign lesions and require surgical resection. Malignant neoplasms of the ovary include the granulosa-thecal cell tumors (often present with signs of precocious puberty) and Sertoli-Leydig tumors (often present with symptoms of androgen excess). These lesions also require surgical excision.

Other Abdominal Masses

When examining the pubertal female one should never forget the possibility that an enlarging abdominal mass might be the result of pregnancy (either tubal or intrauterine). A β-hCG should be obtained to confirm or exclude this diagnosis in the appropriate clinical settings. Functional constipation in children is very common. In more severe cases, a fecal impaction may occur, resulting in a palpable abdominal mass (stool in the colon and rectum) and abdominal pain. A plain film of the abdomen may demonstrate a large amount of retained stool. Treatment with enemas and reexamination should establish this diagnosis. Urinary retention can present as a suprapubic mass. If not clear on examination, an ultrasound will demonstrate a full bladder. Decompression of the urinary bladder with a Foley catheter will confirm the diagnosis. The etiology of the retention is then sought. Retention can be secondary to compression of nerves or mass effect from pelvic tumors, posterior urethral valves, and loss of bladder wall contractility from visceral myopathy, as well as spinal tumors.

APPROACH TO THE CASE

A CT scan of the abdomen and pelvis was obtained (Fig. 1-2). The CT scan demonstrates a very large mass emanating from the left retroperitoneum with displacement and encasement of the abdominal aorta and its branches. The mass displaces the left kidney and pancreas as well. There was bulky adjacent adenopathy. The findings were felt to be most consistent with neuroblastoma. Alternate diagnoses included a Wilms' tumor and rhabdomyosarcoma. A bone scan demonstrated possible osseous metastases in the spine and pelvis. A metaiodobenzylguanidine (MIBG) scan was obtained (Fig. 1-3), demonstrating a large tracer-avid mass in the left side of the abdomen. Head and chest CT scans demonstrated no evidence of metastatic disease. The patient was taken to the operating room and underwent an open biopsy of the mass, bilateral bone marrow aspirates, and placement of a central venous access catheter. The biopsy demonstrated neuroblastoma with unfavorable histology. The bone marrow

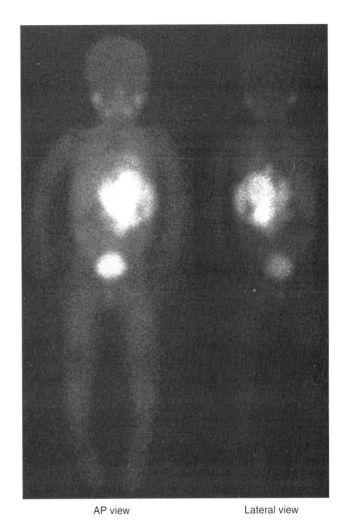

Figure 1-3 MIBG scan demonstrating radionuclide-avid tumor in the left side of the abdomen.

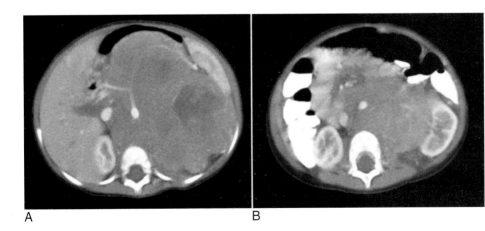

Figure 1-2 Contrast-enhanced abdominal/pelvic computed tomography (CT) scan demonstrating large mass. **A,** Homogeneous mass with central hemorrhage displacing the aorta and celiac artery. **B,** Extension of mass into renal hilar region with displacement of the kidney.

biopsies demonstrated metastatic disease. The patient was placed on a high-risk neuroblastoma protocol.

SUMMARY

In summary, abdominal masses in children are manifestations of a wide range of disease processes. The clinician is obligated to distinguish those patients who require emergent medical attention from those requiring further evaluation. Appropriate medical workup with imaging studies is undertaken in patients with nonemergent medical conditions with involvement of the appropriate medical or surgical subspecialties.

MAJOR POINTS

Abdominal masses in pediatrics typically come to medical attention only after they have achieved a size sufficient to palpate or observe externally.

The most important step in assessment of the patient with an abdominal mass is distinguishing the patient with a process in need of urgent or emergent intervention.

The location of the mass is typically helpful in establishing a differential diagnosis.

The plain film of the abdomen may demonstrate calcifications (e.g., neuroblastoma, meconium peritonitis), mass effect, or abnormal bowel gas pattern.

Ultrasound is particularly useful in evaluating the hepatobiliary system, pancreas, and pelvic structures in the female.

Cross-sectional imaging, such as CT or MRI may provide detailed information about the origin and extent of the mass as well as its relation to other intra-abdominal structures.

Fluoroscopic studies such as a UGI or contrast enema will provide anatomic details about the bowel.

SUGGESTED READINGS

Altman RP, Randolph JG, Lilly JR: Sacrococcygeal teratoma: American Academy of Pediatrics Surgical Section Survey—1973. J Pediatr Surg 9:389-398, 1974.

Baldassano RN, Piccoli DA: Inflammatory bowel disease in pediatric and adolescent patients. Gastroenterol Clin North Am 28:445-458, 1999.

Chandler JC, Gauderer MWL: The neonate with an abdominal mass. Pediatr Clin North Am 51:979-997, 2004.

Emre S, McKenna GJ: Liver tumors in children. Pediatr Transplant 8:632-638, 2004.

Kwok MY, Kim MK, Gorelick MH: Evidence-based approach to the diagnosis of appendicitis in children. Pediatr Emerg Care 20:690-698, 2004.

Meyers RL, Scaife ER: Benign liver and biliary tract masses in infants and toddlers. Semin Pediatr Surg 9:146-155, 2000.

Shamberger RC: Pediatric renal tumors. Semin Surg Oncol 16:105-120, 1999.

Achalasia

MANU R. SOOD
COLIN D. RUDOLPH

Disease Description
Case Presentation
Etiology
Pathophysiology
Differential Diagnosis
Diagnostic Testing
　Radiography
　Manometry
　Endoscopy
　Radionuclide Tests
Treatment
　Drug Therapy
　Botulinum Toxin Injection
　Pneumatic Dilatation
　Surgery
Approach to the Case
Summary
Major Points

DISEASE DESCRIPTION

Achalasia is a motor disorder of the esophagus characterized by loss of esophageal peristalsis, increased lower esophageal sphincter pressure, and absent or incomplete relaxation of the lower esophageal sphincter with swallows.

CASE PRESENTATION

A 6-year-old girl presented with an 8-month history of vomiting, nighttime cough, and weight loss. The vomiting was effortless and the vomitus contained undigested food. Recently she has been reluctant to eat solid foods and takes a long time to finish her meals, with resultant weight loss. Her parents reported hearing a gurgling noise in her chest at night, and she was waking up many nights coughing, followed by vomiting of clear, frothy fluid.

ETIOLOGY

Esophageal achalasia is a relatively uncommon condition, with an estimated incidence between 0.4 and 1.1 in 100,000 and prevalence of 7.9 to 12.6 per 100,000 population. A study of 129 children determined an incidence rate of 0.1 to 0.3 cases per 100,000 children per year in the United Kingdom. Less than 5% of all patients with achalasia present with symptoms in childhood. Most cases of achalasia are idiopathic and sporadic. Familial achalasia represents less than 1% of all achalasia cases, with the majority horizontally transmitted and presenting in childhood. Most occur following consanguineous union, suggesting an autosomal recessive inheritance. Vertically transmitted achalasia is rare and usually occurs in an older age-group.

PATHOPHYSIOLOGY

In early disease, histologic changes may be minimal and confined to inflammation of the myenteric plexus with normal ganglion cell numbers. As the disease progresses, reduced ganglion cell numbers, a decrease in varicose nerve fibers in the myenteric plexus of the esophagus, and degenerative changes in the vagus nerve may be seen.

Autoimmune, infectious, and environmental causes have been implicated in the etiopathogenesis of idiopathic achalasia. Round cell infiltration of ganglion cells in association with class II histocompatibility antigen, DQw1, supports the autoimmune hypothesis. It has been suggested that infectious or toxic inflammatory processes stimulate interferon-γ release, inducing the class II antigen expression on neural tissue. T lymphocytes recognize the neural tissue as foreign antigens and destroy it. Serum antibodies to neurons of the myenteric plexus are seen in 39% to 64% of patients with achalasia. Antibodies to measles virus and varicella zoster also have been reported, and varicella zoster virus has been identified in the esophageal tissue using deoxyribonucleic acid (DNA) hybridization technique. However, studies using more sensitive and specific polymerase chain reaction did not find herpes, measles, or human papillomavirus in myotomy specimens of patients with achalasia.

Quantitative and qualitative changes in the dorsal motor nucleus of the vagus, as well as a decrease in vasoactive intestinal peptide (VIP) and neuropeptide Y also have been reported. VIP is postulated as the major inhibitory transmitter released at the intramural postganglionic neurons of the lower esophageal sphincter (LES), and low levels may be responsible for the lack of LES relaxation during swallowing. The intermediate mechanism by which VIP induces LES relaxation is not well understood. In animal studies, VIP and dopamine have been shown to activate adenylate cyclase and increase intracellular 3'5'-cyclic adenosine monophosphate (cAMP) concentration, which results in LES relaxation. Human studies have demonstrated the absence of nitric oxide synthase (NOS) in the LES of patients with achalasia, and physiologic studies showed LES relaxation when nitric oxide (NO) was added to the muscle strips. Similar pathologic findings are present in patients with triple-A syndrome.

DIFFERENTIAL DIAGNOSIS (TABLE 2-1)

A good history is very important. Infants and toddlers usually present with choking episodes, cough, recurrent chest infections, feeding aversion, and failure to thrive. Clinical clues in older children include history of vomiting, dysphagia, weight loss, respiratory symptoms, and slow eating (Table 2-2). Dysphagia initially may be confined to solids but usually progresses to involve liquids and solids. Stress usually aggravates the symptoms. The child complains of food getting stuck in the chest and may have to make repeated attempts at swallowing or drink fluids to wash down the food. Later, when the esophagus dilates, regurgitation of undigested, nonbilious and nonacidic food eaten hours or days earlier is reported. The child or the parents may notice a gurgling sound in the chest, from the fluid sloshing in the dilated esophagus.

The initial evaluation for these symptoms begins with an upper gastrointestinal imaging study. In most cases, this will identify the location and likely cause of the obstruction and direct further evaluation. If extrinsic obstruction appears likely, cross-sectional imaging with chest computed tomography (CT) or magnetic resonance imaging (MRI) is useful. If the lumen is obstructed or if there appears to be a functional disorder, esophagoscopy is useful to better identify the lesion and possible dilation of a stricture. Even when the upper gastrointestinal (UGI) contrast study demonstrates an obstruction at the lower esophageal sphincter suggestive of achalasia, esophagoscopy is indicated to be certain that there is not a stricture such as a Schatzki ring or congenital cartilaginous stricture. If the endoscopy is normal, esophageal manometry confirms a diagnosis of achalasia.

Leiomyomas of the distal esophagus can be confused with achalasia in children. Reluctance to eat because of swallowing difficulty and associated weight loss can mimic anorexia nervosa in a teenage girl. Careful history and investigations to exclude achalasia should be undertaken if symptoms are suggestive of esophageal obstruction. If vomiting and weight loss are the predominant symptoms, the clinical presentation may mimic bulimia. Children with rumination syndrome learn to voluntarily relax the lower esophageal sphincter and, by simultaneously contracting the abdominal muscles, regurgitate gastric contents; this can also be confused with achalasia. The diagnosis of rumination is usually made on clinical presentation, sometimes antroduodenal manometry can be useful. Esophageal motility abnormalities in Chagas' disease resulting from *Trypanosoma cruzi* infection are similar to achalasia. This must be excluded in patients who have lived or traveled to Latin America. A transient achalasia-like motility

Table 2-1 Differential Diagnosis of Esophageal Achalasia

Esophageal stricture
Leiomyomas
Anorexia nervosa
Rumination
Chagas' disease
Candida esophagitis

Table 2-2 Common Symptoms of Achalasia in Children

Vomiting
Dysphagia
Weight loss
Cough and aspiration pneumonias
Chest pain
Failure to thrive
Nocturnal regurgitation

Table 2-3 Conditions Associated with Achalasia
Triple-A or Allgrove's syndrome
Rozycki syndrome
Other associations:
Chagas' disease
Sarcoidoisis
Hirschsprung's disease
Down syndrome
Hodgkin's disease
Operative and nonoperative trauma

disorder also has been reported in association with candidal esophagitis.

Patients presenting with symptoms from early childhood should be carefully investigated to exclude Allgrove's or triple-A syndrome and associated glucocorticoid deficiency. This disorder appears to be inherited in an autosomal recessive manner, and the gene has been localized to chromosome 12q13 in the *AAAS* gene. Alacrima is present from birth—the majority of children present with hypoglycemia and addisonian skin pigmentation before they are 5 years of age. Neurologic abnormalities, including hyperreflexia, muscle weakness, dysarthria, and ataxia, also have been reported. Children with Rozycki syndrome have achalasia associated with autosomal recessive deafness, short stature, vitiligo, and muscle wasting. This child had none of these features or other conditions associated with achalasia (Table 2-3).

DIAGNOSTIC TESTING

Radiography

A plain chest x-ray may show a widened mediastinum and an air fluid level with an absent gastric air bubble. Barium swallow study shows a dilated esophagus with tapering at the distal end (Fig. 2-1), absent peristalsis, or tertiary contractions. As barium fills the dilated esophagus and the pressure generated by the barium column exceeds LES pressure, partial emptying of the barium is seen. Contrast study may also help to evaluate the response to therapy; the height of the barium column 5 minutes after barium ingestion in the upright position predicts outcome following therapeutic interventions.

Manometry

The characteristic manometry findings include increased LES pressure, absent peristalsis usually involving the entire length of the esophagus, incomplete or absent LES relaxation, and elevated intra-esophageal pressure.

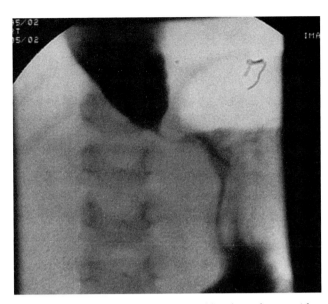

Figure 2-1 Barium x-ray showing a dilated esophagus with a typical beak-like narrowing at the lower end.

Manometric abnormalities have been reported in babies as young as 2 weeks of age. As a result of distal obstruction, the esophageal luminal pressure may be higher than the gastric fundal pressure. Upper esophageal sphincter (UES) abnormalities, including increased pressure, a short duration of relaxation with swallows, and a more rapid onset of pharyngeal contractions after UES relaxation also have been reported, although the clinical significance is unclear.

Endoscopy

The dilated esophagus appears patulous, and esophagitis secondary to food stasis and fermentation may be seen. The LES does not open with insufflation of air into the distal esophagus. Often, resistance is noted with passage of the endoscope through the gastroesophageal junction, which yields to gentle pressure. Particular attention should be paid to the presence of a hiatal hernia, which can increase the risk of perforation during dilatation. Endoscopy also helps to exclude esophageal mucosal infection, carcinoma, and leiomyoma.

Radionuclide Tests

A solid or liquid meal labeled with technetium-99m sulfur colloid can be used to measure esophageal emptying. Patients with achalasia retain the tracer longer in the upright position. The test may help to differentiate achalasia from other conditions such as scleroderma, because of the differing retention pattern. However, the usefulness of the test to assess patient response to therapy is debatable.

TREATMENT

Drug Therapy

Isosorbide dinitrate, a smooth muscle relaxant, reduces LES pressure and may improve esophageal emptying in achalasia. However, headache and hypotension are common side effects, and drug resistance may develop with prolonged treatment. Nifedipine, a calcium channel blocker, has been shown to reduce LES pressure and decreases the amplitude of esophageal contractions in achalasia; however, very limited data are available in children. Drug treatment is a temporizing measure and dilatation or surgical myotomy is ultimately required in most patients.

Botulinum Toxin Injection

In achalasia, loss of inhibitory neurons in the myenteric plexus results in unopposed excitation of the smooth muscles of the lower esophageal sphincter. This excitatory effect is probably mediated through acetylcholine. The botulinum toxin is a neurotoxin that binds to the presynaptic cholinergic terminals, thereby inhibiting the release of acetylcholine at the neuromuscular junction and creating a chemical denervation. In adults, botulinum toxin treatment of achalasia is reported as a safe and simple therapeutic option. The toxin is injected endoscopically into the LES, and adult studies have reported a good initial response in 90% of the patients. However sustained response beyond 2 to 3 months was reported in only 64%, and subsequent therapy was not as effective. Khoshoo and colleagues have reported results of botulinum toxin treatment in three children—all had immediate resolution of symptoms, but only one had a sustained response beyond 10 months. Hurwitz and colleagues treated 23 children with botulinum toxin; 19 responded to initial treatment for a mean of 4.2 ± 4 months. However, 74% of the patients ultimately required dilatation and/or myotomy. The transient response makes botulinum therapy only a temporizing measure rather than a definitive treatment for achalasia. Many surgeons believe that previous botulinum toxin injection increases the difficulty for performing surgical therapy, which may lead to reticence to use this temporizing measure.

Pneumatic Dilatation

The objective of forceful esophageal dilatation is to stretch and rupture enough LES muscle to allow the passage of solids and liquids. Care must be taken not to cause complete rupture of the esophagus or induce post-dilatation gastroesophageal reflux. Very few studies have reported long-term outcomes following dilatation. In a review of all published studies of approximately 151 pediatric patients, overall improvement was reported in 58% ($n = 88$), dysphagia persisted in 20% ($n = 31$), and 25% ($n = 38$) required myotomy because of unsuccessful dilatation. Perforation during dilatation occurred in 5.3% of the patients. It has been suggested that children older than 9 years respond better to dilatation. If symptoms reappear within 6 months following dilatation, surgery is required. With the introduction of minimally invasive surgical techniques, the role of dilatation therapy with its inherent risk of perforation has been challenged.

The main complications of pneumatic dilatation are esophageal perforation, fever, and pleural effusion. Esophageal perforation is accompanied by severe chest pain, fever, dysphagia, mediastinal and subcutaneous emphysema, or a pleural effusion. Post-dilatation water-soluble contrast studies can identify perforation and some centers perform this routinely. In general, asymptomatic linear tears require no therapy. If symptoms occur, conservative treatment with intravenous antibiotics and nothing by mouth is usually adequate. Immediate surgery and drainage are recommended for free perforation; however, medical treatment with intravenous antibiotics and parenteral nutrition also has been used successfully.

Rare complications following dilatation include persistent esophageal pain, aspiration pneumonia, and bleeding. Gastroesophageal reflux is a late complication following dilatation with incidence ranges from 5% to 12%.

Surgery

Prior to the introduction of laparoscopic techniques, surgical treatment for achalasia was reserved for patients who developed perforation during dilatation, had residual dysphagia after dilatation, or were poor candidates for dilatation. Most modern surgical procedures are variations of the Heller myotomy, which was first performed in 1914. The length of the myotomy is debatable, but the aim is to relieve obstruction without inducing reflux. The incidence of post-myotomy reflux ranges from 7% to 50%. In adult patients, performing an antireflux procedure is shown to reduce the risk of acid reflux without worsening post-surgical dysphagia. In a worldwide survey of 164 children with achalasia who underwent myotomy by a variety of approaches, good outcomes were reported in 74%. The best results were following transabdominal myotomy with an antireflux procedure.

With the advent of laparoscopic techniques, the morbidity of achalasia surgery has reduced significantly, and the majority of achalasia surgery in adults is now performed laparoscopically. In a multicenter survey of

22 children who underwent minimally invasive myotomy either laparoscopically ($n = 18$) or via a transthoracic route ($n = 4$), the mean hospital stay was less than 2 days and the majority of patients were able to restart oral feeding within 2 days after surgery. These results are better than those after open surgery. One study suggests that the use of intraoperative esophageal manometry to document a complete reduction in LES pressure may be useful. The decreased morbidity and more rapid discharge from the hospital support the laparoscopic approach as the preferred method in children and adults.

APPROACH TO THE CASE

The patient's history of apparent difficulty in eating—which seemed greater with solids than liquids—and vomiting of undigested food following meals and saliva-like fluid at night suggests a diagnosis of esophageal obstruction. A careful history often finds that the vomitus is of relatively small volume and that it lacks the sour smell or yellowish coloration of gastric vomitus. Nighttime coughing and vomiting of saliva also are common because of swallowed saliva accumulating above the obstruction and triggering coughing with vomiting when it is regurgitated into the pharynx during sleep.

Possible causes of acquired esophageal obstruction include luminal obstruction due to a stricture (either from gastroesophageal reflux, eosinophilic esophagitis, or caustic ingestion), extrinsic obstruction (from a tumor or esophageal duplication), or functional obstruction as seen with achalasia.

The symptoms in children with achalasia can be subtle, and retrosternal discomfort and dysphagia may mimic reflux esophagitis. Our patient had a pH study that showed increase reflux index, probably as a result of esophageal stasis and fermentation of swallowed food. Symptoms did not improve after 4 weeks of acid-suppressant therapy. A subsequent barium swallow examination showed a dilated esophagus with a beak-like narrowing at the lower end. Esophageal manometry confirmed the diagnosis and showed low-amplitude simultaneous esophageal contractions with high LES resting pressure and incomplete relaxation. Upper gastrointestinal endoscopy revealed a patulous esophagus with increased resistance to passage of the scope into the gastric fundus.

Following discussion with family, an elective laparoscopic Heller's procedure was performed 4 weeks later. Postoperative recovery was uneventful, and within 48 hours the patient was drinking and eating semisolid foods. At the 6-month follow-up she was eating a wide variety of foods, and her weight gain and linear growth had improved; however, she had mild persistent dysphagia when eating dry, lumpy food.

SUMMARY

As illustrated by the patient's history, the usual symptoms of achalasia in children include dysphagia, slow feeding, weight loss, and vomiting. Congenital achalasia is rare and usually presents in early infancy. A majority of patients have idiopathic achalasia for which the exact pathogenesis is unknown but autoimmune, infectious, and environmental causes have been implicated. Useful investigations include a barium swallow, esophageal manometry, and upper gastrointestinal endoscopy. Drug therapy and *Botulinum toxin* injection into the lower esophageal sphincter may temporarily improve symptoms, but often this is temporary. The majority of patients require dilatation therapy or lower esophageal sphincter myotomy for long-term relief of symptoms. With laparoscopic myotomy facilities available in most pediatric centers, this is now the treatment of choice.

MAJOR POINTS

Achalasia is an uncommon condition in children.
Dysphagia may initially be confined to solids, but usually progresses to involve both liquids and solids.
The child or the parents may notice a gurgling sound in the chest, from the fluid sloshing in the dilated esophagus.
A plain chest x-ray may show a widened mediastinum and an air fluid level with an absent gastric air bubble.
Barium swallow study shows a dilated esophagus with tapering at the distal end, absent peristalsis, or tertiary contractions.
Characteristic manometry findings include increased LES pressure, absent peristalsis usually involving the entire length of the esophagus, incomplete or absent LES relaxation, and elevated intraesophageal pressure.
Treatment includes pneumatic dilatation, injection of *Botulinum* toxin, drug therapy (isosorbide dinitrate), or surgery.

SUGGESTED READINGS

Azizkhan RG, Tapper D, Eraklis A: Achalasia in childhood: A 20-year experience. J Pediatr Surg 15:452-456, 1980.

Boyle JT, Cohen S, Watkins J: Successful treatment of achalasia in childhood by pneumatic dilatation. J Pediatr 99:35-40, 1981.

Cassella RR, Brown AL Jr, Sayre GP, et al: Achalasia of the esophagus: Pathologic and etiologic considerations. Ann Surg 160:474-487, 1964.

Chapman JR, Joehl RJ, Murayama KM, et al: Achalasia treatment: Improved outcome of laparoscopic myotomy with operative manometry. Arch Surg 139:508-513, 2004.

Hurwitz M, Bahar RJ, Ament ME, et al: Evaluation of the use of botulinum toxin in children with achalasia. J Pediatr Gastroenterol Nutr 30:509-514, 2000.

Khoshoo V, LaGarde DC, Udall JN: Intrasphincteric injection of Botulinum toxin for treating achalasia in children. J Pediatr Gastroenterol Nutr 24:439-441, 1997.

Maksimak M, Perlmutter DH, Winter HS: The use of nifedipine for the treatment of achalasia in children. J Pediatr Gastroenterol Nutr 5:883-886, 1986.

Mayberry JF, Mayell MJ: Epidemiological study of achalasia in children. Gut 29:90-93, 1998.

Mehra M, Bahar RJ, Ament ME, et al: Laparoscopic and thoracoscopic esophagomyotomy for children with achalasia. J Pediatr Gastroenterol Nutr 33:466-467, 2001.

Nakayama DK, Shorter NA, Boyle JT, et al: Pneumatic dilatation and operative treatment of achalasia in children. J Pediatr Surg 22:619-622, 1987.

Nurko S: Other motor disorders. In Walker WA, Durie PR, Hamilton JR, et al (eds): Pediatric Gastrointestinal Disease, Pathophysiology, Diagnosis and Management, 3rd ed. St Louis, Mosby, 2000, pp 317-350.

Pasricha PJ, Rai R, Ravich WJ, et al: Botulinum toxin for achalasia: Long-term outcome and predictors of response. Gastroenterology 110:1410-1415, 1996.

Richards WO, Torquati A, Holzman MD, et al: Heller myotomy versus Heller myotomy with Dor fundoplication for achalasia: A prospective randomized double-blind clinical trial. Ann Surg 240:405-412, 2004.

Russell CO, Bright N, Schmidt G, Sloan J: Achalasia of the oesophagus: Results of treatment. Aust N Z J Surg 61:43-48, 1991.

Wong RKH, Maydonovitch CL: Achalasia. In Castella DO, Richter JE (eds): The Esophagus, 3rd ed. Philadelphia, Lippincott Williams & Wilkins, 1999, pp 185-213.

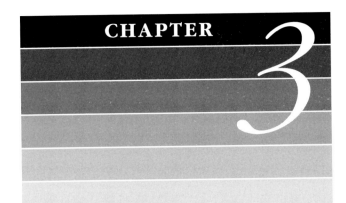

Caustic Ingestions

JONATHAN FLICK

Disease Description
Case Presentation
Epidemiology
Pathophysiology
Signs and Symptoms
Evaluation
Diagnostic Testing
Treatment
Approach to the Case
Summary
Major Points

DISEASE DESCRIPTION

Caustic substances burn, dissolve, or eat away organic tissue by chemical action. Caustic ingestions in children are almost always accidental and include acids and alkalis in solid and liquid forms. They can result in burns, perforations, and strictures of the esophagus and stomach. Accurate initial assessment of the child, including determination of the ingested substance, evaluation of the degree and extent of injury, and initiation of appropriate therapy may decrease the risk of immediate as well as long-term complications.

CASE PRESENTATION

A 2-year-old previously healthy boy was brought to the emergency department (ED) by his mother with the chief complaint of inability to swallow. The child had been playing alone when his mother found him crying and gagging. An open container of liquid drain cleaner was found next to the child. In the ED, the child was irritable with stable vital signs. He was drooling significantly, he refused to drink, and he appeared unable to handle his secretions. He had no visible burns in his mouth; chest and abdominal examinations were normal.

EPIDEMIOLOGY

In 2004, poison control centers reported more than 2.4 million poison exposures. Children younger than the age of 3 were involved in 39% of exposures, and 51% of poison exposures occurred in children younger than the age of 6. The substances most frequently involved in pediatric exposures were cosmetics and personal care products (such as hair relaxers) (13.4%), cleaning substances (including drain openers and oven cleaners, 10.0%), analgesics (7.9%), and foreign bodies (7.3%). Although children younger than 6 are the most likely to be exposed to poisons, they represent just 2.3% of poison fatalities. About 30 children die from poisonings each year, compared with 450 per year in the 1960s.

Caustic injuries are caused overwhelmingly by alkaline substances, vespecially by liquid drain cleaners. Although the liquid lye drain cleaners responsible for a rash of pediatric ingestions in the early 1970s are now sold in reduced alkali concentrations and packaged in child-resistant containers, a variety of household agents remain caustic enough to cause injury if ingested. The moderately concentrated (<10%) liquid drain cleaners available today are still strong enough to occasionally cause esophageal stricture or visceral perforation. Other hazardous household products include cosmetics, alkaline "button" batteries, bleaches, detergents, oven cleaners, concentrated ammonia, paint strippers, and others. Farm and industrial caustic agents continue to be sold without poison prevention safeguards and are a particular hazard to children living in rural areas. Most household detergents are only mildly alkaline, but nonphosphate detergents may contain silicates and carbonates that increase the pH. Liquid automatic dishwashing detergents and liquid laundry detergents may have a pH of greater than 12. Ammonia solutions in excess of 4% concentration are caustic, but most household ammonia products are of lower concentrations. Liquid household bleaches contain 5.25% or less of sodium hypochlorite and have only rarely been reported to cause serious injuries. Granular or powdered household bleaches are more injurious, in part because they remain in contact with the mucosa longer than liquid preparations and in part because they are more concentrated.

PATHOPHYSIOLOGY

On contact with the oral and gastrointestinal (GI) mucosa, alkalis produce an almost immediate liquefaction necrosis by saponification of cellular fats with protein degradation that can penetrate deeply into tissues, leading in some cases to frank perforation. The severity of the injury depends on a number of factors, including the concentration of the product, the duration of contact, and the volume ingested. Alkaline injury typically affects the oral and esophageal mucosa, leaving the stomach relatively uninvolved. Neutralization of the alkaline material by stomach acid may contribute to this gastric sparing. The immediate injury is quickly followed by the onset of an acute inflammatory response, with thrombosis of vessels and invasion by bacteria and inflammatory cells.

A subacute phase begins 3 to 5 days after ingestion and is characterized by intense inflammation, further vascular thrombosis, neovascularization, and sloughing of the superficial layers of mucosa with ulceration and granulation tissue formation. At this phase, esophageal intubation, either by endoscopy or nasogastric tube placement, carries a high risk of perforation. Beginning about 3 weeks after ingestion, a chronic phase is entered, characterized by fibrosis and re-epithelization of the mucosa. With relatively mild injury, healing may occur without sequelae; more severe cases may be complicated by esophageal stricture formation. Alkaline ingestions are reported to be associated with a 1000- to 3000-fold increased risk of esophageal squamous cell carcinoma, developing 15 to 20 years after ingestion.

In contrast, acid ingestions produce a superficial coagulation necrosis with heat generation and eschar formation that provides some protection against mucosal penetration. Maximal damage is to the stomach, pylorus, and duodenum. The esophagus is relatively spared, although perforations following acid ingestion have been reported. After entry into the small bowel, acids are well absorbed and can cause red blood cell hemolysis and a systemic metabolic acidosis.

Caustic ingestion may be associated with respiratory damage from inhalation or direct aspiration; upper airway lesions have been reported to occur in more than 40% of children following caustic ingestion. Although the presence of respiratory symptoms should be viewed with caution, respiratory involvement requiring intervention is not common.

SIGNS AND SYMPTOMS

Signs and symptoms of caustic ingestion are listed in Table 3-1. Unfortunately, multiple studies have failed to show a reliable correlation between signs and symptoms and the extent or severity of the esophageal or gastric injury.

In particular, it has been demonstrated that failure on physical examination to find visible burns of the oropharyngeal mucosa does not rule out the presence of significant esophageal and/or gastric injury at endoscopy. Some children may have no symptoms on presentation and are likely to have no, or minimal, lesions.

EVALUATION

It is important to establish the type and quantity of the caustic substance that the child is suspected of ingesting. Frequently, parents can provide only the name of the substance, and if they did not bring the container, the composition can be found by contacting a poison control center. A careful history should include questions on the amount ingested and whether the child has vomited.

After assessment of vital signs and stabilization of the child, evaluation for oral and pharyngeal burns can be performed, and any ocular or skin burns also should be assessed. Patients in significant respiratory distress may require emergency airway intubation in the ED. Abdominal examination should be performed for signs of peritonitis or perforation.

Table 3-1 Signs and Symptoms of Caustic Ingestion

Edema of the lips, tongue, or palate
Oropharyngeal burns
Drooling, increased salivation
Refusal to drink
Dysphagia
Nausea
   Vomiting
   Abdominal pain
   Tachypnea
   Stridor
Cough
Shortness of breath
   Hematemesis

The initial laboratory evaluation of the child with a caustic ingestion does not need to be extensive, but should include a complete blood count, chest and abdominal x-rays (to assess for perforation, aspiration), and serum electrolytes.

DIAGNOSTIC TESTING

Upper GI endoscopy allows for the detection of esophageal and gastric injury; determination of the extent and severity of involvement is therefore valuable in planning the appropriate course of therapy. Some controversy exists in the literature regarding the necessity of performing endoscopy in the asymptomatic child following accidental caustic ingestion. Although there are documented instances of significant esophageal burns in the absence of oral injury or abdominal complaints, this appears to be a rare event, based on several retrospective and prospective studies in children and adults. The decision whether to perform upper GI endoscopy in the asymptomatic child is best made by an experienced pediatric gastroenterologist after discussion with the referring physician, emergency medicine physician, and the child's family.

Several grading systems for the classification of the severity of injury have been used in the medical literature; a commonly used scheme is presented in Table 3-2.

If the initial assessment suggests that the child has experienced a potentially significant caustic ingestion, endoscopic evaluation should be performed within the first 24 hours to determine the extent and degree of injury (Table 3-3). Endoscopy delayed beyond 24 to 48 hours carries an increased risk of causing perforation because the mucosal injury may by that time have penetrated the wall of the esophagus or stomach. Endoscopy should be performed by a skilled pediatric endoscopist. Excessive air insufflation and retroflexion should be avoided to minimize the risk of iatrogenic damage. Endoscopy is performed with flexible fiberoptic instruments, usually with the patient intubated and anesthetized.

TREATMENT

Induction of emesis following caustic ingestion is contraindicated because it may result in repeated esophageal/hypopharyngeal exposure to the caustic substance with increased severity of burns. An attempt at neutralization of the ingested substance with either mildly acidic or alkaline solutions also is contraindicated because the reaction may generate heat and gas that can cause additional injury. Oral burns can be flushed with water, but large amounts of fluid may prompt emesis, which should be avoided.

Table 3-2 Endoscopic Grading of Esophageal Injury

Grade 0: Normal endoscopic appearance
Grade 1: Superficial esophageal edema, erythema
Grade 2: Focal or linear areas of ulceration, exudate
Grade 3: Circumferential ulceration, obliteration of lumen, perforation

The use of corticosteroids to prevent esophageal stricture formation following caustic ingestion is controversial. Published data are conflicting, and steroids have not been proved to prevent stricture formation. Steroids may promote infection, tissue weakening, and perforation. If the decision is made to initiate steroids, broad-spectrum antibiotics also should be started. Steroids may be helpful if there is upper airway involvement, including edema or bronchospasm.

It is crucial to provide the patient with adequate nutrition to promote healing and reduce the risk of complications. Until oral feedings can be resumed, feedings can be delivered by either the enteral or parenteral route. If the caustic injury is extensive or severe, a nasogastric tube can be placed under direct vision at the time of the initial diagnostic endoscopy. This will allow for administration of intragastric feedings, and the tube may help maintain the patency of the esophageal lumen during stricture formation.

Endoscopic dilation of esophageal strictures may need to be repeated many times and has a success rate of 41% to 100%, depending on the number and extent of stenoses. Dilation failures will require esophageal reconstruction procedures such as colonic interposition. Other techniques for esophageal replacement include gastric interposition and gastric tube formation. Endoscopic application of topical mitomycin-C, an antifibrotic agent, has been used as an adjunct to dilation therapy and may reduce the rate of restenosis. Successful endoscopic balloon dilation of gastric outlet obstruction caused by caustic ingestions has been reported in children and adults, but surgical bypass may be necessary.

Table 3-3 Complications of Caustic Ingestion

Esophageal perforation
Stricture formation
Tracheoesophageal fistula
Pyloric stenosis
Esophageal dysmotility
Increased risk of esophageal carcinoma

APPROACH TO THE CASE

While the child was being assessed in the ED, a call to the poison control center determined that the ingested product had a pH of greater than 12 and contained sodium hydroxide, sodium silicate, and sodium hypochlorite in sufficient concentrations to cause significant mucosal injury. A chest x-ray was obtained and was normal, as were the serum electrolytes, complete blood count (CBC), and pulse oximetry. Pediatric GI consultation was obtained and upper GI endoscopy was recommended. The child was taken to the operating room, and endotracheal general anesthesia was administered. Endoscopy (Figs. 3-1 and 3-2) demonstrated focal areas of esophageal ulceration and exudate (grade 2 injury). A nasogastric (NG) tube was placed; after 48 hours, during which the patient remained afebrile, enteral nutrition was started through the NG tube, and the patient was discharged to home. A barium swallow obtained 3 weeks after the ingestion showed areas of mucosal ulceration and stricture formation (Fig. 3-3).

The child subsequently underwent six bougie dilations of the esophagus, at monthly intervals. On completion of the dilations, he was able to swallow without difficulty and was tolerating an unrestricted diet. Follow-up barium esophagogram obtained 1 year after the

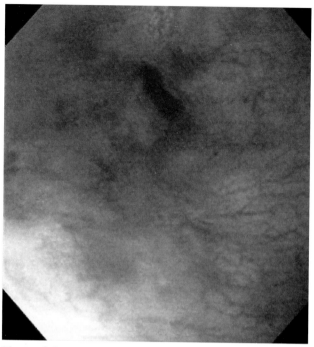

Figure 3-2 *(See also Color Plate 3-2.)* The distal esophagus demonstrates coagulation necrosis and areas of scattered hemorrhage.

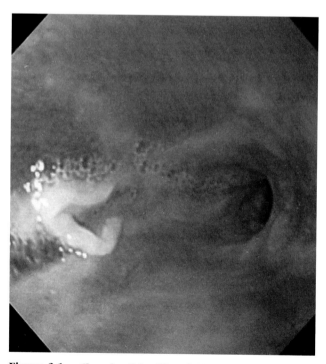

Figure 3-1 *(See also Color Plate 3-1.)* Upper gastrointestinal endoscopy performed approximately 8 hours after ingestion of liquid drain cleaner reveals focal areas of mid-esophageal mucosal ulceration and intra-luminal exudate.

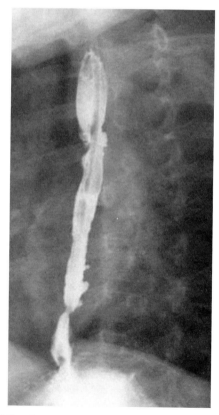

Figure 3-3 Barium esophagogram obtained 3 weeks after caustic ingestion demonstrates mild narrowing of the distal two thirds of the esophagus with mucosal irregularity, areas of focal ulceration, and a focal stricture located just above the gastroesophageal junction.

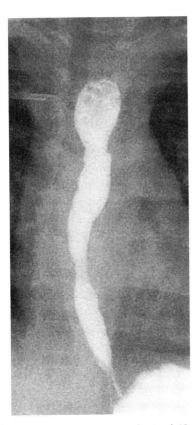

Figure 3-4 Barium esophagogram obtained 12 months after ingestion shows an area of short segmental narrowing in the proximal esophagus, at the level of the aortic arch. There is a second area of narrowing in the more distal esophagus and slight irregularity of the esophageal mucosal contour.

ingestion showed areas of nonrestrictive narrowing and mild mucosal irregularities of the esophagus (Fig. 3-4).

SUMMARY

Caustic ingestions continue to be a cause of significant morbidity in children. The initial evaluation should include determination of the substance ingested and assessment of the degree and extent of injury. Clinical signs and symptoms do not accurately predict the severity of injury and upper GI endoscopy may be required. Corticosteroids do not reduce the risk of stricture formation and should not be routinely administered. Esophageal stricture formation is the most common adverse outcome of caustic injury and may require repeated dilations.

MAJOR POINTS

Caustics include both alkalis and acids.
Ingestions by children are almost always accidental.
It is essential to establish the nature and amount of the ingested substance.
Significant esophageal or gastric injury is unusual, but can occur in the absence of signs or symptoms.
Induction of emesis following caustic ingestion is contraindicated.
Early endoscopy can establish the degree of injury and the appropriate course of treatment.
Steroids have not been proven to prevent esophageal stricture formation.
Late sequelae of caustic ingestions include esophageal stricture formation, upper GI dysmotility, and increased risk of esophageal cancer.

SUGGESTED READINGS

Anderson KD, Rouse TM, Randolph JG: A controlled trial of corticosteroids in children with corrosive injury of the esophagus. N Engl J Med 323:637-640, 1990.

Aronow SP, Aronow HD, Blanchard T, et al: Hair relaxers: A benign caustic ingestion? J Pediatr Gastroenterol Nutr 36:120-125, 2003.

de Jong AL, Macdonald R, Ein S, et al: Corrosive esophagitis in children: A 30-year review. Int J Pediatr Otorhinolaryngol 57:203-211, 2001.

Gupta SK, Croffie JM, Fitzgerald JF: Is esophagogastroduodenoscopy necessary in all caustic ingestions? J Pediatr Gastroenterol Nutr 32:50-53, 2001.

Kay M, Wyllie R: Caustic ingestions and the role of endoscopy. J Pediatr Gastroenterol Nutr 32:8-10, 2001.

Lamireau T, Rebouissoux L, Denis D, et al: Accidental caustic ingestion in children: Is endoscopy always mandatory? J Pediatr Gastroenterol Nutr 33:81-84, 2001.

Mamede RC, De Mello Filho FV: Treatment of caustic ingestion: An analysis of 239 cases. Dis Esophagus 15:210-213, 2002.

Nagi B, Kochhar R, Thapa BR, Singh K: Radiological spectrum of late sequelae of corrosive injury to upper gastrointestinal tract: A pictorial review. Acta Radiol 45:7-12, 2004.

Ozcan C, Ergun O, Sen T, Mutaf O: Gastric outlet obstruction secondary to acid ingestion in children. J Pediatr Surg 39:1651-1653, 2004.

Poley JW, Steyerberg EW, Kuipers EJ, et al: Ingestion of acid and alkaline agents: Outcome and prognostic value of early upper endoscopy. Gastrointest Endosc 60:372-377, 2004.

Turner A, Robinson P: Respiratory and gastrointestinal complications of caustic ingestion in children. Emerg Med J 22:359-361, 2005.

Wilsey MJ Jr, Scheimann AO, Gilger MA: The role of upper gastrointestinal endoscopy in the diagnosis and treatment of caustic ingestion, esophageal strictures, and achalasia in children. Gastrointest Endosc Clin North Am 11:767-787, vii-viii, 2001.

Celiac Disease

EDWARD J. HOFFENBERG
ELIZABETH UTTERSON
ANALICE S. HOFFENBERG

Disease Description
Case Presentation
Epidemiology
Pathophysiology
Differential Diagnosis
Diagnostic Testing
Treatment
Approach to the Case
Summary
Major Points

DISEASE DESCRIPTION

Celiac disease (CD) is an immune-mediated enteropathy caused by intolerance to the ingestion of gluten, a component of wheat, barley, and rye. The presence of celiac disease is confirmed by demonstration of small intestinal villous atrophy and increased numbers of intraepithelial lymphocytes. The disease process normalizes with lifelong avoidance of gluten in the diet.

CASE PRESENTATION

An 18-month-old white female of northern European descent presents to her pediatrician's office because of her mother's concern about poor weight gain and persistent loose, foul stools. After exclusive breastfeeding, pureed baby food, multi-grain infant cereal, and teething biscuits were introduced around 6 months of age. As the diet changed, the yellow-green seedy stools became dark brown, loose, and foul smelling, averaging five per day. The abdomen would "get big and tight" after meals, and was associated with irritability.

Physical examination revealed a slightly fussy toddler in no acute distress. She was afebrile with stable vital signs and her weight had dropped from the 75th percentile at 6 months to the 15th percentile, but her length remained stable at the 50th percentile for her age. Physical examination was remarkable only for a soft but markedly distended tympanic abdomen and fussiness.

Initial laboratory results included a negative test result for fecal occult blood, hematocrit of 28% with mean corpuscular volume of 65 FL. Her electrolytes, calcium, magnesium, and phosphorus levels, were all within normal limits.

EPIDEMIOLOGY

From population-based studies, the prevalence of celiac disease in the United States and Europe is between 3 and 13 cases per 1000 children 2.5 and 15 years of age (1 in 300 to 1 in 80). Most individuals have little or no symptoms and are identifiable only by screening. Some individuals, who initially test negative, later develop evidence of celiac disease.

Specific conditions are associated with an increased risk for celiac disease (Table 4-1). These include dermatitis herpetiformis (virtually all), type 1 diabetes (4% to 10%), autoimmune thyroid disease, trisomy 21 (Down syndrome) (5% to 12%), Turner syndrome, Williams syndrome, immunoglobulin A (IgA) deficiency (3%), and having a family member with celiac disease, type 1 diabetes, or autoimmune thyroid disease.

PATHOPHYSIOLOGY

Celiac disease is unique among autoimmune disorders in that an interaction between an environmental trigger (dietary gluten) and a genetic predisposition

Table 4-1 Conditions Associated with Celiac Disease
Dermatitis herpetiformis (a chronic intensely pruritic rash)
Type 1 diabetes
Autoimmune thyroid disease
Genetic disorders
Trisomy 21
Turner syndrome
Williams syndrome
Selective IgA deficiency
First-degree relative with celiac disease or type 1 diabetes

(HLA-DQ2 or HLA-DQ8) has been characterized. However, most individuals with both prerequisites (dietary gluten and HLA-DQ2 or HLA-DQ8) do not develop celiac disease. Therefore, these environmental and genetic conditions are necessary, but not sufficient, for the development of celiac disease. The additional factors important in the development of celiac disease are not known.

The current theory of pathogenesis is that a particular HLA-DQ heterodimer, encoded by the DQA1*0501 and DQB1*02 alleles on chromosome 6, forms a T-cell receptor on antigen-presenting cells. This particular receptor binds peptides from wheat, rye, and barley (gluten derived peptides or gliadin peptides). In addition, peptides that have been modified by the intestinal enzyme tissue transglutaminase are also bound with increased affinity to this DQ2 molecule peptide-binding groove. The DQ2 peptide binding is believed to induce T-cell activation, cytokine production, and intestinal injury by activating both the humoral and cellular immune systems.

Although attractive, this theory does not explain the role of anti-tissue transglutaminase antibodies. The lack of an animal model has limited research on the immunopathogenesis of celiac disease. Currently, all patients are treated with lifelong dietary restrictions, but this does not take into account the varying severity of the disease, and highlights the limited understanding of the pathogenesis of this disorder.

Long-term risks of untreated celiac disease include decreased bone mineralization and increased risks for fractures, intestinal malignancy, anemia, and nutritional deficiencies.

DIFFERENTIAL DIAGNOSIS

The differential diagnosis of CD depends on the age and mode of presentation. These include infants and toddlers with diarrhea, vomiting, failure to thrive, gas, or constipation; school-age children with abdominal pain; and adolescents with abdominal pain, growth, and pubertal delay. Table 4-2 shows typical presentations and common differential diagnoses.

DIAGNOSTIC TESTING

Guidelines from the North American Society for Pediatric Gastroenterology, Hepatology, and Nutrition recommend that children with a clinical suspicion of celiac disease be screened using the IgA antitissue transglutaminase antibody test, or as an alternative, the IgA antiendomyseal antibody test, although this test requires technician interpretation (Fig. 4-1). Antigliadin antibody testing should no longer be performed. Children with IgA deficiency should be screened using the IgG antitissue transglutaminase antibody test.

Children with a positive screening test should then have the diagnosis confirmed by small bowel biopsy, usually obtained by flexible endoscopy. The findings of villous atrophy with increased numbers of intraepithelial lymphocytes are typical and confirm the diagnosis (Fig. 4-2). This algorithm should lead to the correct diagnosis and correctly exclude celiac disease in over 95% of cases.

Table 4-2 Age, Clinical Presentation, and Common Differential Diagnoses for Celiac Disease		
Age	Presentation	Differential Diagnoses
Infant–toddler	Diarrhea, vomiting, abdominal distention, gas, irritability, constipation, rarely edema	Malabsorption conditions, constipation, milk protein allergy, *Giardia lamblia* infection
School-age	Abdominal pain, vomiting, diarrhea	Functional abdominal pain, acid-peptic disease Lactose intolerance, intestinal infection, inflammatory bowel disease
Adolescence	Growth and pubertal delay, diarrhea, anorexia, rash, anemia	Crohn's disease, growth hormone deficiency, hypothyroidism, eating disorders
Childhood on	Risk group, no symptoms	

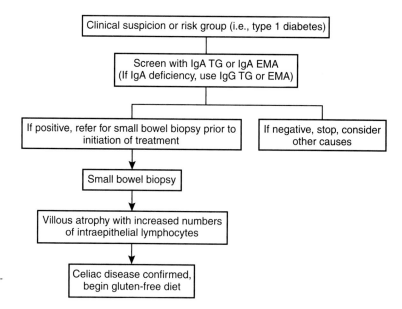

Figure 4-1 Algorithm for evaluating a child for celiac disease. EMA, antiendomyseal antibody; TG, antitissue transglutaminase antibody.

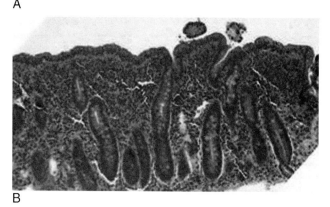

Figure 4-2 *(See also Color Plate 4-2.)* Hematoxylin and eosin stain of duodenal biopsy obtained by grasp forceps during esophagogastroduodenoscopy. **A,** Normal, long slender villi (200×). **B,** Villous atrophy with increased numbers of intraepithelial lymphocytes, characteristic of celiac disease (100×).

Screening at-risk children is more problematic because of the possibility of a normal biopsy despite seropositivity. Whether this represents a false-positive test or a mild or early disease state, remains unclear.

Making the diagnosis after beginning treatment with a gluten-free diet may be difficult because of intestinal healing, the difficulties with gluten-challenge, and recurrent symptoms.

TREATMENT

The treatment of celiac disease is the lifelong maintenance of a gluten-free diet. This dietary restriction includes the avoidance of all foods, supplements, skin care and personal hygiene products that contain gluten, a protein found in wheat, rye, and barley. Unfortunately, gluten is added to many products to thicken or change their consistency. Many preservatives contain wheat, barley, or rye components. Therefore, the diet requires considerable time and effort to learn and adhere to. Table 4-3 lists many gluten-containing grains, whereas Table 4-4 shows select common sources and potential sources of gluten.

Table 4-3 Gluten-Containing Grains

Wheat	Einkorn*	Emmer*
Barley	Malt	Farro*
Rye	Durum*	Triticale
Semolina	Filler	Bran
Spelt	Graham flour	Farina
Bulgur	Kamut*	Orzo
Couscous	Matzo	

*Types of wheat.

Table 4-4 Select Obvious and Potential Sources of Gluten

Obvious Sources	Potential Sources
Breads	Candy and gum
Cereals	Processed meat products/imitation seafood
Pastries	
Pies	Drink mixes
Cakes/cookies	Soy sauce/sauces/marinades
Pastas	Self-basting turkeys
Communion wafers	Modified food starch, seasonings, flavorings
	Hydrolyzed plant and vegetable proteins
	Caramel color
	Lipsticks/balms/glosses, mouthwash/toothpaste
	Prescription medications
	Vitamin/mineral/herbal preparations
	Play-Doh
	Stamp/envelope glues

Grains and starches considered safe for consumption by patients with celiac disease are listed in Table 4-5 and include: amaranth, buckwheat, corn, arrowroot, flax, millet, Montina (Indian rice grass), oats, potato, rice, quinoa, sorghum, soy, tapioca, teff, and flours from nuts, beans and seeds. A combination of these flours is often used to create a consistency that is closely compatible with that of gluten-containing breads and sweet carbohydrates.

Although pure oats are probably safe for the vast majority of celiac disease patients, the purity of the oats often is not guaranteed because processing plants also handle wheat, barley, and rye products, leading to potential contamination.

Health care providers and patients should be aware that many prescription medications contain gluten as an inactive ingredient. It is recommended that patients contact the specific pharmaceutical company for information about the inactive ingredients included in all of their products, as well as information regarding the potential for gluten contamination. Often one preparation of a particular medication will be safe (for example, suppository vs. oral tablet).

Lactose intolerance secondary to intestinal injury usually is temporary and resolves within a few weeks of treatment. However, as the gluten-free diet is begun, a few weeks of a low-lactose diet or lactase supplementation may improve some gastrointestinal symptoms.

A common issue is the degree to which a gluten-free diet needs to be followed; in other words, how good is good enough? There is wide variation in the ability of individual patients to tolerate re-exposure to gluten. Some patients develop significant recurrence of symptoms within hours of even small exposures (e.g., soy sauce), whereas others may not have symptoms at all. In the absence of predictors of long-term outcome, recommendations are for all patients to comply as best as possible with a strict gluten-free diet.

Table 4-6 lists some resources for families. Support groups provide information and support as well as practical regional advice, such as local shopping and restaurants that are "gluten friendly." Some support groups have camps for children.

Table 4-5 Gluten-Free Grains and Starches

Amaranth	Oats*
Arrowroot	Potato
Buckwheat	Quinoa
Corn	Rice (white, wild, brown, basmati, etc.)
Flax	
Flours from nuts/seeds/beans	Sorghum
	Soy
Millet	Tapioca (also called cassava or manioc)
Montina (Indian rice grass)	
	Teff

*Oats are often cross-contaminated with gluten at the time of processing; thus, they are considered gluten free only if their purity can be guaranteed.

APPROACH TO THE CASE

Celiac disease is typically diagnosed between 6 and 24 months of age in infants/toddlers who present with characteristic gastrointestinal symptoms. The onset of gastrointestinal (GI) symptoms (malabsorption-type stools, abdominal distention, poor weight gain) with the initiation of dietary gluten (multi-grain cereal and teething biscuits), and irritability is the typical toddler presentation of celiac disease.

Initial laboratory results reveal a microcytic anemia suggestive of iron deficiency, which is a well-described complication of celiac disease. Screening for celiac disease should be considered early in the evaluation of this child. The recommended screening test is the IgA antitissue transglutaminase antibody test, and if positive, small bowel biopsy to confirm the diagnosis and exclude other causes.

SUMMARY

About 1% of the population may have evidence of celiac disease. This disease has many different clinical manifestations and may present throughout childhood

Table 4-6	Select Resources
Children's Digestive Health and Nutrition Foundation/North American Society for Pediatric Gastroenterology, Hepatology and Nutrition (NASPGHAN)	www.celiachealth.org
National Digestive Diseases Information Clearinghouse	http://digestive.niddk.nih.gov/ddiseases/pubs/celiac
Celiac Sprue Association of America P.O. Box 31700 Omaha, NE 68131-0700 1-877-CSA-4CSA or (402) 558-0600	www.csaceliacs.org
Celiac Disease Foundation 13251 Ventura Blvd #1 Studio City, CA 91604 (818) 990-2354	www.celiac.org
Gluten Intolerance Group 15110 10th Avenue, SW Suite A Seattle, WA 98166 (206) 246-6652	www.gluten.net Email: info@gluten.net
American Celiac Society—Dietary Support Coalition P.O. Box 23455 New Orleans, LA 70183 (504) 737-3293	Email: amerceliacsoc@netscape.net
American Dietetic Association 120 South Riverside Plaza, Suite 2000 Chicago, IL 60606-6995 1-800-366-1655 or 1-800-877-1600	www.eatright.org Email: hotline@eatright.org

MAJOR POINTS

Celiac disease is an enteropathy caused by ingestion of gluten in the diet.

About 1% of the general population may have celiac disease.

Risk factors include type 1 diabetes, family history of type 1 diabetes or celiac disease, Down syndrome, Turner syndrome, Williams syndrome.

Virtually all individuals with celiac disease express DQ2 or DQ8.

There are many clinical presentations of celiac disease; intestinal manifestations include diarrhea, distention, gas, and constipation; extraintestinal manifestations include growth and pubertal delay, the rash of dermatitis herpetiformis, and anemia; asymptomatic form

Screen for celiac disease using the IgA antitissue transglutaminase antibody test.

Confirm the diagnosis of celiac disease with small bowel biopsy.

Treatment is a lifelong gluten-free diet.

Support groups provide resources for long-term adherence to the gluten-free diet.

and adolescence, once gluten is introduced in the diet. Certain groups have a higher risk for celiac disease. Screening involves testing blood for IgA antitissue transglutaminase antibodies. If these are elevated, the diagnosis should be confirmed by small bowel biopsy. Treatment with a gluten-free diet is recommended only *after* a biopsy is obtained. The treatment is lifelong. Support groups are important resources to help achieve successful therapy.

SUGGESTED READINGS

Bonamico M, Vania A, Monti S, et al: Iron deficiency in children with celiac disease. J Pediatr Gastroenterol Nutr 6: 702-706, 1987.

Book L, Hart A, Black J, et al: Prevalence and clinical characteristics of celiac disease in Down's syndrome in a US study. Am J Med Genet 98:70-74, 2001.

Catassi C, Fabiani E, Ratsch IM, et al: Celiac disease in the general population: Should we treat asymptomatic cases? J Pediatr Gastroenterol Nutr 24:S10-S12, 1997.

Dieterich W, Ehnis T, Bauer M, et al: Identification of tissue transglutaminase as the autoantigen of celiac disease. Nat Med 3:797-780, 1997.

Fabiani E, Taccari LM, Ratsch IM, et al: Compliance with gluten-free diet in adolescents with screening-detected celiac disease: A 5-year follow-up study. J Pediatr 136:841-843, 2000.

Farrell RJ, Kelly CP: Celiac sprue. N Engl J Med 346:180-188, 2002.

Fasano A, Berti I, Gerarduzzi T, et al: Prevalence of celiac disease in at-risk and not-at-risk groups in the United States: A large multicenter study. Arch Intern Med 163:286-292, 2003.

Freemark M, Levitsky LL: Screening for celiac disease in children with type 1 diabetes: Two views of the controversy. Diabetes Care 26:1932-1939, 2003.

Hill ID, Dirks M, Liptak G, et al: Guideline for the diagnosis and treatment of celiac disease in children: Recommendations of the North American Society for Pediatric Gastroenterology, Hepatology, and Nutrition. J Pediatr Gastroenterol Nutr 40:1-19, 2005.

Hoffenberg EJ, Haas J, Drescher A, et al: A trial of oats in children with newly diagnosed celiac disease. J Pediatr 137:361-366, 2000.

Hoffenberg EJ, MacKenzie T, Barriga KJ, et al: A prospective study of the incidence of childhood celiac disease. J Pediatr 143:308-311, 2003.

Maki M, Collin P: Coeliac disease. Lancet 349:1755-1759, 1997.

Maki M, Mustalahti K, Kokkonen J, et al: Prevalence of celiac disease among children in Finland. N Engl J Med 348:2517-2524, 2003.

Not T, Horvath K, Hill I, et al: Celiac disease risk in USA: High prevalence of antiendomyseum antibodies in healthy blood donors. Scand J Gastroenterol 33:494-498, 1998.

Partanen J: Major histocompatibility complex and coeliac disease. In Maki M, Collin P, Visakorpi J (eds): Coeliac Disease. Tampere: Coeliac Disease Study Group, Institute of Medical Technology, 1997, pp 253-264.

Rewers M, Liu E, Simmons J, et al: Celiac disease associated with type 1 diabetes mellitus. Endocrinol Metab Clin North Am 33:197-214, 2004.

Sollid LM: Coeliac disease: Dissecting a complex inflammatory disorder. Nat Rev Immunol 2:647-655, 2002.

Wershil B, Hoffenberg EJ, Winter HS: Research Agenda for Pediatric Gastroenterology, Hepatology and Nutrition: Allergy and Immunology: Report of the North American Society for Pediatric Gastroenterology, Hepatology and Nutrition for the Children's Digestive Health and Nutrition Foundation. J Pediatr Gastroenterol Nutr 35:S291-S295, 2002.

Constipation and Irritable Bowel Syndrome

JOSEPH M. CROFFIE

JOSEPH F. FITZGERALD

Disease Description: Constipation
  Case Presentation
  Epidemiology
  Pathophysiology
  Differential Diagnosis
  Diagnostic Testing
  Treatment
  Approach to the Case
Disease Description: Irritable Bowel Syndrome
  Case Presentation
  Epidemiology
  Pathophysiology
  Differential Diagnosis
  Diagnostic Testing
  Treatment
  Approach to the Case
Summary
Major Points

DISEASE DESCRIPTION: CONSTIPATION

Simply defined, constipation describes infrequent or difficult evacuation of feces. It is a common symptom in infants and children, and a source of anxiety for many parents worried that this symptom may be a harbinger of a serious underlying disease process.

Case Presentation

A 3-year-old boy is brought to the office by his parents who are worried about his abnormal bowel habits. He has had this problem since birth and they are convinced there is something seriously wrong.

He was the product of an uncomplicated term pregnancy and weighed 7 pounds 8 ounces. He did not suffer any perinatal problems and passed meconium shortly after delivery. He was initially fed Enfamil formula with iron, but because of a perceived intolerance to the formula, described as regurgitation with each feeding, he was switched to ProSobee formula at 2 months of age. His regurgitation improved, but his stool frequency decreased from an average of six per day to one every other day within 2 weeks of starting this formula. His stool texture changed from soft and mushy to hard pellets, and he began straining to pass stool, often stiffening his whole body, turning red in the face and screaming. His physician suggested glycerin suppositories as needed. This problem did not resolve when fruits and vegetables were introduced into his diet at 4 months of age, as suggested by the physician.

Currently, he passes large "grapefruit-sized" stools about once a week. He refuses to sit on the toilet and only passes stool in his pull-up diaper while standing in a corner of the house. His whole body stiffens and he is quite red in the face during these times. He is a happy, playful boy until a few days before he passes stool, when he becomes very fidgety and irritable and loses his appetite. He is back to his normal self as soon as the ordeal of passing stool is over. He has not experienced any abdominal distention or vomiting and has not had any blood in his stool. The family history is negative for chronic gastrointestinal diseases, including Hirschsprung's disease, celiac disease, and cystic fibrosis. He has been growing well and has maintained height and weight at the 75th percentile for his age and sex. His physical examination is normal except for a palpable fecal mass in the left lower quadrant of the abdomen. He was quite frightened by the rectal examination but allowed it to continue after persuasion by his parents. His gluteal muscles were tightened throughout the examination, making the examination difficult, but the tip of the examining finger encountered hard stool in the rectal vault.

Epidemiology

The true prevalence of constipation in childhood is not known. Some clinicians have estimated that 0.3% to 8% of the pediatric population is affected. The problem accounts for approximately 3% of visits to the general pediatric outpatient clinic and 10% to 25% of visits to a pediatric gastroenterology clinic. Although constipation is more common in adult women than men, it probably occurs equally in boys and girls.

Pathophysiology

The unabsorbed waste product of digestion entering the large intestine is propelled to the rectum by high-amplitude propagated contractions occurring several times per day over varying lengths of colon. Once the stool reaches the rectum and a certain threshold of rectosigmoid distention is attained, an urge to defecate develops. Defecation then becomes a voluntary process whereby the individual making the decision to evacuate in response to this urge relaxes the pelvic floor and increases intra-abdominal pressure to evacuate the rectum. If the decision is made not to evacuate the rectum, the individual can defer defecation by squeezing the external anal sphincter; the rectum then stretches to accommodate its contents and the urge to defecate dissipates. Constipation results from any condition that disturbs the normal process. Thus, constipation can result from disordered transit, abnormal sensation, or disordered anorectal function (outlet obstruction).

Differential Diagnosis

The differential diagnosis for constipation is discussed in relation to pathophysiology in Table 5-1. In the vast majority of children with constipation, no specific anatomic, biochemical, or metabolic abnormality is found, and these patients are said to have functional or idiopathic constipation as opposed to organic constipation in which a biochemical, metabolic, or anatomic abnormality is present. Functional constipation accounts for up to 95% of cases of chronic constipation seen in general pediatric clinics. In many of these children, unresolved acute constipation results in intentional stool-withholding, which leads to chronic constipation. Risk factors that predispose to intentional stool-withholding are discussed in Table 5-2.

Diagnostic Testing

Because organic constipation accounts for only about 5% of cases of constipation in children, most children with chronic constipation do not need any diagnostic testing. A thorough history (Table 5-3) and physical examination

Table 5-1 Causes of Constipation in Children

Causes of Impaired Transit:
Diet
Inadequate fiber intake
Inadequate fluid intake
Underfeeding
Cow's-milk allergy

Metabolic and Endocrine Conditions:
Hypercalcemia
Hypokalemia
Hypocalcemia
Hypothyroidism
Cystic fibrosis
Diabetes mellitus
Multiple endocrine neoplasia type 2B

Disorders of Intestinal Nerves and Muscles:
Chronic intestinal pseudo-obstruction
Hirschsprung's disease
Neuronal intestinal dysplasia

Drugs:
Opiates
Anticholinergics
Antidepressants
Anticonvulsants
Antihypertensives
Antacids
Bismuth
Iron supplements

Others:
Irritable bowel syndrome
Celiac disease
Lead toxicity
Vitamin D toxicity
Genetic predisposition

Causes of Impaired Sensation:
Spinal cord injury
Tethered cord
Myelomeningocele

Causes of Disordered Anorectal Function:
Intentional stool-withholding
Anismus
Imperforate anus
Anteriorly displaced anus
Anal stenosis
Inflammatory strictures of rectum or anus
Tumors of the pelvis (e.g., sacral teratoma)
Painful anal lesions (anal fissure, streptococcal anusitis)

(Table 5-4) will, for the most part, identify red flags for organic disease (Table 5-5), and these will dictate the necessary diagnostic tests (Table 5-6) (Figs. 5-1 through 5-4).

Treatment

Patients with an identifiable organic cause for constipation should have the underlying cause treated.

Table 5-2	Risk Factors Predisposing to Intentional Stool-Withholding in Infants and Children

Infants:
Change from breast milk to formula (soy formulas produce firmer stools)
Change from formula to regular cow's milk (may produce firmer stools)
Perianal irritation (diaper rash, anal fissure)

Toddlers:
Coercive toilet training
Inappropriately early toilet training
Perianal irritation (diaper rash, anal fissure)

Older Children:
Travel (unfamiliar toilets, unappealing toilet facilities)
School (rules about going to bathroom, lack of privacy)
Perianal irritation (streptococcal anusitis)
Sexual abuse

Table 5-3	Pertinent History in Child Presenting with Constipation

Demographics:
Age
Sex

Present History:
Duration of symptoms
Notable circumstances preceding onset of symptoms
Frequency of bowel movements
Consistency of stools
Withholding behavior
Fecal soiling
Urinary symptoms
Abdominal pain
Abdominal distention
Vomiting
Blood in/on stool
Weight loss
Treatments tried
    Diet
    Current other medications

Past History:
Pregnancy complication
Birthweight
Perinatal course
Age at passage of meconium
Major illnesses
Hospitalizations
Surgeries

Family History:
Constipation
Thyroid disease
Cystic fibrosis
Celiac disease
Hirschsprung's disease
Other illnesses

Social History:
Family dynamics
Occupations of parents (explore potential for exposure to toxins)
School dynamics
Interaction with peers
Source of drinking water

In the infant with simple chronic constipation, dietary measures such as an increase in fluid and carbohydrate intake may resolve the problem. Juices that contain sorbitol, such as prune, pear, and apple juices, are recommended. Barley malt extract, lactulose, or sorbitol may be used as stool softeners if juices are not helpful. Glycerin suppositories may be used in the acute setting, including acute relapses, but should not be used for maintenance therapy. In more severe cases, polyethylene glycol solution without electrolytes may be considered. We must point out that some normal breastfed infants may go many days without a bowel movement and experience no symptoms. Table 5-7 outlines the normal frequency of bowel movements in infants and children.

In the older child with no history of stool-withholding but who passes stool infrequently, increasing fluid and dietary fiber intake and the intake of sorbitol-containing fruit juices may be beneficial.

The approach to the child with stool-retentive constipation should begin with the education of the child and parents on the physiology of defecation in very simple language. Specific explanation should be given as to why fecal retention leads to constipation and fecal soiling. This process, termed demystification by Levine and Bakow, is most effectively done with illustrations. If a fecal impaction is present on physical examination, it should be removed with enemas, large-dose lavage solution, or, in some cases, manual disimpaction under anesthesia. The child is then prescribed a laxative (Table 5-8) to maintain soft stools and instructed to sit on the toilet (with proper foot support) for 3 to 10 minutes, at least two times per day, preferably after a meal in order to take advantage of the gastrocolic reflex. The goal is to establish a regular pattern of defecation. The child should then be followed closely with adjustment of the laxative dose. The parents should be informed that the process of establishing a regular pattern of defecation may take several months. The child who does not respond to medical treatment despite being compliant, or the child who is unable to wean off laxatives after several months, should undergo an evaluation to exclude an organic cause for constipation.

Approach to the Case

What is the most likely cause for constipation in this patient?

Table 5-4 Physical Examination of the Child with Constipation

Anthropometric Measurements:
Failure to thrive

Complete Examination of Head and Neck, Lungs, and Heart:
Systemic illness complicated by constipation

Abdominal Examination:
Distention
Palpable masses
Hepatosplenomegaly
Bowel sounds

Anorectal Examination:
Anal position
Perianal lesions
Fecal soiling
Anal tone
Size of rectal vault
Amount and character of feces in rectum
Masses
Decompression on withdrawal of examining finger
Occult blood in stool

Back and Spine Examination:
Unusual lesions
Sacral dimple
Other evidence suggesting myelodysplasia

Skin Examination:
Café-au-lait spots
Eczema/other rashes

Neurologic Examination of Lower Extremities:
Normal tone
Normal strength
Normal deep tendon reflexes
Normal cremasteric reflex in males

Table 5-5 "Red Flags" Suggesting Organic Etiology for Constipation

Poor weight gain/weight loss
Abdominal distention with or without vomiting
Anteriorly displaced anus
Tight anus
Patulous anus
Asymmetry or flattening of the glutei
Nevi or sinus in the lumbosacral region
Multiple café-au-lait spots
Abnormal tone and strength
Abnormal lower extremity reflexes
Presence of gross or occult blood in stool

Begin by reviewing the patient's history. The history indicates that the patient had an uneventful perinatal course and passed meconium prior to discharge from the hospital. He was passing stool several times a day until 2 months of age, when his formula was changed from Enfamil to ProSobee. Transition from breast milk

Table 5-6 Diagnostic Tests	
Test	Indications and Special Features
Serum thyroxine and thyroid-stimulating hormone	To exclude hypothyroidism
Serologic test for celiac disease (antiendomysial/antigliadin antibodies)	To exclude celiac disease
Basic metabolic panel	To exclude electrolyte and metabolic abnormalities
Serum lead level	To exclude lead toxicity
Abdominal x-ray	To exclude fecal impaction in child whose obesity precludes a thorough rectal examination or who refuses digital rectal examination (see Fig. 5-1)
Barium enema	To screen for Hirschsprung's disease (see Fig. 5-2). Should be performed on an unprepared colon to detect transition from aganglionic to ganglionic bowel
Anorectal manometry	To diagnose Hirschsprung's disease or anal achalasia, characterized by absence of relaxation of internal anal sphincter on rectal distention. Also provides information on rectal sensation, the anal sphincters during rest and squeeze, and defecation dynamics (normal vs. anismus) (see Fig. 5-3).
Rectal biopsy	To diagnose Hirschsprung's disease, characterized by absence of submucosal ganglion cells, and neuronal intestinal dysplasia, characterized by abnormal and ectopic ganglion cells.
Radiopaque marker transit studies	To diagnose colonic inertia or segmental colonic transit abnormalities. Patient should be able to swallow gelatin capsule containing markers. The transit of the markers through the gastrointestinal tract is monitored by x-ray 4 days after ingestion. Less than 20% of the markers should be in the colon on day 4.
Colonic manometry	To diagnose other colonic neuromuscular diseases besides Hirschsprung's disease. Contractile responses of colon to food and stimulants, such as bisacodyl, are examined. The presence of high-amplitude, propagated contractions is normal. Absence indicates myopathy; disordered propagation indicates neuropathy (see Fig. 5-4)
Lumbosacral magnetic resonance imaging	To diagnose occult spinal dysraphism, e.g., lipoma, tethered cord, anterior sacral meningocele

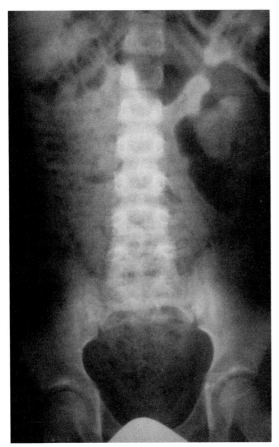

Figure 5-1 Plain x-ray of the abdomen (kidney, ureter, and bladder [KUB]) revealing significant fecal impaction in child with constipation.

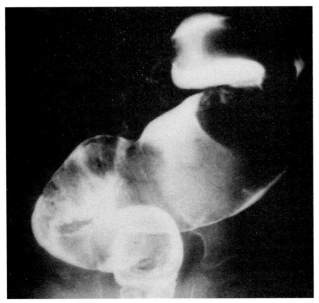

Figure 5-2 Barium enema in a child with Hirschsprung's disease showing a significantly dilated sigmoid colon with a relatively normal size rectum.

to formula or from formula to pasteurized cow's milk may lead to acute constipation, presumably because of a change in the ratio of protein to carbohydrate in these food items, which promotes firmer, smaller stools that may be evacuated with discomfort. The change from a cow's milk-based formula to a soy-based formula may have been the trigger for constipation in this patient. In fact, in a study of the effect of infant formulas on stool characteristics, Hyams and colleagues showed that infants receiving soy formulas produce firmer and harder stools than their counterparts receiving breast milk and non-soy formulas.

Could this patient have Hirschsprung's disease?

Hirschsprung's disease must be considered in the differential diagnosis of children presenting with constipation in infancy. This disorder, which results from absence of submucosal ganglion cells in varying lengths of large intestine and rectum, occurs in 1 per 5000 live births. It is more common in males and accounts for 20% to 25% of neonatal intestinal obstructions. Seven percent of affected infants have a family history, and 94% fail to pass meconium within the first 24 hours of life. The usual presentation is abdominal distention, vomiting, constipation with pencil-thin stools, and poor growth. Greater than 90% of affected children are diagnosed by 1 year of age. This patient passed meconium within the first 24 hours of life and had normal bowel movements until 2 months of age. He has no family history of Hirschsprung's disease, he passes large-diameter stools, has not had abdominal distention or vomiting, and is growing well.

Does the patient need any tests?

This patient clearly has functional retentive constipation. He demonstrates stool-withholding behavior and has an essentially normal physical examination except for the large amount of hard stool on abdominorectal examination. His medical history and physical examination are enough to make the diagnosis of functional constipation, and testing is not indicated at this time. He should be treated for functional retentive constipation.

When is testing necessary?

If there is no improvement in symptoms despite compliance and despite a change to a different laxative, testing is warranted. This should begin with blood tests to exclude occult organic disease such as hypothyroidism and hypocalcemia, and proceed to anorectal manometry to exclude anal achalasia (ultrashort segment Hirschsprung's disease), the diagnosis of which can only be made at manometry. Although manometry is best performed in the awake patient so that sensation and defecation dynamics can be examined, it can be performed under general anesthesia to examine the rectoanal inhibitory reflex only in the uncooperative patient. Other testing such as colonic manometry may

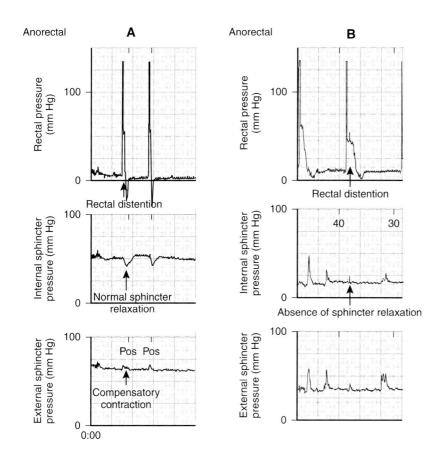

Figure 5-3 **A,** Anorectal manometry tracing showing normal relaxation of internal anal sphincter on rectal distention. **B,** Anorectal manometry tracing in a patient with Hirschsprung's disease.

be considered if symptoms are unrelenting despite a normal anorectal manometry.

What is the role of fiber in this patient?

A high-fiber diet is not advisable in this patient, who is actively withholding stool, because the bulky stool may be retained in the rectum and the fiber may serve as substrate for colonic bacteria, with resultant gas production and a possible worsening of symptoms. Once the fear of defecation is overcome with laxative stool softeners and the patient is no longer withholding stool, a high-fiber diet may be beneficial.

DISEASE DESCRIPTION: IRRITABLE BOWEL SYNDROME

Irritable bowel syndrome, one of the causes of nonretentive constipation, is a common chronic disorder of the gastrointestinal tract characterized by abdominal pain or discomfort and an irregular bowel pattern in the absence of structural or biochemical abnormalities.

Case Presentation

A 10-year-old girl presents with a 4-month history of recurrent abdominal pain. The symptoms began after a visit to the state fair. She and her grandmother ate homemade ice cream from a vendor's stand. They are the only ones in the family who ate the ice cream, and they both became ill with diarrhea and vomiting that lasted 2 days. The grandmother recovered completely from this illness. The patient's diarrhea improved after 2 days, but the abdominal pain never completely resolved. She now has abdominal pain that is localized to the lower abdomen several times a week. She describes this pain as crampy. It is sometimes associated with the passage of loose, mucous stool and other times with hard scybalous stools. Food, particularly pizza, greasy foods, and chocolate milk or chocolate candy appear to trigger pain, the intensity of which is decreased after she passes stool. Tight clothes and stress also seem to trigger her pain. The pain may last a few hours or persist throughout the day, but usually resolves when she manages to go to sleep. Although the pain may sometimes prevent sleep, it does not wake her from sleep. She has missed several days of school or has been sent home early because of abdominal pain. She has lost about 10 pounds since the symptoms began. She and her parents believe this is because she has been afraid to eat and has not been eating much. She denies chronic fever, blood in her stool, joint swelling or pain, and recurrent mouth ulcers. Her mother carries a diagnosis of irritable bowel syndrome. There is no family history of celiac disease, cystic fibrosis, or inflammatory bowel disease. Despite

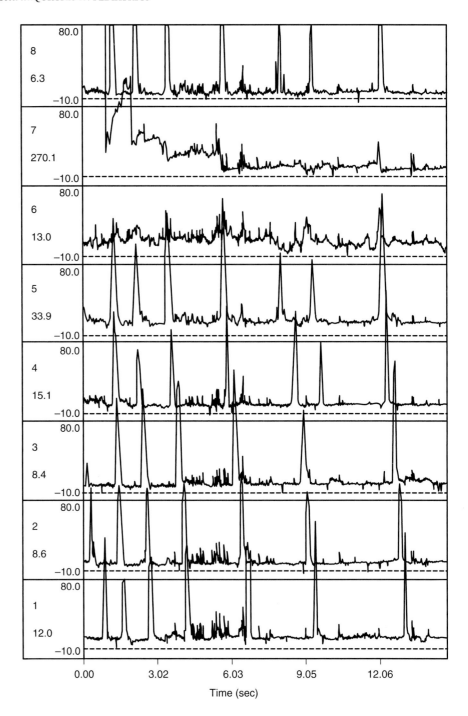

Figure 5-4 Colonic manometry tracing showing normal high amplitude propagated contractions (HAPC) in the colon.

the reported weight loss, her body mass index is in the 75th percentile and her physical examination, including rectal examination with testing of stool for occult blood, is completely normal.

Epidemiology

It is estimated that up to 20% of the adult population of Western countries has irritable bowel syndrome. In a community-based study of middle school and high school students in a mid-size suburban Connecticut town, 17% of the high school students and 8% of the middle school students reported symptoms consistent with irritable bowel syndrome. In a group of patients referred to our tertiary care center for evaluation of recurrent abdominal pain, 25% had symptoms consistent with irritable bowel syndrome. The condition probably occurs at all ages and may present in infancy as colic and in the toddler as nonspecific toddler's diarrhea. It probably occurs with

Table 5-7	Normal Frequency of Bowel Movements in Children*	
Age	Average Daily Movements	Range
0-3 months	2.9	0.7-5.7
6-12 months	1.8	0.7-4.0
1-3 years	1.4	0.6-3.0
> 3 years	1.0	0.4-2.0

*Modified from Baker SS, Liptak GS, Colletti RB, et al: Constipation in infants and children: Evaluation and treatment. J Pediatr Gastroenterol Nutr 29: 612-626, 1999.

Table 5-8 Laxatives Used in the Treatment of Constipation in Children

Bulking Agents:
Psyllium
Calcium polycarbophil

Lubricant:
Mineral oil (15-45 mL bid)

Emollient:
Docusate sodium (< 3 years = 10-40 mg/day, 3-6 years = 20-60 mg/day, 6-12 years = 40-150 mg/day, >12 years = 50-400 mg/day)

Osmotic Agents:
Lactulose (1-3 mL/kg/day divided)
Barley malt extract (2-10 mL/240 mL of formula/day)
Sorbitol (1-3 mL/kg/day divided)
Magnesium hydroxide (1-3 mL/kg/day of 450 mg/5 mL)
Magnesium citrate (<6 years = 2-4 mL/kg/day, 6-12 years = 100-150 mL/day, >12 years = 150-300 mL/day)
Polyethylene glycol 3350 (1-2 g/kg/day)
Stimulants (use short term only)
Senna (8.8 mg/5 mL syrup; <2 yr old = 1.25-2.5 mL/day; 2-6 yr old = 2.5-7.5 mL/day; 6-12 yr old = 5-15 mL/day; >12 yr old = 10-30 mL/day)
Bisacodyl (0.3 mg/kg/day, maximum 20 mg/day)

equal prevalence in males and females in early childhood and shifts to a female predominance in adolescence. In adults, irritable bowel syndrome (IBS) is clearly much more common in females, affecting three times as many females as males. In adults, IBS accounts for about $8 billion in direct medical costs and up to $25 billion in indirect costs annually in the United States, according to some estimates.

Pathophysiology

The pathophysiology of IBS is multifactorial. Familial and genetic epidemiologic studies suggest that heredity plays a role in the pathogenesis of IBS. Psychosocial factors and infection also have been implicated. Anorectal manometric studies have identified enhanced rectal sensitivity in some patients with IBS. Gastrointestinal motility studies have identified specific motor abnormalities in some patients with IBS, and there is accumulating evidence to support a role for serotonin in the motor function of the gastrointestinal tract. It is reasonable to conclude from the evidence that genetic predisposition, coupled with environmental factors and social learning, lead to the visceral hypersensitivity and disordered gastrointestinal motility that characterizes IBS, most likely through an effect on serotonin in the gastrointestinal tract.

Differential Diagnosis

IBS may mimic many gastrointestinal disorders that have an organic basis. These conditions must therefore be considered in patients in whom a diagnosis of IBS is contemplated. Table 5-9 lists several conditions that must be considered in the patient with suspected IBS.

Diagnostic Testing

In the absence of a structural or biochemical abnormality, there is no disease marker for IBS. The diagnosis of this condition therefore is based on recognition of the constellation of symptoms that characterize the syndrome and excluding other gastrointestinal or extraintestinal disorders that might present with similar symptoms through a thorough history and physical examination. To improve diagnostic accuracy, an international group of physicians and researchers meeting in Rome developed symptom-based criteria (Table 5-10) to aid in the diagnosis of the disorder. The intent is to encourage physicians to make a diagnosis of IBS confidently with minimal testing in patients with the classic symptoms and no signs to suggest an organic disease. Clues in the history or physical examination that should prompt testing to exclude organic disease are outlined in Table 5-11; tests that might be performed to screen for organic disease are discussed in Table 5-12. There are no reported long-term studies on the natural history of IBS in children. In a long-term study (10 to 13 years) of 75 adults diagnosed with IBS from symptom-based criteria, Adeniji and coworkers found that 92% did not consider their symptoms resolved and none of the 75 had the diagnosis of IBS refuted, even though 11 patients (15%) had been diagnosed with other conditions, such as diverticulitis, uterine fibromyoma, cholelithiasis, and cholecystitis during the years following the initial diagnosis, suggesting that for most patients diagnosed with IBS based on the established symptom-based criteria, the diagnosis does not change with time as long as the symptoms do not change and new symptoms do not develop.

Table 5-9 Other Causes of Abdominal Pain That Must Be Considered in the Patient with Suspected IBS

Inflammatory Bowel Disease:
Crohn's disease
Ulcerative colitis

Acid-Peptic Disease:
Esophagitis
Gastritis
Duodenitis

Urinary Tract Disease:
Kidney stones
Urinary tract infection

Carbohydrate Malabsorption:
Lactose
Fructose
Sorbitol

Other Malabsorption:
Celiac disease

Hepatobiliary Disease:
Hepatitis
Choledocholithiasis
Chronic cholecystitis
Gallbladder dyskinesia

Pancreatic Disease:
Chronic pancreatitis
Sphincter of Oddi dysfunction

Parasitic Infections:
Giardia
Cryptosporidium

Bacterial Infections:
Clostridium difficile
Yersinia
Salmonella
Campylobacter

Miscellaneous:
Acute intermittent porphyria
Thyroid disease
School avoidance behavior
Laxative abuse

Table 5-10 Rome II Criteria for the Diagnosis of IBS*

At Least 12 Weeks of the Following Symptoms in the Preceding 12 Months:
Abdominal pain or discomfort associated with at least two of the following:
  Change in the frequency of stool
  Change in the consistency of stool (loose, lumpy, or both)
  Resolution of pain or discomfort with defecation

Absence of Structural or Metabolic Abnormalities:
Other common features:
  Mucus in stool
  Sensation of abdominal bloating

*Rasquin-Weber A, Hyman PE, Cucchiara S, et al: Childhood functional gastrointestinal disorders. Gut 45:II60-II68, 1999.

Table 5-11 Historical Clues That Might Suggest the Likelihood of an Organic Cause for Abdominal Symptoms

Pain that awakens patient from sleep
Weight loss or growth failure
Delayed puberty
Gross or occult blood in the stool
Joint swelling or joint pain
Chronic fever
Family history of celiac disease, inflammatory bowel disease, peptic ulcer disease
History of overseas travel preceding onset of symptoms

Table 5-12 Laboratory Studies to Screen for Organic Disease in Patients with Suspected Irritable Bowel Syndrome

Complete blood count with platelets and differential count (anemia, inflammation, infection)
ALT, AST, GGT, bilirubin, albumin (hepatobiliary disease)
Serum amylase and lipase (pancreatic disease)
ESR, CRP (chronic inflammation)
Stool for occult blood, white blood cells, enteric pathogens, *Clostridium difficile*, ova and parasites (inflammation, infection)
Lactose/fructose breath hydrogen test (lactose/fructose malabsorption)

ALT, alanine aminotransferase; AST, aspartate transaminase; CRP, C-reactive protein; ESR, erythrocyte sedimentation rate; GGT, gamma-glutamyl-transferase.

Treatment

The absence of randomized controlled trials examining treatment modalities for IBS in children means that there is no uniformity in the treatment of this disorder in children. Although fiber, anticholinergics, and antidepressants have been used, there are no data confirming their efficacy in children with IBS. A meta-analysis of randomized controlled trials in adults, however, has suggested that some adults with IBS might benefit from tricyclic antidepressants and anticholinergics.

The treatment of IBS should begin with education of the patient and parents about IBS, followed by reassurance that the disorder, although real and sometimes associated with severe, debilitating symptoms, is a benign condition. Although the patient may not be cured, one could set realistic goals to decrease the frequency and intensity of symptoms to enable the patient to function in society. Because many patients have postprandial symptoms, we advise our patients to avoid foods that trigger or aggravate symptoms and suggest avoidance or limitation of highly seasoned foods, caffeine, carbonated beverages, and fatty foods. For patients whose symptoms are mild and constipation is predominant, we recommend a high-fiber diet or fiber supplements (the equivalent, in grams, of the patient's age in years plus 5 daily). For those with mild symptoms and diarrhea predominance, we place the emphasis on diet. In addition to the avoidance of caffeine, highly seasoned foods, greasy foods, and carbonated beverages, we advise patients to avoid foods, beverages, and candy or gum containing sorbitol and other artificial sweeteners. We perform a lactose breath hydrogen test and treat those with lactose intolerance with supplemental lactase. Any psychosocial factors that might trigger or aggravate symptoms are addressed, including referral for counseling when indicated.

For patients with mild symptoms not responding to dietary restrictions and fiber, and for patients with moderate to severe symptoms (patients who are missing school and whose day-to-day activities are impaired), we prescribe pharmacologic agents in addition to dietary restrictions and fiber. Our first-line pharmacologic agent is dicyclomine, although hyoscyamine also may be used. Dicyclomine is prescribed at a dose of 30 to 80 mg/day in three or four divided doses, starting with the lowest dose and increasing if necessary, as tolerated. Side effects include dry mouth and constipation and rarely, blurred vision and dizziness. Patients are encouraged to increase their consumption of water and fiber to offset the dry mouth and constipating effects of the medication. For patients failing to respond to anticholinergics, we prescribe either a tricyclic antidepressant (TCA) or a selective serotonin reuptake inhibitor (SSRI). Tricyclic antidepressants have been shown, at low doses, to improve symptoms of IBS in adults; however, side effects may limit their use in many patients. In a randomized controlled study of desipramine versus placebo in 216 adults with IBS, Drossman and colleagues did not find a statistically significant benefit of desipramine over placebo in the intention-to-treat analysis; however, in the per-protocol analysis, desipramine was superior to placebo. The reason for the discrepancy was because 28% of patients on desipramine failed to complete the study because of side effects. A recent double-blind, randomized controlled study of paroxetine versus placebo in adults with IBS showed improvement in general well-being in patients on paroxetine compared with placebo, although abdominal pain and bloating were not significantly improved over placebo. SSRIs are better tolerated than TCAs and are certainly helpful when anxiety plays a significant role in symptom generation. In general, antidepressants of either class may be beneficial in patients with obvious psychological comorbidities affecting their IBS.

Other pharmacologic agents approved for treatment of IBS in adult women are tegaserod, a 5HT4 partial agonist that has been shown to be superior to placebo in the treatment of women with constipation-predominant IBS, and alosetron, a 5HT3 antagonist that has been shown to be superior to placebo in the treatment of diarrhea-predominant IBS. Alosetron was voluntarily withdrawn from the U.S. market in 2000 following a link to ischemic colitis and other serious side effects. It was recently reintroduced for use, under very strict guidelines, in the treatment of women with severe diarrhea-predominant IBS who failed with other therapies. There are no data on the use of these medications in children with IBS; they certainly may be considered in teenage girls with severe IBS failing other therapies (Table 5-13 lists medications used in the treatment of IBS). It is important in the treatment of the child with IBS to maintain a close relationship with the patient and family, seeing them at follow-up until symptoms are well managed and the patient is functioning in society. Maintaining such a close relationship provides a sense of security for the patient and family and assurance that they are not being abandoned. If severe symptoms persist, symptoms change in character, or new symptoms develop, a limited evaluation should be performed to exclude organic disease.

Approach to the Case

What is the cause of this patient's symptoms?

In reviewing the history, it is noted that this patient was a healthy child until the trip to the state fair. She and

Table 5-13 Drugs Commonly Used to Treat IBS

Anticholinergics:
Dicyclomine
Hyoscyamine

Antidepressants:

TCAs
  Amitriptyline
  Nortriptyline
  Desipramine

SSRIs:
  Fluoxetine
  Paroxetine

Serotonin Agonists/Antagonists:
Alosetron (diarrhea-predominant irritable bowel syndrome [IBS] in women)
Tegaserod (constipation-predominant IBS in women) (Temporarily withdrawn from the market in March 2007 due to concerns about cardiac side effects)

her grandmother ate ice cream at the fair and became ill afterward, suggesting that they might have been stricken with acute food poisoning. Her grandmother recovered completely, but the patient continued to have abdominal symptoms. The history she provides and her normal physical examination satisfy established symptom-based criteria for the diagnosis of IBS. The history of IBS in the mother is certainly helpful in making the case for this diagnosis. This patient most likely suffers from postinfectious IBS.

What about the history of weight loss?

Although there is a logical explanation, weight loss is not part of the symptom complex of IBS and should be a "red flag."

How should this patient be managed?

The suspected diagnosis of IBS, the pathophysiology, and the compelling reasons for this diagnosis should be discussed at the initial evaluation, and realistic goals of therapy set. Because of the weight loss, a negative screening test for inflammatory bowel disease, infectious enterocolitis, celiac disease, and thyroid disease would be reassuring to the patient, parents, and physician. Blood tests for complete blood count (CBC), erythrocyte sedimentation rate (ESR), thyroxine (T_4), thyroid-stimulating hormone (TSH), and antiendomysial and antigliadin antibodies; and stool for *Clostridium difficile* and ova and parasites should be obtained. The patient should be advised to avoid foods that aggravate her symptoms and to increase her dietary fiber intake to 15 g per day. An anticholinergic such as dicyclomine at a dose of 10 mg four times per day (30 to 60 minutes before meals and at bedtime) would be a reasonable choice for a pharmacologic agent. A follow-up appointment should be scheduled within 4 to 6 weeks, and the parents should be encouraged to call the physician if symptoms do not improve.

When would further testing be indicated in this patient?

If symptoms do not improve on fiber and antispasmodics, a trial of an antidepressant should be considered. If symptoms do not improve on both antispasmodics and antidepressants or if new symptoms develop at any time, further testing to include endoscopic evaluation is indicated.

SUMMARY

Constipation and abdominal pain, often due to IBS, are two of the most common conditions for which children are referred to a pediatric gastroenterologist, and account for a substantial fraction of general health care costs. Although many organic disorders may manifest with abdominal pain and/or constipation, most children presenting with these symptoms do not have an organic etiology. Being able to separate out, through a thorough history and physical examination, patients with a potential organic etiology who require extensive evaluation from those who clearly have a functional disorder and do not require extensive testing prevents unnecessary and costly evaluations. In this chapter, we have discussed the pathophysiology, clinical features, and management of constipation and IBS in children, and have demonstrated an approach to patients using two real case studies. We highlighted what we believe to be a logical approach to the management of patients presenting with similar complaints that takes into consideration cost issues and optimal patient care.

▶ MAJOR POINTS ◀

Constipation and IBS are common disorders of the gastrointestinal tract seen in children and they account for a substantial portion of annual health care costs.

Ninety-five percent of children with constipation have a functional etiology for their symptoms. Many demonstrate stool-withholding behavior.

If a history of stool-withholding behavior is elicited in a child presenting with constipation, a functional etiology should be assumed and the patient treated as such without testing.

Treatment of childhood functional constipation begins with education of the child and parents, and includes the use of laxatives to maintain soft stools and behavioral modification to establish a regular bowel habit. Several months of treatment with a nonstimulant laxative may be necessary to achieve a successful outcome.

The diagnosis of IBS can be made positively in a child with abdominal pain and a normal physical examination if other aspects of the history meet established symptom-based criteria for diagnosis of the disorder.

The treatment of IBS in children should begin with education and reassurance of the patient and parents, and should include a discussion of dietary and psychosocial triggers. Fiber, anticholinergics, and antidepressants, though not studied for efficacy in children, may be beneficial. It is important to establish and maintain a good relationship with the patient and parents.

In the absence of a change in symptoms or the appearance of new symptoms, the diagnosis of IBS does not change over time in most patients who have a normal physical examination and meet the established symptom-based criteria for the diagnosis.

SUGGESTED READINGS

Adeniji OA, Barnett CB, DiPalma JA: Durability of the diagnosis of irritable bowel syndrome based on clinical criteria. Dig Dis Sci 49:572-574, 2004.

Baker SS, Liptak GS, Colletti RB, et al: Constipation in infants and children: Evaluation and treatment. J Pediatr Gastroenterol Nutr 29:612-626, 1999.

Croffie JM, Fitzgerald JF, Chong SKF: Recurrent abdominal pain in children: A retrospective study of outcome in a group referred to a pediatric gastroenterology practice. Clin Pediatr 39:267-274, 2000.

Drossman DA: Irritable bowel syndrome. Gastrointest Dis Today 4:9-18, 1995.

Drossman DA, Toner BB, Whitehead WE, et al: Cognitive-behavioral therapy versus education and desipramine versus placebo for moderate to severe functional bowel disorders. Gastroenterology 125:19-31, 2003.

Gwee KA, Graham JC, McKendrick MW, et al: Psychometric scores and persistence of irritable bowel after infectious diarrhea. Lancet 347:150-153, 1996.

Horwitz BJ, Fisher RS: The irritable bowel syndrome. N Engl J Med 344:1846-1850, 2001.

Hyams JS, Burke G, Davis PM, et al: Abdominal pain and irritable bowel syndrome in adolescents: A community-based study. J Pediatr 129:220-226, 1996.

Hyams JS, Treem WR, Etienne NL, et al: Effect of infant formula on stool characteristics of young infants. Pediatrics 95:50-54, 1995.

Imseis E, Gariety C: Hirschsprung's disease. In Walker WA, Goulet O, Kleinman RE, et al (eds): Pediatric Gastrointestinal Disease: Pathophysiology, Diagnosis, Management, 4th ed. Hamilton, Ontario, BC Decker, 2004, pp 1031-1043.

Jailwala J, Imperiale TF, Kroenke K: Pharmacologic treatment of the irritable bowel syndrome: A systematic review of randomized, controlled trials. Ann Intern Med 133:136-147, 2000.

Levine MD, Bakow H: Children with encopresis: A study of treatment outcome. Pediatrics 58:845-852, 1976.

Levy RL, Jones KR, Whitehead WE, et al: Irritable bowel syndrome in twins: Heredity and social learning both contribute to etiology. Gastroenterology 121:799-804, 2001.

Loening-Baucke V: Constipation in early childhood: Patient characteristics, treatment, and longterm follow up. Gut 34:1400-1404, 1993.

Loening-Baucke V: Functional constipation. Sem Pediatr Surg 4:26-34, 1995.

Pata C, Erdal ME, Derici E, et al: Serotonin transporter gene polymorphism in irritable bowel syndrome. Am J Gastroenterol 97:1780-1784, 2002.

Rasquin-Weber A, Hyman PE, Cucchiara S, et al: Childhood functional gastrointestinal disorders. Gut 45:II60-II68, 1999.

Roma E, Adamidis D, Nikolara R, et al: Diet and chronic constipation in children: The role of fiber. J Pediatr Gastroenterol Nutr 28:169-174, 1999.

Tabas G, Beaves M, Wang J, et al: Paroxetine to treat irritable bowel syndrome not responding to high-fiber diet: A double-blind, placebo-controlled trial. Am J Gastroenterol 99:921-923, 2004.

Taitz LS, Wales JK, Urwin OM, et al: Factors associated with outcome in management of defecation disorders. Arch Dis Child 61:472-477, 1986.

CHAPTER 6

Eosinophilic Esophagitis

EDWIN DeZOETEN
JONATHAN E. MARKOWITZ

Disease Description
Case Presentation
Epidemiology
Pathophysiology
Differential Diagnosis
Diagnostic Testing
Treatment
Approach to the Case
Summary
Major Points

DISEASE DESCRIPTION

Eosinophilic esophagitis (EoE) is a disease of children and adults characterized by an isolated, severe eosinophilic infiltration of the esophagus manifested by gastroesophageal reflux (GER)-like symptoms—regurgitation, epigastric and chest pain, vomiting, heartburn, feeding difficulties, dysphagia—unresponsive to acid-suppression therapy. Initially, eosinophilia of the esophagus was believed to be the sole evidence of GER; recently it has been defined as a separate entity.

CASE PRESENTATION

A 7-year-old male with a history of asthma presents to a gastroenterologist's office with a 1-year history of epigastric pain and frequent regurgitation of sour-tasting food and liquid. He was seen by his primary care physician, diagnosed with reflux, and started on an H₂-receptor antagonist without improvement. He was given a proton pump inhibitor, which also provided no relief after a 1-month trial. He was then referred to a gastroenterologist.

On further evaluation he complains of the sensation of food getting stuck in his esophagus. He also complains of occasional vomiting that is nonbloody and nonbilious. There is a history of reflux as well as multiple environmental allergies in his family. Esophagogastroduodenoscopy (EGD) with biopsy was performed. Visually the esophagus appeared to have deep linear furrows and whitish plaques on the surface. The stomach and duodenum were visually normal. Biopsies revealed high numbers of eosinophils in the mucosa of the esophagus, with normal histology of the stomach and duodenum.

EPIDEMIOLOGY

EoE occurs in children and adults. Whereas food allergy in infancy often manifests with diarrhea, abdominal pain, and a bloody colitis, the presentation of EoE in children is similar to the symptoms associated with GER. There are many more reports in the literature of children with this disease compared with adults. This may reflect a higher incidence of food allergies in children, but likely also reflects the practice in the field of pediatric gastroenterology of taking biopsies of all tissues, regardless of visual appearance. This practice is not common among adult gastroenterologists.

There are currently very few national epidemiologic data about the incidence and prevalence of EoE, yet the gastroenterology community in adults and children has noted a significant upward trend. This may be in part due to increased awareness and identification of the disease, but current evidence suggests a true increasing incidence as well. One study performed in Hamilton County, Ohio, defined the incidence of EoE as approximately 1 in 10,000 children from birth to 19 years old between 2000 and 2003. In that study, the prevalence of the disease was 4.3 per 10,000 children by the end of 2003. Interestingly, the investigators noted that only 2.8% of the total cases were identified prior to 2000, with almost 97% discovered between 2000 and 2003.

Boys develop EoE more frequently than girls, with approximately 70% of the reported cases occurring in males. The typical symptoms include nausea, vomiting, regurgitation, epigastric abdominal pain, and poor eating. Young children more commonly demonstrate food refusal, whereas adolescents often experience dysphagia. Adults present with similar symptoms; however, dysphagia occurs much more commonly and can be associated with esophageal strictures. Less common symptoms include growth failure, hematemesis, globus, and water brash. The clinical features of EoE may evolve over years. Symptoms such as abdominal pain and heartburn occur regularly; however, patients with vomiting or dysphagia may display these symptoms sporadically, complaining only once or twice a month. Approximately 50% of affected children also exhibit atopic signs and symptoms including bronchospasm, allergic rhinitis, and eczema. Frequently, there is a strong family history of food allergies or similar allergic disorders.

PATHOPHYSIOLOGY

EoE appears to be caused by an abnormal immunologic response to specific food antigens. A large proportion of EoE patients have evidence of food and aeroallergen hypersensitivity, as defined by skinprick tests, radioallergosorbent tests (RASTs), or patch testing. Although several studies have documented resolution of EoE with the strict avoidance of food antigens, in 1995 Kelly and colleagues published the original paper on the resolution of EoE with an elemental diet. Each patient with refractory reflux symptoms was treated with a strict elimination diet, which included an amino acid–based formula. Patients were also allowed clear liquids, corn, and apples. Seventeen patients were initially offered a dietary elimination trial, with 10 patients adhering to the protocol. Symptomatic improvement was seen within an average of 3 weeks after the introduction of the elemental diet (resolution in 8 patients, improvement in 2). In addition, all 10 patients demonstrated a significant improvement in esophageal eosinophilia. Subsequently, all patients reverted to previous symptoms on reintroduction of foods. Pre- and post-dietary trial evaluations demonstrated a significant improvement in clinical symptoms and an almost complete resolution in esophageal eosinophilia, from a mean of 41 eosinophils per microscopic high-powered field (HPF) to less than 1 per HPF. Open food challenges were then conducted in which a return of symptoms was noted with a challenge to milk (7 patients), soy (4), wheat (2), peanut (2), and egg (1).

Although an exact etiology was not determined, in 1995, Kelly and coworkers suggested an immunologic basis, secondary to a delayed hypersensitivity or a cell-mediated hypersensitivity response, as the cause for EoE. A study by Spergel and associates confirmed that foods that cause EoE are often not based on an immediate hypersensitivity reaction. By using a combination of traditional skin testing and patch testing, he established that a delayed cellular-mediated allergic response might be responsible for many cases of EoE. Recently, $CD8^+$ T lymphocytes have been identified as the predominant T cell within the squamous epithelium of patients diagnosed with EoE. Studies by Mishra and associates demonstrated that in *Aspergillus fumigatus*-induced eosinophilic infiltration of the esophagus, interleukin-5 (IL-5), the most specific growth factor for eosinophil lineage expansion, was necessary for this infiltration. In addition, the chemokine eotaxin-1 has been implicated as an eosinophil-trafficking molecule necessary for homing of eosinophils to the gastrointestinal tract. A study of eight patients with EoE further supported the involvement of IL-5 in this disease process, in which they identified increased expression of IL-5 and tumor necrosis factor-alpha (TNF-α) from biopsy specimens. Finally, although other causes of EoE have been suggested, such as aeroallergens or infectious agents, only food antigens thus far have been extensively tested.

Previous studies have established the link between eosinophilic esophagitis and atopy. It was these initial links between atopy and EoE that suggested food allergies might play a role in the pathogenesis of this disease. The role of food allergy was confirmed as patients improved on elemental diets. Elimination of the responsible food usually does not lead to rapid resolution of the symptoms. Rather, improvement of symptoms occurs approximately 1 to 2 weeks after the removal of the causative antigen. Also, in patients with EoE, symptoms may not occur immediately after reintroduction to the foods. It commonly takes several days for symptoms to develop, suggesting either a mixed IgE and T-cell–mediated allergic response or strictly a T-cell–delayed mechanism in the pathogenesis of this disease. Both IgE and T-cell–mediated reactions have been identified as possible causative factors, but T-cell–mediated reactions seem to be the main mechanism of disease.

Not all patients' disease processes suggest a food allergen. Aeroallergens may also play a role in the development of EoE. Mishra and Rothenberg used a mouse model to show that the inhalation of aspergillus caused EoE. They found that the allergen-challenged mice developed elevated levels of esophageal eosinophils and features of epithelial cell hyperplasia that mimic EoE, even when the allergen was delivered directly to the lung. In addition, Spergel and coworkers reported a case of a 21-year-old female with asthma and allergic rhinoconjunctivitis who also had EoE. The patient's EoE became symptomatic with exacerbations during pollen seasons, followed by resolution during winter months.

DIFFERENTIAL DIAGNOSIS

The differential diagnosis is broad prior to performing the diagnostic tests for eosinophilic esophagitis. After endoscopy the differential decreases significantly.

Differential diagnosis at presentation:
1. Gastroesophageal reflux disease (GERD)
2. Eosinophilic esophagitis
3. Gastritis
4. Peptic ulcer disease
5. Esophageal dysmotility
6. Esophageal stricture
7. Infection, such as *Helicobacter pylori*
8. Inflammatory bowel disease
9. Connective tissue disease

Differential diagnosis after biopsy proved eosinophilia in the esophagus:
1. Eosinophilic esophagitis
2. Eosinophilic gastroenteritis
3. GERD
4. Recurrent vomiting
5. Parasitic or fungal infections
6. Inflammatory bowel disease
7. Esophageal leiomyomatosis
8. Myeloproliferative disorder

DIAGNOSTIC TESTING

The definitive diagnosis of EoE is made endoscopically in patients who have reflux-like symptoms and normal (or borderline-normal) pH probes and are unresponsive to acid inhibition. A few patients may experience a modest symptomatic response to acid blockade; however, their biopsy findings do not change. This fact underscores the importance of obtaining esophageal biopsies whenever questions arise regarding the disease process. The performance of esophageal pH monitoring may also be useful because significant acid reflux disease should be excluded before confirming the diagnosis. In EoE, pH probes often reveal frequent, brief reflux episodes but normal esophageal acid clearance and a normal reflux index. The number of esophageal eosinophils per HPF is the strongest marker of EoE. A review of multiple studies suggests that the vast majority of patients with EoE present with more than 20 eosinophils per HPF.

In 1999, Ruchelli and colleagues studied 102 patients who presented with symptoms of GERD and who had evidence of esophagitis and at least one intraepithelial eosinophil on endoscopic biopsy. These patients were treated with H_2-receptor blockers and prokinetic agents. If the patient's symptoms persisted after 3 months of therapy with H_2-blockers, a proton pump inhibitor was begun, and these patients were re-evaluated 3 months later by endoscopy with biopsy. The treatment response was classified into three categories: (1) clinical improvement without relapse; (2) improvement with relapse of clinical symptoms; and (3) failure of medical treatment. All but two patients had isolated esophageal involvement. The number of esophageal eosinophils predicted the type of response, with group 1 having the lowest number (1.1 eosinophils/HPF), group 2 an intermediate number (6.4 eosinophils/HPF), and group 3 having the highest number (24.5 eosinophils/HPF). Although an isolated, severe, esophageal eosinophilia unresponsive to acid blockade is necessary for the diagnosis of EoE, several reports have detailed the macroscopic appearance of the esophagus in patients with EoE.

Orenstein reported on a series of children with probable EoE and suggested that the endoscopic appearance revealed a granular, subtle, furrowed ringed appearance. In addition, a recent report by Teitelbaum and associates suggested that in patients successfully treated for EoE, a furrowed, ringed esophagus may persist despite normal biopsies. However, a ringed esophageal appearance also can be appreciated in patients who have other causes of severe esophagitis. Additionally, Fox and colleagues performed endoscopic ultrasound on patients with EoE and compared them with a control group. He demonstrated that the mucosa to submucosa ratio and muscularis propria thickness were greater in EoE patients when compared with a control group. However, no comparison was made with patients who had esophagitis secondary to other disorders.

EoE can occur in both the mid- and distal portions of the esophagus. Several previous adult reports demonstrated mid-esophageal involvement associated with stricture formation. Most adults with EoE have been reported to have a significant number of eosinophils in the mid-esophagus; however, many of these patients did not have their distal esophagus biopsied. In contrast, Liacouras established that even in those cases of proximal esophageal involvement that the distal esophageal was also involved, typically to a higher degree than the midesophagus. A peripheral eosinophilia and increased IgE levels have been reported in 20% to 60% of patients with EoE, but these findings alone are neither sensitive nor specific for EoE.

TREATMENT

The identification and removal of allergic dietary antigens are mainstays of treatment for EoE. Although removal of the offending food(s) reverses the disease process in patients with EoE, in many cases, the isolation of these foods is extremely difficult. Often, patients with EoE cannot correlate their gastrointestinal symptoms with the ingestion of a specific food because of a delayed hypersensitivity response. Several reports have demonstrated that it takes several days for symptoms to recur on ingestion of antigens that cause EoE. Furthermore, allergy testing using skin tests and RAST tests are of limited value in many patients with EoE. Even when a particular food causing EoE has been isolated, it may take days or weeks for the symptoms to resolve. In addition, although one food may be identified, there may be several others (not easily identified) that could also be contributing to EoE. Finally, upper endoscopy with biopsy is the only diagnostic test that has been shown to document resolution of the disease.

Although attempts should be made to identify and eliminate potential food allergens through a careful history and the use of allergy testing, the administration of a strict diet, using an amino acid–based formula, is often necessary. As established by Kelly and colleagues, as well as by Markowitz and coworkers, the use of an elemental diet rapidly improves clinical symptoms and histology in patients with EoE. Because of poor palatability, continuous nasogastric feeding is commonly employed to administer the elemental formula. The diet may be supplemented with water, one fruit (typically apples or grapes), and the corresponding pure fruit juice, provided allergy testing to these fruits is negative. In EoE, the response to this diet confirms the diagnosis. Reversal of symptoms typically occurs within 10 days, with histologic improvement in 4 weeks. Although the strict use of an amino acid–based formula may be difficult for patients (and parents) to accept initially, its benefits outweigh the risks of other treatments.

First, because food allergens have thus far been the most consistently implicated factor in the etiology of EoE, removal of these allergens provides a long-term remission of the disease. In contrast, the use of other medications such as corticosteroids may improve the disease, but on their discontinuation the disease recurs, which in turn necessitates recurrent courses of medications that commonly have undesirable side effects. Finally, because it is difficult to determine the allergic foods by history, and allergy testing or random elimination of suspected foods is successful in only a proportion of cases, the use of an elemental diet ensures and proves that food allergy is the cause of EoE. Once the esophagus is healed, foods may be reintroduced systematically, allowing for identification of the causative foods.

Treatment of EoE with aggressive acid blockade, including medical and surgical therapy, is not effective. Several published reports have demonstrated the failure of H_2-blocker and proton pump therapy in patients with EoE. Although acid blockade may improve clinical symptoms by improving acid reflux that occurs secondary to the underlying inflamed esophageal mucosa, it does not reverse the esophageal histologic abnormality. Furthermore, Liacouras published findings on two patients found to have an isolated eosinophilic infiltration of the esophagus who failed medical therapy and underwent Nissen fundoplication. In both cases, the patients continued to have clinical symptoms and evidence of an isolated esophageal eosinophilia by biopsy after fundoplication. Each responded to oral corticosteroids with resolution of their clinical symptoms and a return to normal of their esophageal mucosa. In one patient, symptoms recurred on discontinuation of corticosteroids; however, the patient subsequently responded to the introduction of an elemental diet.

Before 1997, reports suggested that systemic corticosteroids improved the symptoms of EoE in adults identified with a severe eosinophilic esophagitis. In 1997, Liacouras was the first to publish the use of oral corticosteroids in 20 children diagnosed with EoE. These patients were treated with oral methylprednisolone (average dose 1.5 mg/kg/day; maximum dose 48 mg/day) for 1 month. Symptoms were significantly improved in 19 of 20 patients by an average of 8 days. A repeat endoscopy with biopsy, 4 weeks after the initiation of therapy, demonstrated a significant reduction of esophageal eosinophils, from 34 to 1.5 eosinophils per HPF. However, on discontinuation of corticosteroids, 90% had recurrence of symptoms.

In 1999, Faubion and colleagues reported that swallowing a metered dose of inhaled corticosteroids was also effective in treating the symptoms of EoE in children. Four patients diagnosed with EoE manifested by epigastric pain, dysphagia, and a severe esophageal eosinophilia unresponsive to aggressive acid blockade were given fluticasone, four puffs twice a day. Patients were instructed to use inhaled corticosteroids but to immediately swallow after inhalation in order to deliver the medication to the esophagus. Histologic improvement was not determined. Within 2 months, all four patients responded with an improvement in symptoms. Two patients required repeat use of inhalation therapy. This therapy was recently confirmed. Although this therapy can improve EoE, the side effects can include esophageal candidiasis and growth failure. In addition, symptoms recur on discontinuation of the therapy.

The mast cell–stabilizing agent cromolyn sodium has also been used to treat children with EoE. In similar fashion to its use for children with EoG, oral cromolyn has been given to patients with a severe esophageal eosinophilia in conjunction with other systemic signs and symptoms of allergic disease. However, no controlled reports have been performed, and no efficacy for oral cromolyn has been established for treating EoE. Finally, there has been recent evidence as to the efficacy of anti–IL-5 (mepolizumab) in the therapy of generalized hypereosinophilic syndromes as well as in eosinophilic disorders and atopic asthma. In one of these studies a patient with severe EoE had a ten-fold reduction in tissue eosinophils, lending hope that this drug may be another potential treatment for EoE in the future.

APPROACH TO THE CASE

Patients with chronic symptoms of vomiting, regurgitation, epigastric abdominal pain, dysphagia, or symptoms of gastoresophageal reflux unresponsive to medical therapy should be evaluated for EoE. Every evaluation should include a radiographic upper gastrointestinal series to rule out anatomic abnormalities and an upper endoscopy with biopsy. In a patient with normal anatomy, the presence of an isolated, severe esophageal eosinophilia (>20 eosinophils/HPF), obtained while the patient is receiving adequate gastric acid blockade with a proton pump inhibitor, strongly suggests the diagnosis of EoE. The diagnosis can be further supported with pH probe monitoring. Although the pH probe may reveal frequent, brief reflux episodes (up to three episodes per hour), the probe should demonstrate normal esophageal acid clearance and a normal reflux index. Patients with severely abnormal pH probe findings should undergo further evaluation for refractory gastroesophageal reflux disease.

SUMMARY

Eosinophilic esophagitis is an increasingly recognized disease in children and adults. Patients with EoE can present with a range of symptoms, ranging from those similar to GERD to dysphagia and stricture. The symptoms are generally not responsive to antiacid therapy. Evidence indicates that this is an immunologic disorder that is characterized by a food sensitivity. With that in mind, initiation of an elemental diet followed by selective dietary expansion has been the best proved long-term therapy. Medications used in this disease tend to relieve symptoms in the short term or not at all and may be associated with significant side effects.

MAJOR POINTS

EoE can mimic the symptoms of GERD.
EoE has a strong male predominance.
Younger children with EoE are more likely to present with reflux symptoms.
Adolescents with EoE are more likely to present with dysphagia or food impaction.
Esophageal pH monitoring is typically normal in EoE, as opposed to GERD.
EoE is likely an allergic response to a food antigen.
Patients with symptoms similar to GERD yet unresponsive to sufficient acid blockade should be evaluated by EGD and tissue biopsies
EoE is typified by greater than 20 eosinophils per HPF on esophageal biopsies.
EoE is increasing in incidence.
EoE is best treated by an elimination diet
Modulation of the immune system with corticosteroids is not the long-term treatment of choice in EoE.
Interleukin-5 is the cytokine most correlated with eosinophilic infiltration, and is the target of experimental biologic agents for EoE.

SUGGESTED READINGS

Bousvaros A, Antonioli DA, Winter HS: Ringed esophagus: An association with esophagitis. Am J Gastroenterol 87:1187-1190, 1992.

Dobbins JW, Sheahan DG, Behar J: Eosinophilic gastroenteritis with esophageal involvement. Gastroenterology 72:1312-1316, 1977.

Faubion WA Jr, Perrault J, Burgart LJ, et al: Treatment of eosinophilic esophagitis with inhaled corticosteroids. J Pediatr Gastroenterol Nutr 27:90-93, 1998.

Fogg MI, Ruchelli E, Spergel JM: Pollen and eosinophilic esophagitis. J Allergy Clin Immunol 112:796-797, 2003.

Fox VL, Nurko S, Teitelbaum JE, et al: High-resolution EUS in children with eosinophilic "allergic" esophagitis. Gastrointest Endosc 57:30-36, 2003.

Furuta GT: Eosinophilic esophagitis: An emerging clinicopathologic entity. Curr Allergy Asthma Rep 2:67-72, 2002.

Garrett JK, Jameson SC, Thomson B, et al: Anti-interleukin-5 (mepolizumab) therapy for hypereosinophilic syndromes. J Allergy Clin Immunol 113:115-119, 2004.

Gupta SK, Fitzgerald JF, Chong SK, et al: Vertical lines in distal esophageal mucosa (VLEM): A true endoscopic manifestation of esophagitis in children? Gastrointest Endosc 45:485-489, 1997.

Hogan SP, Mishra A, Brandt EB, et al: A pathological function for eotaxin and eosinophils in eosinophilic gastrointestinal inflammation. Nat Immunol 2:353-360, 2001.

Kelly KJ, Lazenby AJ, Rowe PC, et al: Eosinophilic esophagitis attributed to gastroesophageal reflux: Improvement with an amino acid-based formula. Gastroenterology 109:1503-1512, 1995.

Lee RG: Marked eosinophilia in esophageal mucosal biopsies. Am J Surg Pathol 9:475-479, 1985.

Liacouras CA: Failed Nissen fundoplication in two patients who had persistent vomiting and eosinophilic esophagitis. J Pediatr Surg 32:1504-1506, 1997.

Liacouras CA, Markowitz JE: Eosinophilic esophagitis: A subset of eosinophilic gastroenteritis. Curr Gastroenterol Rep 1:253-258, 1999.

Liacouras CA, Wenner WJ, Brown K, et al: Primary eosinophilic esophagitis in children: Successful treatment with oral corticosteroids. J Pediatr Gastroenterol Nutr 26:380-385, 1998.

Lucendo Villarin AJ, Carrion Alonso G, Navarro Sanchez M, et al: Eosinophilic esophagitis in adults, an emerging cause of dysphagia: Description of 9 cases. Rev Esp Enferm Dig 97:229-239, 2005.

Markowitz JE, Spergel JM, Ruchelli E, et al: Elemental diet is an effective treatment for eosinophilic esophagitis in children and adolescents. Am J Gastroenterol 98:777-782, 2003.

Menzies-Gow A, Flood-Page P, Schmi R, et al: Anti-IL-5 (mepolizumab) therapy induces bone marrow eosinophil maturational arrest and decreases eosinophil progenitors in the bronchial mucosa of atopic asthmatics. J Allergy Clin Immunol 111:714-719, 2003.

Mishra A, Hogan SP, Brandt EB, et al: An etiological role for aeroallergens and eosinophils in experimental esophagitis. J Clin Invest 107:83-90, 2001.

Mishra A, Hogan SP, Brandt EB, et al: IL-5 promotes eosinophil trafficking to the esophagus. J Immunol 168:2464-2469, 2002.

Noel RJ, Putnam PE, Rothenberg ME: Eosinophilic esophagitis. N Engl J Med 351:940-941, 2004.

Orenstein SR, Shalaby TM, Di Lorenzo C, et al: The spectrum of pediatric eosinophilic esophagitis beyond infancy: A clinical series of 30 children. Am J Gastroenterol 95:1422-1430, 2000.

Ruchelli E, Wenner W, Voytek T, et al: Severity of esophageal eosinophilia predicts response to conventional gastroesophageal reflux therapy. Pediatr Dev Pathol 2:15-18, 1999.

Simon MR, Houser WL, Smith KA, et al: Esophageal candidiasis as a complication of inhaled corticosteroids. Ann Allergy Asthma Immunol 79:333-338, 1997.

Spergel JM, Beausoleil JL, Mascarenhas M, et al: The use of skin prick tests and patch tests to identify causative foods in eosinophilic esophagitis. J Allergy Clin Immunol 109:363-368, 2002.

Straumann A, Bauer M, Fisher B, et al: Idiopathic eosinophilic esophagitis is associated with a T(H)$_2$-type allergic inflammatory response. J Allergy Clin Immunol 108:954-961, 2001.

Straumann A, Simon HU: Eosinophilic esophagitis: Escalating epidemiology? J Allergy Clin Immunol 115:418-419, 2005.

Teitelbaum JE, Fox VL, Twarug FJ, et al: Eosinophilic esophagitis in children: Immunopathological analysis and response to fluticasone propionate. Gastroenterology 122:1216-1225, 2002.

Vitellas KM, Bennett WF, Bova JG, et al: Radiographic manifestations of eosinophilic gastroenteritis. Abdom Imaging 20:406-413, 1995.

Walsh SV, Antonioli DA, Goldman H, et al: Allergic esophagitis in children: A clinicopathological entity. Am J Surg Pathol 23:390-396, 1999.

CHAPTER 7

Failure to Thrive

ASIM MAQBOOL

Disease Description
Case Presentation
Definitions
Anthropometric Measurements of Nutritional
   and Growth Status
   Normal Growth
Pathophysiology
Differential Diagnosis
Management
History
Physical Examination
Diagnostic Testing
Laboratory Evaluation
Additional Diagnostic Considerations
Treatment
Approach to the Case
Summary
Major Points

DISEASE DESCRIPTION

The term "failure to thrive" denotes a degree of malnourishment and undernutrition in children. It is a symptom or manifestation of underlying processes that result in growth faltering or failure in children. During the first eight months of 2005, 2342 children presented for outpatient evaluations for failure to thrive.

CASE PRESENTATION

A 9-month-old white child is referred from her primary care physician for a history of failure to thrive. She has been difficult to feed since about 3 months of age, with frequent arching, spitting up, and irritability during feeds. She spits up nearly one ounce at a time, immediately following meals. She does not sleep well through the night and is described as being gassy and flatulent. Her mother reports bowel movements occur up to five times per day and are often watery and with mucus, and she is distressed about blood streaks in the stool noted for the past 3 weeks.

The child was the product of an uneventful term pregnancy: birthweight was 3810 g (75th percentile), length 51 cm (75th percentile), and head circumference of 35.5 cm (50th to 75th percentile); Apgar score was 9 at 1 minute and at 5 minutes. She has never been hospitalized, has congestion intermittently, and has not had any surgeries. She is not on any medications, and does not have any known drug or food allergies. The mother has used an over-the-counter gas remedy without much success. Her immunizations are up to date, and her developmental history is age appropriate.

The physical examination reveals a heart rate of 100, respiratory rate 20, blood pressure 90/60 mm Hg temperature 37.6° C, weight 7.38 kg (5th to 10th percentile), length 69 cm (25th to 50th percentile), and head circumference 44 cm (50th percentile). Her weight for height is 89%, and her standard length for weight is 99%.

She is fussy but consolable in her mother's lap. Pertinent findings are a slightly distended abdomen that is tympanetic to percussion without hepatosplenomegaly or vascular prominence, with normal deep tendon reflexes, rectal examination, and extremity examination. Eczema has been noted in a bimalar fashion, as well at the flexor creases, and scattered about the torso, with no diaper area involvement. There is no suggestion of a sacral dimple or of gluteal wasting. The perianal examination does not reveal erythema, skin tags, fissures, or tears. Deep tendon reflexes are normal and there is normal range of motion. The extremity examination does not reveal digital clubbing, but there is decreased muscle mass about the thighs.

You call the pediatrician's office and obtain a growth chart, which is as displayed in Figure 7-1. How do you proceed?

DEFINITIONS

A universally acceptable definition of failure to thrive remains elusive, given that it is the manifestation of a multitude of factors and illnesses in pediatrics. Quantification of degree of growth faltering or failure to thrive has been proposed in increasing the index of suspicion for this finding, and the two most current commonly used criteria depend on the use of anthropometric data and indices and reference data provided by normative growth charts by the National Center for Health Statistics (NCHS). In particular, the following two criteria are employed:

- Weight (weight for height) fewer than two standard deviations below age and gender means.
- Crossing of two or more growth curve percentile lines along the NCHS growth charts after having achieved a stable pattern.

The latter criterion is of additional significance if the weight velocity trends below the fifth percentile, and as per the most recent Centers for Disease Control and Prevention (CDC) growth charts, below the third percentile. To further quantify the degree of weight velocity, use of weight for age Z scores (a Z score is an expression of a standard deviation of anthropometric data from age- and gender-specific means). Use of Z scores confers a greater degree of precision than simply referring to values being below the fifth percentile; for example, a Z score of -1.0 is of less significance than one of -2.5.

The difficulty of solely relying on anthropometric data and NCHS growth charts to "diagnose" failure to thrive stems from multiple factors. The NCHS growth charts represent a national survey and a normal distribution; hence, 3% of normal, healthy children will fall below the third percentile. Additional considerations must include errors in anthropometric measurement, differential growth patterns in subpopulations not adequately reflected by growth charts, and the observation that children who are breastfed do not necessarily exhibit the same growth velocity as formula-fed infants, which is not to say they are any less healthy or robust. Lastly, it is important to recognize that some crossing of growth percentile lines—or fluctuations—is normal; each point on the growth chart represents a cross-sectional mathematical average, and children may not grow exactly longitudinally along a particular line; in fact, in a study by Smith and Rogers, 30% of normal, healthy, white children crossed at least one growth percentile line, and 23% crossed two lines as they moved from birth to 2 years. In this study, the shift between growth percentiles occurred between 3 and 13 months of age.

ANTHROPOMETRIC MEASUREMENTS OF NUTRITIONAL AND GROWTH STATUS

Weight in kilograms (also referred to as the ponderal component), length (in children younger than 2 years of age) and height (the linear component), and the head circumference in centimeters form the core set of anthropometric measurements that need to be obtained at regularly set intervals and plotted on appropriate growth curves. Ponderal growth is usually easier to assess in children, and should be performed with the child in a state of undress with a scale sensitive to detect errors as small as 0.1 kg; regular calibration of measuring equipment is recommended. Determination of mid–upper arm circumference and skinfold thickness also comprises the ponderal component, although these are less commonly employed in routine general clinical practice.

Linear growth poses more of a challenge to accurately and consistently measure. For children younger than 2, a supine recumbent length is obtained using a baby board with a fixed, superior portion and a perpendicular free-moving distal portion. Proper positioning by holding the child's head in firm contact with the headboard and the eye socket perpendicular (Frankford plane), with straightened legs and ankles, and feet flat against the moving plate (perpendicular to the base), are critical in obtaining a measurement to the nearest 0.1 cm. This technique requires a minimum of two operators to perform correctly. A stadiometer is employed for children older than 2 years, and should be performed with the child barefoot, heels together, both buttocks and shoulder blades in contact with the rear wall, and the sliding plate perpendicular to the wall and pressed firmly against the head with the hair flattened. Length or height also is recorded to the nearest 0.1 cm; note that the measurement error may be as high as 0.5 cm, despite good measurement technique. Recumbent lengths are more accurately obtained than heights in children younger than 5 years of age, and if the former is obtained for children older than 2, then 1.0 cm should be subtracted. The transition point between recumbent length and height measurements should be recorded on the growth chart. Additionally, this method of measurement signals the need for transition to the next growth chart. Head circumference should be measured for all children younger than 3 years of age, using a flexible nonstretch tape measure about the maximum head circumference (above the supraorbital ridge around to the occiput) recorded to the nearest 0.1 cm.

Additional anthropometrics used to assess nutritional status include the mid–upper arm circumference, which can be used to approximate energy and protein stores. The measurement is obtained at the midpoint of the arm, approximately midway between the lateral tip of

50 PEDIATRIC GASTROENTEROLOGY: THE REQUISITES IN PEDIATRICS

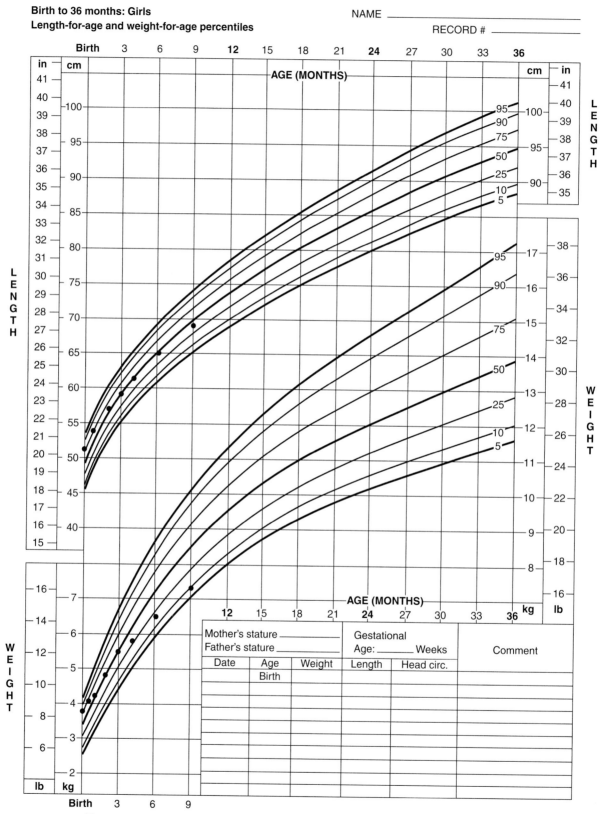

Figure 7-1 Growth curves for patient presenting with failure to thrive for evaluation.

(Continued)

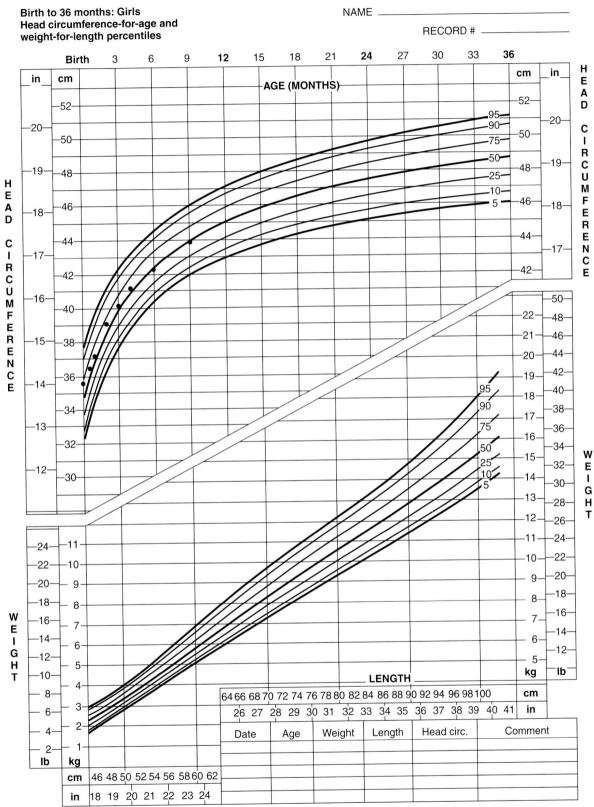

Figure 7-1, cont'd Growth curves for patient presenting with failure to thrive for evaluation.

the acromion and the olecranon, with the arm in a 90-degree flexed angle. The measurement is obtained with the patient seated upright, arm relaxed at the side, and by flexible nonstretch tape; the measurement is recorded to the nearest 0.1 cm.

Anthropometric measurements can then be plotted and tracked over time on the growth chart and are a valuable tool in screening for children at risk for malnutrition. Appropriate growth charts for the specific patient should be employed, such as premature growth charts, those for trisomy 21, Prader-Willi syndrome, Cornelia de Lange syndrome, and so on, which may more accurately reflect growth trends. Neonates born prematurely should be tracked on specific neonatal growth charts. Infants with a history of prematurity should have their chronologic ages corrected according to the gestational age. For these premature infants and children, weight measurements are adjusted until 24 months, for 40 months for the length, and until 18 months for head circumference.

The same personnel should employ measurements over time using consistency in terms of state of undress, equipment, and technique. Accuracy and precision in obtaining these measurements are critical, and small errors in measurement can lead to erroneous conclusions that can be amplified when measurements are used to calculate indices.

Growth is thus measured by a combination of anthropometric measurements on the growth chart and by combinations of measurements to form indices, such as weight for height and body mass index (BMI; kg/m^2), and against each other, such as by weight for age and height for age. These indices can also be compared with reference data and expressed as Z scores, for example. Growth is the rate of change in weight, height, head circumference compared with reference data and norms. In addition to using growth charts, reference data for rate of weight change by percentiles also may be used, particularly for short-term or frequent measurements (Tables 7-1 and 7-2). The most commonly used indices are weight for age, weight for height, and height for age, and are expressed as percentage deviations from the mean. This schema, as proposed by Gomez and Waterlow (Table 7-3), is very useful in defining wasting (low weight for age), which reflects acute malnutrition, stunting (which reflects low height for age), and reflecting slowing of skeletal growth, suggestive of chronic malnutrition. Weight for height is a combination of the two indices and reflects proportionality, but has its own limitations.

Each of these indices changes by age, reflecting changes in body composition and normal patterns of growth. A ratio of the mid–upper arm circumference to the head circumference is an older technique employed to estimate nutritional status, used when proper apparatuses to measure weight and length are not available. The midarm circumference approximates the subcutaneous fat and is prone to fluctuate with the total body weight, whereas the head circumference parallels linear growth. A ratio of greater than 0.30 is considered normal, with a value of less than 0.27 suggestive of severe malnutrition in neonates. For older children up to 3 years of age, a ratio of greater than 0.31 is considered normal, and a ratio of less than 0.25 is indicative of severe malnutrition, with varying degrees of malnutrition between these two values. After 3 years of age, the decline in head circumference velocity precludes use of this measurement for estimation of nutritional status.

Tracking weight velocity is an important additional manner with which to track growth faltering. Devia-

Table 7-1 Percentiles for 1-Month Increments in Weight Gain from Birth to 6 Months

Age (Months)	Infants (n)	Mean (g/Day)	SD	Percentiles (g/day)						
				5th	10th	25th	50th	75th	90th	95th
Males										
Birth to 1	580	30	9.4	15	18	24	30	36	42	45
1-2	580	35	8.5	22	25	29	35	40	46	50
2-3	580	27	7.9	15	18	22	26	31	36	41
3-4	298	20	3.6	15	16	18	20	22	24	26
4-5	298	17	3.4	12	14	15	17	19	21	23
5-6	298	16	3.5	11	12	14	15	17	19	21
Females										
Birth to 1	562	26	8.4	11	16	20	26	32	36	39
1-2	562	29	7.7	18	20	24	29	34	39	42
2-3	562	23	7.2	12	14	19	23	28	32	35
3-4	298	19	5.3	13	15	17	19	21	23	26
4-5	298	16	5.0	11	13	14	16	18	20	22
5-6	298	15	4.7	10	11	13	14	16	18	18

SD, standard deviation.
Adapted from Guo S, Roche AF, Fomon SJ, et al: Reference data for gains in weight and length during the first 2 years of life. J Pediatr 119:355-362, 1991.

Table 7-2 Select Percentiles for 2-Month Increments in Length from Birth to 6 Months

				Percentiles (mm/day)						
Age (Months)	Infants (n)	Mean (g/Day)	SD	5th	10th	25th	50th	75th	90th	95th
Males										
Birth to 2	580	1.10	0.15	0.87	0.90	1.00	1.10	1.18	1.28	1.34
1-3	580	1.08	0.14	0.85	0.90	0.98	1.08	1.17	1.26	1.31
2-4	65	0.93	0.75	—	0.75	0.82	0.95	1.02	1.07	—
3 to 5	255	0.73	0.09	0.60	0.63	0.68	0.73	0.79	0.86	0.90
4 to 6	255	0.64	0.08	0.49	0.54	0.59	0.63	0.69	0.74	0.78
Females										
Birth to 2	562	1.03	0.13	0.80	0.87	0.92	1.03	1.11	1.20	1.25
1-3	562	0.99	0.13	0.79	0.84	0.93	0.98	1.07	1.15	1.18
2-4	74	0.89	0.13	—	0.72	0.80	0.90	0.97	1.05	—
3-5	241	0.71	0.10	0.57	0.60	0.66	0.71	0.77	0.82	0.87
4-6	241	0.62	0.08	0.48	0.52	0.57	0.63	0.67	0.70	0.73

SD, standard deviation.
Adapted from Guo S, Roche AF, Fomon SJ, et al: Reference data for gains in weight and length during the first 2 years of life. J Pediatr 119:355-362, 1991.

Table 7-3 Waterlow Criteria for Categorizing Type and Chronicity of Malnutrition

	Normal	Mild	Moderate	Severe
Weight for height (acute malnutrition)	>90	80-90	70-80	<70
Height for age (chronic malnutrition; stunting)	>95	90-95	85-90	<95

Adapted from Waterlow JC: Nutrition and growth. In Protein Energy Malnutrition. London, Edward Arnold; 1992.
Reproduced with permission from the American Academy of Pediatrics Nutrition Handbook, 5th Edition, 2004.

Calculation:

$$\% \text{ of median} = \frac{\text{Actual Weight}}{\text{Median Weight}} \times 100$$

tion by two standard deviations from the median value warrants closer examination and workup; three standard deviations from the median value indicate the need for aggressive investigation and intervention. Changes in growth velocity occur for each of the aforementioned measurements and are included in Table 7-4.

The usefulness of measurements and growth indices is aiding to predict subsequent health problems, which, in addition to morbidity and mortality can address future risks to growth and development. The first 2 years of life mark a continuation of central nervous system (CNS) development that began in utero; the first 3 years are the period during which head circumference velocity is also at its highest. A sizable body of literature exists pertaining to these growth trends in children with intrauterine growth retardation, with respect to intel-

Table 7-4 Minimal Time Interval to Measure Changes in Growth Velocity

Measurement	Interval
Weight	7 days
Length*	4 weeks
Stature	8 weeks
Head circumference	7 days (in infants)
	4 weeks (for children up to 4 years old)
Midarm circumference	4 weeks

*Length is measured for children up to 2 years of age, after which stature may be assessed.
Reproduced with permission from the American Academy of Pediatrics Nutrition Handbook, 5th Edition, 2004.

lectual development, to future risk of stunting and attainment of adult height.

Normal Growth

Normal growth patterns are influenced by a number of factors, beginning with maternal prepregnancy weight and height, illnesses, placental factors and the intrauterine environment, use of tobacco, alcohol, recreational drugs and medications, and nutrition throughout the pregnancy. Interruptions in nutritional status during pregnancy have been hypothesized to effect changes in metabolic imprinting on the fetus, which may confer an increased lifetime risk of noncommunicable diseases to the unborn child. Intrauterine growth restriction (IUGR) can be either asymmetric or symmetric. Asymmetric IUGR is defined as decreased weight/age (using maturation), and children with this form of IUGR are more able to recover the weight and resume normal postnatal growth as compared with those who may have symmetric IUGR stunting and wasting. Although wasting in general is more readily correctable with caloric supplementation, stunting may take more time to correct; the timing of these phenomena have profound implications on growth potential.

An appreciation for what constitutes normal growth patterns and the factors that influence growth are of critical importance to comprehend, a departure from which would indicate the need and would attribute a degree of urgency to investigate, intervene early to prevent malnutrition when recognized deviation from normal growth occurs, and treat failure to thrive when it occurs. The three major phases of growth are those of infancy, childhood, and puberty.

Although birthweight is more dependent on maternal factors, height potential is contributed by both parents; genetic growth percentile is thus determined by calculation of a midparental height (MPH), which takes on greater significance if there is considerable disparity between parental heights. This is based on older Fels Institute and NCHS data, and therefore should be used with the 1979 growth charts. The calculations are as follows:

$$\text{MPH (girls)} = \frac{(\text{father's height} - 5 \text{ inches}) + \text{mother's height}}{\text{Age}}$$

$$\text{MPH (boys)} = \frac{\text{father's height} + (\text{mother's height} + 5 \text{ inches})}{\text{Age}}$$

PATHOPHYSIOLOGY

The effects of growth potential are most prominent *during the first 3 years of life.* Crossing of percentile values occurs commonly, with children usually settling about a curve at approximately 2 years onward.

Infancy marks a continuation of rapid fetal growth, and prematurely born children with adequate nutritional support can grow at the same rate as expected in the intrauterine environment. This growth phase rapidly declines until about 3 years of age, at which time the *childhood phase* is noted, with maternal and fetal influences on growth giving way to more genetic determinants of growth potential, and with nutrition forming the underlying fabric supporting these changes. Growth hormone influences this phase in growth. The age at onset of this phase is variable, but it is of critical importance in determining the eventually obtained height. The later onset of this phase is seen more in malnourished populations and/or in children with chronic diseases. Although truncal growth dominates the infancy phase, long bone growth mediated by growth hormone dominates this phase. Growth faltering preceding this phase can have a profound effect on future growth, thereby indicating a need to intervene before 3 years of age to facilitate the childhood phase of growth to proceed on time and normally. Whereas the childhood phase reflects a relatively slower rate of growth, it contributes two thirds of overall postnatal growth, and sets the stage for the pubertal phase of growth.

The *pubertal phase* constitutes the final phase of growth and is marked by development of secondary sexual characteristics, changes in body composition, and rapid growth. Sex differences are noted, with the female growth spurt occurring on average 6 months before that of males (at the G2 Tanner stage) and ending with the onset of menarche. The male growth spurt occurs later (at the G3 Tanner stage), with later peak height velocity and continuing growth potential after secondary sexual development is complete. The male growth spurt contributes more to the attainment of final adult height than it does in females. Malnutrition can affect this phase of growth, with undernutrition typically delaying the onset of puberty, and in obese children undergoing perhaps an earlier growth spurt and skeletal maturation, but not the ultimate magnitude of linear growth per se. Growth hormone is the main hormonal influence during the childhood and pubertal stages, with insulin-like growth factor-1 (IGF-1) and the sex hormones playing important roles in the latter as well.

Recognition of critical periods for intervention may facilitate resumption of normal growth in accordance to growth and development potential, with interventions in the first 2 years being most pressing. In a study by Martorell and associates, nutritional interventions during the first 3 years of life facilitated catch-up growth and reversal of stunting; Guatemalan children from 3 to 7 years old did not benefit from the nutritional supplementation. Additional considerations of malnutrition, then, of environmental factors, illness, and disease, particularly in the developing world, need to be enter-

DIFFERENTIAL DIAGNOSIS

Impairments in growth can occur from a multitude of causes, with inadequate oral intake being the most common. The underlying medical causes can be diverse and encompass the breadth of pediatrics, are often multifactorial, can be a combination of both primary causes and adaptive as well as maladaptive physiologic behavioral consequences of this process, and must be viewed in this context. It is often difficult to establish a clear cause-and-effect relationship that is exclusively contributory to failure to thrive. Therefore, dichotomous classification of causality into organic versus nonorganic may be inadequate and limiting or misleading. The transactional model encompasses and considers interactions between medical, behavioral, and developmental characteristics of the infant, as well as the familial, psychosocial, and the economic components.

Medical risk factors include those involving digestive diseases resulting from decreased oral intake, increased metabolic rate or turnover, and maldigestion and malabsorption. Neurologic impairments and developmental delays likewise confer additional risk factors. Environmental factors extend beyond those of nutrition and encompass those of the family's socioeconomic status and ability to provide for the patient, stressors, stability, structure of the home environment, support for caregivers, consistency in the approach to and ritual of mealtimes, pleasurable experiences associated with eating, abuse and neglect, as well as factitious disorders.

MANAGEMENT

Determining the etiology of failure to thrive in a patient relies heavily on the quality and comprehensive approach to the history and physical examination. The maximum diagnostic yield is obtained by a good history and physical examination, which must also include a determination of nutritional status. Nutritional rehabilitation must not be delayed while a diagnosis is sought, given its implications on growth and development. In many cases, a response to nutritional supplementation can in itself yield a diagnosis of inadequate nutrition to meet caloric needs for maintenance and catch-up growth. The yield from laboratory testing in general is very poor, of limited use, and should be minimized, directed by diagnostic clues obtained in the history and on physical examination. In a study by Sills, for 185 children younger than 3 years of age admitted for failure to thrive, only 36 of 2607 laboratory tests performed (1.4%) aided in confirming a clinically suspected diagnosis. A growth curve from the primary care physician's office is a valuable tool in guiding the initial interaction with the patient, and probably of more value than any initial laboratory test. The growth chart can indicate the timing and the differential magnitudes of affected growth indices, as well as their relative patterns, which may help guide the approach to the patient.

The gastroenterologist's approach to failure to thrive often centers around the general notion that unless adequate calories are provided, absorbed, or correctly used for growth, growth will not occur at an expected rate or along an anticipated trend (Fig. 7-2). Hence, the "too little in, too little absorbed, or too much burnt off approach," which belies a useful initial approach, in conjunction with patterns of growth reflected on growth charts. The investigative approach will depend on what is indicated by the history and physical examination, and in the absence of any gastrointestinal symptoms, evaluations of malabsorption and maldigestion are thus guided in the context of the presentation (approaches to the evaluation of chronic diarrhea, gastroesophageal reflux, and so on are provided elsewhere in this text).

Inadequate caloric intake relative to needs will often reflect in the weight initially, height next, and ultimately head circumference of an infant; decline in height velocity must be interpreted in the context of the weight trend. If the weight velocity declines before the height velocity, this may indicate acute malnutrition. If the height velocity is affected before the height, or if in isolation, underlying chronic disease (often inflammatory, such as in Crohn's disease or cystic fibrosis), endocrinopathies, and skeletal dysplasias also must be entertained. When weight, height, and head circumference are all decreased, perinatal/intrauterine insults and chromosomal, metabolic, and CNS abnormalities should be investigated (see Fig. 7-3 for examples of growth chart patterns). In all cases, nutritional rehabilitation should not be delayed until a diagnosis is made, thereby potentially preventing further deterioration in growth status and effects on head circumference and neurologic development. Isolated macrocephaly should be evaluated both in the contexts of family history and development and feeding difficulties.

HISTORY

The history should be as broad and comprehensive as possible to help guide the subsequent evaluation, if any, beyond the physical examination. The timing and onset, as well as the nature of growth faltering obtained early in the history are very important diagnostic clues. The adequacy of intake—both in terms of calories and of

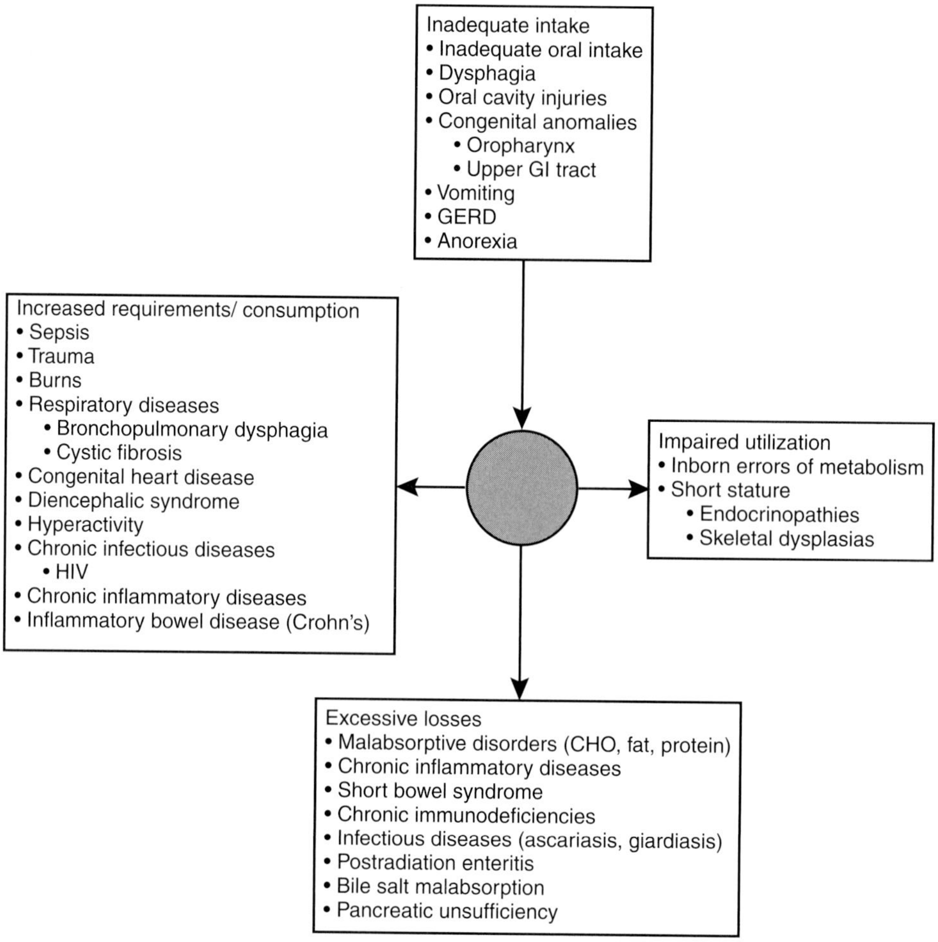

Figure 7-2 Conceptual framework: failure to thrive from a gastroenterologist's perspective. CHO, carbohydrate; GI, gastrointestinal; HIV, human immunodeficiency virus; GERD, gastroesophageal reflux disease.

```
Inadequate intake
• Inadequate oral intake
• Dysphagia
• Oral cavity injuries
• Congenital anomalies
    • Oropharynx
    • Upper GI tract
• Vomiting
• GERD
• Anorexia

Increased requirements/ consumption
• Sepsis
• Trauma
• Burns
• Respiratory diseases
    • Bronchopulmonary dysphagia
    • Cystic fibrosis
• Congenital heart disease
• Diencephalic syndrome
• Hyperactivity
• Chronic infectious diseases
    • HIV
• Chronic inflammatory diseases
• Inflammatory bowel disease (Crohn's)

Impaired utilization
• Inborn errors of metabolism
• Short stature
    • Endocrinopathies
    • Skeletal dysplasias

Excessive losses
• Malabsorptive disorders (CHO, fat, protein)
• Chronic inflammatory diseases
• Short bowel syndrome
• Chronic immunodeficiencies
• Infectious diseases (ascariasis, giardiasis)
• Postradiation enteritis
• Bile salt malabsorption
• Pancreatic unsufficiency
```

micronutrients—deserves particular attention, as do details regarding formula or meal composition, preparation (for example, how is the formula prepared? Is it premixed or is water added? Is the prepared formula diluted?), mealtime structure, and dynamics. Inquiry as to the amount of juice intake and its displacement of milk or formula intake also should be ascertained. Changes in food intake coincident to the onset of growth faltering warrant close scrutiny. In the child who is not exclusively breast- or formula fed, a 3-day dietary recall should be entertained.

Prenatal history revolving around maternal nutrition and intake, dietary limitations, illnesses, and peripartum infections should be taken. The gestational age and birth measurements, as well as complications revolving around birth itself should be determined.

Symptoms coincident to or preceding growth faltering can provide important clues to underlying disease processes. Inquire about intakes, volumes, defecatory pattern, frequency, and consistency. Likewise, past medical history and history of prior surgeries involving the gastrointestinal (GI) tract and otherwise may be helpful in establishing a diagnosis. A history of recurrent infectious illnesses and of persistent illnesses also raises the question of immunodeficiency (note that malnutrition is the leading worldwide cause of death in children younger than 5) human immunodeficiency virus (HIV) and tuberculosis should be entertained in this setting of increased susceptibility to infection.

A thorough review of medications is also useful. Drug-nutrient interactions should be taken into consideration, both for macronutrients and micronutrients, which may influence growth (Table 7-5).

The family history, in addition to providing some context of illnesses that may occur in higher frequency in families, should be expanded to determine the growth patterns of any siblings as well as those of the parents. Parental heights should be recorded and used to generate a midparental height, which should be to estimate an expected height for the patient; reference values have been published. In particular, questioning regarding the onset of puberty and of parental growth spurts may be of value when evaluating the child with short stature.

Consideration of geographic location and travel history may aid in alluding to underlying primary illnesses and disease processes that may manifest as failure to thrive. Splenomegaly in a child residing in the tropics where malaria is endemic has different connotations to splenomegaly in an African American child with sickle cell anemia, for example.

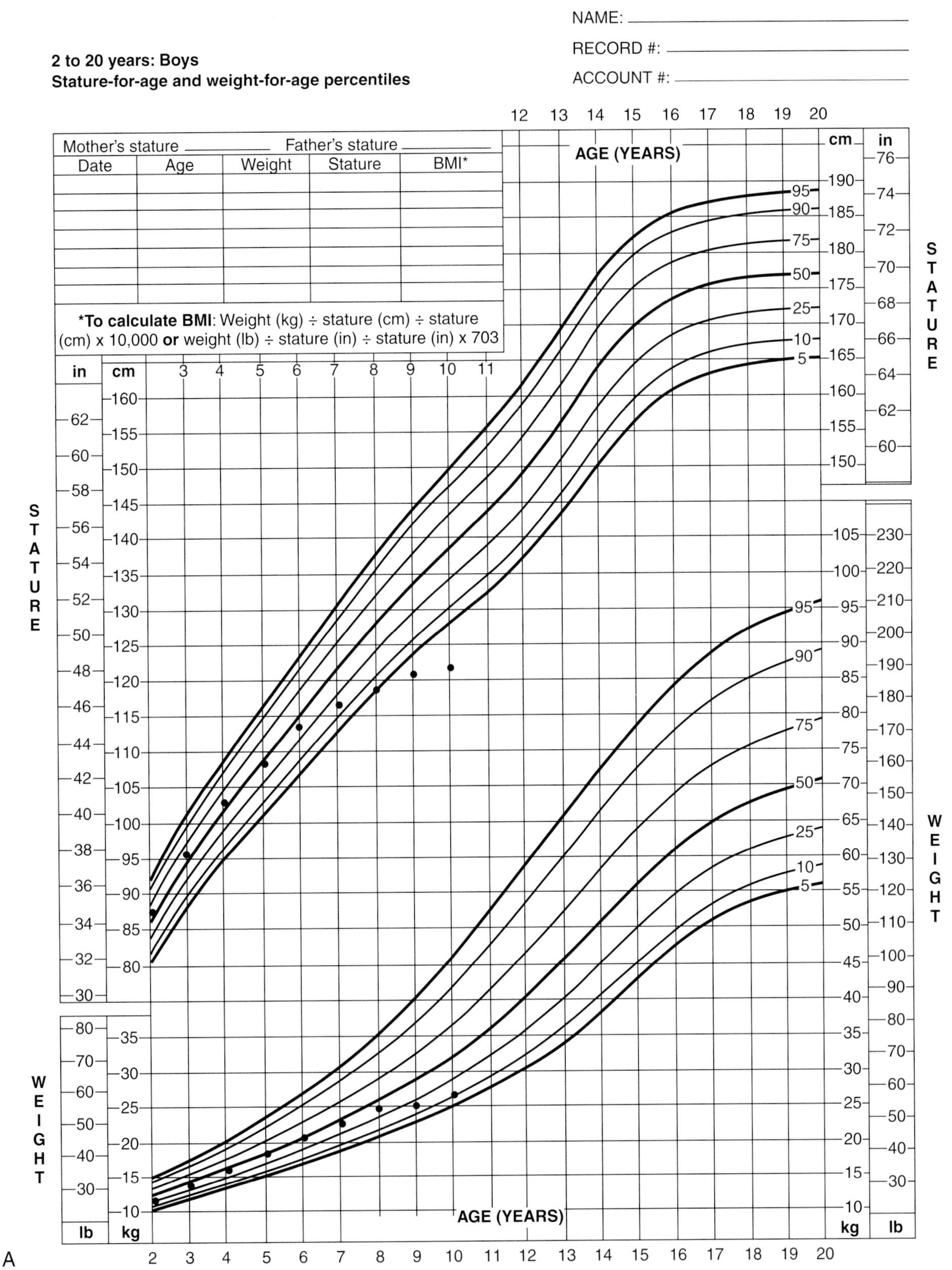
NAME:
RECORD #:
ACCOUNT #:
2 to 20 years: Boys
Stature-for-age and weight-for-age percentiles
Mother's stature
Father's stature
Date
Age
Weight
Stature
BMI*
*To calculate BMI: Weight (kg) ÷ stature (cm) ÷ stature (cm) x 10,000 or weight (lb) ÷ stature (in) ÷ stature (in) x 703
AGE (YEARS)
STATURE
WEIGHT
in
cm
kg
lb
95
90
75
50
25
10
5

A

Figure 7-3 Growth chart examples. *(Continued)*

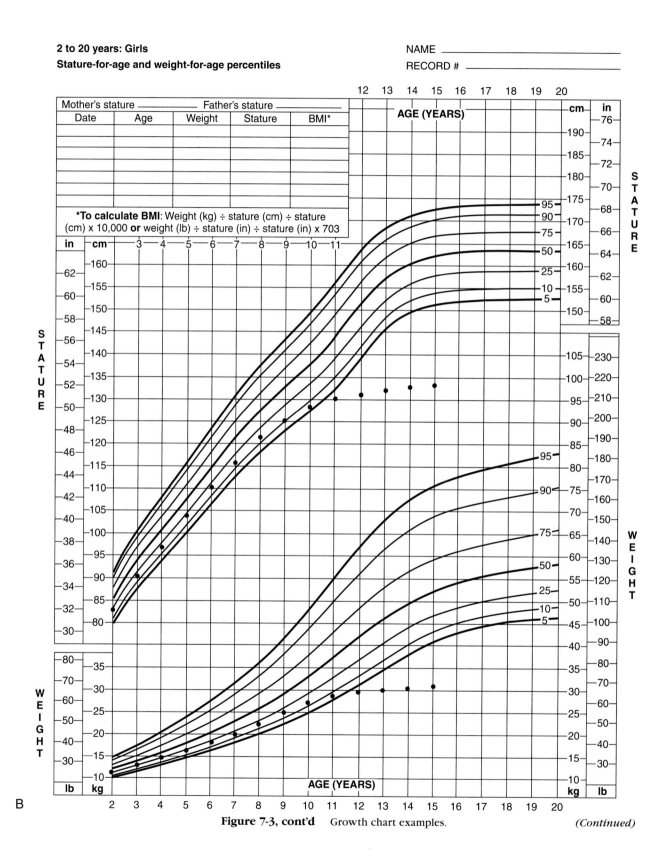

Figure 7-3, cont'd Growth chart examples. *(Continued)*

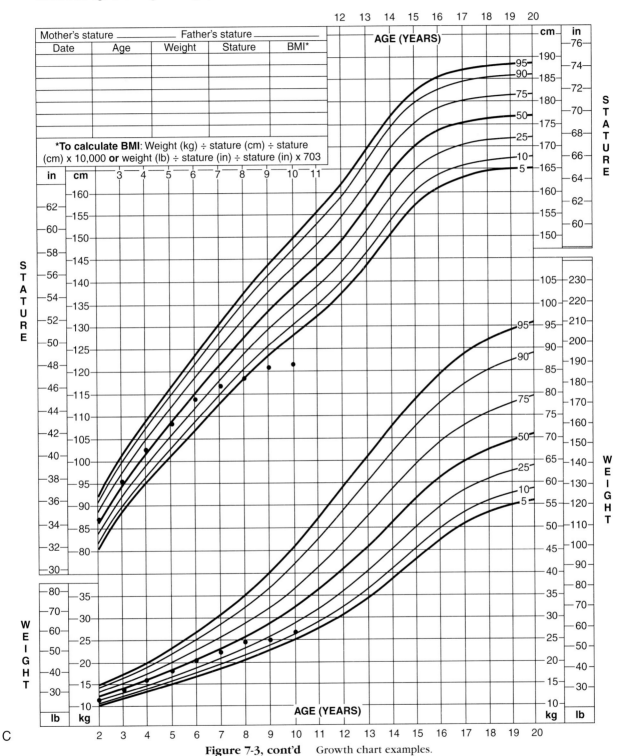

Figure 7-3, cont'd Growth chart examples.

Table 7-5	Select Common Drug–Nutrient Interactions
Drug	**Nutrient**
Acid Blockade	
Antacids	Vitamin D deficiency
	Iron deficiency
	Hypophosphatemia
H$_2$-blockers	Iron deficiency
Sucralfate	Hypophosphatemia
Other Intraluminal Agents	
Cholestyramine	Fat-soluble vitamin malabsorption (A, D, E, and K)
Sulfasalazine	Folate deficiency
Immunosuppressives	
Cyclosporine	Elevated triglycerides
	Hypokalemia
	Hypomagnesemia
Methotrexate	Folate deficiency
Corticosteroids	Hyperglycemia
	Hypophosphatemia
Antiepileptics	
Phenytoin	Folate deficiency
Phenobarbital	Vitamin D deficiency

The review of symptoms should be as broad and comprehensive as possible in this setting, given the enormous differential diagnosis for failure to thrive, with particular attention to gastrointestinal, developmental, metabolic, and constitutional symptoms as well as the presence of fever. Note that a disease process can have multiple manifestations, such as emesis, diarrhea, anorexia, growth failure, skin lesions, hair changes, occasional stigmata of autoimmune disease, and mood disturbances such as in celiac disease, the suspicion for and diagnosis of which can be aided by a thorough review of systems. In addition, children with celiac disease are prone to nutritional deficiencies related to the location of the primary inflammatory lesion, which includes iron deficiency (Fig. 7-4).

The social history, with close attention to any socioeconomic stressors, the environment in which feeding occurs, the consistency of feeding technique, and caregivers, is important. The risk of environmental contamination, most notably as it relates to water and to risk of lead exposure, also should be considered.

PHYSICAL EXAMINATION

The dual purpose of the physical examination is to provide diagnostic clues as well as to assess the nutritional and growth status of the patient. As previously outlined, anthropometrics and growth reference data are important assessment tools. The patterns of growth failure can help in narrowing the focus of further investigation (examples of some relevant physical findings are in Fig. 7-5).

DIAGNOSTIC TESTING

As mentioned, laboratory evaluations are of limited diagnostic value outside of confirming a clinically suspected diagnosis. Among the initial evaluations, a trial of caloric supplementation is recommended; the patient's response to age- and gender-adequate calories to meet assessed needs, resulting in adequate growth response, limits the need for an exhaustive, broad workup.

LABORATORY EVALUATION

The history and physical examination guide the laboratory evaluation. A complete blood count (CBC) with differential, comprehensive metabolic panel, erythrocyte sedimentation rate, lead level, and a urinalysis form a reasonable initial screen. Predominant short stature may prompt an endocrinopathic workup and a bone age to screen for skeletal dysplasias. A more exhaustive review of the workup for chronic diarrhea, persistent vomiting, and other GI disease processes can be found elsewhere in this book.

ADDITIONAL DIAGNOSTIC CONSIDERATIONS

A multidisciplinary approach can be beneficial in some settings. Careful assessment of the family dynamic as it revolves about feeding, such as conducted by a feeding disorders team, can be of great value in the setting for which an organic pathology cannot be ascertained readily, if at all. Socioeconomic stressors can be explored, and support and resources provided by a social worker; note that 13% of patients in a series of failure to thrive were homeless. Endocrinology and genetics referrals also may be indicated.

TREATMENT

The therapy of failure to thrive revolves around the underlying diagnosis when one can be ascertained. Nutritional rehabilitation should be implemented immediately, providing adequate calories to meet current needs as well as those for catch-up growth, and can be estimated by the following formula:

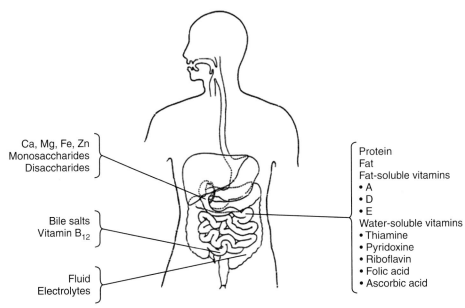

Figure 7-4 Sites of nutrient absorption.

$$\text{Kcal/kg required} = \frac{\text{Recommended Dietary Allowances (RDA) for age (kcal/kg)} \times \text{ideal weight for height}}{\text{Actual weight}}$$

The ideal weight for height can be determined by median values from the NCHS weight for height curves. Frequently, caloric supplementation on the order of 110-120% RDA are sufficient to effect improved growth. Younger infants may require 120-150% RDA for calories to achieve desired growth response, and in some clinical scenarios, up to 1.5 to 2 times the RDA calories for age may be required to meet needs for catch-up growth. Once an initial reasonable goal for caloric intake is employed, depending on the growth response of the patient, caloric intake can be adjusted, as indicated. More recent approaches to estimating caloric needs derive from the estimated energy requirements (EER), which are based on age, weight, height, and level of physical activity, and are addressed in detail in the Dietary Reference Intakes.

The child with failure to thrive may require additional calories to resume growth, with weight velocity recovering within a few days of adequate caloric supplementation. Linear growth usually takes longer to respond, and may take several weeks to months to resume normal velocity, predicated on underlying diagnoses, ages at which diagnoses occurred and interventions were initiated; sustained nutritional support is usually required. Once a more specific diagnosis has been made and a more detailed assessment of nutritional status and adequacy of dietary intake (macronu-

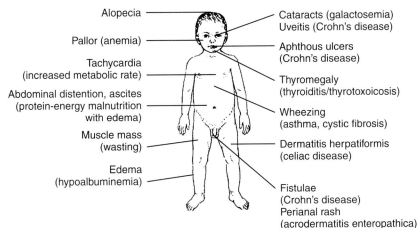

Figure 7-5 Examples of relevant findings during the physical examination.

trients and micronutrients) have been determined, appropriate nutritional therapy can be tailored. It is imperative to initiate early nutritional rehabilitation regardless of the eventual diagnosis, given the potential sequelae of intellectual development, attainment of adult height capacity, and work capacity as an adult.

Supplemental calories can be administered on an outpatient basis by means of substitutions in favor of calorically more dense foods/ingredients, substitutions, and supplemental high-caloric foods and drinks. Overnight supplemental nasogastric drip-feeding is a commonly used technique, which is practical in an outpatient setting. Prolonged requirements for supplemental tube feeds may be facilitated by a gastrostomy tube. Both the nasogastric and gastrostomy tubes have the advantage of bypassing the issues of patient compliance with orally consuming large quantities of supplements as well as palatability preferences. Supplemental feeding of semi-elemental diets, particularly as in the case of Crohn's disease, in itself is considered an adjuvant therapy and may improve growth failure associated with the condition.

Intestinal failure is among the diagnoses for which enteral feedings may not be effective, necessitating parenteral nutrition therapy and prompting hospital admission. Severe malnutrition also warrants hospitalization for initial management, to monitor for refeeding syndrome during initial nutritional rehabilitation. Failure of outpatient nutritional therapy also should be considered as an indication to admit the patient for inpatient treatment and observation of the parent-child dynamic, with an increased index of suspicion for abuse, neglect, and Munchausen syndrome by proxy. During these admissions, care should be taken to avoid unnecessary procedures and tests and to avoid interruptions in the consumption of calories.

Nutritional rehabilitation goals for children with symmetric IUGR are a matter of debate; given the suggestion of an increased incidence of noncommunicable diseases in adulthood, such as diabetes and cardiovascular disease; it is unclear how aggressively and to what level nutritional rehabilitation should be pursued for these children. Should these children be allowed to grow along their own growth curves and patterns, according to their intrinsic growth potential?

APPROACH TO THE CASE

On obtaining a diet history, the mother had nursed the child until 3 months of age, after which the infant had been on a cow's-milk formula for the next 3 weeks. The cow's-milk formula was discontinued secondary to increased fussiness and regurgitation. The baby was then introduced to soy-based formula, which she tolerated well for the first month or so, then with progressive feeding intolerance. The baby is also consuming stage II foods, 2 ounces three times per day. On closer examination of the volume, frequency, and calories per ounce of the formula as prepared, you ascertain that the child has been receiving about 70 kcal/kg/day.

You decide to proceed conservatively, and have a complete blood count with differential, comprehensive metabolic panel, and urinalysis, as well as an erythrocyte sedimentation rate (ESR) drawn. These tests results are as shown:

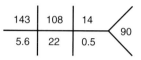

Mg 2.2 mg/dL, Ca 10 mg/dL, Phos 2.2 mg/dL

u/a: yellow/ clear/ sp. grav 1.028/ pH 6.0/ 0 WBC/ 0 RBC

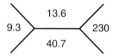

WBC differential: N 39%, B 0.4%, E 11%, L 41.6%, M 9.2%
Total protein 8 g/dL, albumin 4.8 g/dL, Alkaline phosphatase 277 U/L, ALT 24 U/L, AST 30 U/L, GGT 21 U/L, Conjugated bilirubin 0 mg/dL, Unconjugated bilirubin 0.5 mg/dL

Your differential diagnosis includes gastroesophageal reflux (GER), anatomic abnormalities, cow's-milk protein allergy, and eosinophilic gastroenteropathy.

Based on the information above, you do the following:

- You change the formula to a protein hydrolysate.
- Given the current weight, and estimating the calories required for current needs, regular growth needs and for catch-up growth are calculated as follows:

$$\frac{8.3 \text{ kg (Median weight)} \times 98 \text{ kcal/kg (RDA)}}{7.38 \text{ kg (actual weight)}} = 110 \text{ kcal/kg}$$

- You recommend that the formula be concentrated to either 24 kcal/ounce, with 34 ounces per day required to meet her needs, or to concentrate the formula to 27 kcal/ounce, with 27 calories required per day to meet her needs.
- You start an H_2RA at the age-appropriate dose.
- You ask the mother to obtain weekly weights, and if symptoms do not improve or if the child loses weight within the next 3 weeks, she is to return for follow-up.
- You ask the mother to contemplate food allergy testing if the child does not respond with adequate growth as anticipated.

The mother calls back in 3 weeks, stating her daughter is less fussy and doing better, with slowly improving growth in terms of weight gain; her height continues to follow the 50th percentile, and her weight has moved to between the 10th and 25th percentiles. There is no further blood in the stool. You recommend continuing weight checks and readjusting the formula intake based on her new weight and current deficits.

SUMMARY

Failure to thrive is a symptom of poor growth in children, and is often indicative of inadequate oral intake versus an underlying illness or disorder precluding normal growth. The diagnostic approach to failure to thrive relies on a thorough history and physical examination to place the proposed workup in the proper context. An understanding of caloric requirements by age of normal growth patterns and stages is essential for diagnosis and management. Diagnosis and treatment of the underlying cause, when identifiable, are indicated. Regardless of the underlying cause, adequate calories should be provided to the patient to achieve growth according to the child's genetic potential. Growth should be assessed by performing routine anthropometric assessments and tracking on appropriate growth charts.

MAJOR POINTS

Failure to thrive is a symptom, not a diagnosis.
Knowledge of nutritional requirements by age is relevant and an important aspect of the assessment.
An understanding of growth patterns in children through various stages is important in terms of diagnosis, timing of intervention, and gauging response to therapy.
Routine accurate anthropometric measurements and the use of age- and sex-appropriate growth charts is recommended to assess growth against reference standards.
Regardless of the underlying diagnosis, adequate nutrition is required to achieve growth along predictable patterns.

SUGGESTED READINGS

Barker DJ: Fetal growth and adult disease. Br J Obstet Gynaecol 99:275-276, 1992.

Barker DJ, Gluckman PD, Godfrey KM, et al: Fetal nutrition and cardiovascular disease in adult life. Lancet 341:938-941, 1993.

Belli DC, Seidman E, Bouthillier L, et al: Chronic intermittent elemental diet improves growth failure in children with Crohn's disease. Gastroenterology 94:603-610, 1998.

Bithoney WG, Dubowitz H, Egan: Failure to thrive/growth deficiency. Ped Rev 13:453-445, 1992.

Frank DA, Zeisal SH: Failure to thrive. Ped Clin North Am 35:1187-1200, 1988.

Garn SM, Rohman CC: Interaction of nutrition and genetics in timing of growth. Ped Clin North Am 13;353, 1996.

The Global Burden of Disease 2000 Project Aims, Methods, and Data Sources. Global Programme on Evidence for Health (EIP) policy discussion paper no. 36. Geneva, World Health Organization, 2001.

Gomez F, Ramos Galvan R, Frenk S, et al: Mortality in second and third degree malnutrition. In: Bull World Health Organ 78:1275-1280, 2000. J Trop Ped Afr Child Health 2:77, 1956.

Gordon CC, Chumlea WC, Roche AF: Stature, recumbent length and weight. In Lohman TG, Roche AF, Martorell R (eds): Anthropometric Standardization Reference Manual. Champaign, Ill, Human Kinetic Books, 1988.

Guo S, Roche AF, Fomon SJ, et al: Reference data for gains in weight and length during the first 2 years of life. J Pediatr 119:355-362, 1991.

Hack M: Effects of intrauterine growth retardation on mental performance and behavior: Outcomes during adolescence and adulthood Eur J Clin Nutr 52:s65-s71, 1988.

Hamill PVV, Drizd TA, Johnson CL, et al: Physical growth: National Center for Health Statistics percentiles. Am J Clin Nutr 32:607-629, 1979.

Hass JD, Murdoch S, Rivera J, Martorell R: Early nutrition and later physical work capacity. Nutr Rev 54:S41-S48, 1996.

Institute of Medicine. Energy. In: Dietary reference intakes for energy, carbohydrate, fiber, fat, fatty acids, cholesterol, protein, and amino acids. Washington, DC: National Academy Press; 2002.

Kanawati AA, McLaren DS: Assessment of marginal malnutrition. Nature 228:573-575, 1970.

Kleinman RE (ed): The Pediatric Nutrition Handbook, 5th ed, American Academy of Pediatrics. 2004.

Martorell R., Ramikrishnan U, Schroeder DG, et al: Intrauterine growth retardation, body size, body composition, and physical performance in adolescence. Eur J Clin Nutr 52(Suppl): S43-S45, 1998.

Sasanow SR, Georgieff MK, Pereira GR: Mid-arm circumference and midarm/head circumference ratio: Standard curves for anthropometric assessment of neonatal nutritional status. J Pediatr 109:311-315, 1986.

Schroeder DG, Martorell R, Rivera JA, et al: Age differences in the impact of nutritional supplementation on growth. J Nutr 125:1051S-1059S, 1995.

Sills RH: Failure to thrive: The role of clinical and laboratory evaluation. Am J Dis Child 132:967-969, 1978.

Smith DA, Rogers JE: Shifting linear growth during infancy: Illustration of genetic factors in growth from fetal life until infancy. J Pediatr 89:225-230, 1976.

U.S. Department of Health and Human Services, Center for Disease Control. National Center for Health Statistics, Hyattsville, Md, 2000. www.cdc.gov/nchs/about/major/nhanes/growthcharts/clinical_charts.htm.

Waterlow JC: Nutrition and growth. In Protein Energy Malnutrition. London, Edward Arnold, 1992, pp 187-211.

CHAPTER 8

Foreign Bodies and Bezoars

MARSHA KAY

ROBERT WYLLIE

Disease Description
Case Presentation
Epidemiology
Pathophysiology
    Symptoms
    Natural History
Diagnostic Testing and Management
    Coins
    Battery Ingestions
    Sharp Foreign Bodies
    Long or Large Objects
    Magnets and Lead
    Food Impactions
    Pediatric Body Packing
    Bezoars
Approach to the Case
Summary
Major Points

DISEASE DESCRIPTION

Ingestion of foreign bodies is a common pediatric problem, with more than 100,000 cases occurring each year in the United States. In pediatric patients the vast majority of ingestions are accidental, with an increasing incidence of intentional ingestions starting during the teenage years. In the United States the most common foreign body ingestion in children is coins, followed by a variety of other objects, including toys and toy parts, sharp objects, batteries, bones, and food. In adolescents and adults, meat or food impactions represent the most common accidental foreign body ingestion. Bezoars are a relatively uncommon problem in pediatric patients. There are four types of bezoars: phytobezoars, which are composed of plant or vegetable material; trichobezoars, which are composed of hair or other fibers; lactobezoars, which derive from milk; and medication bezoars.

CASE PRESENTATION

A 23-month-old male is brought to the emergency department (ED) following a button battery ingestion. The battery was part of a hearing aid that belonged to the toddler's 6-year-old brother. The ingestion was witnessed by the 6-year-old, who reported it to his mother. The ingestion occurred approximately 4 hours before the ED evaluation. The patient has been asymptomatic with no evidence of pain or respiratory distress, is eating normally, and last ate 2 hours ago. The patient is afebrile on initial examination with normal vital signs, and his examination is otherwise unremarkable. An anteroposterior (AP) and lateral chest x-ray is obtained. The battery is located in the midesophagus, but the x-ray is otherwise normal.

What is the recommended management for this patient?

EPIDEMIOLOGY

Foreign body ingestion is primarily a pediatric problem, with more than 80% of cases occurring in childhood and the majority in patients under 3 years of age. There is a significant difference in the type of foreign body ingested by children compared with adults, with differences in the complication rates following ingestion based on the type of the foreign body. Foreign body ingestion is a worldwide phenomenon, but the relative frequency of each type of foreign body ingested varies geographically. There were more than 107,000 cases of foreign body ingestions by children and adolescents alone in the United States in 2000, according to data collected from the American Association of Poison Control Centers, the overwhelming majority of which were accidental. Intentional foreign body ingestions in adults are a result of a variety of factors including underlying psychiatric disorders, mental retardation, alcohol ingestion, and seeking of secondary gain such as transfer to the hospital in cases of incarcerated individuals. In the United States and Europe coins are the most common ingested foreign body in children. A variety of other objects, including toys and toy parts, sharp objects such as needles and pins, batteries, chicken and fish bones, and food each account for 5% to 30% of ingestions in children. In Asia and other countries, where fish represent a significant component of the diet, fish bone ingestions and impactions are common and account for a greater percent of foreign body ingestions in children and adults. Coins are the second most frequently ingested objects in those areas, followed by toys, needles, and so on.

In adults, meat impaction is the most frequent cause of accidental foreign body ingestion in the United States. Meat impactions usually occur in patients with underlying esophageal pathology, including esophageal strictures or eosinophilic esophagitis. Intentional and accidental foreign body ingestions in adults include toothbrushes or other implements used to induce vomiting in anorexic and bulimic patients, and miscellaneous sharp, large, or numerous foreign bodies in prisoners or psychiatrically impaired individuals. Some adolescent gangs have adopted the practice of foreign body ingestion as part of their initiation ritual.

PATHOPHYSIOLOGY

Symptoms

The symptoms of a foreign body ingestion vary based on the type, location of the foreign body, relative patient size, and the duration of impaction. Symptoms may be on the basis of the location of the foreign body; its nature, that is, the caustic nature of a battery; or from complications that arise as a result of the foreign body ingestion such as obstruction or perforation. Pediatric patients may present with a variety of symptoms including choking, drooling, and poor feeding in younger patients; dysphagia, odynophagia, and chest pain in older patients, or respiratory symptoms, especially in younger patients due to tracheal compression or erosion of an esophageal foreign body. Size-related symptoms, drooling, feeding difficulty, and respiratory symptoms are more common in younger patients due to the size of the foreign body in relation to the normal esophageal caliber and compressibility of the trachea in small patients. Occasionally, retained esophageal foreign bodies present with massive life-threatening gastrointestinal (GI) hemorrhage due to development of an aortoesophageal fistula from an unsuspected foreign body; exsanguination has been reported. Fever is a worrisome presenting complaint because it may suggest deep ulceration or perforation. On occasion, foreign body ingestion is unsuspected until the foreign body is passed through the stool in the diaper or toilet.

Natural History

Of the foreign bodies that come to medical attention, 80% to 90% pass spontaneously, 10% to 20% require endoscopic removal, and less than 1% require surgery. Serious complications, including obstruction and perforation are significantly more common with large, long, or sharp foreign bodies. In cases of ingestion of sharp objects, the complication rate increases from less than or equal to 1% to more than 15-35% depending on the number, type of ingestion and the gastrointestinal contact time. Unusual complications reported following foreign body ingestion include lead intoxication following ingestion of lead toys, a single case of systemic lithium absorption following ingestion of a lithium button battery, appendicitis without perforation due to impaction of a foreign body (tongue stud), and intestinal perforation with or without fistula development. Historically, perforation has occurred following ingestion of sharp objects and bones. Recently, this complication is being increasingly reported after ingestion of multiple nonsharp magnets due to attraction between the magnets, with subsequent perforation or fistula development. This complication may become increasingly common with the widespread availability of magnetized objects such as earrings, beads, and toys.

DIAGNOSTIC TESTING AND MANAGEMENT

Coins

An x-ray should be obtained in every case of suspected coin or other radiopaque foreign body ingestion. Coins in the esophagus will assume an enface appearance on AP view, with the edge of the coin seen on the lateral view. On occasion, coins in the esophagus will demonstrate a lateral edge on AP x-ray. In addition to noting the position of the ingested coin, the trachea should also be assessed on x-ray because coins and other foreign bodies may impinge on the trachea (or be located within the trachea). Unsuspected esophageal coins are sometimes found on the x-rays of children undergoing evaluation of wheezing or other respiratory symptoms. In these cases, if the symptoms are prolonged, the possibility of erosion of the coin into the esophageal wall should be considered. These coins may be harder to remove endoscopically, and additional preprocedure, evaluations, such as computed tomography may be indicated.

Coins lodge in the esophagus in three common locations: approximately 60% to 70% lodge in the proximal esophagus at the upper esophageal sphincter or thoracic inlet, 10% to 20% lodge in the midesophagus at the level of the aortic notch, and 20% are located just above the lower esophageal sphincter. Patients at increased risk of a retained esophageal coin include those indicated in Table 8-1.

Emergent endoscopic removal of esophageal coins should be performed in symptomatic patients unable to swallow their secretions or in those who are experiencing acute respiratory symptoms. Procedures in patients who have not been nothing per mouth (NPO) and who are experiencing acute symptoms may be associated with a higher risk of aspiration of gastric contents, and appropriate pre-cautions should be observed. Symptomatic patients with esophageal coins who are able to handle their secretions or asymptomatic patients can undergo an endoscopy within 12 to 24 hours to allow an appropriate pre-anesthetic fasting interval. If there is a significant delay in the procedure, consideration should be given to repeating the x-ray immediately before the procedure to determine if the coin has passed to the stomach. Glucagon has not been shown to date to be effective in facilitating esophageal coin passage in pediatric patients. In distinction to esophageal coins, in the majority of patients with gastric or distally located coins who are asymptomatic, a "wait and see" approach can be used. Symptomatic patients with pain, vomiting, feeding intolerance, or other symptoms warrant endoscopic removal. On occasion, the coin can come to overlie the pylorus, causing intermittent obstruction, and endoscopic removal is warranted if this occurs. Except in younger children, those with underlying disease or prior surgery, or with very large coins, once in the stomach, most coins will pass through the remainder of the GI tract uneventfully. In patients who are being observed for coin passage, parents can strain the stool to document passage. A repeat kidney, ureter, and bladder x-ray (KUB) can be obtained at 2 to 3 weeks and again at 4 to 6 weeks if the coin has not been observed to pass, and if still present, endoscopic removal then performed. In cases of ingestion of multiple coins, the coins may adhere to one another, which may decrease the likelihood of transpyloric passage (Fig. 8-1). In 1982, the composition of pennies changed from a copper-predominant coin to a zinc-predominant coin. Concern has been raised in the literature about the potential for zinc toxicity from retained post-1982 gastric pennies. At this time, most centers do not advocate early removal of gastric pennies compared with other coins. Once having traversed the pylorus, the vast majority of coins will negotiate the remainder of the GI tract uneventfully.

Battery Ingestions

Battery ingestions are common among young children, in impaired individuals, and in those with underlying psychiatric disorders. Batteries are readily available in a variety of sizes and are not perceived as an object at risk for ingestion (Table 8-2). In children, button batteries are ingested more frequently than cylindrical batteries. Sources include a child's own hearing aid or other common household products. The management of battery

Table 8-1 Patients at Increased Risk of a Retained Esophageal Coin
Small patient
Large coin
Underlying esophageal disease
Esophageal stricture
Status post caustic ingestion
Prior esophageal or cardiac surgery
Repair of TEF
Repair of esophageal atresia
Fundoplication
Simultaneous ingestion of multiple coins

TEF, tracheoesophageal fistula.

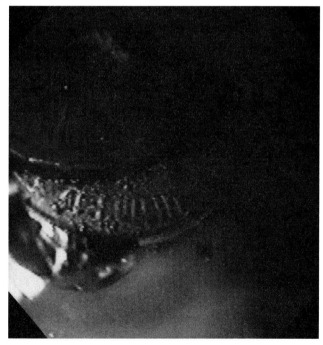

Figure 8-1 *(See also Color Plate 8-1.)* Retained gastric quarter and a penny in a 4-year-old with autism. Note the eroded appearance of the penny. The coins were believed to be in place for 6 weeks. The coins adhered to each other at the time of endoscopy, which may have contributed to their nonpassage but were easily removed endoscopically using alligator forceps.

Table 8-2	Representative Battery Sizes		
Type	Diameter (mm)	Height (mm)	Weight (g)
AAAA	8.3	42.5	6.5
AAA	10.5	44.5	11.5
AA	14.5	50.5	23
C	26.2	50	66.2
D	34.2	61.5	141.9
Disk	4.8-24.5	1.65-6.1	0.12-6.9

Disk batteries are available in a wide range of sizes. Please consult manufacturer's data for technical information and specifications. Information derived from the energizer.com website, June 2005.

ingestion is significantly different from coin ingestion despite their similar size. Symptoms following battery ingestion are uncommon, occurring in only 3% to 10% of cases. Symptoms correlate poorly with clinical outcome. An immediate x-ray to locate the battery is warranted in every case of suspected battery ingestion, even in asymptomatic patients. Significant morbidity is associated with batteries lodged in the esophagus. Because of this, immediate endoscopic removal of esophageal batteries is warranted, recognizing the increased risk of aspiration in a patient who has not been NPO. Retained esophageal batteries result in complications for three reasons: the nature of the battery, the caustic material within it, and the potential for discharge of current. Batteries often contain concentrated solutions of sodium or potassium hydroxide, both of which are alkalis. Leakage following ingestion and impaction in the esophagus may result in burns that cause injury similar to that seen following caustic ingestion of a product such as lye (sodium hydroxide pH > 11.5). Esophageal injury following ingestion of alkali occurs due to liquefaction necrosis, which may result in deep penetration and perforation of the esophagus, as liquefied tissue provides no barrier to further injury.

Complications may arise very early following battery impaction in the esophagus and have occurred within 6 to 10 hours (reported complications are indicated in Table 8-3). The majority of serious esophageal injuries

Table 8-3	Reported Complications from Retained Esophageal Batteries

Esophageal perforation (within 6 hours)
TEF development
Esophageal stricture
Esophageal stenosis (within 10 hours)
Perforation
Death

TEF, tracheoesophageal fistula.

follow ingestion of large batteries (20 to 23 mm in diameter), although complications have been reported following ingestion of smaller batteries (8 to 11 mm in diameter). When compared with esophageal batteries, batteries in the stomach require a less urgent approach. If patients are asymptomatic and the battery is in the stomach, especially in older children, it is likely to pass through the remainder of the GI tract uneventfully. In this circumstance, 80% will pass within 48 hours. Batteries larger 15 mm that do not pass the pylorus within 48 hours in an adolescent, generally require removal because of a higher likelihood of being retained. Size modifications are required in younger and smaller patients, in those with prior intestinal surgery, or in those with other conditions that would decrease the intestinal lumen size. For example, an AA battery (14 mm $\times$ 5 cm) would be unlikely to pass the pylorus in a 1-year-old child, and early endoscopy after an appropriate period of preanesthetic fasting would be indicated. Symptomatic patients with gastric batteries of any size warrant prompt endoscopic removal. Complications from gastric batteries include gastric ulceration, which has been reported, the theoretical but unreported complication of mercury poisoning, and a single case report of lithium absorption.

Sharp Foreign Bodies

A variety of sharp foreign bodies are ingested both accidentally and intentionally (Fig. 8-2). In pediatric patients, sharp ingestions are frequently accidental. In adults, fish and chicken bones are usually accidentally ingested in distinction to the majority of sharps such as pins, razor blades, nails, and so on that are usually intentionally ingested. There is a significant increase in the risk of complications following ingestion of sharp foreign bodies, both at the time of ingestion and also during removal of the foreign body, with complication rates increasing to 35% or more.

Most ingested bones lodge in the oropharynx. Patients are almost universally symptomatic. Lodged bones can frequently be removed using Magill forceps; sedation may be required. Bones located more distally in the esophagus can result in esophageal perforation or life-threatening hemorrhage if erosion through the esophageal wall occurs. Distally impacted bones require endoscopic removal if within reach of the endoscope. Unsuspected fish and chicken bone ingestions may result in perforation distally, often in the region of the ileum, ileocecal (IC) valve, or rectosigmoid. This is due to a combination of reduction in lumen caliber (ileum, IC valve) and change in directional transit between mobile portions of the mesocolon and fixed positions in the retroperitoneum. Specialized computed tomography may aid in the diagnosis.

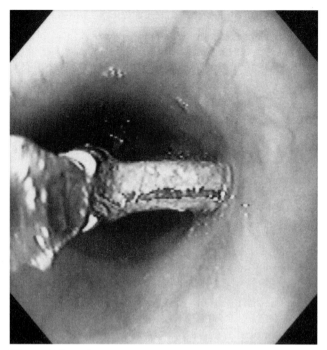

Figure 8-2 *(See also Color Plate 8-2.)* Withdrawal of a swallowed key using alligator forceps. Note the key is withdrawn parallel to the axis of the esophagus.

Straight pin ingestions are unique compared with other sharp foreign bodies. Straight pins tend to follow Jackson's axiom that "advancing points perforate and trailing points don't." Straight pins usually do not require endoscopic removal and pass uneventfully through the GI tract. This is because the blunt head usually passes first, with the sharp end trailing. Gastric impaction of a straight pin with penetration has been reported. Ingestion of a large number of straight pins may increase the risk of perforation.

Non–straight-pin sharps require endoscopic, or in some cases, surgical removal. If not removed, perforation is likely, which can be associated with extraluminal migration of the foreign body. The majority of perforations occur in the region of the IC valve, although they may occur anywhere in the GI tract. A variety of strategies have been developed to optimize removal of sharp foreign bodies. These include placement of an endoscopic overtube through which the foreign body can be retracted to reduce esophageal mucosal damage, although pediatric-sized overtubes are not currently available, and size permitting, use of a latex hood or friction fit adaptor at the tip of the endoscope to minimize injury with removal of the sharp object. Safety pin ingestion remains a relatively common accidental sharp ingestion in children. Some cultures attach safety pins to young children's clothing for cultural or religious reasons, increasing the risk of accidental ingestion. Following ingestion, safety pins frequently lodge in the esophagus or stomach, although they may impact in the duodenal C loop or distally. Pins require removal either with Magill forceps if proximally located or with a variety of endoscopic forceps and techniques that have been developed to deal with an ingested open pin. If closure of the pin is not possible, the goal is to remove the open pin with the open end trailing to reduce the risk of further esophageal injury.

Long or Large Objects

Although not usually sharp, objects that are long or large may be associated with a significant risk of complications following ingestion. However, there are scattered case reports of long-standing ingestions of long foreign bodies that have followed relatively uncomplicated courses. These likely represent the exception rather than the rule. Ingestions of these types of objects are primarily intentional but may be accidental as is the case with dental instruments, dentures, and toothbrushes or spoons used to induce vomiting. Other long or large objects that have been swallowed include a variety of toys, tools such as screwdrivers, knives, and chopsticks. The primary sites of impaction for long or large objects are the esophagus; the pylorus, which may not allow passage of objects greater than 15 mm in diameter; and the duodenal C loop, which represents the primary impediment to the passage of long objects and will not allow passage of objects greater than 10 cm long. In patients with a normal bowel rotation, the ileocecal valve is typically the final location where ingested objects become impacted.

A combination of length and caliber may preclude passage of a large object. Ovoid objects greater than 5 cm in length and 2 cm in thickness have a decreased likelihood of passing the pylorus in an adolescent. Size criteria require modification in younger and smaller patients. In asymptomatic patients who have swallowed a nonsharp long or large object, endoscopy may be performed after an appropriate period of preanesthetic fasting. Symptomatic patients require more urgent endoscopy despite the risks of aspiration and the additional risk of impaired visualization at the time of endoscopy. A variety of endoscopic tools are used to remove large or long objects. These include polypectomy snares in a number of sizes, and the Roth Net retrieval device (US Endoscopy, Mentor, Ohio). Long objects should be removed parallel to the axis of the esophagus. Orientation of long objects may be difficult and a double snare technique via a two-channel endoscope can be helpful. All standard toothbrushes need to be removed because their size precludes passage through the duodenal C loop. Other techniques to remove long or large objects include the suture technique described elsewhere. Complications of retained large or long foreign bodies include pressure necrosis, perforation, and obstruction.

Magnets and Lead

Accidental ingestion of magnets is increasing in pediatric patients. The number of magnets ingested is extremely important because ingestion of a single magnet is less likely to result in complications due to magnetic issues although it may result in size- or sharpness-related complications (Fig. 8-3). Ingestion of more than one magnet may be exceedingly hazardous because the magnets may attract each other and result in fistulization (gastroenteric, enteroenteric), obstruction, and perforation. Magnets are generally not perceived as dangerous and are increasingly ubiquitous as parts of toys, jewelry, and common household objects. Although there are no formal recommendations following a suspected magnet ingestion, an x-ray should be performed to localize the magnet(s). If more than one magnet is present, early endoscopic intervention would seem warranted if the magnets are within reach. If the magnets are not large and are beyond the reach of the endoscope, careful monitoring for evidence of continued passage through the GI tract and surgical consultation for removal are therapeutic options that should be made on a case-by-case basis.

Lead intoxication has been reported following accidental ingestion of lead-based toys or products such as weights, fishing sinkers, lead shot/pellets, and clothing accessories. Symptoms may be related to the foreign body and from lead intoxication. Early endoscopic removal is indicated if feasible following ingestion of a known or suspected lead-based product. If unable to be removed endoscopically, a combination of serial examinations, serial radiography, blood lead–level monitoring, chelation therapy, and bowel irrigation may be required to reduce the likelihood of complications.

Food Impactions

Meat and other food impactions are the most common causes of accidental "foreign body ingestion" in adolescents and adults. Patients frequently have a history of similar episodes or of a feeling that "food gets stuck." If thoroughly investigated, approximately 95% of cases of meat impaction are associated with underlying esophageal pathology, including esophageal strictures, or narrowing from a variety of etiologies including acid-peptic disease, following a caustic ingestion or postoperatively. Eosinophilic esophagitis is increasingly being recognized as a contributing factor to food impactions. Circular esophageal rings that cause the esophagus to resemble the trachea and linear furrowing and white specks on the esophageal mucosa are characteristic (Fig. 8-4). Food impactions may also be associated with underlying motility disorders.

In patients with a suspected food impaction, a plain x-ray may be obtained. Administration of contrast is contraindicated because contrast may pool above the

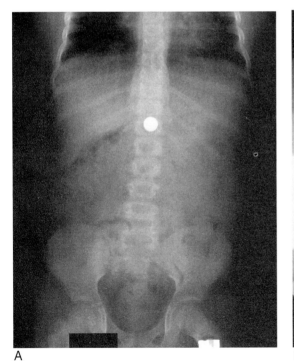
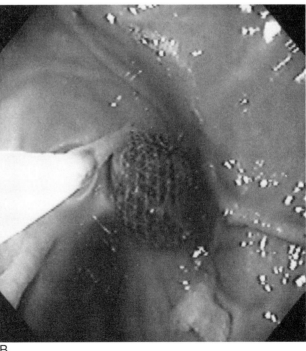

Figure 8-3 *(See also Color Plate 8-3.)* **A** and **B,** Magnetic marble demonstrated on KUB and in the stomach at the time of endoscopic retrieval using the Roth Net. The marble was part of a toy game and weighed 12 g.

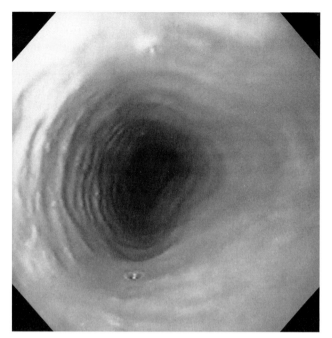

Figure 8-4 *(See also Color Plate 8-4.)* Ringed esophagus in a teenager with a meat impaction. Note that the mucosal appearance of the esophagus resembles that of the trachea. The patient had eosinophilic esophagitis on endoscopic biopsy.

impaction and result in aspiration. Symptomatic patients who are unable to handle their secretions require urgent endoscopy for removal of the impaction. Symptomatic patients able to handle their secretions should undergo endoscopy within 12 hours. In all cases, oral administration of "meat tenderizers" to dissolve the impaction should be avoided because this practice has been associated with hypernatremia and injury to the esophagus. At endoscopy, attempts should be made to remove the impaction rather than advance it blindly into the stomach due to the high rate of underlying esophageal pathology, which may be located distal to the impaction and not immediately apparent. Removal is typically performed with a protected airway to avoid aspiration. Endoscopic equipment used for removal of meat impactions includes the tripod or pentapod forceps, the Roth Net retrieval device, and the friction fit adaptor. Once a portion of the meat is removed, the remainder may pass into the stomach. In patients without evidence of underlying esophageal pathology, endoscopic biopsies of the distal and midesophagus should be considered in order to rule out eosinophilic esophagitis.

Pediatric Body Packing

Body packing is the practice of swallowing drug-filled balloons, condoms, fingercots, or plastic kitchen wrap in order to smuggle drugs. With increased awareness of this practice in adults and teenagers and increased security following the events of September 11, 2001, younger children are being used as "mules" to smuggle drugs. Drugs smuggled by this method include cocaine, heroin, amphetamines, and ecstasy. Patients may be asymptomatic, seek medical attention because they become apprehensive, present with symptoms of intestinal obstruction (usually gastric outlet obstruction), or present with specific drug toxicity due to rupture of one or more packets. Endoscopy is contraindicated, because it could result in rupture of intact packages with subsequent drug release. Asymptomatic patients can be observed for passage of the packets. Some centers will administer non–oil-based oral cathartics to speed condom passage and administer activated charcoal repetitively to delay drug absorption if a condom has accidentally ruptured. Patients who are symptomatic due to drug toxicity and/or obstruction require stabilization and surgical therapy.

Bezoars

Bezoars represent retained foreign material within the gastrointestinal tract that is generally indigestible. Symptoms vary based on the size of the bezoar and include no symptoms, epigastric discomfort, dyspepsia, abdominal bloating, vomiting, gastric outlet or distal obstruction, weight loss, ulceration or bleeding, and perforation. Diagnosis is usually established by KUB or upper GI (UGI), and the diagnosis may be confirmed endoscopically. Anemia, steatorrhea, and protein-losing enteropathy may be present. Bezoars may arise from a variety of substances; the relative frequency of each type varies by patient age and predisposing factors. Lactobezoars occur primarily in premature infants although they also occasionally occur in term infants. The etiology is not known, but risk factors may include the high casein content of some premature formulas, early initiation of feeding in sick or ill patients, calorically dense formulas or those with a high calcium content, and impaired gastric motility. Some patients do not require treatment for this condition, whereas others respond to being NPO and receiving intravenous fluids for 24 to 48 hours. Phytobezoars are derived from plant and vegetable materials.

The most frequent cause of phytobezoars is persimmons, although a variety of plant products may result in their formation. Oranges are a frequent cause in patients with prior gastric surgery. Other common causes include celery, pumpkin, grape skins, prunes, raisins, leeks, beets, and grass. In addition to prior gastric surgery or alterations of gastric anatomy or motility, other risk factors include poor chewing and hypochlorhydria. Phytobezoars may be amenable to physical disruption at the time of endoscopy and dissolution using cellulase, an enzyme that cleaves leucoanthocyanidin-hemicellulose-cellulose bonds. Some physicians have used a combination of gastric lavage with cola beverages with an acid pH and physical disruption of the phytobezoar. Administration of papain that was used in the past may be associated with significant hypernatremia and is currently not recommended. Trichobezoars are composed usually of swallowed hair, which in many cases is the patient's own, but also may be a variety of fibers from blankets, doll's hair, animal hair, or carpet fibers (Fig. 8-5). Symptoms are as indicated above and may include patchy baldness and halitosis. Trichobezoars may be slow growing and result in a gastric cast, which may extend into the small bowel, resulting in obstruction, obstructive jaundice, or nutrient malabsorption. Trichobezoars may not be amenable to endoscopic disruption and may require surgical therapy. Various medications also may result in bezoar formation. Common agents include antacids, sucralfate, and calcium channel blockers. The majority of pharmacobezoars occur with extended-release products. Pharmacobezoars can also occur due to medication vehicles and casings, especially in patients with impaired gastric motility or prior surgery, and there are rare cases of bezoars of swallowed toilet paper, intestinal worms, and a combination of products (trichophytobezoars).

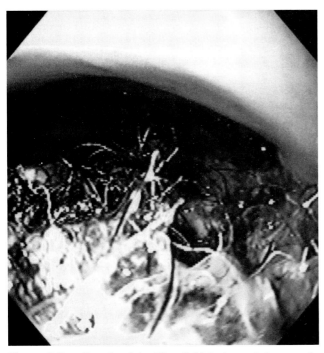

Figure 8-5 *(See also Color Plate 8-5.)* Endoscopic images of a massive trichobezoar in a 3-year-old patient who presented with acute abdominal pain and a palpable abdominal mass. The patient also had anorexia and significant iron deficiency anemia. The bezoar was composed of hair and a variety of fibers and required surgical removal because of its size and extension into the small intestine. Image courtesy of Vera Hupertz, M.D. and Franziska Mohr, M.D.

APPROACH TO THE CASE

Batteries lodged in the esophagus are associated with a significant risk of injury even if patients are asymptomatic. Injury may be due to the nature of the battery itself, discharge of current, or leakage of caustic contents of the battery. The spectrum of injury in the esophagus ranges from no injury to burns, which may be superficial or deep, to esophageal perforation, which may be associated with fistula formation or hemorrhage. Burns may result in scarring, which manifests as esophageal stenosis or narrowing or esophageal stricture. Larger batteries are more likely to be retained than smaller batteries, but any retained battery may result in complications. In our patient, immediate endoscopic removal is warranted to reduce the likelihood of developing complications. This is done with special precautions even if the patient has not fasted, because complications have been reported as early as 6 to 12 hours following battery ingestion. The absence of symptoms following an ingestion of a battery that is located in the esophagus does not preclude early removal because the lack of symptoms does not correlate with a reduced complication rate. Patients who have symptoms such as respiratory distress, and inability to handle their secretions following a retained esophageal foreign body warrant early endoscopy, even with non-battery ingestions.

SUMMARY

Children and adolescents accidentally or intentionally ingest a variety of foreign objects. The timing and need for endoscopic removal are based on the type and size of foreign body ingested, its location, and the symptoms the patient is experiencing. Some objects require observation only and will pass on their own. In some patients, surgery is required because of the location of the foreign body or actual or anticipated complications. A variety of tools is available to the pediatric endoscopist to assist with foreign body removal and to reduce the need for surgical intervention. Although not strictly speaking, a "foreign body" meat impaction is the most common accidental ingestion in adults. The majority of cases are associated with underlying esophageal pathology, and eosinophilic esophagitis is increasingly recognized as an important contributing factor. Bezoars are retained undigested foreign material that usually present with symptoms of gastric outlet obstruction. They can be derived from plant or vegetable material, hair or other fibers, milk, or medication. Some bezoars can be managed conservatively, but depending on the etiology, endoscopic or surgical therapy may be required.

MAJOR POINTS

The majority of foreign body ingestions occur in childhood, usually in patients younger than age 3.

Foreign body ingestions in adolescents and adults are more likely to be nonaccidental.

There is a higher rate of sharp or large foreign body ingestions in adolescents and adults due to their nonaccidental nature and a higher rate of associated complications.

Coins are the most common foreign body ingested in children.

If coins are located in the esophagus, they require removal within 24 hours.

Distally located coins may not require immediate removal in some cases, and management is patient specific according to current guidelines based on patient age, size, type of coin, location, and duration of impaction.

Batteries located in the esophagus always require early endoscopic removal.

Gastrically or distally located batteries require management individually as indicated above for coins.

Management of other foreign body ingestions is based on the nature of the object ingested, patient age, size, location, and duration of impaction.

Ingestion of sharp foreign bodies increases the complication rate significantly both at the time of ingestion and at the time of removal.

A variety of endoscopic techniques and accessories are available to assist with removal of particular foreign bodies. Accessories include specialized forceps, baskets, and snares.

Meat impaction is the most common accidental foreign body ingestion in adolescents and adults. In the majority of cases there is underlying esophageal pathology. Symptomatic patients require early endoscopy to relieve the impaction. Use of meat tenderizers is contraindicated.

Several bezoars can form in pediatric patients. Phytobezoars and lactobezoars can often be managed medically or with endoscopic therapy. Trichobezoars often require surgical therapy.

SUGGESTED READINGS

Aoyagi K, Maeda K, Morita I, et al: Endoscopic removal of a spoon from the stomach with a double-snare and balloon. Gastrointest Endosc 57:990-991, 2003.

Bulstrode N, Banks F, Shrotria S: The outcome of drug smuggling by "body packers": The British experience. Ann Royal Coll Surg Engl 84:35-38, 2002.

Byard RW: Mechanisms of unexpected death in infants and young children following foreign body ingestion. J Forensic Sci 41:438-441, 1996.

Cauchi JA, Shawis RN: Multiple magnet ingestion and gastrointestinal morbidity. Arch Dis Child 87:539-540, 2002.

Chaves DM, Ishioka S, Felix VN, et al: Removal of a foreign body from the upper gastrointestinal tract with a flexible endoscope: A prospective study. Endoscopy 36:887-892, 2004.

Chung JH, Kim JS, Song YT: Small bowel complication caused by magnetic foreign body ingestion of children: Two case reports. J Pediatr Surgery 38:1548-1550, 2003.

Coulier B, Tancredi MH, Ramboux A: Spiral CT and multidetector-row CT diagnosis of perforation of the small intestine caused by ingested foreign bodies. European Radiol 14:1918-1925, 2004.

Fischer CD, Mukherjee A: Appendicitis due to tongue stud ingestion: A case study and review of management plans. S D J Med 57:19-22, 2004.

Fox VL, Nurko S, Furuta GT: Eosinophilic esophagitis: It's not just kids' stuff. Gastrointest Endosc 56:260-270, 2002.

Gilchrist BF, Valerie EP, Nguyen M, et al: Pearls and perils in the management of prolonged, peculiar, penetrating esophageal foreign bodies in children. J Pediatr Surg 32:1429-1431, 1997.

Gun F, Salman T, Abbasoglu L, et al: Safety-pin ingestion in children: A cultural fact. Pediatr Surgery Int 19:482-484, 2003.

Jackson C, Jackson CL: Disease of the Air and Food Passages of Foreign Body Origin. Philadelphia, Saunders, 1937.

Karaman A, Cavusoglu YH, Karaman I, et al: Magill forceps technique for removal of safety pins in upper esophagus: A preliminary report. Int J Pediatr Otorhinolaryngol 68:1189-1191, 2004.

Karjoo M, Kader H: A novel technique for closing and removing an open safety pin from the stomach. Gastrointest Endosc 57:627-629, 2003.

Kay M, Wyllie R: Techniques of foreign body removal in infants and children. Tech Gastrointest Endosc 4:188-195, 2002.

Lao J, Bostwick HE, Berezin S, et al: Esophageal food impaction in children. Pediatr Emerg Care 19:402-407, 2003.

Litovitz TL, Klein-Schwartz W, White S, et al: 2000 Annual report of the American Association of Poison Control Centers Toxic Exposure Surveillance System. Am J Emerg Med 19:337-395, 2001.

Litovitz T, Schmitz BF: Ingestion of cylindrical and button batteries: An analysis of 2382 cases. Pediatrics 89:747-75, 1992.

Mallon PT, White JS, Thompson RL: Systemic absorption of lithium following ingestion of a lithium button battery. Hum Experiment Toxicol 23:193-195, 2004.

Miller RS, Willging JP, Rutter MJ, Rookkapan K: Chronic esophageal foreign bodies in pediatric patients: A retrospective review. Int J Pediatr Otorhinolaryngol 68:265-272, 2004.

Ohno Y, Yoneda A, Enjoji A, et al: Gastroduodenal fistula caused by ingested magnets. Gastrointest Endosc 61:109-110, 2005.

Sanders MK: Bezoars: from mystical charms to medical and nutritional management. Pract Gastroenterol 28:37-50, 2004.

Sica GS, Djapardy V, Westaby S, Maynard ND: Diagnosis and management of aortoesophageal fistula caused by a foreign body. Ann Thorac Surg 77:2217-2218, 2004.

Tay ET, Weinberg G, Levin TL: Ingested magnets: The force within. Pediatr Emerg Care 20:466-467, 2004.

Traub SJ, Kohn GL, Hoffman RS, Nelson LS: Pediatric "body packing." Arch Pediatr Adolesc Med 157:174-177, 2003.

VanArsdale JL, Leiker RD, Kohn M, et al: Lead poisoning from a toy necklace. Pediatrics 114:1096-1099, 2004.

Yin WY, Lin PW, Huang SM, et al: Bezoar manifested with digestive and biliary obstruction. Hepatogastroenterology 44:1037-1045, 1997.

CHAPTER 9

Gastroesophageal Reflux

ANDREW B. GROSSMAN

CHRIS A. LIACOURAS

Disease Description
Case Presentation
Epidemiology
Clinical Presentation
Pathophysiology
Differential Diagnosis
Diagnostic Testing
   Empiric Therapy
   Upper Gastrointestinal Series
   Nuclear Scintigraphy
   Upper Endoscopy
   Esophageal pH Probe Monitoring
   Wireless pH Monitoring
   Multichannel Intraluminal Impedance
Treatment
   Dietary Changes
   Positioning Therapy
   Other Lifestyle Management
   Pharmacologic Therapy
     Acid Suppression
     Prokinetic Therapy
   Surgical Therapy
Approach to the Case
Summary
Major Points

DISEASE DESCRIPTION

Gastroesophageal reflux (GER), which is the intermittent regurgitation of gastric material into the esophagus, is a normal physiologic process that affects children and adults of all ages. Gastroesophageal reflux disease (GERD), or the clinical symptoms that result from GER, is one of the most frequent complaints seen by primary care pediatricians and the most common diagnosis for which infants are referred to a pediatric gastroenterologist. Clinical manifestations can include frequent crying, regurgitation or emesis, poor weight gain, epigastric or chest pain, chronic cough, respiratory distress, and esophagitis. Complications such as esophageal strictures, Barrett's esophagus, and adenocarcinoma occur more commonly in adult patients and are rarely reported in childhood. Treatment options include lifestyle changes, dietary manipulation, various pharmacologic therapies, and surgery.

CASE PRESENTATION

The patient is a 3-month-old boy who presents with fussiness and nonbloody, nonbilious vomiting after feeds. He was born full term via a normal spontaneous vaginal delivery with no complications. He has been fed only a cow's milk–based infant formula; solid foods have not yet been introduced. His mother reports that he has always been an "excellent feeder" and these symptoms have not affected his interest in feeding. She informs you that since approximately 6 weeks of age, the patient has vomited "a large amount" within 15 minutes after most feeds. He is described as a "happy baby." He has four normal bowel movements daily, with no blood or diarrhea noted. From a developmental standpoint, he has been progressing as expected.

On physical examination, the infant appears active, playful, well nourished, and healthy. Plotting his measurements on the growth curve reveals that he continues to track at the 75th percentile for weight, the 50th percentile for height, and the 75th percentile for head circumference. His entire physical examination, including head, eyes, ears, nose, and throat (HEENT), pulmonary, cardiac, abdominal, and neurologic examinations, is normal.

The patient's mother is concerned that the frequency and volume of his emesis have resulted in an inadequate intake. She wonders if he would benefit from a change to a soy-based formula. Additionally, she asks if he should be prescribed medication for his symptoms.

EPIDEMIOLOGY

GER is a normal physiologic process that occurs to some degree in all people. Identifying the incidence of GERD is complicated by a nebulous delineation between physiologic and pathologic refluxes, as well as the lack of a gold standard for diagnosing this disorder. Additionally, numerous other medical conditions can manifest with either secondary GERD or with similar symptoms to GERD.

In infancy, GERD most often presents with emesis. Recurrent emesis is reported in 50% of infants between birth and 3 months, peaks at 67% at 4 months, and decreases to 5% by 10 to 12 months of age. GERD symptoms such as heartburn, epigastric pain, and regurgitation are reported in 2% to 8% of children and adolescents. GERD is more common in babies born prematurely as well as in infants and children with concomitant medical disorders. The incidence of GERD is estimated at greater than 50% for children moderately or severely affected by neurologic disorders or developmental delay. Additionally, studies have demonstrated a greater incidence of GERD in patients with primary respiratory disease such as asthma and cystic fibrosis.

CLINICAL PRESENTATION

Regurgitation is the classic symptom of GERD in infants but is rarely the presenting complaint for children and adolescents. Most commonly, an infant will present as a "happy spitter," characterized by repeated regurgitation that does not appear to cause any discomfort and is not accompanied by other symptoms such as frequent crying, feeding refusal, or poor weight gain. Parents often do not perceive this as problematic unless the volume of the vomitus is large. Improvement of symptoms is typically observed over the first year of life, and symptoms usually abate by 12 months of age.

Less commonly, infants develop GERD, with the reflux resulting in additional symptoms such as esophagitis, which can manifest as crying or feeding refusal, back arching during feeds, or painful emesis. If feeding refusal or fussiness results in inadequate caloric intake, failure to thrive can result. Occasionally, infants will present with chronic respiratory problems such as reactive airway disease, recurrent stridor, or pneumonia.

With toddlers, GERD often manifests as recurrent emesis. Older children, however, rarely report vomiting and more often experience adult-like symptoms such as chronic heartburn or regurgitation without emesis. Because the airway is larger and not as sensitive in toddlers and older children, apnea and stridor do not typically occur; hoarseness, laryngitis, and acute episodes of croup can be observed. Rarely, either infants or children can present with atypical repetitive movements due to esophageal pain that are often mistaken for seizures, tics, or dystonia. These stereotypic arching and stretching movements, called Sandifer's syndrome, generally involve the patient extending the neck to one side and legs in the opposite direction with a stretched-out appearance. Generally, the patient will remain in a stiff, tonic position, as opposed to seizure or tic activity, which usually presents with more rapid, repetitive movements.

Complications from GERD are less common in the pediatric population as compared with adults. Chronic esophageal inflammation can result in the formation of an esophageal stricture. Barrett's esophagus, or the replacement of the distal esophageal mucosa with metaplastic epithelium, and esophageal adenocarcinoma are rarely encountered in pediatrics, although there are questions regarding whether infant or childhood reflux predisposes to GERD later in life and a higher risk for developing these complications. GERD has also been associated with apparent life-threatening events (ALTEs) in infants. The infant's proximal airway is small and at high risk for regurgitation-related laryngospasm and obstruction. It should be noted, however, that although reflux-associated apnea has been described and studies have demonstrated that a high percentage of ALTE patients do suffer from GER, a temporal relationship between apneic episodes and instances of regurgitation has not been well established. The contribution of reflux to symptoms of asthma has been demonstrated and the pharmacologic treatment of GERD can result in an improvement in asthma symptoms. Recently, GERD has been implicated in children who develop feeding refusal or who have behavioral issues surrounding the act of feeding.

PATHOPHYSIOLOGY

The distal portion of the esophagus is composed of involuntary smooth muscle that functions to propel food particles from the mouth into the stomach after ingestion. The lower esophageal sphincter (LES) is the tonically contracted specialized muscle located at the gastroesophageal junction (GEJ) that helps prevent the reflux of stomach contents into the distal esophagus. The LES is supposed to remain tonically closed except when relaxing in response to swallowing, during periods of esophageal distention, and with esophageal contractions in the absence of deglutition. A high-pressure zone exists in the region of the distal esophagus, consisting of the tonic LES pressure, the diaphragmatic crura, and the pressure transmitted to the intra-abdominal portion of the distal esophagus. This high-pressure zone functions to prevent GER.

Tonic LES pressure is maintained at greater than 4 mm Hg, which is generally adequate to prevent reflux. Most reflux occurs during spontaneous transient LES relaxations. In patients with GERD, transient relaxations occur too frequently, allowing for GER. Transient LES relaxations are mediated via the vagal pathway, probably initiated by gastric fundus distention. The crural diaphragm bolsters the tone of the LES. With a hiatal hernia, the LES pressure can be overcome by intragastric pressure even in the absence of transient LES relaxations.

Familial clustering of a variety of esophageal disorders, including hiatal hernia, severe GERD, Barrett's esophagus, and adenocarcinoma suggests a genetic predisposition. A gene for "severe pediatric GERD," which was observed in five families with a hereditary pattern with high penetrance, has been linked to a locus on chromosome 13 (13q14). This gene has, however, been excluded for infantile esophagitis.

DIFFERENTIAL DIAGNOSIS

The patient in the above case presentation presented with frequent regurgitation but was otherwise asymptomatic. Although this presentation is suggestive of a diagnosis of GER, there are many other disorders that need to be considered with a similar presentation or when additional symptoms are present. The differential diagnosis for entities that have similar symptoms to GERD is quite vast and comprehensive. By obtaining a thorough history, the practitioner can elicit various clues to help diagnose GERD or direct attention toward an alternative diagnosis (Table 9-1). This should include a comprehensive ascertainment of the feeding history, patterns of symptoms, and past medical history.

When an infant or child is experiencing only acute symptoms, GERD is less likely and the workup should focus on other causes of emesis. The presence of fever often suggests an infectious etiology, projectile emesis could be due to pyloric stenosis, and bilious emesis requires an investigation for an obstruction. For infants with chronic symptoms, it is important to obtain very specific details regarding the feeding history, including how much they are consuming, what they are being fed, and how the formula is prepared. One of the most common reasons for infant GER symptoms is overfeeding, which can easily be elicited.

For all children with reflux symptoms, the specific nature and frequency of the reported symptoms must be determined, including how often emesis occurs, how these episodes are related to feeds, what type of distress the patient is experiencing, and if there are any exacerbating or relieving factors. Postprandial right up-

Table 9-1 Comprehensive History for Pediatric GERD

Feeding
Frequency/amount of intake? Overfeeding?
How is the formula being mixed?
What type of formula/food?
Does there seem to be a great deal of air swallowing during feeds?
What is the body positioning during and after feeds?
Any symptoms of choking, gagging, or arching during or after the feed?
Symptoms
When did the symptoms begin?
Does the patient complain of regurgitation into the oropharynx?
Is the patient vomiting?
    How frequently?
    How forcefully?
    Any bilious emesis? Any hematemesis?
    Has there been emesis of completely undigested food?
Has the patient exhibited feeding refusal?
Has the patient suffered apnea associated with symptoms?
Does the patient experience pain or discomfort?
    Any exacerbating/relieving factors?
    Location of the pain?
    Temporally related to feeding?
    Any specific foods that make symptoms worse?
Is the patient unusually fussy or irritable?
Any respiratory problems?
Medical History
Patient born prematurely?
Growth and development?
Any other medical problems?
    Does the patient suffer from recurrent illness?
    Is there an intercurrent acute illness?
    Any infectious symptoms such as fever or diarrhea?
        Asthma, cystic fibrosis (CF), or other primary respiratory disease?
        Neuromuscular disease?
        Metabolic disease? (Was the newborn screen normal?)
        Eczema or other allergic symptoms?
Any past surgeries?
Physical Examination
Height/weight
Is head circumference normal? Evidence of hydrocephalus or intracranial pathology?
General appearance and activity level?
Any evidence of dehydration?
    Does patient appear malnourished?
    Normal respiratory examination?
    Any abnormal abdominal findings?
    Normal neurologic examination?

per quadrant pain might suggest gallbladder disease, whereas abdominal pain relieved by eating might prompt consideration of peptic ulcer disease. Non-GI complaints, such as eczema or other allergic symptoms, should prompt an investigation for food allergies. Recently, eosinophilic esophagitis (EoE), a disorder characterized by a severe eosinophilic infiltrate of the esophagus that does not respond to acid blockade but improves with the removal of dietary antigens, has been recognized as a prevalent pediatric disorder. Because at least 70% of those diagnosed with EoE present with reflux symptoms, this should always be considered in the differential diagnosis of GERD, particularly if the symptoms are not responding to appropriate acid-suppression therapy. Other possibly contributory medical problems, such as chronic respiratory disease, also should be elicited.

On physical examination, height, weight, and head circumference should be assessed and compared with previous recordings on an age-appropriate growth curve. The examiner should investigate for any evidence of decreased activity level, dehydration, malnutrition, respiratory disease, or neurologic disease (e.g., hypotonia). For infants with recurrent emesis, there are various red flags on history, physical examination, and laboratory testing that should prompt the clinician to expand the differential diagnosis and initiate a workup for disorders other than GERD (Table 9-2).

The best method for organizing the differential diagnosis is to categorize these disorders by primary presentation. When a patient presents with emesis, the practitioner must consider other sources such as an obstruction, food allergy, other GI disorders, neurologic or intracranial pathology, infection, and toxic ingestions (Table 9-3). Although sternal pain and symptoms suggestive of esophagitis often are indicative of GERD, other considerations including allergy, primary gastric pathology, and non-GI sources, such as cardiac disease should be ruled out (Table 9-4). GERD must also be considered with other presentations, including respiratory symptoms and neurobehavioral abnormalities (Table 9-5).

DIAGNOSTIC TESTING

For the infant with uncomplicated emesis who first presents before 6 months of age, a thorough history and physical examination without further diagnostic testing should be adequate to diagnose GER. If indicated, radiographic or laboratory testing for other sources of vomiting should be performed. Similarly, for older children with symptoms limited to regurgitation and heartburn, a standard history and physical examination should allow the practitioner to diagnose GERD. However, when patients are not responding to typical conservative treatments used to treat GER or have findings such as poor weight gain, excessive irritability, feeding or respiratory problems, diagnostic testing should commence. Different methods include empiric treatment, radiographic testing, upper endoscopy with biopsies, pH probe monitoring, and impedance techniques (Table 9-6).

Empiric Therapy

One of the most frequently employed methods for diagnosing uncomplicated GERD is to treat empirically, most commonly with either an H_2-receptor antagonist or a proton pump inhibitor. Additionally, empiric therapy is sometimes employed when GER is believed to be contributing to other medical conditions such as cough or persistent asthma that have proved refractory to appropriate treatment. Although no studies have supported empiric therapy as a valid diagnostic method, it is a safe and noninvasive method that often can be effective.

Upper Gastrointestinal Series

An upper GI series (upper GI) is a barium contrast radiographic study in which contrast is swallowed by the patient and followed fluoroscopically while passing through the esophagus, stomach, and duodenum until it passes the ligament of Treitz. This test should be employed to exclude anatomic abnormalities or obstructive conditions that could provide an alternative explanation for vomiting or complicated reflux symptoms. Such conditions that can be diagnosed by upper GI include malrotation, pyloric stenosis, antral web, intestinal atresia, esophageal stricture, or achalasia. However, upper GI is neither sensitive nor specific for episodes of reflux and is not the appropriate test for detecting the presence or absence of GERD.

Table 9-2 Red Flags in the Vomiting Infant
Bilious emesis
Hematemesis or hematochezia
Onset of emesis at age 6 months or older
Feeding refusal
Poor weight gain/failure to thrive
Macrocephaly or microcephaly
Bulging fontanelle
Seizures
Respiratory distress
History of apnea
Diarrhea
Fever
Lethargy
Hepatosplenomegaly
Abdominal tenderness or distention
History of genetic disorders
Other chronic illnesses
Electrolyte abnormalities

Adapted from Rudolph, CD, Mazur LJ, Liptak, GS, et al: Guidelines for evaluation and treatment of gastroesophageal reflux in infants and children: Recommendations of the North American Society for Pediatric Gastroenterology and Nutrition. J Pediatr Gastroenterol Nutr 32: S1-S31, 2001.

Table 9-3	Differential Diagnosis of Pediatric Gastroesophageal Reflux Disease (GERD): Emesis

Gastrointestinal (GI) obstruction
  Malrotation/volvulus
  Pyloric stenosis
  Intermittent intussusception
  Intestinal duplication
  Esophageal atresia or stricture
  Gastric outlet obstruction
  Antral or duodenal web/stenosis
  Bezoar
  Adhesions
  Foreign body
  Incarcerated hernia
  Meconium ileus
  Annular pancreas
Other GI disorders
  GERD
  Hiatal hernia
  Achalasia
  Enteritis
  Pseudo-obstruction
  Gastroparesis
  Peptic ulcer disease/gastritis
  Pancreatitis
  Hepatobiliary disease (e.g., cholelithiasis)
  Appendicitis
  Cyclic vomiting syndrome
  Rumination
  Toxic ingestion
Food intolerance/allergy
  Celiac disease
  Milk protein/soy allergy
  Eosinophilic esophagitis/enteritis
  Nonspecific food allergy
	Infectious
	  Gastroenteritis
	  Helicobacter pylori
	  Sepsis
	  Meningitis/encephalitis
	  Urinary tract infection
	  Pneumonia
	  Upper respiratory infection
	  Hepatitis
	  Parasitic infection
	Neurologic
	  Encephalopathy
	  Tumor/mass lesion
	  Hydrocephalus
	  Intracranial bleed
	  Intracranial injury/concussion
	  Migraines
	  Vestibular disease
	Extragastrointestinal
	  Metabolic disorders
	  Congenital adrenal hyperplasia
	  Adrenal insufficiency
	  Ureteropelvic junction obstruction
	  Uremia
	  Lead poisoning
	  Vascular ring
	  Pregnancy
	  Eating disorder/bulimia
	  Munchausen syndrome by proxy
	  Medications

Table 9-4	Differential Diagnosis of Pediatric Gastroesophageal Reflux Disease (GERD): Esophagitis/Pain

GERD
Eosinophilic esophagitis
Gastritis/peptic ulcer disease
Celiac disease
Colic
Hepatobiliary disorders
Pancreatitis
Cardiac pain
Costochondritis
Mediastinal mass
Malingering

Nuclear Scintigraphy

Gastroesophageal scintigraphy, commonly referred to as a "milk scan" or "gastric emptying study," is a nuclear scan performed by oral ingestion of technetium-labeled formula/milk or food. After ingestion of the radiolabeled meal, the child is placed supine on a table, and repeated images are obtained for 2 hours. The esophagus, stomach, and lungs are assessed for the presence of radiotracer. These images can detect a delay in the rate of gastric emptying, which could be contributing to the pathophysiology of GER. The rate of gastric emptying varies depending on the patient's age as well as the composition of the meal, so the recorded values are compared with established norms. The number of episodes of GER and whether radiotracer reaches the upper esophagus also can be assessed. Additionally, episodes of aspiration can be noted by nuclear scintigraphy, although a negative test does not rule out infrequent aspiration.

The main purpose of nuclear scintigraphy is to detect delayed gastric emptying, which could focus future therapy. An advantage of this method is that it measures postprandial acid and non-acid reflux. However, nuclear scintigraphy is not sensitive for the presence of GER that is not postprandial. Additionally, although this is currently the test of choice for detecting aspiration, it has poor sensitivity.

Table 9-5	Differential Diagnosis of Pediatric Gastroesophageal Reflux Disease (GERD): Other Presentations

Dysphagia
    Achalasia
    Eosinophilic esophagitis
    Vascular ring
    Esophageal stricture
Failure to thrive
    Metabolic disorder
    Feeding disorder/inadequate intake
    Malabsorption
    Celiac disease/other food allergy
    Genetic disorder
    Neglect
Respiratory symptoms
    Extrinsic compression (vascular ring)
    Foreign body
    Reactive airway disease
    Pneumonia
    Cystic fibrosis
    Central apnea
    Sinusitis
    Infection
    Tracheomalacia
    Laryngomalacia
Neurobehavioral
    Seizures
    Sandifer's syndrome
    Vestibular disorders

Upper Endoscopy

Esophagogastroduodenoscopy (EGD) allows for visualization as well as biopsies of the esophageal, gastric, and duodenal epithelium. This is the most sensitive method for detecting esophageal mucosal inflammation or damage secondary to GERD; EGD is also the best method for detecting gastritis, duodenitis, *Helicobacter pylori* infection, celiac disease, antral webs, and eosinophilic or infectious esophagitis. Visually, the physician can assess for the presence of ulcers, gross evidence of inflammation, and hiatal hernia (Fig. 9-1).

When an EGD is performed, biopsies should routinely be collected from the distal esophagus, antrum, and third portion of the duodenum as well as from any areas that appear visually abnormal. Typically, with esophagitis secondary to reflux, the mucosa of the distal esophagus will demonstrate an infiltrate of inflammatory cells (Fig. 9-2). Biopsies of patients with GERD may reveal neutrophils, eosinophils, increased lymphocytes, basal cell hyperplasia, and papillary lengthening. The presence of greater than 15 or 20 eosinophils per high-powered field is generally diagnostic of eosinophilic esophagitis; however, these findings can rarely be consistent with reflux esophagitis. If these results are obtained from a patient who has not been treated with aggressive acid suppression, then the child should be prescribed high-dose proton pump inhibitors (PPIs) for 4 to 6 weeks before a repeat EGD. Persistence of the eosinophilic infiltrate confirms a diagnosis of EoE, whereas resolution would suggest that the prior pathologic findings were secondary to GERD.

There are no standard indications for when EGD should be performed as a component of the workup for GERD. Endoscopy should be considered when the patient is not responding to standard therapy, when severe esophagitis is suspected, if failure to thrive results from feeding difficulties, or when symptoms concerning for the presence of food allergy or eosinophilic esophagitis are evident. The advantage of EGD is the ability to visualize the GI tract and obtain tissue for histologic analysis. The primary disadvantage is that this is an invasive test that, although generally well tolerated, requires the patient to be sedated and is not without risk.

Esophageal pH Probe Monitoring

Esophageal pH monitoring measures the frequency and duration of episodes of acid reflux. The probe, which is placed transnasally, usually has a pH electrode near or at the distal tip; other designs have multiple sensors so that measurements can be simultaneously recorded in the distal and more proximal esophagus. A recording device measures the pH every 4 to 8 seconds and stores the information. The patient or a parent is asked to record any change in activity, positioning, or level of arousal as well as when the patient is feeding. An event record is maintained to temporally correlate symptoms with episodes of acid reflux. Most studies record for 16 to 24 hours. Patients are able to feed during a pH probe study. For routine pH probe monitoring, the patient should not receive acid suppression medication for 48 to 72 hours before the test. However, there are clinical indications, such as assessing response to pharmacologic therapy or the presence of unusual symptoms (cough, hoarseness) when the pH probe should be performed while the child is still receiving medications.

On completion of the study, the data are transferred from the recording device to a computer program, where they are analyzed. The reflux index, which is the percentage of time that the esophageal pH is less than 4, is considered the most valid measure of reflux because it reflects the duration of esophageal acid exposure. Other common measures include the frequency of reflux episodes, the number of episodes greater than 5 minutes, acid clearance time, and the duration of the longest episode of reflux.

Esophageal pH probe was previously considered the gold standard in the diagnosis of GER. The advantages include the ability to detect acid reflux in all phases of activity and correlate symptoms with GER. However,

Table 9-6 Diagnostic Methods for Gastroesophageal Reflux Disease (GERD)

Method	Use	Advantages	Disadvantages
Upper gastrointestinal (GI) series	Assess for anatomic abnormalities	Useful to rule out anatomic abnormalities as source of emesis	Not a reliable indicator of gastroesophageal reflux (GER)
Nuclear scintigraphy (milk scan or gastric emptying scan)	Measure postprandial acid and non-acid reflux. Assess for aspiration. Detect abnormalities in rate of gastric emptying	Detects postprandial GER. Detects delayed gastric emptying	Poor sensitivity for esophagitis/gastritis. Moderate sensitivity for GERD and aspiration. Tests only postprandial period. Expensive
Endoscopy with biopsies	Visualization of mucosa of the upper GI tract. Documentation of gross ulceration or erosion. Histopathologic analysis of the epithelium	Most sensitive indicator of esophageal inflammation. Rule out eosinophilic esophagitis, celiac disease, gastritis, *Helicobacter pylori*, peptic ulcer disease	More invasive with increased risk. Requires sedation. Expensive
pH probe	Document the frequency and duration of acid reflux episodes	Quantifies acid reflux. Correlation between acid reflux and symptoms or behaviors (e.g., arching, apnea). Good for assessing treatment failures	Poor for reflux at pH >4. Cannot distinguish between acid reflux and ingestion of acidic contents. Short duration. Poor sensitivity for brief, clinically significant GER
Wireless pH monitoring	Radiotelemetry pH sensor placed in the distal esophagus	No transnasal wire. Capsule in fixed location. 48-hour duration	Only detects acid reflux events. Occasional discomfort. Requires esophagogastroduodenoscopy (EGD) for accurate placement
Multichannel intraluminal impedance	Document the presence of non-acid reflux episodes. Also performs functions of pH probe	Documents acid and non-acid reflux	No standard data for the "normal" amount of non-acid reflux
Empiric pharmacologic therapy	Demonstrate whether certain symptoms improve when GER is treated	Noninvasive. Potential amelioration of symptoms	Negative response to therapy does not rule out GER

there are multiple limitations to this method, most notably the inability to discern non-acid reflux, which is a common postprandial finding in infants. Additionally, this method measures a limited period and is not sensitive for very short episodes of reflux, which can have clinically significant consequences. Lastly, many patients find the pH probe uncomfortable; infants and toddlers commonly remove it before completion of the study. A pH probe can be quite beneficial for assessment of poor response to treatment or antireflux surgery, establishment of a temporal relationship between acid reflux and non-GI symptoms (e.g., arching, apnea), and investigation for the presence of occult or "silent" reflux as an etiology for chronic respiratory or otolaryngologic complaints such as chronic cough and hoarseness.

Wireless pH Monitoring

Wireless pH monitoring has recently been introduced as an alternative to traditional pH probe testing. With the Bravo system, a radiotelemetry pH-sensing capsule is attached to the esophageal mucosa approximately 5 cm proximal to the gastroesophageal junction. Usually an EGD is performed before placement in order to accurately determine the optimal location for placement. The obvious advantage to this method is the lack of an intranasal catheter, which is often bothersome to the patient. Additionally, the Bravo records pH measurements for approximately 48 hours, which is longer than most pH probe studies. The Bravo capsule is well tolerated,

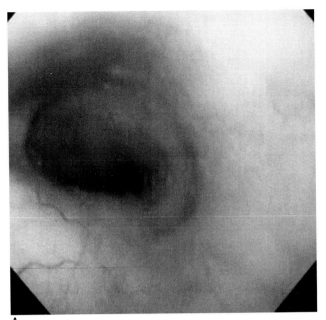 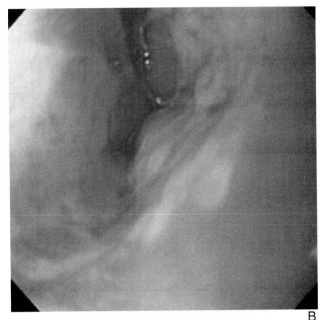

Figure 9-1 *(See also Color Plate 9-1.)* **A,** Smooth endoscopic appearance of normal esophageal mucosa. **B,** Erythematous, inflamed, irregular appearance of distal esophageal mucosa from patient with gastroesophageal reflux disease (GERD). No discrete ulcers are noted.

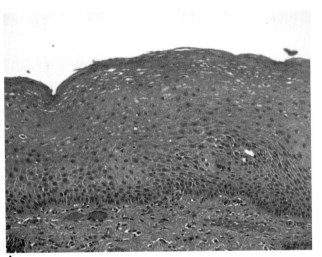 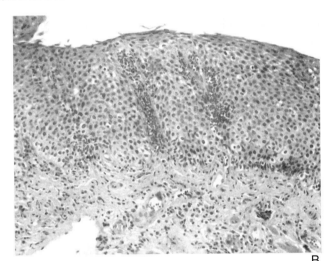

Figure 9-2 *(See also Color Plate 9-2.)* **A,** Normal esophageal mucosa. **B,** Reflux esophagitis as shown by expanded basal cell layer and scattered inflammatory cells. (**A** and **B** × 100). (**A** and **B** courtesy E. Ruchelli, MD, Division of Pathology, Children's Hospital of Philadelphia and the University of Pennsylvania School of Medicine.)

although there are occasional patients who experience chest discomfort, and it disassociates from the esophageal mucosa after approximately 48 hours. Like the pH probe, though, the Bravo only detects acid reflux and is not reliable for the detection of non-acid GER.

Multichannel Intraluminal Impedance

Multichannel intraluminal impedance (MII) has been introduced as an alternative method for detecting GERD. Because air, fluid, and solid material in the esophagus each has a characteristic impedance, intraluminal bolus movement, size, and character can be detected by an intraesophageal catheter based on differences in conductivity to alternating current. MII catheters also have pH sensors, allowing for the concomitant measurement of acid reflux. The obvious theoretical advantage of this method is that both acid and non-acid reflux can be detected, which should render this a more sensitive method of diagnosing reflux. Pediatric studies have demonstrated that this method does identify additional non-acid reflux events that would not have been diagnosed by pH probe alone, particularly in children who are being treated by acid suppression but are still having symptoms.

TREATMENT

Most infants with uncomplicated GERD will experience resolution of symptoms some time during the first year of life without any specific therapeutic intervention. For infants with GER who are not excessively fussy, feeding well and thriving, and not experiencing any respiratory sequelae, the parents can be educated regarding the pathophysiology and the natural history of the disorder and should be reassured. However, for children and adolescents who have been diagnosed with GERD as well as for infants with additional symptoms, multiple treatment options can be considered, including conservative measures such as feeding and lifestyle changes, pharmacologic therapy, and surgery.

Dietary Changes

For most infants, changing the formula fails to result in an improvement in reflux symptoms. Infrequently, cow's-milk–protein allergy, however, can manifest as emesis, although additional symptoms such as irritability, diarrhea, blood in the stool, or poor weight gain also usually are noted. Elimination of milk protein from the diet is a reasonable measure if there is concern that GER is secondary to allergy. Typically, symptoms will improve within the first 24 to 48 hours after eliminating milk protein from the diet. Because of a high cross-reactivity with soy, formula-fed infants with milk-protein allergy should probably be transitioned directly to a hydrolyzed formula. There is no evidence to support the discontinuation of breastfeeding for infants with GERD.

Thickening of feeds is another common dietary treatment of infantile GER. In the United States, this is usually accomplished by adding rice cereal to the formula. Although thickened feeds can decrease the incidence of emesis, there is evidence that reflux still may occur. When thickened feeds are employed, the nipple should be cross-cut to allow for adequate flow.

Dietary manipulation is often suggested for children and adolescents as a first-line management for GERD. The most common recommendations include avoidance of caffeine, chocolate, high-fat foods, spicy foods, carbonated beverages, citrus fruits and juices, and alcohol. Anecdotal evidence suggests that these factors can contribute to individual symptoms of GERD, and some studies have provided evidence supporting an improvement in esophageal pH after discontinuation of some of these substances. However, a recent evidence-based review of the adult GERD literature reports that no evidence has ever been published establishing that removal of any of the above has resulted in an abatement or improvement in reflux symptoms. Empiric dietary manipulation should not be recommended, although it would be prudent to discontinue any food or beverage that the patient or parent feels is causing an exacerbation of the child's individual symptoms.

Positioning Therapy

Infants clearly have a decreased incidence of GER when placed in the prone position as compared with the supine or seated position. However, because of the associated increased risk of sudden infant death syndrome (SIDS), the American Academy of Pediatrics has recommended non-prone positioning for all sleeping infants. Prone positioning should not be endorsed as an appropriate treatment for infantile GERD except in those circumstances when the risk of death from GERD is believed to outweigh the risk of SIDS. Although placement of an infant in a car seat or seated position after feeds is often advocated, there is evidence that this type of positioning could actually contribute to reflux by increasing abdominal pressure. Upright positioning is helpful.

For children and adolescents with nocturnal GERD symptoms, elevation of the head of the bed is often recommended as a method to decrease the frequency and duration of reflux episodes. There is evidence that this is an effective treatment method. Additionally, although not well investigated in children, reflux has been shown to occur significantly less frequently in adults sleeping in the left lateral decubitus position as compared with the right lateral decubitus position.

Other Lifestyle Management

Alcohol and tobacco use is associated with an increase in GERD, although there is no clear evidence that cessation of these activities results in an improvement in symptoms. Many practitioners advocate for avoidance of a late evening meal because of increased postprandial reflux, but the timing of dinner has not been demonstrated to have an effect on reflux symptoms. Patients suffering from obesity do have an increased incidence of reflux, and weight loss has been demonstrated to result in an improvement in symptoms.

Pharmacologic Therapy

Acid Suppression

Acid-lowering agents, in order of potency, include antacids, histamine-2 receptor antagonists (H_2-antagonist), and proton pump inhibitors (PPIs) (Table 9-7). Antacids, such as magnesium hydroxide, calcium carbonate, or aluminum hydroxide, neutralize gastric acid, thereby reducing esophageal acid exposure and ameliorating heartburn symptoms. The safety of these medications in children has not been well studied. Antacids can be effective

Table 9-7 Pharmacotherapy for Pediatric Gastroesophageal Reflux Disease (GERD)

Medication	Recommended Dose	Adverse Effects
H_2-Receptor Antagonists		
Cimetidine (Tagamet)	20-40 mg/kg/day divided tid-qid Adult: 800-1200 mg/dose bid-tid	Headache, diarrhea, pancytopenia, gynecomastia, nausea, vomiting, drowsiness, rash, dizziness, reduces hepatic metabolism of other medications, bradycardia, hypotension, transaminitis central nervous system (CNS) toxicity/psychiatric disturbances (rare)
Famotidine (Pepcid)	0.5-1 mg/kg/day divided bid Adult: 20-40 mg bid	Headache, dizziness, constipation, diarrhea, taste changes, nausea, CNS toxicity/psychiatric disturbances (rare)
Nizatidine (Axid)	4-6 mg/kg/day divided bid Adult: 150 mg bid	Headaches, dizziness, constipation, diarrhea, abdominal pain, nausea, dizziness, emesis, anemia, urticaria, constipation, CNS toxicity/psychiatric disturbances (rare)
Ranitidine (Zantac)	4-6 mg/kg/day divided bid Adult: 150 mg bid	Headache, dizziness, constipation, diarrhea, fatigue, thrombocytopenia, transaminitis, rash, dry mouth, dry skin, CNS toxicity/psychiatric disturbances (rare)
Proton Pump Inhibitors		
Lansoprazole (Prevacid)	1-2 mg/kg/day Adult: 15-30 mg daily	Headache, diarrhea, constipation, abdominal pain, nausea
Omeprazole (Prilosec)	1-2 mg/kg/day Adult: 20-40 mg daily	Headache, diarrhea, constipation, abdominal pain, nausea, vitamin B_{12} deficiency, rash
Esomeprazole (Nexium)	Pediatric dose not defined Adult: 20-40 mg daily	Headache, diarrhea, abdominal pain, nausea
Pantoprazole (Protonix)	Pediatric dose not defined Adult: 40 mg daily-bid	Headache, diarrhea, abdominal pain, nausea
Rabeprazole (Aciphex)	Pediatric dose not defined Adult: 20 mg daily-bid	Headache, diarrhea, abdominal pain, nausea
Prokinetics		
Metoclopramide (Reglan)	0.1 mg/kg/dose qid	Fatigue, anxiety, insomnia, headache, dizziness, nausea, diarrhea, extrapyramidal symptoms, hyperprolactinemia, urinary frequency, rash, acute dystonia, tardive dyskinesia, pancytopenia, bradycardia
Erythromycin	1-5 mg/kg/dose tid-qid	Diarrhea, vomiting, abdominal pain, potential bacterial resistance, pyloric stenosis, dysrhythmias, transaminitis
Bethanechol (Urecholine)	0.1-0.2 mg/kg/dose tid-qid Adult: 25 mg qid	Hypotension, bronchospasm, cholinergic side effects

*Not U.S. Food and Drug Administration (FDA) approved for use in the United States except for a limited access program.

for symptomatic relief but should not be used as chronic therapy.

H_2-antagonists reduce acid production by competitive inhibition of the H_2-receptor of gastric parietal cells. In the past, they have been considered a first-line therapy for pediatric GERD because of their effectiveness and excellent safety profile. All have been shown to reduce acid reflux, improve symptoms, and assist in healing of the esophageal mucosa. Tachyphylaxis has been described after 1 week of daily dosing of H_2-antagonists. Nizatidine, the newest H_2-antagonist, also has been shown to have prokinetic properties.

PPIs are the most effective acid-suppression medications and function by covalently bonding to and deactivating the H^+-K^+-ATPase pumps. Because they require acid in the parietal cell canaliculus for activation, PPIs are most effective when administered 15 to 30 minutes before a meal, which stimulates the parietal cell. Concomitant administration of an H_2-antagonist can decrease the efficacy of the PPI. Nocturnal acid breakthrough has been a noted problem with PPIs, which has been addressed with twice daily dosing or a dose of an H_2-antagonist before bedtime. Lansoprazole and omeprazole have been approved for use in children; both can be compounded as a liquid, and lansoprazole is available as a powder as well as a soluble tablet.

There are two main approaches to the implementation of acid-suppression therapy in pediatric GERD. The *step-up approach* introduces an H_2-antagonist as initial therapy, escalating from low- to high-dose therapy followed by replacement with a PPI if symptoms have been refractory to the prior step. The *step-down approach* begins with a high-dose PPI to initiate improvement and then weans to a lower dose of PPI or H_2-antagonist for maintenance of remission. Neither approach has been adequately studied for pediatric GERD. Although both categories of medications rarely cause adverse effects, there have been recent reports of an increased risk of gastroenteritis, community-acquired pneumonia, and small bowel bacterial overgrowth in patients who are being treated with these medications.

Prokinetic Therapy

Theoretically, prokinetic agents should have an important role in GERD therapy (see Table 9-7). Metoclopramide is a dopamine antagonist that enhances the response of the upper GI tract to acetylcholine, thereby increasing motility and improving gastric emptying. Placebo-controlled studies have failed to demonstrate the effectiveness of this medication as a treatment for GERD. Additionally, metoclopramide has numerous adverse effects, most notably extrapyramidal reactions such as dystonia and tardive dyskinesia that sometimes do not immediately resolve with discontinuation of the medication. Erythromycin is a macrolide antibiotic that increases GI motility by acting as an agonist to motilin, a hormone secreted by the GI tract that contributes to smooth muscle contraction. Erythromycin has been proved an effective and relatively safe medication for patients with motility disorders, but has not been well studied in pediatric GERD. Bethanechol is a cholinergic agonist that has not been shown to effectively decrease the risk of GERD. Cisapride, a serotonergic agent that enhances myenteric plexus acetylcholine release, thereby promoting gastric motility, is the only prokinetic medication that has been demonstrated to be effective for GERD. Unfortunately, cisapride has been associated with prolonged QT interval and an increase in the incidence of dysrhythmias and is only available in the United States through a limited-access program requiring frequent cardiac monitoring by the prescribing physician.

Surgical Therapy

Antireflux surgery is considered for children with persistent reflux that has proved refractory to maximal medical therapy as well as for those who have suffered severe complications of GERD, such as recurrent aspiration. The most frequently used surgical technique is the Nissen fundoplication, which entails wrapping the gastric fundus around the gastroesophageal junction, preventing the reflux of gastric contents in the distal esophagus. This surgery has become less prevalent with the implementation of PPIs in the management of pediatric GERD but is still one of the three most common procedures performed by pediatric surgeons. Over the past decade, fundoplication is increasingly being performed laparoscopically; this less invasive approach has resulted in decreased hospital stays and decreased risks of scarring and infection. A success rate of Nissen fundoplication between 57% and 92% has been reported and is similar for open and laparoscopic methods. Reflux symptoms tend to persist if the wrap is not tight enough.

Unfortunately, complications from Nissen fundoplication are not uncommon and are similar for open and laparoscopic methods (Table 9-8). Medical management should be maximized before considering surgical treatment of GERD. Additionally, a thorough diagnostic workup

Table 9-8 Common Complications of Nissen Fundoplication

Complication	Description	Treatment
Dysphagia	Complications from wrap being too tight	Investigate for other causes of symptoms, surgical release of wrap
Small bowel obstruction	Direct surgical complication from adhesions	Lysis of adhesions
Paraesophageal hernia	Direct surgical complication	Symptomatic relief Surgical correction if necessary
Gas-bloat syndrome	Persistent postoperative gagging, retching, nausea, abdominal distention, and sometimes food refusal	Venting gastrostomy tube can help partially relieve symptoms
Dumping syndrome	Postprandial nausea, retching, diaphoresis, diarrhea, initial hyperglycemia followed by hypoglycemia Symptoms related to rapid discharge of gastric contents into the duodenum	Dietary management: smaller, more frequent meals; increase complex carbohydrates and avoid simple sugars; increase fat and protein in diet; avoid liquid with meals; restrict lactose Acarbose, octreotide can be effective therapies

should be performed to ensure that the symptoms are due to GERD and not other entities that would not be relieved by surgery, such as cyclic vomiting, eosinophilic esophagitis, gastroparesis, and rumination.

APPROACH TO THE CASE

The patient is a 3-month-old boy who suffers from frequent postprandial nonbloody and nonbilious emesis. He is not suffering from symptoms of irritability, fussiness, or feeding refusal. His physical examination is reassuring and he continues to gain weight appropriately. Based on this clinical presentation, the patient can be categorized as having uncomplicated GER. The patient's mother was reassured and told to call if the emesis intensified or if new symptoms arose.

The patient's mother returns 3 weeks later and reports that the emesis has become more frequent and that he now seems to be more fussy and at times difficult to console. Additionally, his formula intake has decreased. His growth has been unaffected but on examination he is crying and seems uncomfortable. Now that the patient is symptomatic, he is diagnosed with GERD. At this point, the patient is started on ranitidine at a dose of 3 mg/kg/dose twice daily. The patient demonstrates some mild improvement but continues to have daily significant symptoms. An upper GI is performed to determine that he does not have an anatomic abnormality, such as malrotation, contributing to this frequent emesis. The results of the upper GI are normal. Subsequently, lansoprazole is prescribed. After 2 weeks of PPI therapy, his mother states that the patient's symptoms are vastly improved; although he still is experiencing occasional emesis, he seems more comfortable and the episodes are less voluminous and less frequent. She is instructed to continue the lansoprazole and follow-up is arranged in 2 months, at which point a decision will be made regarding whether to wean this medication.

SUMMARY

GERD is a common complaint that affects patients of all ages. When GERD is suspected, the pediatrician should perform a thorough history and physical examination that will either consolidate the diagnosis or elicit other symptoms that might suggest another etiology. GERD can usually be diagnosed by history and physical examination as well as response to empiric treatment. When vomiting is persistent, an upper GI should be performed to rule out malrotation and other anatomic abnormalities. Most cases of GERD can be treated via conservative measures and pharmacologic therapy with either an H_2-receptor antagonist or proton pump inhibitor.

MAJOR POINTS

- GER, the intermittent regurgitation of gastric material into the esophagus, is a normal physiologic process.
- GERD describes the clinical symptoms that occur secondary to GER.
- Recurrent emesis is reported in up to 67% of infants but generally resolves by 12 months.
- The classic presentation of GERD is recurrent emesis in infants, and heartburn and regurgitation in children and adolescents.
- A thorough history and physical examination focusing on feeding details, frequency and characterization of symptoms, growth parameters, and additional medical problems is usually sufficient to diagnose GERD or suggest a need to consider other disorders.
- An acute presentation of emesis, bilious emesis, fever, ALTE, abnormal neurologic findings, poor feeding/growth, respiratory distress, hepatosplenomegaly, and lethargy warrant workup for other diagnoses in addition to GERD.
- An upper GI should be performed in any patient with persistent emesis to rule out malrotation.
- Esophageal pH monitoring, although helpful in measuring the degree of acid reflux, has limitations, including an inability to detect non-acid reflux.
- A trial of empiric acid-suppression therapy is a reasonable diagnostic and therapeutic method for a patient with symptoms suggestive of uncomplicated GERD.
- Conservative treatment measures such as dietary manipulation, positioning therapy, and lifestyle changes can be implemented on an individual basis.
- EGD with biopsies should be performed when the symptoms suggest severe esophagitis or if the patient is not responding to therapy. This can help distinguish between GERD and eosinophilic esophagitis.
- Prokinetic agents should be considered as a treatment for pediatric GERD only if dysmotility or a delay in gastric emptying has been demonstrated.
- Surgical management should be reserved for patients with severe GERD that has been refractory to maximal medical therapy or who have experienced severe complications.

SUGGESTED READINGS

Arad-Cohen N, Cohen A, Tirosh E: The relationship between gastroesophageal reflux and apnea in infants. J Pediatr 137: 321-326, 2000.

Canani RB, Cirrillo P, Roggero P, et al: Therapy with gastric acidity inhibitors increases the risk of acute gastroenteritis and community-acquired pneumonia in children. Pediatrics 117:e817-e820, 2006.

Chicella MF, Batres A, Heesters MS, et al: Prokinetic drug therapy in children: A review of current options. Ann Pharmacother 39:706-711, 2005.

Condino AA, Sondheimer J, Pan Z, et al: Evaluation of infantile acid and nonacid gastroesophageal reflux using combined pH monitoring and impedance measurement. J Pediatr Gastroenterol Nutr 42:16-21, 2005.

Di Lorenzo C, Orenstein SR: Fundoplication: Friend or foe. J Pediatr Gastroenterol Nutr 34:117-124, 2002.

Kahrilas PJ, Pandolfino JE: Review article: Oesophageal pH monitoring: Technologies, interpretation, and correlation with clinical outcomes. Aliment Pharmacol Ther 22:2-9, 2005.

Kaltenbach T, Crockett S, Gerson LB: Are lifestyle measures effective in patients with gastroesophageal reflux disease? An evidence-based approach. Arch Intern Med 166:965-971, 2006.

Kiljander TO, Harding SM, Field SK, et al: Effects of esomeprazole 40 mg twice daily on asthma: A randomized placebo-controlled trial. Am J Respiratory Crit Care Med 173:1091-1097, 2006.

Liacouras CA, Spergel JM, Ruchelli E, et al: Eosinophilic esophagitis: A 10-year experience in 381 children. Clin Gastroenterol Hepatol 3:1198-1206, 2005.

Nelson SP, Chen EH, Synair GM, et al: Prevalence of symptoms of gastroesophageal reflux during infancy: A pediatric practice-based survey. Arch Pediatr Adolesc Med 151:569-572, 1997.

Nelson SP, Chen EH, Synair GM, et al: Prevalence of symptoms of gastroesophageal reflux during childhood: A pediatric practice-based survey. Arch Pediatr Adolesc Med 154:150-154, 2000.

Orenstein SR, Izadnia F, Khan S: Gastroesophageal reflux in children. Gastroenterol Clin 28:948-969, 1999.

Orenstein SR, Khan S: Gastroesophageal reflux. In Walker WA, Goulet O, Kleinman R, et al (eds): Pediatric Gastrointestinal Disease, 4th ed, Hamilton, Ontario, BC Decker, 2004.

Rosen R, Lord C, Nurko S: The sensitivity of multichannel intraluminal impedance and the pH probe in the evaluation of gastroesophageal reflux in children. Clin Gastroenterol Hepatol 4:167-172, 2006

Rudolph CD, Mazur LJ, Liptak GS, et al: Guidelines for evaluation and treatment of gastroesophageal reflux in infants and children: Recommendations of the North American Society for Pediatric Gastroenterology and Nutrition. J Pediatr Gastroenterol Nutr 32:S1-S31, 2001.

Shaffer SE: Gastroesophageal reflux. In Altschuler SM, Liacouras, CA (eds): Clinicial Pediatric Gastroenterology, Philadelphia, Churchill Livingstone, 1998.

CHAPTER 10

Gastrointestinal Bleeding

BINITA M. KAMATH

PETAR MAMULA

Disease Description
Case Presentation
Epidemiology
Pathophysiology
Differential Diagnosis
Diagnostic Testing
Treatment
Approach to the Case
Summary
Major Points

DISEASE DESCRIPTION

Gastrointestinal (GI) bleeding in the pediatric population can occur from any location in the intestinal tract. The bleeding may manifest as hematemesis, melena, or hematochezia, or it may be occult. The etiology of GI bleeding is broad, and the frequency of common diagnoses varies with age. Whereas some etiologies are not clinically significant, other even minor bleeding episodes may herald a massive hemorrhage or indicate an underlying serious disease. GI bleeding in children always warrants careful consideration. Endoscopy and colonoscopy are invaluable tools for diagnosis and therapy.

CASE PRESENTATION

A 7-year-old boy presents with a history of bright red bleeding per rectum for 3 days. The child was previously fit and well and was taking no regular medications. The bleeding was painless and he had no history of diarrhea or constipation. The blood was bright red and sufficient to coat the toilet bowl. On presentation, he is hemodynamically stable and he has an unremarkable physical examination, except for soft heme-positive stool on rectal examination. His hemoglobin is 11.6 g/dL.

A 4-year-old girl presents with hematemesis. She is an ex-premature baby born at 31 weeks' gestation, but had had a relatively benign neonatal intensive care course. She is taking no regular medications and is in a mainstream school. She had acute onset of profuse bright red hematemesis with no preceding illness. At presentation she is pale, tachycardic, and sweaty. Her hemoglobin is 6.4 g/dL.

EPIDEMIOLOGY

GI is a common symptom in the pediatric population. Significant acute GI bleeding is a relatively uncommon problem, although epidemiologic data are sparse. The overall incidence is not known because the majority of available data come from the sick pediatric intensive care population, with reported incidences ranging from 10% to 25%. A prospective 1-year study described incidence of upper GI bleeding in the intensive care unit setting at 6%. In a retrospective case series of pediatric patients seen in an urban tertiary emergency department (ED) during a 10-month period, 0.3% of visits were for chief complaint of blood in the stool. Fortunately, in most cases presenting to the ED, the etiology is nonsignificant, management is predominantly conservative, and mortality is low.

PATHOPHYSIOLOGY

Broadly speaking, the processes underlying GI bleeding originate from the intestinal mucosa, involve structural or vascular anomalies, or are consequences of systemic disease. Regardless of the mechanism for the bleeding, the most important issue is to determine the severity of the bleeding and to identify signs of hemorrhagic shock. Detailed reviews of resuscitation algorithms have been widely published. Briefly, significant bleeding may lead to hypovolemic shock, decrease in preload, cardiac output, and blood pressure. The decrease in mean arterial pressure triggers a sympathetic response, causing vasoconstriction, increase in heart rate, and redirection of the blood to the brain and heart with improved cardiac output and blood pressure. However, if the shock is left untreated it may lead to tissue ischemia, organ failure, and ultimately death. Fortunately, a fatal outcome in GI bleeding is extremely rare in children and adolescents.

Because estimates of blood loss are difficult to make based on history alone, it is important to rely on vital signs, physical examination, symptoms, and laboratory results. Vital signs should be taken in lying, sitting, and standing positions. If orthostatic signs are noted (with an increase in pulse rate and a decrease in blood pressure when going from lying to sitting or standing positions), significant loss of intravascular volume should be suspected. Additionally, tachycardia is one of the most sensitive indicators of shock, and in adult patients an increase in heart rate of 10% to 20% corresponds to decrease in intravascular volume of 10% to 15%. Due to redirection of blood to the brain and heart, the skin is less well perfused, leading to a decrease in surface body temperature and cyanosis. When the decrease in intravascular volume exceeds 25%, capillary refill is prolonged. Further depletion results in decreased urine output, indicating renal hypoperfusion with urine output in children of less than 1 mL/kg/hour. Hyperventilation also may be noted because of acidosis as a result of tissue hypoperfusion. Further volume compromise may lead to decrease in cerebral perfusion manifested by lethargy, change in mental status, and coma.

DIFFERENTIAL DIAGNOSIS

When evaluating a child with a history of GI bleeding the first question should be, is it really blood? If so, it should be taken into consideration that the blood may have originated from a source outside the GI tract or that it may not belong to the patient. Red food coloring in cereals, or in Jell-O or Kool-Aid may mimic blood, particularly in toddlers with rapid intestinal transit. Other foods or drinks like tomato or cranberry juice, fruit punch, beets, spinach, berries, licorice, and chocolate, as well as certain medications, can also mimic blood. In children wearing diapers *Serratia marcescens* in stool may cause red discoloration.

The nasopharynx is a common source of bleeding in a child, but hemoptysis is very rarely an underlying cause of GI bleeding. Swallowed maternal blood should be excluded in a breastfed infant. Maternal and fetal hemoglobin can be distinguished using the Apt-Downey test. Denatured maternal hemoglobin turns filter paper yellow or rusty, whereas pink or red indicates fetal hemoglobin. Finally, the blood may not be human, as has been seen in rare cases of Munchausen syndrome by proxy.

Several tests are used for detection of blood in the GI tract. They are based on guaiac or leukodye (Gastroccult, Hemoccult), fluorescent antibody to porphyrin, or antihemoglobin antibody. Reagents using guaiac are very reliable and have the advantage of allowing parents to use them at home, although the sensitivity varies. For the detection of blood in an acid environment like the stomach, the Gastroccult (SmithKline Diagnostics, San Jose, CA) test should be used instead of a Hemoccult test. A comparison study was performed in children to detect the presence of occult GI bleeding in 100 patients. The tests used included Hemoccult II (Beckman Coulter, Inc., Brea, CA), Hemoccult SENSA (Beckman Coulter, Inc., Brea, CA), and HemeSelect (SmithKline Diagnostics, San Jose, CA). Forty-two children had upper GI and 58 had lower GI sources of bleeding. The authors concluded that fecal occult blood tests vary, depending on the origin of bleeding. The results favored use of Hemoccult SENSA slides for suspected upper GI and HemeSelect slides for lower GI bleeding.

Several substances may interfere with occult blood tests. False-positive results may be caused by meat, horseradish, turnips, iron preparations, tomatoes, and fresh red cherries, and ingestion of vitamin C, or long storage of tests may produce false-negative results.

Once it has been established that the blood loss is indeed real and from the GI tract, one of the most helpful factors in narrowing the differential diagnosis is the patient's age (Table 10-1). Certain conditions, such as cow's milk protein allergy, and intussusception are almost exclusively seen in infants up to the age of 2 years. Variceal bleeding or hematochezia from inflammatory bowel disease is usually seen later in childhood and adolescence. Many conditions such as esophagitis, peptic ulcer disease, and infectious colitis are commonly encountered across all age-groups. Finally, establishing whether the bleeding is acute or chronic may help in the differential diagnosis.

Upper GI bleeding is defined as originating proximal to the ligament of Treitz and it usually manifests with vomiting of blood (hematemesis). The blood may appear bright red, or a "coffee ground" color due to denatured hemoglobin, which has been exposed to gastric acid and secretions. The color of the blood may be helpful in distinguishing blood loss from a briskly bleeding source such as esophageal varices or a large peptic ulcer, which may manifest as bright red hematemesis, or from gastritis, which usually presents with coffee-ground emesis.

Table 10-1 Differential Diagnoses of Gastrointestinal Bleeding		
	Upper Gastrointestinal Bleeding	**Lower Gastrointestinal Bleeding**

Infant	*Mucosal*
	    Esophagitis
	    Gastritis
	    Peptic ulcer disease
	    Mallory-Weiss tear
	    Gastric heterotopia
	Structural
	    Gastric or intestinal duplication
	Other
	    Hemorrhagic disease of the newborn
	    Vascular anomalies
	    Swallowed maternal blood
		Mucosal
		    Peptic ulcer disease
		    Necrotizing enterocolitis
		    Infectious colitis
		    Eosinophilic/allergic colitis
		    Hirschsprung's enterocolitis
		Structural
		    Intestinal duplication
		    Meckel's diverticulum
		    Intussusception

Child	*Mucosal*
	    Esophagitis
	    Gastritis
	    Peptic ulcer disease
	    Mallory-Weiss tear
	Other
	    Esophageal varices
	    Hereditary telangiectasia
	    Vascular anomalies
	    Hemobilia
	    Foreign body
	    Tumor
		Mucosal
		    Peptic ulcer disease
		    Infectious colitis
		    Ulcerative colitis/Crohn's disease
		    Anal fissure
		    Juvenile polyp
		    Solitary rectal ulcer
		    Hemorrhoid
		    Lymphonodular hyperplasia
		Structural
		    Intestinal duplication
		    Meckel's diverticulum
		    Intussusception
		    Volvulus
		    Visceral artery aneurysm
		Other
		    Hemolytic-uremic syndrome
		    Henoch-Schönlein purpura
		    Dieulafoy's malformation
		    Munchausen syndrome by proxy
		    Arteriovenous malformation

Finally, in cases of intussusception or Meckel's diverticulum the stool may have a "currant jelly" or dark maroon color. It is important to realize that infants and young children with upper GI bleeding may present with hematochezia because of their accelerated intestinal transit time. However, in most cases, bleeding from the upper GI tract will be dark colored due to blood exposure to oxygen during the passage through intestine.

Lower GI bleeding is characterized either by bright red blood (hematochezia), or dark tarry stool (melena). In lower GI bleeding, three factors may be helpful—the color of the blood, the nature of the stool, and the presence or absence of pain. Bright red blood with normal or hard stool implies an anal or rectal source. The presence of pain may suggest a fissure, whereas its absence may indicate a juvenile polyp. Bright red blood mixed with mucus and loose stools, associated with crampy abdominal pain and tenesmus, is suggestive of an infectious or inflammatory process. Profuse painless bleeding is typical of Meckel's diverticulum. Intussusception is classically heralded by red currant jelly stool and colicky abdominal pain.

DIAGNOSTIC TESTING

The initial diagnostic step in investigating GI bleeding is a detailed history and careful physical examination. On physical examination multiple findings could point to the etiology of bleeding (Table 10-2). This will narrow the differential diagnosis considerably and target further tests appropriately, avoiding unnecessary extensive investigation.

Nasogastric tube placement and gastric irrigation with normal saline are invaluable tools in the evaluation of GI hemorrhage and should be considered a mandatory test in significant upper GI bleeding. The presence of fresh blood in the stomach aids in determining the site of bleeding and indicates bleeding from a site proximal to the ligament of Treitz, although a negative test

Table 10-2 Physical Examination Findings in Conditions Associated with a Risk of Gastrointestinal (GI) Bleeding

	Findings	Conditions
Skin	Purpura on buttocks and legs	Henoch-Schönlein purpura
	Petechiae, purpura	Coagulopathy, thrombocytopenia, intense vomiting
	Hemangioma, telangiectasia	Vascular anomalies
	Caput medusae, spider angioma	Chronic liver disease
	Jaundice	Chronic liver disease
Head/Neck	Epistaxis	Nose bleeding
	Webbed neck	Turner's syndrome
	Blood in hypopharynx	Adenoid or tonsillar disorders
	Hyperpigmented lesions on lips and gums	Peutz-Jeghers syndrome
	Lesions on buccal mucosa	Trauma
Lungs	Hemoptysis	Tuberculosis, pulmonary hemosiderosis
Abdomen	Organomegaly and/or ascites	Chronic liver disease
	Hyperactive bowel signs/borborygmi	Upper GI bleeding
	Palpable and tender loops of intestine	Inflammatory bowel disease, intussusception
Anal/Rectal	Abscess, fistula, skin tags	Inflammatory bowel disease
	Fissure	Constipation
	Polyp	Polyp
	Erythema	A beta-hemolytic streptococcus cellulitis
	Hemorrhoids	Hemorrhoids, portal hypertension

does not exclude an upper GI source. Nasogastric irrigation is a useful method for determination of the extent of blood loss and monitoring of ongoing losses. Nasogastric aspirate was shown to predict high-risk bleeding lesions, especially in hemodynamically stable patients with no hematemesis. Based on aspirate color, early endoscopy was shown not to be needed in bleeding peptic ulcer patients with clear or coffee-grounds nasogastric aspirate; the patients benefited from early endoscopy in cases of bloody aspirate. In an adult study, the combined score consisting of signs of hemodynamic instability, low hemoglobin, high white blood count, and presence of bright red blood on nasogastric irrigation, was predictive of a need for urgent endoscopy with a high sensitivity and specificity of 96% and 98%, respectively. However, another study suggested that it is not clear if there is a value for a nasogastric aspirate in determining presence of bleeding and its location, and if endoscopy is necessary. Laboratory studies are important in the assessment of the severity and duration of the bleeding, and may point to an etiology such as chronic liver disease and variceal hemorrhage. The blood urea nitrogen to creatinine ratio is believed to discriminate upper from lower GI bleeding with a higher ratio seen in upper GI bleeding. In a study of 952 adult patients this was confirmed, but significant degree of overlap existed, especially in patients without hematemesis. Studies routinely ordered for the evaluation of bleeding severity and etiology include complete blood count with differential and reticulocyte count, comprehensive metabolic panel, and coagulation studies (Table 10-3). Blood type and screen are obtained if it is anticipated that the patient will require blood products.

Plain x-ray films are generally of limited value in GI bleeding but are valuable if obstruction or perforation is suspected. In particular, plain films may identify pneumatosis intestinalis, which is characteristic of necrotizing enterocolitis in infants. The x-rays of the neck, the chest, and the abdomen also may be useful in foreign body ingestion if the object is radiopaque (Fig. 10-1).

Contrast x-ray studies are usually not the first line of diagnostic radiologic testing unless the history and physical examination point toward a source, which can be best detected through contrast investigation. Upper GI contrast study can detect ulceration, radiolucent foreign body, malrotation with or without volvulus, duplication cyst, Meckel's diverticulum, and inflammatory bowel disease (IBD). Barium enema can be used for diagnosis of IBD and diagnosis and therapy of intussusception. A computed tomography (CT) scan is also not frequently used in the investigation of GI bleeding, although in cases of abdominal trauma it is considered to be the modality of choice.

Nuclear medicine studies include technetium-99m (Tc-99m) radiolabeled red blood cell (RBC) scan, Tc-99m sulfur colloid, and Tc-99m pertechnetate Meckel's scan. The Meckel scan detects accumulation of radiopharmaceuticals in ectopic gastric mucosa within the Meckel's diverticulum with more than 90% accuracy. If clinical suspicion is still strong despite a negative scan, use of a histamine (H_2)-blocker may improve enhancement at the time of a repeat scan. Because contrast studies and

Table 10-3 Diagnostic Tests in Gastrointestinal Bleeding

	Studies
Laboratory study	Complete blood count and differential, erythrocyte sedimentation rate, reticulocyte count, prothrombin time and partial thromboplastin time, chemistry panel, liver function tests, blood type and crossmatching
Gastric irrigation	Nasogastric tube irrigation
Radiographic imaging	Neck, chest, and abdominal plain x-rays and obstruction series Computed tomography (CT) Contrast studies: upper gastrointestinal (UGI) series with small bowel follow-through (SBFT) and barium enema (BE) Magnetic resonance imaging (MRI) Magnetic resonance angiography/venography (MRA/MRV)
Nuclear medicine	Technetium-labeled Meckel's scan Technetium-labeled bleeding scan
Endoscopy	Diagnostic and/or therapeutic
Angiography	Diagnostic and/or therapeutic
Surgery	Explorative laparoscopy or laparotomy

angiography can interfere with a Meckel's scan, those tests should be performed after the scan in order to minimize the chance of a false-negative result. The radiolabeled RBC scan can detect bleeding as low as 0.1 mL/minute, which is more sensitive than angiography. However, if non–blood-pooling sulfur colloid is used, extravasating particles can be detected in a relatively short interval of 15 to 20 minutes after the time of contrast injection. If the patient is not actively bleeding during that time, the study may be false-negative. A radiolabeled RBC scan can be used in patients who are bleeding more slowly or intermittently.

Abdominal ultrasound with Doppler examination is performed in cases of suspected portal hypertension, and may reveal splenomegaly and reversal of the flow in the portal vein. The study may be diagnostic, in cavernous transformation of the portal vein, as described in the clinical vignette above, or in vascular anomalies.

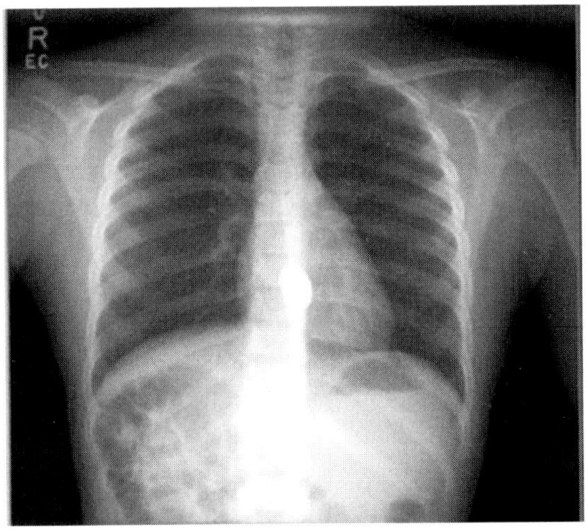

Angiography can detect bleeding at a rate of approximately 0.5 mL/minute and greater. In a pediatric study it detected the source of acute bleeding in 71% and chronic bleeding in 55%. The advantage of this technique is that it allows for a therapeutic intervention at the same time. Magnetic resonance imaging (MRI) may identify mass lesions and magnetic resonance angiography and venography (MRA/MRV) may be useful noninvasive tools to target vascular lesions.

Video capsule endoscopy is increasingly being used for detection of GI bleeding in children. Currently, the limitations are the size of the device, which requires endoscopic placement under general anesthesia in small children and the risk of obstruction, especially in patients with Crohn's disease.

Endoscopy is the preferred diagnostic procedure in GI bleeding because it offers diagnostic and therapeutic opportunities. Emergency upper endoscopy can determine the source of bleeding in upper GI hemorrhage in the vast majority of patients. It is particularly useful in detecting mucosal lesions such as Mallory-Weiss tears, erosive esophagitis, or gastritis (Fig. 10-2). Although upper endoscopy can usually be easily accomplished with intravenous sedation, in acute upper GI hemorrhage in children it may be necessary to administer general anesthesia in order to prevent complications like aspiration, ensure success of the procedure, and allow the use of a larger therapeutic endoscope. It is important to realize, however, that upper endoscopy is not mandatory in all cases of upper GI hemorrhage, and conservative management may be appropriate in cases in which the bleeding is not associated with anemia or hemodynamic

Figure 10-1 Coin in the esophagus.

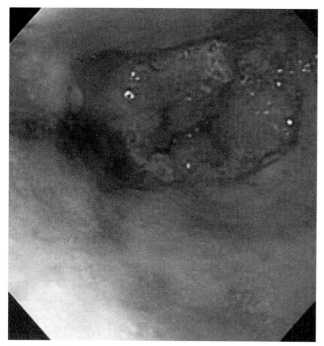

Figure 10-2 *(See also Color Plate 10-2.)* Erosive esophagitis.

instability and is self limited. The risk of major complications in emergency endoscopy is 0.59% and potential complications include perforation (0.26%), aspiration (0.2%), and hemorrhage (0.13%).

Colonoscopy is indicated early in the diagnostic testing for hematochezia. Colonoscopic examination is superior to contrast radiology in detecting lesions such as polyps, and it allows for therapeutic intervention. Age-appropriate colon clean-out needs to be performed in order to complete the procedure safely, examine the colon in its entirety, and perform the therapeutic procedure.

Finally, surgery may be employed in select cases for definitive diagnosis and therapy if other studies did not reveal the source of bleeding. Often the surgeon and endoscopist will work in tandem to examine the intestine in its entirety and identify the source of bleeding.

TREATMENT

The initial management of a child with acute GI bleeding involves basic resuscitative measures. Resuscitation must provide adequate oxygen delivery, repletion of circulating volume, and correction of any coagulopathy or electrolyte abnormalities. Because the total blood volume of a child is relatively small, resuscitation has to be aggressive; however, children rarely have comorbid illnesses, and therefore mortality from GI bleeding in pediatrics is generally quite low. Basic fluid resuscitation with limited laboratory studies should be initiated without delay. Overexpansion of intravascular volume is potentially dangerous in case of bleeding from esophageal varices, and volume replacement should match ongoing losses after correction of shock.

The empiric use of acid-suppressing medications is justified in the pediatric population, based on the most common etiologies (see Table 10-1). Intravenous acid suppression has been shown to improve ulcer healing and decrease rebleeding while not causing a change in morbidity or mortality in patients with significant hematemesis. Intravenous omeprazole was shown to have similar pharmacokinetic parameters in children as in adults, and it was well tolerated. Sucralfate, a basic aluminum salt of sulphated sucrose, which binds directly to the ulcer site, has been effectively used for treatment of peptic ulcer disease. In cases of bleeding secondary to *Helicobacter pylori* infection, combination antibiotic therapy in addition to acid suppression is used. Other therapies may include antifungal and antiviral treatment or avoidance of food allergens. Inflammatory bowel disease is a rare cause of major GI bleeding and it occurs most commonly in Crohn's disease. Endoscopically treatable lesions are uncommon, and surgery is required in almost 40% of patients.

The most commonly used form of medical therapy in pediatric patients with severe upper GI bleeding secondary to a vascular lesion (varices, bleeding ulcer) is octreotide or vasopressin. Vasopressin is given by a separate infusion in a carefully monitored setting. The dose is 0.1 to 0.4 units/minute and there is no "per kilogram" dose. Typically, a dose of 0.1 to 0.2 units/minute is begun. The blood pressure, serum electrolytes and osmolarity, urine output, and digital perfusion must be frequently monitored for side effects of the therapy, which include syndrome of inappropriate antidiuretic hormone secretion and peripheral vasoconstriction. Intravenous somatostatin has been shown to be as effective as vasopressin with fewer side effects in patients with cirrhosis.

Endoscopy, both esophagogastroduodenoscopy (EGD) and colonoscopy, is the mainstay of therapy in GI bleeding. Endoscopic therapies can be broadly thought of as variceal and nonvariceal, and several techniques for endoscopic control of GI bleeding exist (Table 10-4). The hemostatic endoscopic therapies have often been validated for the treatment of nonvariceal bleeding in the adult population and then applied to pediatrics. The specific mode of treatment for nonvariceal bleeding may be limited by the small size of pediatric endoscopes, which cannot accommodate larger therapeutic catheters. However, the great majority of therapeutic procedures can be successfully and safely performed in children of any age.

Several studies have demonstrated the effectiveness of direct injection therapy. The most commonly used agent is epinephrine, although others like thrombin and

Table 10-4	Endoscopic Therapies for Gastrointestinal Bleeding

Nonvariceal
Bipolar electrocoagulation
Thermal coagulation
Injection therapy
Laser photocoagulation
Hot biopsy forceps

Variceal
Injection sclerotherapy
Variceal band ligation

Polyp
Snare polypectomy with electrocautery

ethanol have been used too. Several adult studies have established that the use of epinephrine, injected into and near the periphery of oozing lesions, is as effective as the use of heater probe coagulation. Some endoscopists use injection therapy to slow vigorous bleeding lesions so that coagulation therapy can be attempted.

The most common coagulation methods available for treating bleeding lesions of the GI tract involve bipolar and thermal (heater probe) coagulation. The probe, which is attached to an electrosurgical unit, is passed through the endoscopic biopsy channel. Usually, a large-channel endoscope is required not only for passage of the cautery catheter but also to enable adequate water irrigation and suction in cases of excessive bleeding. With bipolar electrocoagulation, the potential for deep tissue injury seen with monopolar probes is reduced because the electrodes are limited to the area of the probe; however, a larger number of applications are usually needed to stop bleeding. Currently, the most commonly used bipolar electrode systems are Gold Probe (Microvasive, Milford, MA) and BICAP (Circon-ACMO, Stamford, CT). Finally, direct-heat thermal cautery units or heater probes transfer energy to tissue by thermal conduction. The energy is diffused at a relatively low temperature (250° C), thereby limiting the potential for acute tissue erosion. In cases of small vascular lesions, especially in the colon, hot biopsy forceps may be used. In this case, electrocoagulating current is passed through the forceps while the mucosa is lifted from the muscular layer, which then allows for both preservation of histology specimen and bleeding control.

One of the most common indications for the use of endoscopic coagulation is to stop active bleeding from gastric or duodenal ulcers, a focal area of gastritis, and severe Mallory-Weiss tear. In addition, coagulation therapy can be used to prevent bleeding from lesions that are at high risk for bleeding. Contraindications to coagulation therapy are a hemodynamically unstable patient, massive bleeding from arterial lesions (secondary to obscured visual field), bleeding from esophageal varices and arteriovenous malformations greater than 1 cm.

The therapy for esophageal variceal bleeding (Fig. 10-3) consists of injection sclerotherapy and variceal ligation with elastic bands. The preferred method depends on endoscopist's expertise and experience, and it may be guided by a patient's age, size, severity of bleeding, and medical history. During sclerotherapy, a sclerosing agent is injected into a varix during upper endoscopy, starting above the gastroesophageal junction and progressing in a circumferential and ascending fashion. A review study describing the success rate and side effects of sclerotherapy in a large number of pediatric patients has been published. After successful initial therapy, patients are scheduled for repeat procedures until varices are eradicated. For prevention of bleeding, propranolol therapy can be safely used in children. However, the efficacy depends on adherence to treatment regimen and appropriate dosing, which most likely requires a reduction in heart rate of more than 25%. Developed 20 years ago, the variceal banding technique uses a hollow transparent cylinder mounted at the tip of the endoscope. After applying suction, the wire releasing the rubber band is triggered, strangulating the varix (Fig. 10-4). Variceal ligation in children was first reported in 1988, and since then multiple case series with more than 100 patients have been published. Two techniques used for the treatment of variceal bleeding were compared for the first time in children

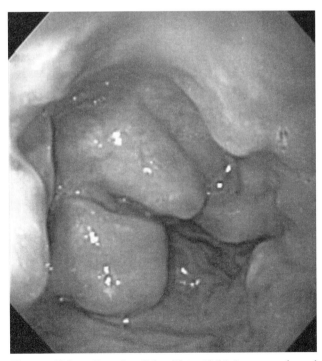

Figure 10-3 *(See also Color Plate 10-3.)* Large esophageal varices.

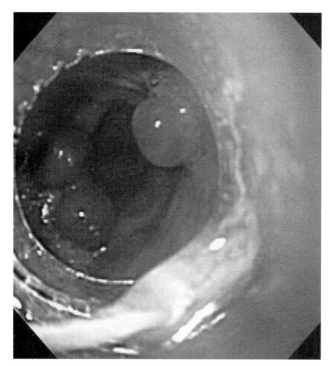

Figure 10-4 *(See also Color Plate 10-4.)* Postligation appearance of banded esophageal varices.

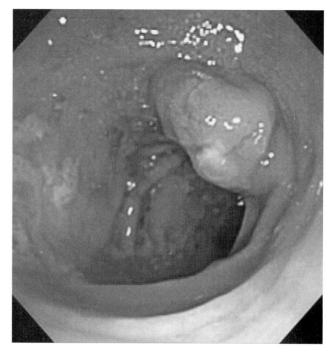

Figure 10-5 *(See also Color Plate 10-5.)* Large polyp in the descending colon.

with extrahepatic portal venous obstruction. Forty-nine children were randomized to receive either sclerotherapy or ligation therapy. The control of bleeding was achieved at a similar rate in both groups. However, the ligation therapy showed lower rate of rebleeding with fewer complications, and the eradication of varices was achieved in fewer sessions.

Laser photocoagulation therapy has been increasingly used for active bleeding, particularly from vascular malformations. Two different systems are available. The argon laser's energy is absorbed by hemoglobin, thus causing superficial coagulation. In contrast, the neodymium-yttrium-aluminum-garnet laser penetrates the mucosa to a greater depth, thus surface bleeding does not interfere with its use. The use of laser therapy requires significant expertise in order to avoid complications. Khan and colleagues used argon laser in 13 pediatric patients with history of upper GI bleeding and were able to achieve good bleeding control with minor side effects in 2 of the 13 patients who developed submucosal argon gas and scar formation.

Polyp removal using snare and electrocautery is the most common therapeutic procedure for control of bleeding at the time of colonoscopy (Figs. 10-5 and 10-6). Other methods have been used for vascular colonic anomalies (Fig. 10-7). Full colonoscopy to the terminal ileum should be performed in order to evaluate for presence of multiple polyps, which could be associated with polyposis syndrome and may require surveillance colonoscopy, or other investigations. The majority of pediatric polyps are pedunculated, and their removal is fairly straightforward. However, the adverse event rate is higher than that of diagnostic colonoscopy, and complications include intestinal per-

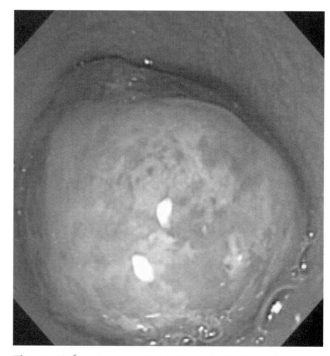

Figure 10-6 *(See also Color Plate 10-6.)* Postpolypectomy appearance of a juvenile polyp.

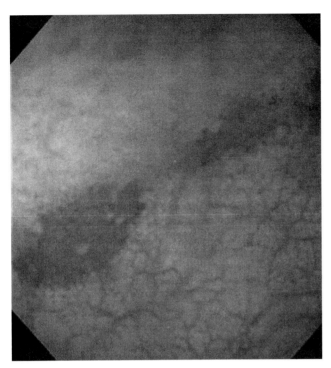

Figure 10-7 *(See also Color Plate 10-7.)* Hemangioma in the colon.

foration, persistent bleeding, and postpolypectomy coagulation and distention syndromes.

Finally, although EGD or colonoscopy and angiography should be considered in the majority of cases in children with significant GI bleeding, in certain cases, surgical therapy remains the best option. For example, patients with a perforated bleeding ulcer or volvulus should undergo emergency surgery. In addition, whenever a congenital abnormality is present, such as an enteric duplication, surgery is indicated. For patients with blue rubber bleb nevus lesion, endoscopic therapy can be attempted, but in cases in which multiple sites are involved, surgery is the therapy of choice. In situations in which the diagnostic workup has not revealed an etiology of the bleeding, panendoscopy at the time of laparoscopy or laparotomy should be considered. In cases that require aggressive resuscitation therapy, the surgical team should be involved from the onset of evaluation, and it is often prudent to have a surgeon available during endoscopy.

APPROACH TO THE CASE

This 7-year-old boy presented with acute painless hematochezia with no associated change in bowel movements. He was not hemodynamically compromised or anemic, implying that the bleeding was not severe or chronic. A colonoscopy revealed a polyp in the rectosigmoid colon, which was successfully snared and removed. The histology demonstrated a benign juvenile polyp. The remainder of the colon was entirely normal.

This 4-year-old girl presented with severe hematemesis, resulting in hemodynamic compromise and severe anemia. The initial objective in this situation was resuscitation with administration of oxygen and fluids. A gastric irrigation demonstrated copious amounts of fresh blood in the stomach, which cleared to pink after administration of 400 mL of normal saline. Within 10 minutes of the lavage, the nasogastric tube drainage was bloody again. An upper endoscopy under general anesthesia was emergently performed after fluid and blood resuscitation was completed and revealed three large esophageal varices. There was fresh blood in the stomach but no other gastric or duodenal abnormalities visualized. Sclerotherapy was performed with sodium morrhuate injections into the varices. The bleeding was successfully stopped and the child stabilized. Following the endoscopy she underwent additional studies to investigate the etiology of the esophageal varices. An abdominal ultrasound revealed cavernous transformation of the portal vein with splenomegaly. It is most likely that she developed portal vein thrombosis as a result of umbilical vein catheterization during her neonatal intensive care course.

SUMMARY

The causes of upper and lower GI bleeding in children and adolescents are numerous. Thorough history and physical examination need to be performed universally in order to assess the bleeding severity and urgency of treatment. The majority of patients require baseline laboratory workup, which consists of complete blood count and, in select cases, liver function tests and coagulation studies. The great majority of patients do not require extensive testing or admission to the hospital. However, in cases of serious GI bleeding diagnostic workup needs to occur on an expeditious basis. Most commonly used investigational radiologic studies include plain and contrast x-rays and nuclear medicine bleeding scan or Meckel's scan, as well as endoscopic studies, EGD, and/or colonoscopy depending on the presumptive source of bleeding. Endoscopy can serve as a diagnostic tool as well as therapy for GI bleeding. A wide variety of therapeutic procedures including injection and coagulation therapy, variceal sclerotherapy and ligation, foreign body removal (Fig. 10-8), polypectomy, and others can be employed at the time of endoscopy. Fortunately, serious complications or a fatal outcome are rare in the pediatric population. Lately, video capsule endoscopy is being used to investigate areas of the intestine that cannot be reached at the time of endoscopy.

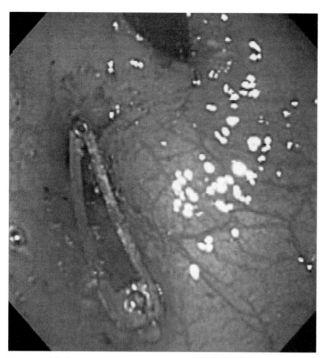

Figure 10-8 *(See also Color Plate 10-8.)* Foreign body (hairpin) in the stomach.

MAJOR POINTS

A history of GI bleeding in a child or adolescent requires prompt investigation.

Severe bleeding with serious consequences is uncommon.

Initial evaluation of GI bleeding should concentrate on rapid detection of severity and location of bleeding, which will guide further diagnostic evaluation and treatment.

Nasogastric tube irrigation is useful for determining and monitoring of upper GI bleeding.

Endoscopy and colonoscopy are invaluable tools in diagnosis and therapy of GI bleeding.

SUGGESTED READINGS

Adamopoulos AB, Baibas NM, Efstathiou SP, et al: Differentiation between patients with acute upper gastrointestinal bleeding who need early urgent upper gastrointestinal endoscopy and those who do not: A prospective study. Eur J Gastroenterol Hepatol 15:381-387, 2003.

Aljebreen AM, Fallone CA, Barkun AN: Nasogastric aspirate predicts high-risk endoscopic lesions in patients with acute upper-GI bleeding. Gastrointest Endosc 59:172-178, 2004.

Casson D, Williams HJ: Radionuclide diagnosis. In Walker A, Goulet O, Kleinman RE, et al (eds): Pediatric Gastrointestinal Disease. Hamilton, Ontario, BC Decker, 2004, pp 1906-1922.

Chalasani N, Clark WS, Wilcox CM: Blood urea nitrogen to creatinine concentration in gastrointestinal bleeding: A reappraisal. Am J Gastroenterol 92:1796-1799, 1997.

Cox K, Ament ME: Upper gastrointestinal bleeding in children and adolescents. Pediatrics 63:408-413, 1979.

Cuellar RE, Gavaler JS, Alexander JA, et al: Gastrointestinal tract hemorrhage: The value of a nasogastric aspirate. Arch Intern Med 150:1381-1384, 1990.

Fox VL: Gastrointestinal bleeding in infancy and childhood. Gastroenterol Clin North Am 29:37-66, v, 2000.

Gilbert DA, DiMarino AJ, Jensen DM, et al: Status evaluation: Hot biopsy forceps. American Society for Gastrointestinal Endoscopy. Technology Assessment Committee. Gastrointest Endosc 38:753-756, 1992.

Hall RJ, Lilly JR, Stiegmann GV: Endoscopic esophageal varix ligation: Technique and preliminary results in children. J Pediatr Surg 23:1222-1223, 1988.

Jaffe RM, Kasten B, Young DS, MacLowry JD: False-negative stool occult blood tests caused by ingestion of ascorbic acid (vitamin C). Ann Intern Med 83:824-826, 1975.

Khan K, Schwarzenberg SJ, Sharp H, Weisdorf-Schindele S: Argon plasma coagulation: Clinical experience in pediatric patients. Gastrointest Endosc 57:110-112, 2003.

Latt TT, Nicholl R, Domizio P, et al: Rectal bleeding and polyps. Arch Dis Child 69:144-147, 1993.

Leung AK, Wong AL: Lower gastrointestinal bleeding in children. Pediatr Emerg Care 18:319-323, 2002.

Marshall JB: Acute gastrointestinal bleeding: A logical approach to management. Postgrad Med 87:63-70, 1990.

O'Hara SM: Acute gastrointestinal bleeding. Radiol Clin North Am 35:879-895, 1997.

Olson A, Hillemeier AC: Gastrointestinal Hemorrhage. In Wyllie R, Hyams J (eds): Pediatric Gastrointestinal Disease. Philadelphia, WB Saunders, 1993, pp 251-270.

Orellana P, Vial I, Prieto C, et al: 99mTc red blood cell scintigraphy for the assessment of active gastrointestinal bleeding. Rev Med Child 126:413-418, 1998.

Racadio JM, Agha AK, Johnson ND, Warner BW: Imaging and radiological interventional techniques for gastrointestinal bleeding in children. Semin Pediatr Surg 8:181-192, 1999.

Sanowski RA: Thermal application for gastrointestinal bleeding. J Clin Gastroenterol 8:239-244, 1986.

Seidman EG, Sant'Anna AM, Dirks MH: Potential applications of wireless capsule endoscopy in the pediatric age group. Gastrointest Endosc Clin North Am 14:207-217, 2004.

Squires RH Jr: Gastrointestinal bleeding. In Altschuler SM, Liacouras C (eds): Clinical Pediatric Gastroenterology. Philadelphia, Churchill Livingstone, 1998, pp 31-42.

Teach SJ, Fleisher GR: Rectal bleeding in the pediatric emergency department. Ann Emerg Med 23:1252-1258, 1994.

Treem W: Gastrointestinal hemorrhage in children. Practical Gastroenterology 16:21-38, 1997.

Tuggle DW, Bennett KG, Scott J, Tunell WP: Intravenous vasopressin and gastrointestinal hemorrhage in children. J Pediatr Surg 23:627-629, 1988.

Wyllie R, Kay MH: Therapeutic intervention for nonvariceal gastrointestinal hemorrhage. J Pediatr Gastroenterol Nutr 22:123-133, 1996.

Zargar SA, Javid G, Khan BA, et al: Endoscopic ligation compared with sclerotherapy for bleeding esophageal varices in children with extrahepatic portal venous obstruction. Hepatology 36:666-672, 2002.

CHAPTER 11

Helicobacter pylori Infection

BENJAMIN D. GOLD

Disease Description
Case Presentation
Epidemiology
Pathophysiology
Diagnosis
    Gastrointestinal Endoscopy and Histology Evaluation
    Noninvasive Tests for *H. pylori* Infection
        Serology
        Urea Breath Test
        Stool Antigen Test
        Urine Antibody Test
Clinical Manifestations of *H. pylori* Infection
    Gastroduodenal Disease
    Extragastric Disease
    H. pylori Infection and Reflux Disease
Treatment
Approach to the Case
Summary
Major Points

DISEASE DESCRIPTION

Once upon a time, ulcers in the stomach and small intestine were believed to be caused by stress and spicy foods. Those patients diagnosed with an ulcer had to suffer not only the ulcer pain for the remainder of their lives, but the foul medication and blandness of the diet that were believed to help cure the condition. In 1982, when Barry Marshall of Australia and his mentor Dr. Robin Warren demonstrated that a bacterium called *Helicobacter pylori* (called *Campylobacter pyloridis* at the time) was the culprit, they caused quite a stir . . . and eventually made history. The scientific and medical community decided in October of 2005, based on the significant contribution to the fields of gastroenterology, microbiology, and medicine, to award Warren and Marshall the Nobel Prize for medicine and physiology for their discovery of the human gastric pathogen *H. pylori* and its role in gastroduodenal diseases in humans. In particular, the Nobel Prize committee decided that Warren and Marshall's 1982 discovery transformed peptic ulcer disease from a chronic, frequently disabling condition to one that can be cured by a short regimen of antibiotics and other medicines. Thanks to Marshall and Warren's work, it has now been established that *H. pylori* is the most common cause of peptic ulcers worldwide (www.msnbc.msn.com/id/9576387).

This review describes the status of the field of *H. pylori* infection, focusing in particular on research in pediatric *H. pylori* infection, and highlights the scientific advances made in this area.

CASE PRESENTATION

A 10-year-old Asian American boy presents with a 4-month history of abdominal pain. The boy and mother described the pain as localized to the epigastric region. The abdominal pain occurs primarily at night and early in the morning, usually right after awakening, just before leaving for school. The boy's mother denies witnessing any regurgitation or vomiting, and the boy's appetite, although somewhat decreased, has remained about the same. The boy does not seem to experience the abdominal pain in association with any foods, but avoids spicy and greasy foods without really being aware that he does so. The abdominal pain has awakened him at night once every one to two weeks. Past medical history reveals that this boy had a history of frequent regurgitation as an infant. Family history is remarkable for peptic ulcer disease on both the father's and mother's sides of the family (two uncles and one aunt, respectively) and gastric cancer in two cousins who live in Beijing, China. The parents were born in the United States and their respective parents (the boy's grandparents) immigrated to the United States from China. Social history revealed a young fifth-grade boy who does quite well in school and participates on a youth travel soccer team.

Physical examination demonstrates a well-appearing, articulate preadolescent with pale mucous membranes. On examination of the abdomen, no hepatosplenomegaly was discerned, but tenderness was elicited with palpation of the epigastric area. The remainder of the physical examination revealed no abnormal findings. Laboratory workup identifies a normal comprehensive metabolic panel, including liver biochemistries. Upper gastrointestinal series with barium revealed a normal examination, that is, normal anatomy and no evidence of obstruction, mucosal abnormalities, or stricture.

EPIDEMIOLOGY

"Any modality that entails the transfer of the *H. pylori* organism from the stomach of an infected individual to the stomach of an uninfected individual is a potential mode of transmission . . ." (Anonymous). The majority of evidence supports person-to-person transmission via the fecal–oral, oral–oral, or gastro–oral routes. Fecally contaminated uncooked vegetables or grossly contaminated water supplies are important routes of transmission in some countries. Finally, iatrogenic infection in health care personnel has been documented following the use of a variety of inadequately disinfected medical devices such as endoscopes.

PATHOPHYSIOLOGY

H. pylori is largely a childhood-acquired infection with some early onset disease, but typically disease presentation in adult clusters of the infection are within families. One relatively recent and innovative study conducted sequence typing of clinical *H. pylori* isolates exploiting genetic variation in core fragments of three key housekeeping loci (*ure*I, *atp*A, and *ahp*C) within this bacteria's genome. This unique typing methodology was used to determine clonal descent among isolates of 10 members of four families in Northern Ireland and a family with three generations in central England. Transmission has been felt to be facilitated by close contact and is primarily related to poor sanitary conditions, especially by the level of household hygiene. One novel study, in fact, demonstrated the ability to culture *H. pylori* from untreated municipal water, demonstrating that water may in fact be an extra-human reservoir for its infection and transmission.

In one cross-sectional study, 695 healthy people (308 males, 387 females; median age 60 years) participating in a health check-up program in Yamagata were evaluated. *H. pylori* status was determined in all subjects by evaluation of serum anti–*H. pylori* immunoglobulin G antibody. The authors used antibody against hepatitis A virus as a surrogate marker of fecal–oral exposure to assess the correlation between *H. pylori* infection and hepatitis A virus infection. By using multivariate logistic regression analysis, the authors determined that *H. pylori* infection was significantly associated with availability of a sewage system in childhood (odds ratio [OR] = 4.06, 95% confidence interval [CI]: 1.36 to 13.94). Nishise and colleagues also demonstrated that the number of gastrointestinal endoscopies undergone (four or more times) (OR = 3.18, 95% CI: 1.71 to 6.03), ($p < 0.01$ for trend) conferred a significant risk for *H. pylori* infection transmission. The authors concluded that poor hygiene in childhood is related to *H. pylori* infection. In addition, infection with *H. pylori*, like other enteric pathogens, appeared to require contact with gastric secretions (e.g., vomit) or fecally contaminated objects or food.

No studies have yet demonstrated risk from casual contact or even more intimate contact such as kissing or other sexual practices. Studies performed in couples attending infertility clinics demonstrated a low likelihood of the uninfected spouse acquiring the infection unless a baby or child was present in the household. In particular, bed sharing and horizontal transmission recently has been shown to be another mechanism for acquiring this infection. However, a recent, rather unique, study demonstrated that tonsil and adenoid tissues may be an ecologic niche of the mouth without regard to transient or permanent colonization. The authors extracted *H. pylori* deoxyribonucleic acid (DNA) from 3-mm-diameter tissue samples obtained from each tonsil and adenoid tissue specimen. They then performed gene amplifications employing *H. pylori* 16S ribosomal ribonucleic acid (RNA) (rRNA) and *cag*A genes in the samples obtained. Seven (30%) of 23 patients were shown to be positive for *H. pylori* DNA, 5 (71%) of whom also possessed the *Cag*A gene. These authors concluded that oral–oral transmission may be a possible mode of spread of *H. pylori*.

In a recent Japanese study, the major transmission routes of *H. pylori*, oral–oral or fecal–oral, were evaluated. Transfusion transmitted (TT) virus or TTV, a recently discovered microbe that is prevalent in healthy people, is believed to be transmitted mainly by nonparenteral routes. The authors tested the hypothesis that these two microorganisms have a common mode of transmission. The seroprevalence of *H. pylori* and TTV was investigated in a cross-sectional study of 454 healthy Japanese children from birth to age 15 years, living in five different geographic areas. The overall prevalences of *H. pylori* and TTV were 12.2% and 21.6%, respectively. An age-related increase of prevalence was shown for *H. pylori* ($p < 0.001$), but not for TTV ($p = 0.23$); no true correlation between the prevalence of these two organisms was demonstrated (Phi coefficient = −0.02 and P = 0.66). The authors concluded that although Japanese children frequently acquire both *H. pylori* and TTV, especially in early childhood, their acquisition appears to be of independent mechanisms.

Contaminated drinking water also appears to confer higher risk for *H. pylori* infection transmission than intrafamilial transmission. In this study, *H. pylori* prevalence increased with age, and there was a strong relationship between *H. pylori* serologic prevalence and a history of drinking of well water. Among the people who have a history of drinking well water, *H. pylori* prevalence in those at least 10 years old was 85.3%, which is significantly higher than that in those less than 10 years old (25%) and no history of drinking well water (6.3%). There were 5 families with *H. pylori* serologically positive members who drank well water and *H. pylori* DNA was detected from the well water of all five wells. Random amplification of polymorphic DNA (RAPD) fingerprinting of isolated *H. pylori* strains from these family members suggest that the origin of *H. pylori* infection was the well water. The authors speculated that most *H. pylori* transmission in Japan depends on waterborne transmission and the occurrence of its transmission is strongly associated with the duration of the history of drinking well water.

Evidence for the fecal–oral route of transmission was evaluated in a study that, although methodologically limited, nonetheless tested this transmission hypothesis. In developing countries such as Turkey, where the poor hygienic conditions facilitate the transmission of hepatitis A virus (HAV), infection with HAV is transmitted mainly via the enteral route, and thus can be used as a surrogate marker for enteral infection transmission. Of the 90 children enrolled, 33.3% were seropositive for both *H. pylori* and HAV, 33.3% were seronegative for both, 8.9% were seropositive for *H. pylori* only, and 24.4% were seropositive for HAV only. Unlike the study with TTV, the percentage of seropositive children increased with age for both *H. pylori* and HAV. However, there was no significant relationship in seroprevalence between *H. pylori* and HAV when analyzed by logistic regression analysis ($p = 0.178$). The authors concluded that the seropositivity rates of *H. pylori* and HAV increase with age, whereas the fecal–oral route may not be an important mode of transmission for *H. pylori* in children living in western Anatolia (Manisa region).

Our group has recently demonstrated similar observations supporting the potential for waterborne transmission in a study conducted in rural Guatemala. We previously demonstrated presence of *H. pylori* in dental plaque and tongue dorsum of a high proportion (86%) of people living in San Juan la Laguna, an indigenous Mayan population of western Guatemala. In this particular region of Guatemala, no hot running water is available. All households use standing water from rain collection or pipe or carry water from a lake. To determine the presence of *H. pylori* in water or biofilms, we collected water and biofilm samples from households previously surveyed with serology (*H. pylori* antibodies) and polymerase chain reaction (PCR) of dental plaque for *H. pylori* infection. Water sources obtained were from storage vessels, pipes (spout, bend), and biofilm swabs from each source. All samples were tested for coliforms, including *Escherichia coli*. DNA extraction from water samples and swabs by conventional PCR and nested-PCR methods was performed in two independent laboratories for the presence of *H. pylori*. Eight households had *H. pylori*-infected people by serology and oral evaluation; four households evaluated had everyone negative for *H. pylori* serology, and few oral sites contained *H. pylori* DNA. All samples from standing water, pipes, and vessels were positive for fecal coliforms and *E. coli*. Using conventional and nested PCR, a greater proportion of standing water samples (65%) than swab samples (29%) was positive for *H. pylori* DNA ($p < 0.002$), yet swabs from deep pipe sections had more *H. pylori* than pipe spouts. Thus, *H. pylori* appeared to be present in both water and biofilm in households where infected people reside in rural Guatemala.

DIAGNOSIS

In 1999, the Canadian Helicobacter Study Group was the first to publish recommendations regarding aspects of *H. pylori* infection in the pediatric population. These guidelines have now been revised to look at the most relevant data and advances in the field in the past 5 to 6 years. In the year 2000, the European Pediatric Task Force on *H. pylori* and the North American Society for Pediatric Gastroenterology Hepatology and Nutrition (NASPGHN) both proposed guidelines for the management of *H. pylori* infection in children. Both consensus committees reviewed the best available evidence and employed consensus techniques to make recommendations regarding the indication for testing, the optimal methods for detection, the appropriate rationale for therapy, and methods for follow-up of *H. pylori* infection in childhood. Similar consensus guidelines have been published that describe optimal methods for management of *H. pylori* infection in adults.

Gastrointestinal Endoscopy and Histology Evaluation

The upper gastrointestinal endoscopy with biopsies is still the gold standard in diagnosing *H. pylori* in adults and children. However, more recently, the urea breath test (UBT) has been described as the gold standard for both the detection and as a test for the cure of *H. pylori* infection in Europe. Unlike in adult endoscopy in which mucosal biopsies, particularly during upper endoscopy, are an exception, biopsies are routine in pediatric endoscopy. Kori and associates investigated the significance of performing routine duodenal biopsies. Biopsies from 201 pediatric patients were retrospectively reviewed: 79.1% were normal, and 17.4% were abnormal. Findings in abnormal biopsies included, 4.6% *Giardia lamblia*, 6.5% mild chronic inflammation, 3.9% increased intraepithelial lymphocytes, and two biopsies showed mixed acute and chronic inflammation. This investigation demonstrated that the risk for microscopic pathology was higher when *H. pylori* was present (25.98% vs. 12.16%, $P < 0.02$). The authors concluded that routine duodenal biopsies yield additional pathologic findings that otherwise could have been missed.

Recent controversy has waged over the overall decline in gastric cancer and subsequent increase in esophageal and proximal stomach cancers and the association with the overall decline of *H. pylori* prevalence. However, recent attention has been directed at understanding the severity and causes of inflammation of the gastric cardia in children undergoing endoscopy for symptoms of acid peptic disease. In a study by Borrelli and coworkers, 47 children were investigated, and *H. pylori* was detected in cardiac biopsies from 22 children by rapid urease test and histology. No patient had *H. pylori* in gastric corpus and/or antrum without having the organism at the cardia as well. The authors concluded that in children with symptoms of acid-peptic disease, inflammation of the gastric cardia occurs, which is more severe when the cardiac zone is infected with *H. pylori* than in its absence.

An American group studied how frequently atrophy and intestinal metaplasia occur in children, a novel observation, and a disease outcome believed previously to only occur in the adult population. In this study, 4 of 19 *H. pylori*-infected children had mild intestinal metaplasia, in two of whom it appeared to be accompanied by atrophy. Guarner and associates concluded that intestinal metaplasia is associated with *H. pylori* infection in children and because atrophy usually precedes intestinal metaplasia in adults, they suggested that atrophy exists in children. Additional studies have now demonstrated that intestinal metaplasia and atrophy can occur in childhood. Thus, determination of where the gastric histopathology becomes an irreversible lesion following eradication of *H. pylori* remains unclear.

As with many of the disease sequelae resulting from infection with *H. pylori*, ulcer disease is more often seen in adults than in children. However, the mechanisms underlying the different disease phenotypes in any one individual remain poorly characterized. Bontems and colleagues investigated mucosal T-cell responses in *H. pylori*-infected children and compared them with those of adults and negative controls. The results suggest that interferon-gamma (IFN-γ) secretion in the stomach of *H. pylori*-infected patients is lower in children than in adults. This immune phenotype was felt by the authors to potentially confer protection of children from the development of severe gastroduodenal diseases such as ulcer disease. This and other studies may explain why ulcer disease may not be as prevalent in the pediatric population infected by this organism and is more difficult to detect macroscopically, thus requiring biopsies in the child undergoing diagnostic upper endoscopy.

Noninvasive Tests for *H. pylori* Infection

Serology

Despite numerous publications demonstrating variability in *H. pylori*-infected people's immune response, inaccuracy of antibody detection in a variety of populations and inability to correlate antibody presence with active infection, studies continue to be published about serology use for *H. pylori* infection in the clinical setting. A Western blot kit (Helico Blot 2.1; Genelabs Diagnostics, Singapore) was evaluated in 88 children (mean age 9.15 years). The gold standard for the evaluation of this serologic assay accuracy was a histology and rapid urease test. These authors observed that in this cohort, the test was useful for *H. pylori* infection in children older than the age of 6 years. However, the study investigators raised questions about the clinical usefulness of serology in the diagnosis and, more important, as a test for cure of this infection.

In a 2003 study, the association between IgG subclass response to *H. pylori* antigens and recombinant CagA and gastric histology was characterized in symptomatic children. In this study, 75 symptomatic children with histologically confirmed *H. pylori* infection were enrolled. *H. pylori* stimulated an IgG1-predominant response as has been shown for a variety of enteric infections. The subclass IgG2 proved to be a useful predictor of disease phenotype in this cohort. IgG3 titers showed a positive association with peptic ulcer disease, chronicity of antral inflammation, and density of *H. pylori* colonization. CagA appeared to stimulate an IgG1- and IgG3-predominant humoral response. Total CagA IgG titers were higher in children with active and more severe chronic antral inflammation. The Polish group suggested that in children the systemic humoral immune response to *H. pylori* infection may reflect gastroduodenal pathology.

In another more recent study, the prevalence of *H. pylori* in symptomatic Lithuanian children was estimated and the infection correlated with pathologic and serologic analyses: 116 symptomatic children (ages 8 to 16) with gastritis and duodenal ulcer were enrolled and biopsies histologically assessed according to the updated Sydney-System. Serum IgG antibodies against *H. pylori* were detected by an enzyme-linked immunosorbent assay (ELISA), using low molecular mass antigen. The Western blot technique was used to detect serum antibodies against the cytotoxin-associated protein (CagA) using whole-cell antigen. The prevalence of IgG antibodies was significantly higher in patients with duodenal ulcer compared with children with gastritis in this Western European pediatric population. The investigators observed that a high number of false seronegative cases were due to poor immunologic responses in children and poor locally validated tests. The authors concluded that *H. pylori* infection is acquired in early life in this cohort, and more important, as recommended in all of the pediatric evidence-based guidelines, that endoscopy/histology remains a gold standard for diagnosis.

Urea Breath Test

In a recent study, 22 Canadian children were evaluated for *H. pylori* infection by a novel laser associated ratio analysis (LARA)–^{13}C-urea breath test (UBT), and these results were compared with the diagnostic standard of upper endoscopy and biopsy. In this prospective study, 8 of 22 children were *H. pylori* positive by histology or culture of gastric biopsies. Urea breath testing using this novel methodology showed a sensitivity of 75% and a specificity of 100%.

Niv and associates performed urea breath tests (75 mg urea) in 1655 children (ages 1 to 18 years) and demonstrated, unlike other studies which have shown variability in the <5 year old age groups, that the breath test performance was quite consistent across all of the ages evaluated. These authors confirmed that the urea breath test may be performed in children of all age groups. To significantly lower the cost of the urea breath test, Canete and coworkers investigated whether a single 50-mg dose of ^{13}C-urea was sufficient for diagnosing infection. By demonstrating a sensitivity of 91% and a specificity of 97% when compared with upper endoscopy and biopsy, they concluded that 50 mg of urea is sufficient and accurate for the diagnosis of infection in children. Moreover, these authors demonstrated that the use of a small test dose significantly lowers the cost of the test.

In a recent multicenter European study the sensitivity, specificity, and positive and negative predictive values of four noninvasive tests—UBT, stool antigen test, and antibody detection in serum and urine—were characterized in comparison with biopsy-based tests. The participating sites enrolled a total of 503 patients in this multicenter, multicountry pediatric study. Of the patients enrolled, 473 fulfilled the definition of study enrollment criteria—a minimum of two non-invasive tests for *H. pylori* including the "gold standard". Among those 473, 316 had results available for the four noninvasive tests (including 133 *H. pylori*-positive patients). The UBT had the best sensitivity in all age-groups, followed by serology, stool test, and antibody detection in urine. A trend for better sensitivity with an increase in age was observed, except for the stool test. The receiver operating characteristic (ROC) curves showed that sensitivity of serology, stool test, and urine-based immunoassay could be improved by changing the cutoff value. An inadequate storage of the specimens may explain the poor results of the stool test. These authors concluded that the UBT appears to be an excellent test for the diagnosis of *H. pylori* infection for children and adolescents.

Stool Antigen Test

Several studies have been published describing the HpSA (Meridian Diagnostics, Cincinnati, Ohio), which uses polyclonal antibodies to detect *H. pylori* antigens in stool. The overall performance of this assay worldwide has been acceptable. However, in pediatric patients, the stool antigen test has performed inconsistently with varying results depending on the center or geographic region in which the test has been conducted. Gosciniak and colleagues found before therapy, that the stool antigen test for pediatric *H. pylori* infection yielded a sensitivity of 88.7% and a specificity of 95.5%. Four to 6 weeks after eradication therapy, the sensitivity, specificity, positive predictive value, and negative predictive value of the stool antigen (HpSA) test were 88.9%, 96.2%, 80%, and 98%, respectively. A European trial studying 316 children with biopsy-based *H. pylori* status achieved only a sensitivity of 72.7%. This suggests that the polyclonal *H. pylori* antigen test, the HpSA, might have a problem with the lot-to-lot variability.

In adults the stool antigen test has performed quite well, both for the diagnosis of *H. pylori* infection and as a test for cure. A prospective study was conducted at six clinical centers in the United States and Europe, and enrolled 84 *H. pylori*-infected patients who had undergone diagnostic endoscopy for upper abdominal symptoms. At baseline and on day 35 after the completion of triple eradication therapy, all patients underwent endoscopy with histologic examination, rapid urease test and culture, urea breath test, and a stool antigen test. Compared with the gold standard endoscopic tests on day 35 after antimicrobial therapy, the urea breath test had a sensitivity of 94% (95% CI: 71% to 100%) and a specificity of 100% (CI, 94% to 100%). The stool antigen test had a sensitivity of 94% (CI, 71% to 100%) and a specificity of 97% (CI, 89% to 100%). More remarkably, on day 7 after treatment, the stool antigen test was predictive of eradication (positive predictive value, 100% [CI, 69% to 100%]; negative predictive value, 91% [CI, 82% to 97%]).

In a recent pediatric study, the accuracy of the stool antigen test in developing countries and particularly in children younger than 6 years was evaluated. In this investigation, 133 patients (4 months to 17 years old) were enrolled and all underwent stool antigen testing compared with the standard of a positive culture or positive histology and rapid urease test obtained at diagnostic upper endoscopy. The test showed a 94.6% sensitivity (95% CI: 90.6 to 98.5) and a 96.5% specificity (95% CI: 93.3 to 99.7). At ages 2 to 6 years, the specificity was 96.4% (95% CI: 85.1 to 99.2) and the sensitivity was 80% (95% CI: 64.8 to 89.7), at ages 6 to 10 years the sensitivity was 100% and the specificity 95.7%, and at ages more than 10 years, the sensitivity and specificity were 100%. Although these results may be "falsely" elevated, the study demonstrated the potential usefulness of the stool antigen test in pediatric patients living in developing countries.

More recently, a monoclonal stool antigen test (FemtoLab *H. pylori* Cnx, Martinsried, Germany identical to HpStAR, DakoCytomation GmbH, Hamburg, Germany) has been investigated in 302 symptomatic children (ages 0.5 to 18.7 years; 148 girls) and compared with culture, histology, rapid urease test, and urea breath test by Koletzko and coworkers. The sensitivity, specificity, positive predictive value, and negative predictive value in the study cohort, under research conditions were 98%, 99%, 98%, and 99%, respectively. The authors concluded that the monoclonal stool antigen test performed well in diagnosing *H. pylori* infection in symptomatic children. In this study, unlike the aforementioned studies of the polyclonal test in children, accuracy of this monoclonal assay was independent of the laboratory, production lot used, or the child's age. Because only 18 of 116 children younger than 6 years of age were infected with *H. pylori*, further validation of the test was felt to be still critically needed in young infected children.

Urine Antibody Test

There have been few studies that have evaluated the presence or absence of urine antibodies specific for *H. pylori* in children or adults. Okuda and colleagues assessed 100 children (mean age 7 years; range, 2 to 15) in which the urea breath test, HpSA, and urine-HpELISA were performed. In this study, 36 children were *H. pylori* positive by urea breath test and HpSA. Interestingly, the urine-HpELISA test had 94.4% sensitivity and 96.9% specificity, with an accuracy rate of 96%.

CLINICAL MANIFESTATIONS OF *H. PYLORI* INFECTION

Gastroduodenal Disease

Even today, at the writing of this manuscript, a causal relationship between *H. pylori* infection and reportable gastrointestinal symptoms such as recurrent abdominal pain or nonulcer dyspepsia is still not proved. Although there is frequently a relationship or correlation between ulcer disease and abdominal symptoms, it is still unknown whether chronic gastritis causes symptoms in children and adults.

A study from India found a possible association of *H. pylori* with recurrent abdominal pain in 65 *H. pylori*–positive children. In this study of children ages 3 to 12 years old with recurrent abdominal pain, 83% had "complete" relief of their abdominal pain after eradication therapy. There were a number of limitations to this study, however, namely, the study was not randomized or double-blinded and either did not include the patient demographics (e.g., socioeconomic status) or this wasn't assessed; also, the symptom assessment instrument was not validated and follow-up evaluation was variable.

Bode and coworkers analyzed the relationship between social and familial factors, *H. pylori* infection, and recurrent abdominal pain in children in a population-based cross-sectional study among 1221 preschool children ages 5 to 8 years. These German authors found a clear association between recurrent abdominal pain and social or familial factors, but not with *H. pylori* infection. This raises further questions about the role of *H. pylori* and gastrointestinal symptoms.

Moreover, a study performed in Helsinki, Finland, Ashorn and associates demonstrated in a rigorous fashion that symptoms do not respond to eradication of *H. pylori*. In this well-designed prospective study, 20 children with recurrent abdominal pain who were *H. pylori* positive as measured with the UBT were enrolled in a randomized, double-blinded placebo (i.e., antisecretory agent only) controlled trial. In this study the children were randomized either to receive omeprazole, amoxicillin, and clarithromycin ($n = 10$), or omeprazole and two placebos ($n = 10$) for 1 week after gastroscopy. Symptoms were registered before the treatment and at follow-up visits 2, 6, 24, and 52 weeks after stopping the treatment. UBT was performed on all patients 6 weeks post-treatment and again at the 52-week follow-up visit, when re-endoscopy with biopsies was done to all participants. *H. pylori* eradication was achieved in 8 of 10 in the triple treatment group and in none in the placebo group. There was no change in symptom index in either group at 2 weeks post-treatment. At 52 weeks a similar reduction in symptom index was observed in both groups irrespective of the healing of gastritis, and as would be expected, gastritis resolution was more commonly achieved along the eradication. The authors concluded that *H. pylori* eradication and healing of gastric inflammation does not lead to symptomatic relief of chronic abdominal pain in children.

In a rather unique study, Candelli and associates studied 121 children (mean age 15 ± 6 years) with type 1 diabetes mellitus and compared the prevalence of *H. pylori*, CagA–positive strains, and the effects of infection on gastrointestinal symptoms and metabolic control with 147 matched controls. These authors showed that *H. pylori* infection and particularly those with CagA-positive strains did not affect metabolic control in patients with type 1 diabetes mellitus. However, patients with better metabolic control appeared to be only those children in which *H. pylori* infection was eradicated. The clinical relevance of these findings remains unclear.

In an important study by Bedoya and colleagues, the histopathology of the gastric mucosa in infected children from a population at high risk for gastric cancer (Pasto, Colombia) was characterized and compared with that of a lower-risk population (New Orleans, Louisiana). The authors performed histopathologic evaluations of gastric biopsies obtained from the antrum and corpus. Immunohistochemical stains were used to identify B lymphocytes (CD20), T lymphocytes (CD3 and CD8), macrophages (CD68), and polymorphonuclear neutrophil myeloperoxidase. In both pediatric populations infected by *H. pylori*, the inflammatory lesions were seen predominantly in the antrum. Compared with children from the lower-risk populations, children from the higher-risk population exhibited more severe polymorphonuclear neutrophil infiltration, stromal and intraepithelial lymphocyte infiltration, mucus depletion, and *H. pylori* colonization density. Regenerative activity was significantly more marked in the lower-risk population. Morphometric analysis of immunohistochemical stains showed increased representation of T lymphocytes and macrophages in the higher-risk population. Most T lymphocytes stained positive for CD8, a marker of suppressor/cytotoxic cells. B lymphocytes were relatively more abundant in the lower-risk population.

Finally, recent studies over the past 5 years provide compelling evidence for the *H. pylori*–related gastroduodenal disease, in particular, gastric adenocarcinoma being a complex disease; (i.e., influences from bacteria, host, and environment determining disease phenotype). In particular, the gastric physiologic response is influenced by the severity and anatomic distribution of gastritis induced by *H. pylori*. Thus, individuals with gastritis predominantly localized to the antrum tend to retain normal (or even high) acid secretion, whereas individuals with extensive corpus gastritis develop hypochlorhydria and gastric atrophy, which are presumptive precursors of gastric cancer. In a landmark paper published by El-Omar and colleagues, specific host factors/determinants, namely interleukin-1 (IL-1) gene cluster polymorphisms suspected of enhancing production of IL-1β, were found to be associated with an increased risk of both hypochlorhydria induced by *H. pylori* and gastric cancer. Two of these polymorphisms are in near-complete linkage disequilibrium and one is a TATA-box polymorphism (i.e., C to T mutation with a T-allele makes a TATA box) that markedly affects DNA protein interactions in vitro. The association with disease may be explained by the biologic properties of IL-1β, which is an important proinflammatory cytokine and a powerful inhibitor of gastric acid secretion. Thus, host genetic factors that affect IL-1β may determine why some individuals infected with *H. pylori* develop gastric cancer and others do not.

H. pylori was initially classified in 1994 by the World Health Organization (WHO) as a Group 1 carcinogen for gastric cancer. Many believed that this classification of *H. pylori* may have been a bit premature based on the nested case control and case control studies reviewed and available at that time; there is now sufficient evidence to demonstrate that *H. pylori* satisfies Koch's postulates as a causative agent for human gastric adenocarcinoma. Moreover, there is now a reproducible, biologically relevant animal model, the Mongolian gerbil, described and available for the study of *H. pylori*-associated gastric carcinogenesis. In the Mongolian gerbil model, gastric carcinoma of similar histopathology and morphology to the lesions in *H. pylori*–infected humans are highly prevalent after chronic colonization by *H. pylori* (i.e., human strains). Investigators orally challenged the animals with *H. pylori*, and demonstrated consistent infection of all animals that were challenged. By 26 weeks of infection, severe active chronic gastritis, ulcers, and intestinal metaplasia could be observed in infected animals. By 62 weeks, just over 1 year of *H. pylori* infection, adenocarcinoma had developed in the pyloric region of 37% of the infected Mongolian gerbils. All tumors consisted of well-differentiated intestinal-type epithelium, and their development seemed to be closely related to intestinal metaplasia. In one of the more recent animal studies published, the investigators were actually able to significantly reverse the early neoplastic lesions by eradication of the organism. In this study, the tumor incidences were related to the period of inflammatory status induced by *H. pylori* infection. In addition, *H. pylori* infection strongly enhanced gastric carcinogenesis initiated with a chemical carcinogen, and following eradication at an early period, this enhancing effect was effectively reduced. Thus, although human studies to date have been equivocal demonstrating irreversibility of gastric cancer, eradication of *H. pylori* at an early stage of inflammation might be effective in preventing *H. pylori*–related gastric carcinogenesis.

It is estimated that there is between a two- and sixfold increase in the risk of developing gastric cancer among infected patients. Among different populations, the risk of *H. pylori*-infected individuals developing gastric cancer is highly variable, lending to the difficulty in both conducting eradication trials and in initiating surveillance programs. Clearly, gastric cancer is still a significant public health problem—on a worldwide scale, it is the second most common cause of cancer-related death. Therefore, *H. pylori* eradication could help prevent up to 4 million gastric cancer deaths per year. *H. pylori* is usually acquired in childhood; thus, childhood is theoretically an attractive time for *H. pylori* eradication, which could help prevent gastric cancer later in life. However, as *H. pylori* prevalence and the incidence of gastric cancer are falling rapidly in developed nations, widespread population screening programs aimed at the eradication of *H. pylori* in these countries are cost prohibitive until more of the pathobiology is characterized. Therefore, except in groups with a high risk for development of gastric cancer (e.g., Japanese or those with a strong positive family history of gastric cancer), a population-based test-and-treat policy has not yet been advocated.

Extragastric Disease

Although it remains unclear whether there is a causal relationship between *H. pylori* infection and growth retardation in children, recent data suggest that there may in fact be a positive association. A study by Bravo and colleagues prospectively characterized the impact of *H. pylori* infection on growth of children. Of the 347 asymptomatic children (ages 12 to 60 months), who tested negative for *H. pylori* by UBT, and who were monitored for 2.5 years; 105 children became infected during follow-up. Growth velocity in infected children was reduced by 0.042 ± 0.014 cm/month ($P = 0.003$). The authors concluded that among these lower-middle-class children *H. pylori* infection is followed by significant growth restriction.

In another study, the height, weight, and body mass index (BMI) of children presenting with dyspeptic symptoms and *H. pylori* infection were compared with those with dyspepsia but without the infection. This retrospective chart review of 257 children in which the UBT was performed to detect *H. pylori* infection also determined weight and height and BMI of the study cohort. Ninety seven of the 257 children were *H. pylori* positive, and the mean age at diagnosis and the presenting symptoms of infected compared with uninfected patients were similar. The mean weight and height standard deviation (SD) score were significantly lower for children with *H. pylori* infection compared with those without. Although children with dyspepsia and *H. pylori* infection were shorter and lighter than patients with similar symptoms but no infection, the differences in anthropometry may be due to socioeconomic and ethnic factors rather than *H. pylori* infection.

In another recent study, performed in Colombian children, the authors sought to determine if new infection by *H. pylori* in preschool children transiently or permanently affected height and weight. The investigators evaluated a well-powered cohort of 347 children from three daycare centers, and followed up the study group for a median of 494 days. Breath tests and anthropometric measurements of each subject were performed every 2 to 4 months: 105 children (30.3%) became infected during the follow-up period and accumulated 92 person-years of follow-up. Interestingly, a significant decrease in growth velocity was observed during the first 4 months after infection, and there was no height catch-up in infected children. This well-designed, prospective study demonstrated a significant and nontransient effect of *H. pylori* infection on height and weight.

Compelling evidence published in the past few years provides biologic plausibility for an association between *H. pylori* and idiopathic thrombocytopenic purpura (ITP). Eradication of *H. pylori* was associated with platelet recovery in adults with ITP. Rajantie and Klemola studied 17 children (ages 0.3 to 14.3 years) with ITP after *H. pylori* eradication. Serology and urea breath test were used to identify *H. pylori* colonization. *H. pylori* infection was not found in any of the children. Consequently, the authors concluded that idiopathic thrombocytopenic purpura is a disorder with different pathogenetic and clinical features in children and adults, and that *H. pylori* may not be important in the pathogenesis of idiopathic thrombocytopenic purpura in children. In contrast, Jaing and associates investigated 22 patients with ITP with the polyclonal *H. pylori* antigen stool test. Of these children, 9 were infected with *H. pylori*. Serial follow-ups at 4, 12, and 24 months after eradication therapy were performed, and 5 of the 9 patients had increased platelet counts that persisted throughout the follow-up period. The authors concluded that these results should stimulate additional research into the involvement of *H. pylori* infection in chronic ITP in childhood and that this approach may offer an accepted algorithm at least for some of these patients.

A Korean group investigated the correlation between *H. pylori* infection and vitamin C levels in whole blood, gastric juice, and pH of gastric juice in 452 (ages 1 to 15 years) children. Vitamin C levels in whole blood, plasma, and gastric juice exhibited significant negative correlation with the age of patients, the histologic density of *H. pylori*, the degree of active and chronic gastritis, and the severity of *H. pylori* infection (based on urease positivity and histologic density of *H. pylori*). Park and coworkers concluded that vitamin C levels in whole blood, plasma, and gastric juice and the gastric juice pH in Korean children are closely related to the severity of *H. pylori* infection and the histologic changes in the stomach, and that vitamin C supplementation may be an important axis for the management of *H. pylori* infection in children.

A number of studies have shown that *H. pylori* may in fact be associated with anemia, iron deficiency, and iron deficiency anemia. For example, in a retrospective analysis of 283 Japanese children (mean age, 11.5 years) with non-nodular gastritis ($n = 73$), nodular gastritis ($n = 67$), duodenal ulcer ($n = 100$), and gastric ulcer

($n = 43$), clinical symptoms were analyzed with regard to a possible association with the infection. *H. pylori* was significantly linked to duodenal ulcer and gastric ulcers in the age-group of 10 to 16 years, but not in the age-group of 9 years and younger. In addition, *H. pylori* infection was significantly associated with the prevalence of anemia ($P < 0.05$). The authors concluded that as previously demonstrated by others, *H. pylori* is the most important causal factor for the development of duodenal ulcer in this Japanese cohort. Moreover, these investigators observed that chronic infection with *H. pylori* is associated with anemia.

To date, however, few trials of treatment for *H. pylori* infection have been conducted in high-prevalence or pediatric populations, and risk factors for treatment failure are poorly understood. Moreover, outcomes of eradication trials have been both in favor of and against *H. pylori* playing a causative role in iron deficiency and anemia. In a study for the role, a group from Korea, Choe and colleagues, conducted a double-blind, placebo-controlled therapeutic trial in 43 subjects (mean age, 15.4 years) with iron deficiency anemia. Endoscopy was performed, and biopsy specimens were examined by urease test and histologic analysis. The investigators then randomly assigned 22 of 25 *H. pylori*–positive patients to three groups: group A patients were given oral ferrous sulfate and a 2-week course of bismuth subcitrate, amoxicillin, and metronidazole; group B patients were given placebo for iron and a 2-week course of triple therapy, and group C patients were given oral ferrous sulfate and a 2-week course of placebo. Of the 43 subjects with iron deficiency anemia, 25 (58.1%) had *H. pylori* in the antrum. Groups A and B subjects, who received eradication therapy, showed a significant increase in hemoglobin level as compared with group C subjects at 8 weeks after therapy ($p = 0.0086$). Thus, eradication of *H. pylori* infection was associated with a more rapid response to oral iron therapy as compared with the use of iron therapy alone. Such treatment also led to enhanced iron absorption even in those subjects who did not receive oral iron therapy.

With respect to the relationship between *H. pylori* and allergic disorders, even epidemiologic associations have been equivocal. In one study by Corrado and associates, 90 pediatric patients were studied: 30 with food allergy, 30 with atopic asthma, and 30 with inflammatory bowel disease. A nonvalidated immunoassay that detected anti–*H. pylori* IgG and one that detected anti–*H. pylori* CagA IgG were employed in all children enrolled in this study. The anti–*H. pylori* IgG titer was significantly higher in allergic patients than in the other two groups; however, the anti-CagA IgG titer did not differ significantly among the patients. In another study, Cremonini and Gasbarrini reviewed the impact of *H. pylori* infection on allergy development. These authors summarized that novel epidemiologic data from a cross-sectional survey show that in subjects with active *H. pylori* infection the prevalence of asthma, eczema, and allergic rhinitis is lower than in *H. pylori*-negative subjects, although these observations demonstrated a positive association between *H. pylori* infection and food allergy in children. Well-powered case control cohort studies are needed, in addition to eradication of the organism in individuals with allergies, in order to determine true cause and effect and validate biologic plausibility.

H. pylori Infection and Reflux Disease

Conflicting reports have noted a possible association linking eradication of *H. pylori* with aggravation of gastroesophageal reflux disease (GERD). A novel study by Levine and associates evaluated 95 children who were referred for endoscopy for frequency, severity, and nocturnal presence of symptoms related to gastroesophageal reflux (GER) before and 6 months after endoscopy. The distribution of outcomes for each GER symptom (better, worse, unchanged) was similar before and after eradication and did not depend on prior *H. pylori* status. They concluded that eradication therapy is not associated with increased symptoms of GER.

A French group studied the relationship between *H. pylori* infection and GERD in neurologically impaired children retrospectively. Pollet and colleagues recruited 43 children with *H. pylori* infection (determined by culture and/or histology) who had upper gastrointestinal endoscopy between 1990 and 2000. Reflux esophagitis was diagnosed by ulceration of the esophageal mucosa at endoscopy before and 4 to 6 weeks after eradication therapy; of the study cohort, 14 of 43 patients had a macroscopically evident erosive esophagitis. After treatment, esophagitis was still present in 4 of 14 children. Persistent esophagitis was only related to the presence of esophagitis before treatment ($P = 0.02$). In 29 patients with a normal esophagus at the first endoscopy, only 1 case of esophagitis was observed after *H. pylori* eradication. They concluded that eradication therapy in neurologically impaired children is unlikely to either induce or exacerbate peptic esophagitis.

Clearly, GERD is a common problem in childhood and in adults with a significant health care effect, particularly in developed countries. It is not clear why the incidence of GERD is increasing in developed countries; studies demonstrated that the prevalence of *H. pylori* is decreasing particularly in developed populations. Thus, it has been suggested that this infection protects against GERD. Observational data from pediatric studies, in addition to those mentioned, suggest that *H. pylori* eradication does not have a deleterious effect on GERD and this is supported by randomized controlled trials in adults (Moayyedi, 2005). *H. pylori* eradication may also reduce the efficacy of proton pump inhibitor therapy in infected patients; however, at present, there are no data from children, but speculations from randomized controlled trials in adults suggest this effect is likely to be modest and of uncertain clinical significance. As mentioned in this review, *H. pylori* is an important risk factor for distal gastric adenocarcinoma. A meta-analysis of four randomized controlled trials suggests that there is a statistically significant impact on healing of chronic gastritis after 1 year compared with placebo (relative risk [RR] of chronic gastritis: 0.27; 95% CI: 0.23 to 0.32). Thus, in the most recently revised Canadian guidelines on the management of pediatric *H. pylori* infection, eradication of this organism is therefore recommended in children with GERD who are undergoing an endoscopy. However, when the diagnosis of GERD is being made clinically or by pH monitoring, it is not necessary to screen for *H. pylori*.

TREATMENT

There are increasing numbers of reported *H. pylori* eradication trials in adults and children, although very few randomized placebo controlled trials in children. Moreover, those that have been published have had disappointingly low overall eradication rates (i.e., less than 80%). At present, based on the best available evidence per the recently published Canadian Helicobacter Study Group consensus guidelines, population-based screening for *H. pylori* in asymptomatic children to prevent gastric cancer is not warranted. However, unlike previous guidelines and now more consistent with recommendations for infection in adults, testing for *H. pylori* in children should be considered if there is a family history of gastric cancer. As with the previous guidelines, the goal of diagnostic interventions should be to determine the cause of presenting gastrointestinal symptoms and not the presence of *H. pylori* infection. *H. pylori* testing may be considered before the use of long-term proton pump inhibitor therapy for GERD and GERD-related disorders. Unlike the previous guidelines, testing for *H. pylori* infection should be considered in children with refractory iron deficiency anemia when no other cause has been found. First-line therapy for *H. pylori* infection in children is a twice-daily, triple-drug regimen composed of a proton pump inhibitor plus two antibiotics (clarithromycin plus amoxicillin or metronidazole). Unlike the adult guidelines where even a 7-day duration of therapy can be considered, the optimal treatment period for *H. pylori* infection in children is 14 days. Finally, *H. pylori* culture and antibiotic sensitivity testing should be made available to monitor population antibiotic resistance and manage treatment failures.

Because of increasing reports describing antimicrobial resistance, alternative approaches to the treatment of *H. pylori* have been investigated. A novel double-blind, randomized, controlled clinical trial was carried out in schoolchildren from a low socioeconomic area in Santiago, Chile. In this study, 326 asymptomatic children (mean age: 9.7 ± 2.6 years) were screened for *H. pylori* by the urea breath test. *H. pylori*–positive children were distributed into five groups to receive a product containing live *Lactobacillus johnsonii* La1 or *Lactobacillus paracasei* ST11 (groups 1 and 3), heat-killed La1 or ST11 (groups 2 and 4), or vehicle (group 5) every day for 4 weeks. A moderate but significant difference was detected in children receiving live La1, whereas no differences were observed in the other groups. They concluded that regular ingestion of *Lactobacillus* La1 may represent an interesting alternative to modulate *H. pylori* colonization in children.

Antibiotic resistance is still a main factor affecting the outcome of *H. pylori* treatment. During the last years multiple studies showed a high resistance of *H. pylori* to metronidazole and clarithromycin around the world. Until now there has been no resistance to amoxicillin observed in Europe. However, there have been reports from other parts of the world. An Australian group from Melbourne found resistance rates of *H. pylori* to metronidazole and clarithromycin of 43.5% and 8.7%, respectively. No *H. pylori* strains were resistant to amoxicillin or tetracycline.

In a study from Portugal, eradication rates after antibiotic susceptibility testing-based treatment and eradication outcomes were assessed in a cohort of 109 children with a gastric biopsy culture positive for *H. pylori*. The authors implemented initial therapy with amoxicillin, omeprazole, and clarithromycin or metronidazole; this was guided by susceptibility testing (E test), and eradication was assessed by ^{13}C-UBT. As in previous studies, all of the strains tested were susceptible to amoxicillin and tetracycline. However, 39.4% of the organisms were resistant to clarithromycin, 16.5% to metronidazole, and 4.5% to ciprofloxacin. No significant association was found between resistance and sex, age, clinical status, gastritis scores, *H. pylori* density scores, and genotype. Clarithromycin resistance was significantly associated with European origin ([OR], 3.9], previous *H. pylori* empiric therapy [OR 2.8], and amoxicillin minimal inhibitory concentration, 0.016 [OR 6.0]). Eradication rate after susceptibility-based treatment was 74.7% (59 of 79; 95% confidence interval, 65.9 to 82.9), and a significant association was found between eradication failure and presence of resistance to 1 or more antibiotics ($P < 0.05$). The rather disappointing therapeutic success of clarithromycin and metronidazole susceptibility-based regimens suggests that in addition to resistance, other factors may be involved. Susceptibility-based treatment studies in children and of antimicrobial resistance surveillance in high prevalence areas for H. pylori are critically needed.

Finally, in one recent U.S. surveillance study of H. pylori antibiotic resistance conducted by the Centers for Disease Control and Prevention, the Helicobacter pylori Antimicrobial Resistance Monitoring Program (HARP), 347 clinical H. pylori isolates collected from December 1998 through 2002 were evaluated for resistance to four of the most commonly used antibiotics in H. pylori eradication regimens [Duck, 2004]. Of the strains tested, 101 (29.1%) were resistant to one antimicrobial agent, and 17 (5%) were resistant to two or more antimicrobial agents. Eighty-seven (25.1%) isolates were resistant to metronidazole, 45 (12.9%) to clarithromycin, and 3 (0.9%) to amoxicillin. On multivariate analysis, African American race was the only significant risk factor ($p < 0.01$, hazard ratio 2.04) for infection with a resistant H. pylori strain. Clearly, more population-based surveillance systems are needed, and formulating pretreatment screening strategies or providing alternative therapeutic regimens for high-risk populations may be important for future clinical practice.

APPROACH TO THE CASE

Due to the family history, remarkable history of present illness, physical examination and laboratory investigation results, an esophagogastroduodenoscopy (i.e., upper endoscopy) with biopsies was performed. Inspection of the gastric mucosa during the endoscopy demonstrated the presence of small erosions in the antral area, and on duodenal intubation with the endoscope, a small 0.5-cm duodenal ulcer that was not actively bleeding was revealed. The antral mucosa was friable and granular but not overwhelmingly nodular. Histologic evaluation of the gastric biopsies demonstrated chronic active gastritis with prominent lymphoid follicles. Steiner stain revealed numerous organisms consistent with the diagnosis of H. pylori. A rapid urease test was also performed using a gastric biopsy obtained at upper endoscopy and was positive; findings consistent with H. pylori infection.

Following upper endoscopy and assessment of the histopathology and rapid urease test results, after relaying the diagnosis of H. pylori infection and H. pylori-associated gastric erosions and duodenal ulcer disease to the family, the boy was started on triple therapy consisting of a proton pump inhibitor, amoxicillin, and clarithromycin for 2 weeks. After completing the course of antibiotics, the proton pump inhibitor was continued for another 2 months and the patient then brought back for evaluation in the office. At the time of re-evaluation, there was still some residual abdominal pain reported, but overall the patient was markedly improved. Laboratory evaluation at that time revealed improvements in all of the laboratory parameters, MCV, hemoglobin and hematocrit; although they had not completely normalized.

SUMMARY

Helicobacter pylori infections remain one of the most common infections worldwide. Eradication of this important pathogen would lead to virtual elimination of gastric cancer, the second most common cancer worldwide. A variety of accurate diagnostic tests are available, but current therapeutic regimens are generally unsatisfactory, with failure rates between 20% and 40%. The difficulty in curing the infection has led to a three-step approach: diagnosis, therapy, and confirmation of cure. Better studies including head-to-head comparison of different drugs, drug formulations, dosing intervals, dosing in relation to meals, and duration of therapy are needed. The high rates of reinfection and the lack of improvements in standards of living in developing countries make development of a vaccine (although not discussed in this review) a high priority.

There have been major inroads in our understanding of the pathogenesis of gastroduodenal disease since H. pylori first became recognized as a human pathogen. In particular, advances in molecular bacteriology including the complete sequencing of the H. pylori genome provide tools with which to delineate the pathogenesis of disease, and should be applied immediately to multicenter pediatric studies that evaluate disease outcome, and molecular epidemiology and disease associations with the organism. More recent developments indicate that a better understanding of the microbial-host interaction is critical to furthering knowledge with respect to H. pylori–induced disease outcomes. Moreover, only recently has attention been applied to elucidating the roles of the host response and the immunophysiologic reactions both in the pathogenesis of H. pylori infection and as predictors of disease. Multicenter, multinational studies of H. pylori infection in the pediatric population, which include specific, randomized controlled eradication trials, are essential to extend current knowledge and develop better predictors of disease outcome.

MAJOR POINTS

Helicobacter pylori infection remains one of the most common human infections worldwide, with infection prevalence rates higher in developing compared with developed regions of the world.

Transmission of *H. pylori* infection occurs person-to-person via fecal–oral, oral–oral and gastro–oral routes, with fecally contaminated water potentially playing a role in infection transmission in countries with high rates of infection and poor water sanitation.

Childhood still remains the primary period of *H. pylori* acquisition with intra-familial clustering via sibling-to-sibling and parent-to-child transmission (particularly maternal to infant).

H. pylori infection definitely causes childhood gastroduodenal disease, including gastritis, gastric atrophy with and without intestinal metaplasia, gastric and more commonly duodenal ulcers, and also causes MALT lymphoma.

H. pylori infection is associated with extra-gastric diseases in children, in particular iron deficiency and iron-deficiency anemia, and may cause idiopathic thrombocytopenic purpura and growth disturbance.

A number of diagnostic tests are available and validated for the work-up of the suspected *H. pylori*-infected child, including both non-invasive (stool antigen and urea breath tests in particular) and invasive tests (i.e., endoscopy and biopsy), which facilitate diagnosis of infection and mucosal disease.

Treatment of *H. pylori* is increasingly becoming more difficult due to antibiotic resistance, but is best achieved by triple therapy with a proton pump inhibitor and two antibiotics administered for a minimum of two weeks.

Future studies are still critically needed to determine the role of the host-microbial interaction, in addition to environmental co-factors/influences in dictating host-disease phenotype to identify which populations merit early intervention and eradication to decrease overall disease burden.

SUGGESTED READINGS

Annibale B, Capurso G, Delle Fave G: The stomach and iron deficiency anaemia: A forgotten link. Dig Liver Dis 35:288-295, 2003.

Annibale B, Capurso G, Lahner E, et al: Concomitant alterations in intragastric pH and ascorbic acid concentration in patients with *Helicobacter pylori* gastritis and associated iron deficiency anaemia. Gut 52:496-501, 2003.

Ashorn M, Rago T, Kokkonen J, et al: Symptomatic response to *Helicobacter pylori* eradication in children with recurrent abdominal pain: Double blind randomized placebo-controlled trial. J Clin Gastroenterol 38:646-650, 2004.

Bedoya A, Garay J, Sanzon F, et al: Histopathology of gastritis in *Helicobacter pylori*–infected children from populations at high and low gastric cancer risk. Hum Pathol 34:206-213, 2003.

Bergin IL, Sheppard BJ, Fox JG: *Helicobacter pylori* infection and high dietary salt independently induce atrophic gastritis and intestinal metaplasia in commercially available outbred Mongolian gerbils. Dig Dis Sci 48:475-478, 2003.

Blanchard SS, Bauman L, Czinn SJ: Treatment of *Helicobacter pylori* in pediatrics. Curr Treat Options Gastroenterol 7:407-412, 2004.

Bode G, Brenner H, Adler G, Rothenbacher D: Recurrent abdominal pain in children: Evidence from a population-based study that social and familial factors play a major role but not *Helicobacter pylori* infection. J Psychosom Res 54:417-421, 2003.

Bontems P, Robert F, Van Gossum A, et al: *Helicobacter pylori* modulation of gastric and duodenal mucosal T cell cytokine secretions in children compared with adults. Helicobacter 8:216-226, 2003.

Borrelli O, Hassall E, D'Armiento F, et al: Inflammation of the gastric cardia in children with symptoms of acid peptic disease. J Pediatr 143:520-524, 2003.

Bourke B: Will treatment of *Helicobacter pylori* infection in childhood alter the risk of developing gastric cancer? Can J Gastroenterol 19:409-411, 2005.

Bourke B, Ceponis P, Chiba N, et al: Canadian Helicobacter Study Group Consensus Conference: Update on the approach to *Helicobacter pylori* infection in children and adolescents—An evidence-based evaluation. Can J Gastroenterol 19:399-408, 2005.

Bravo LE, Mera R, Reina JC, et al: Impact of *Helicobacter pylori* infection on growth of children: A prospective cohort study. J Pediatr Gastroenterol Nutr 37:614-619, 2003.

Brown LM: *Helicobacter pylori*: Epidemiology and routes of transmission. Epidemiol Rev 22:283-297, 2000.

Cadranel S, Goossens H, De Boeck M, et al: *Campylobacter pyloridis* in children [letter]. Lancet 1:735-736, 1986.

Campbell DI, Pearce MS, Parker L, Thomas J: IgG subclass responses in childhood *Helicobacter pylori* duodenal ulcer: Evidence of T-helper cell type 2 responses. Helicobacter 9:289-292, 2004.

Candelli M, Nista EC, Pignataro G, et al: Idiopathic thrombocytopenic purpura and *Helicobacter pylori* infection. Scand J Gastroenterol 38:569-570, 2003.

Canete A, Abunaji Y, Alvarez-Calatayud G, et al: Breath test using a single 50-mg dose of 13C-urea to detect *Helicobacter pylori* infection in children. J Pediatr Gastroenterol Nutr 36:105-111, 2003.

Chang PS, Ni YH, Chang MH: Household *Helicobacter pylori* antibody survey in children with upper gastrointestinal symptoms. Acta Paediatr Taiwan 44:336-338, 2003.

Choe YH, Kim SK, Son BK, et al: Randomized placebo-controlled trial of *Helicobacter pylori* eradication for iron-deficiency anemia in preadolescent children and adolescents. Helicobacter 4:135-139, 1999.

Choe YH, Lee JE, Kim SK: Effect of *Helicobacter pylori* eradication on sideropenic refractory anaemia in adolescent girls with *Helicobacter pylori* infection. Acta Paediatr 89:154-157, 2000.

Choi JW: Does *Helicobacter pylori* infection relate to iron deficiency anaemia in prepubescent children under 12 years of age? Acta Paediatr 92:970-972, 2003.

Cirak MY, Ozdek A, Yilmaz D, et al: Detection of *Helicobacter pylori* and its CagA gene in tonsil and adenoid tissues by PCR. Arch Otolaryngol Head Neck Surg 129:1225-1229, 2003.

Corrado G, Luzzi I, Lucarelli S, et al: Positive association between *Helicobacter pylori* infection and food allergy in children. Scand J Gastroenterol 33:1135-1139, 1998.

Correa P: New strategies for the prevention of gastric cancer: *Helicobacter pylori* and genetic susceptibility. J Surg Oncol 90:134-138, 2005.

Cremonini F, Gasbarrini A: Atopy, *Helicobacter pylori* and the hygiene hypothesis. Eur J Gastroenterol Hepatol 15:635-636, 2003.

Cruchet S, Obregon MC, Salazar G, et al: Effect of the ingestion of a dietary product containing *Lactobacillus johnsonii* La1 on *Helicobacter pylori* colonization in children. Nutrition 19:716-721, 2003.

Czinn SJ: *Helicobacter pylori* infection: Detection, investigation, and management. J Pediatr 146:S21-S26, 2005.

Czinn S, Carr H, Aronoff S: Susceptibility of *Campylobacter pyloridis* to three macrolide antibiotics (erythromycin, roxithromycin [RU 28965], and CP 62,993) and rifampin. Antimicrob Agents Chemother 30:328-329, 1986.

Czinn SJ, Dahms BB, Jacobs GH, et al: *Campylobacter*-like organisms in association with symptomatic gastritis in children. J Pediatr 109:80-83, 1986.

Das BK, Kakkar S, Dixit VK, et al: *Helicobacter pylori* infection and recurrent abdominal pain in children. J Trop Pediatr 49:250-252, 2003.

Day AS, Veldhuyzen van Zanten S, Otley AR, et al: Use of LARA-urea breath test in the diagnosis of *Helicobacter pylori* infection in children and adolescents: A preliminary study. Can J Gastroenterol 17:701-706, 2003.

de Carvalho Costa Cardinali L, Rocha GA, Rocha AM, et al: Evaluation of [13C]urea breath test and *Helicobacter pylori* stool antigen test for diagnosis of *H. pylori* infection in children from a developing country. J Clin Microbiol 41:3334-3335, 2003.

Dixon MF, Genta RM, Yardley JH, Correa P: Classification and grading of gastritis: The updated Sydney System. International Workshop on the Histopathology of Gastritis, Houston, 1994. Am J Surg Pathol 20:1161-1181, 1996.

Drumm B, Koletzko S, Oderda G: *Helicobacter pylori* infection in children: A consensus statement. Medical position paper: Report of the European Paediatric Task Force on *Helicobacter pylori* on a Consensus Conference, Budapest, Hungary, September 1998. J Pediatr Gastroenterol Nutr 30:207-213, 2000.

Drumm B, O'Brien A, Cutz E, Sherman P: *Campylobacter pyloridis*-associated primary gastritis in children. Pediatrics 80:192-195, 1987.

DuBois S, Kearney DJ: Iron-deficiency anemia and *Helicobacter pylori* infection: A review of the evidence. Am J Gastroenterol 100:453-459, 2005.

Duck WM, Sobel J, Pruckler JM, et al: Antimicrobial resistance incidence and risk factors among *Helicobacter pylori*-infected persons, United States. Emerg Infect Dis 10:1088-1094, 2004.

Dzierzanowska-Fangrat K, Raeiszadeh M, Dzierzanowska D, et al: IgG subclass response to *Helicobacter pylori* and CagA antigens in children. Clin Exp Immunol 134:442-446, 2003.

El-Omar EM, Carrington M, Chow WH, et al: Interleukin-1 polymorphisms associated with increased risk of gastric cancer. Nature 404:398-402, 2000.

Emilia G, Longo G, Luppi M, et al: *Helicobacter pylori* eradication can induce platelet recovery in idiopathic thrombocytopenic purpura. Blood 97:812-814, 2001.

Farrell S, Doherty GM, Milliken I, et al: Risk factors for *Helicobacter pylori* infection in children: An examination of the role played by intrafamilial bed sharing. Pediatr Infect Dis J 24:149-152, 2005.

Farrell S, Milliken I, Murphy JL, et al: Nonulcer dyspepsia and *Helicobacter pylori* eradication in children. J Pediatr Surg 40:1547-1550, 2005.

Gal E, Abuksis G, Fraser G, et al: 13C-urea breath test to validate eradication of *Helicobacter pylori* in an Israeli population. Isr Med Assoc J 5:98-100, 2003.

Gessner BD, Bruce MG, Parkinson AJ, et al: A randomized trial of triple therapy for pediatric *Helicobacter pylori* infection and risk factors for treatment failure in a population with a high prevalence of infection. Clin Infect Dis 41:1261-1268, 2005.

Gold BD: *Helicobacter pylori* infection in children. Curr Probl Pediatr 31:247-266, 2001.

Gold BD: Outcomes of pediatric gastroesophageal reflux disease: in the first year of life, in childhood, and in adults. Oh, and should we really leave *Helicobacter pylori* alone? J Pediatr Gastroenterol Nutr 37(Suppl):S33-S39, 2003.

Gold BD, Colletti RB, Abbott M, et al: *Helicobacter pylori* infection in children: Recommendations for diagnosis and treatment. J Pediatr Gastroenterol Nutr 31:490-497, 2000.

Gold BD, van Doorn LJ, Guarner J, et al: Genotypic, clinical, and demographic characteristics of children infected with *Helicobacter pylori*. J Clin Microbiol 39:1348-1345, 2001.

Goodman KJ, Cockburn M: The role of epidemiology in understanding the health effects of *Helicobacter pylori*. Epidemiology 12:266-271, 2001.

Gosciniak G, Przondo-Mordarska A, Iwanczak B, Blitek A: *Helicobacter pylori* antigens in stool specimens of gastritis children before and after treatment. J Pediatr Gastroenterol Nutr 36:376-380, 2003.

Gottrand F, Kalach N, Spyckerelle C, et al: Omeprazole combined with amoxicillin and clarithromycin in the eradication of *Helicobacter pylori* in children with gastritis: A prospective randomized double-blind trial. J Pediatr 139:664-668, 2001.

Graham DY: *Helicobacter pylori* is not and never was "protective" against anything, including GERD. Dig Dis Sci 48:629-623, 2003.

Graham DY, Shiotani A: The time to eradicate gastric cancer is now. Gut 54:735-738, 2005.

Guarner J, Bartlett J, Whistler T, et al: Can pre-neoplastic lesions be detected in gastric biopsies of children with *Helicobacter pylori* infection? J Pediatr Gastroenterol Nutr 37:309-314, 2003.

Haggerty TD, Perry S, Sanchez L, et al: Significance of transiently positive enzyme-linked immunosorbent assay results in detection of *Helicobacter pylori* in stool samples from children. J Clin Microbiol 43:2220-2223, 2005.

Hassall E, Dimmick JE: Unique features of *Helicobacter pylori* disease in children. Dig Dis Sci 36:417-423, 1991.

Hill R, Pearman J, Worthy P, et al: *Campylobacter pyloridis* and gastritis in children [letter]. Lancet 1:387, 1986.

Hunt R, Fallone C, Veldhuyzan van Zanten S, et al: Canadian Helicobacter Study Group Consensus Conference: Update on the management of *Helicobacter pylori*—An evidence-based evaluation of six topics relevant to clinical outcomes in patients evaluated for *H. pylori* infection. Can J Gastroenterol 18:547-554, 2004.

Jaing TH, Yang CP, Hung IJ, et al: Efficacy of *Helicobacter pylori* eradication on platelet recovery in children with chronic idiopathic thrombocytopenic purpura. Acta Paediatr 92:1153-1157, 2003.

Janulaityte-Gunther D, Kucinskiene R, Kupcinskas L, et al: The humoral immunoresponse to *Helicobacter pylori* infection in children with gastrointestinal symptoms. FEMS Immunol Med Microbiol 44:205-212, 2005.

Jones NL, Sherman P, Fallone CA, et al: Canadian Helicobacter Study Group Consensus Conference: Update on the approach to *Helicobacter pylori* infection in children and adolescents—An evidence-based evaluation. Can J Gastroenterol 19: 399-408, 2005.

Karita M, Teramukai S, Matsumoto S: Risk of *Helicobacter pylori* transmission from drinking well water is higher than that from infected intrafamilial members in Japan. Dig Dis Sci 48:1062-1067, 2003.

Kato S, Konno M, Maisawa S, et al: Results of triple eradication therapy in Japanese children: A retrospective multicenter study. J Gastroenterol 39:838-843, 2004.

Kato S, Okamoto H, Nishino Y, et al: *Helicobacter pylori* and TT virus prevalence in Japanese children. J Gastroenterol 38:1126-1130, 2003.

Kato S, Ozawa K, Koike T, et al: Effect of *Helicobacter pylori* infection on gastric acid secretion and meal-stimulated serum gastrin in children. Helicobacter 9:100-105, 2004.

Kato S, Ozawa K, Okuda M, et al: Accuracy of the stool antigen test for the diagnosis of childhood *Helicobacter pylori* infection: A multicenter Japanese study. Am J Gastroenterol 98:296-300, 2003.

Kato S, Sherman PM: What is new related to *Helicobacter pylori* infection in children and teenagers? Arch Pediatr Adolesc Med 159:415-421, 2005.

Koletzko S, Konstantopoulos N, Bosman D, et al: Evaluation of a novel monoclonal enzyme immunoassay for detection of *Helicobacter pylori* antigen in stool from children. Gut 52:804-806, 2003.

Kori M, Gladish V, Ziv-Sokolovskaya N, et al: The significance of routine duodenal biopsies in pediatric patients undergoing upper intestinal endoscopy. J Clin Gastroenterol 37:39-41, 2003.

Kostaki M, Fessatou S, Karpathios T: Refractory iron-deficiency anaemia due to silent *Helicobacter pylori* gastritis in children. Eur J Pediatr 162:177-179, 2003.

Kowolick MJ, Dowsett SA, Achila L, et al: Water and biofilm transmission of *Helicobacter pylori* (Hp) in rural Guatemalan households. J Pediatric Gastroenterol Nutr 41:554, 2005.

Kurekci AE, Atay AA, Sarici SU, et al: Is there a relationship between childhood *Helicobacter pylori* infection and iron deficiency anemia? J Trop Pediatr 51:166-169, 2005.

Leal-Herrera Y, Torres J, Monath TP, et al: High rates of recurrence and of transient reinfections of *Helicobacter pylori* in a population with high prevalence of infection. Am J Gastroenterol 98:2395-2402, 2003.

Levine A, Milo T, Broide E, et al: Influence of *Helicobacter pylori* eradication on gastroesophageal reflux symptoms and epigastric pain in children and adolescents. Pediatrics 113:54-58, 2004.

Liang S, Redlinger T: A protocol for isolating putative *Helicobacter pylori* from fecal specimens and genotyping using vacA alleles. Helicobacter 8:561-567, 2003.

Lin JT: *Helicobacter pylori* infection in children: The role of intrafamilial clustering. Acta Paediatr Taiwan 44:325-326, 2003.

Lopes AI, Oleastro M, Palha A, et al: Antibiotic-resistant *Helicobacter pylori* strains in Portuguese children. Pediatr Infect Dis J 24:404-409, 2005.

Lu Y, Redlinger TE, Avitia R, et al: Isolation and genotyping of *Helicobacter pylori* from untreated municipal wastewater. Appl Environ Microbiol 68:1436-1439, 2002.

Lui SL, Wong WM, Ng SY, et al: Seroprevalence of *Helicobacter pylori* in Chinese patients on continuous ambulatory peritoneal dialysis. Nephrology (Carlton) 10:21-24, 2005.

Luzza F, Pensabene L, Imeneo M, et al: Antral nodularity identifies children infected with *Helicobacter pylori* with higher grades of gastric inflammation. Gastrointest Endosc 53:60-64, 2001.

Ma F, Misumi J, Zhao W, et al: Long-term treatment with sterigmatocystin, a fungus toxin, enhances the development of intestinal metaplasia of gastric mucosa in *Helicobacter pylori*-infected Mongolian gerbils. Scand J Gastroenterol 38:360-369, 2003.

MacKay WG, Williams CL, McMillan M, et al: Evaluation of protocol using gene capture and PCR for detection of *Helicobacter pylori* DNA in feces. J Clin Microbiol 41:4589-4593, 2003.

Malaty HM, Tanaka E, Kumagai T, et al: Seroepidemiology of *Helicobacter pylori* and hepatitis A virus and the mode of transmission of infection: A 9-year cohort study in rural Japan. Clin Infect Dis 37:1067-1072, 2003.

Malfertheiner P, Megraud F, O'Morain C, et al: Current concepts in the management of *Helicobacter pylori* infection—

The Maastricht 2-2000 Consensus Report. Aliment Pharmacol Ther 16:167-180, 2002.

Malfertheiner P, Megraud F, O'Morain C, et al: Current European concepts in the management of *Helicobacter pylori* infection—The Maastricht Consensus Report. The European *Helicobacter pylori* Study Group (EHPSG). Eur J Gastroenterol Hepatol 9:1-2, 1997.

Malfertheiner P, Sipponen P, Naumann M, et al: *Helicobacter pylori* eradication has the potential to prevent gastric cancer: A state-of-the-art critique. Am J Gastroenterol 100:2100-2115, 2005.

Mayers N, Couzos S, Murray R, Daniels J: Prevalence of *Helicobacter pylori* in indigenous western Australians: Comparison between urban and remote rural populations. Med J Aust 182:544, 2005.

Megraud F: Comparison of non-invasive tests to detect *Helicobacter pylori* infection in children and adolescents: Results of a multicenter European study. J Pediatr 146:198-200, 2005.

Megraud F: On behalf of the Paediatric Task Force of *H. pylori* in children: Evaluation in a multicentric European study. Gut 51:A81, 2002.

Mera RM, Correa P, Fontham EE, et al: Effects of a new *Helicobacter pylori* infection on height and weight in Colombian children. Ann Epidemiol 16:347-351, 2006.

Moayyedi P: Should we test for *Helicobacter pylori* before treating gastroesophageal reflux disease? Can J Gastroenterol 19:425-427, 2005.

Mones J, Gisbert JP, Borda F, Dominguez-Munoz E: Indications, diagnostic tests and *Helicobacter pylori* eradication therapy. Recommendations by the 2nd Spanish Consensus Conference. Rev Esp Enferm Dig 97:348-374, 2005.

Moreira ED Jr, Nassri VB, Santos RS, et al: Association of *Helicobacter pylori* infection and giardiasis: Results from a study of surrogate markers for fecal exposure among children. World J Gastroenterol 11:2759-2763, 2005.

Nijevitch AA, Loguinovskaya VV, Tyrtyshnaya LV, et al: *Helicobacter pylori* infection and reflux esophagitis in children with chronic asthma. J Clin Gastroenterol 38:14-18, 2004.

Nishise Y, Fukao A, Takahashi T: Risk factors for *Helicobacter pylori* infection among a rural population in Japan: Relation to living environment and medical history. J Epidemiol 13:266-273, 2003.

Niv Y, Abuksis G, Koren R: 13C-urea breath test, referral patterns, and results in children. J Clin Gastroenterol 37:142-146, 2003.

Nozaki K, Shimizu N, Ikehara Y, et al: Effect of early eradication on *Helicobacter pylori*–related gastric carcinogenesis in Mongolian gerbils. Cancer Sci 94:235-239, 2003.

Ogunc D, Artan R, Ongut G, et al: Evaluation of a Western blot technique (Helicoblot 2.1) for the diagnosis of *Helicobacter pylori* infection in children. Pathology 35:157-160, 2003.

Okuda M, Nakazawa T, Booka M, et al: Evaluation of a urine antibody test for *Helicobacter pylori* in Japanese children. J Pediatr 144:196-199, 2004.

Owen RJ, Xerry J: Tracing clonality of *Helicobacter pylori* infecting family members from analysis of DNA sequences of three housekeeping genes (ureI, atpA and ahpC), deduced amino acid sequences, and pathogenicity-associated markers (cagA and vacA). J Med Microbiol 52:515-524, 2003.

Park JH, Kim SY, Kim DW, et al: Correlation between *Helicobacter pylori* infection and vitamin C levels in whole blood, plasma, and gastric juice, and the pH of gastric juice in Korean children. J Pediatr Gastroenterol Nutr 37:53-62, 2003.

Peura DA: Proceedings of an international update conference on *Helicobacter pylori*. Gastroenterology 113:S1-S169, 1997.

Pollet S, Gottrand F, Vincent P, et al: Gastroesophageal reflux disease and *Helicobacter pylori* infection in neurologically impaired children: Inter-relations and therapeutic implications. J Pediatr Gastroenterol Nutr 38:70-74, 2004.

Raguza D, Granato CF, Kawakami E: Evaluation of the stool antigen test for *Helicobacter pylori* in children and adolescents. Dig Dis Sci 50:453-457, 2005.

Rajantie J, Klemola T: *Helicobacter pylori* and idiopathic thrombocytopenic purpura in children. Blood 101:1660, 2003.

Rerksuppaphol S, Hardikar W, Midolo PD, Ward P: Antimicrobial resistance in *Helicobacter pylori* isolates from children. J Paediatr Child Health 39:332-335, 2003.

Rowland M, Lambert I, Gormally S, et al: Carbon 13-labeled urea breath test for the diagnosis of *Helicobacter pylori* infection in children [see comments]. J Pediatr 131:815-820, 1997.

Sandler RS, Everhart JE, Donowitz M, et al: The burden of selected digestive diseases in the United States. Gastroenterology 122:1500-1511, 2002.

Schistosomes, liver flukes and *Helicobacter pylori*. IARC Working Group on the Evaluation of Carcinogenic Risks to Humans. Lyon, France, 7-14 June 1994. IARC Monogr Eval Carcinog Risks Hum 61:1-241, 1994.

Sherman P, Hassall E, Hunt RH, et al: Canadian Helicobacter Study Group Consensus Conference on the Approach to *Helicobacter pylori* infection in Children and Adolescents. Can J Gastroenterol 13:553-559, 1999.

Sherman PM, Lin FY: Extradigestive manifestation of *Helicobacter pylori* infection in children and adolescents. Can J Gastroenterol 19:421-424, 2005.

Sinha SK, Martin B, Gold BD, et al: The incidence of *Helicobacter pylori* acquisition in children of a Canadian First Nations community and the potential for parent-to-child transmission. Helicobacter 9:59-68, 2004.

Sood MR, Joshi S, Akobeng AK, et al: Growth in children with *Helicobacter pylori* infection and dyspepsia. Arch Dis Child 90:1025-1028, 2005.

Tatematsu M, Nozaki K, Tsukamoto T: *Helicobacter pylori* infection and gastric carcinogenesis in animal models. Gastric Cancer 6:1-7, 2003.

Tolia V, Brown W, El-Baba M, Lin CH. *Helicobacter pylori* culture and antimicrobial susceptibility from pediatric patients in Michigan. Pediatr Infect Dis J 19:1167-1171, 2000.

Tosun SY, Kasirga E, Ertan P, Aksu S: Evidence against the fecal-oral route of transmission for *Helicobacter pylori* infection in childhood. Med Sci Monit 9:CR489-CR492, 2003.

Tytgat GN: Endoscopic transmission of *Helicobacter pylori*. Aliment Pharmacol Ther 9(Suppl):105-110, 1995.

Uc A, Chong SK: Treatment of *Helicobacter pylori* gastritis improves dyspeptic symptoms in children. J Pediatr Gastroenterol Nutr 34:281-285, 2002.

Uemura N, Okamoto S, Yamamoto S, et al: *Helicobacter pylori* infection and the development of gastric cancer. N Engl J Med 345:784-789, 2001.

Uhlig HH, Tannapfel A, Mossner J, et al: Histopathological parameters of *Helicobacter pylori*-associated gastritis in children and adolescents: Comparison with findings in adults. Scand J Gastroenterol 38:701-706, 2003.

Ukarapol N, Lertprasertsuk N, Wongsawasdi L: Recurrent abdominal pain in children: The utility of upper endoscopy and histopathology. Singapore Med J 45:121-124, 2004.

Vaira D, Vakil N, Menegatti M, et al: The stool antigen test for detection of *Helicobacter pylori* after eradication therapy. Ann Intern Med 136:280-287, 2002.

Warren JR, Marshall BJ: Unidentified curved bacilli on gastric epithelium in active chronic gastritis. Lancet 1:1273-1275, 1983.

Watanabe T, Tada M, Nagai H, et al: *Helicobacter pylori* infection induces gastric cancer in mongolian gerbils [see comments]. Gastroenterology 115:642-648, 1998.

Wong BC, Lam SK, Wong WM, et al: *Helicobacter pylori* eradication to prevent gastric cancer in a high-risk region of China: A randomized controlled trial. JAMA 291:187-189, 2004.

Wu MS, Wang JT, Yang JC, et al: Effective reduction of *Helicobacter pylori* infection after upper gastrointestinal endoscopy by mechanical washing of the endoscope. Hepatogastroenterology 43:1660-1664, 1996.

CHAPTER 12

Hirschsprung's Disease

PETER MATTEI

Disease Description
Case Presentation
Epidemiology
Pathophysiology
Differential Diagnosis
Diagnostic Testing
Treatment
Approach to the Case
Summary
Major Points

DISEASE DESCRIPTION

Hirschsprung's disease is an idiopathic congenital disorder of colorectal motility that usually manifests in infancy and is characterized by the absence of ganglion cells in the myenteric plexuses of the rectum and a variable length of colon. The resulting pseudo-obstruction causes severe constipation and a characteristic dilation of the more proximal normal colon (megacolon). The disease is treated by surgical resection of the aganglionic segment of bowel, with excellent results in most patients.

CASE PRESENTATION

A 2-day-old term male infant in the newborn nursery presents with feeding intolerance and abdominal distention. Although he initially fed normally, he began spitting up formula 12 hours ago and is now vomiting with every feed. The emesis has become progressively more tinged with green bile. The nurses have documented an increase in abdominal girth and describe the abdomen as "distended and firm." He is afebrile, has normal respirations, and remains hemodynamically stable. He is voiding normally. He is 48 hours old and has not passed meconium.

On examination he is alert and his skin is well perfused. Examination of the head, neck, and chest is unremarkable. The abdomen is very distended, but nontender and without masses. The anus is positioned normally on the perineum. Digital rectal examination reveals normal sphincter tone and no masses. After examination, the infant promptly passes a very large meconium stool.

A complete blood count and electrolyte panel are within normal limits. A plain abdominal x-ray reveals multiple dilated loops of bowel. A decubitus abdominal x-ray shows multiple air-fluid levels. There is no evidence of pneumatosis intestinalis or free intraperitoneal air.

EPIDEMIOLOGY

Hirschsprung's disease occurs with an estimated incidence of 1 in 5000 live births. The disease is limited to the rectum and distal sigmoid colon in approximately 85% of cases and involves all or part of the rest of the colon in the remainder of patients. It occurs more frequently in boys, with a male-to-female ratio of nearly 4:1. In patients with total colonic aganglionosis, this ratio is closer to 2:1. Less than 10% of patients with Hirschsprung's disease have a relative with the disease, though nearly one half of patients with total colonic involvement have a positive family history. Several specific genetic mutations have been identified in patients with Hirschsprung's disease, although there is no single genetic defect that characterizes all cases.

Approximately 30% of patients with Hirschsprung's disease have other anomalies. Trisomy 21 occurs in approximately 5% of patients. Cardiac anomalies occur in approximately 5% of patients without trisomy 21 and in 50% of patients with trisomy 21. Hirschsprung's disease also has been described in association with other disorders of neural crest migration, such as Waardenburg-Shah syndrome, Ondine's curse, and multiple endocrine neoplasia type 2, as well as other genetic syndromes, such as Smith-Lemli-Opitz syndrome.

PATHOPHYSIOLOGY

Hirschsprung's disease is a form of intestinal pseudo-obstruction. Peristalsis requires successive segments of the bowel to relax and then contract sequentially. A segment of bowel in which receptive relaxation cannot occur does not permit propagation of the wave and thus acts like a point of obstruction despite the absence of a true physical blockage. The subsequent dilation of the normal bowel proximal to the affected segment completes the classic clinical picture of Hirschsprung's disease: dilated proximal bowel and narrow-caliber distal bowel, separated by a tapered segment known as the transition zone.

Ganglion cells are required to allow receptive relaxation of the bowel. They are derived from the neural crest and populate the plexuses of Auerbach and Meissner within the bowel wall (Fig. 12-1). Neural crest cells originate in the proximal intestine and migrate distally during development, populating the rectum last. It is believed that Hirschsprung's disease results from the arrested cephalocaudal migration of neural crest cells along the intestinal tract. This is consistent with the clinical finding that in nearly all cases it is a single segment of the most distal part of the intestine (the rectum and colon) that is involved, without skip areas or more proximal bowel being affected.

Ganglion cells form an essential part of the enteric nervous system. It is believed that their role is to provide inhibitory signals that allow muscular relaxation through a mechanism that is mediated by nitric oxide. In addition to lack of receptive relaxation of the affected bowel, there is also loss of the rectosphincteric reflex, in which the internal anal sphincter relaxes in response to stimulation of the rectum by the presence of a stool bolus. This forms the basis for the anal manometric studies that were used at some centers in the past to make the diagnosis of Hirschsprung's disease.

Although constipation is the hallmark symptom of classic Hirschsprung's disease, an acute and sometimes recurring diarrheal illness is another. *Enterocolitis* is an affliction that is specific to infants with Hirschsprung's disease, occurs most frequently in the first 2 years of life, and can occur even after a definitive operation has been performed. The pathophysiology of the disease is unclear. Stasis with subsequent bacterial overgrowth has been proposed as a possible cause; however, the fact that it is almost never seen in patients with other forms of obstruction would argue against this theory. There appears to be something very specific about patients with Hirschsprung's disease that makes them susceptible to this process. Some have postulated that there is a specific immunologic abnormality or mucosal barrier defect that accompanies the absence of ganglion cells in patients with Hirschsprung's disease, but the nature of such a defect has yet to be defined.

DIFFERENTIAL DIAGNOSIS

The differential diagnosis for patients with severe constipation varies somewhat depending on the age at presentation (Table 12-1). In the newborn period, the classic

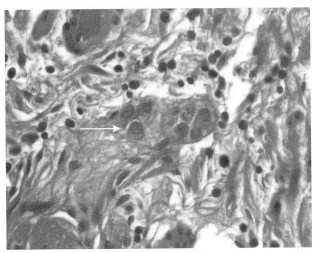

Figure 12-1 *(See also Color Plate 12-1)* Ganglion cells within the myenteric plexus of the rectum *(arrow)*. (Hematoxylin and eosin stain, × 400.)

Table 12-1 Differential Diagnosis of Constipation

Age	Diagnosis
Newborn	Imperforate anus
	Meconium plug syndrome
	Intestinal atresia/stenosis
	Small left colon syndrome
	Meconium ileus
	Intestinal duplication
	Incarcerated hernia
	Intestinal volvulus
Toddler/school age	Functional constipation
	Milk protein allergy
	Intestinal neuronal dysplasia
	Intestinal pseudo-obstruction
	Intestinal duplication
	Rectal duplication
	Pelvic tumor
Adolescent/adult	Functional constipation
	Dietary constipation
	Intestinal pseudo-obstruction
	Chagas' disease

presentation includes failure to pass meconium in the first 48 hours of life, abdominal distention, feeding intolerance, and bilious emesis. This clinical picture can be the result of other forms of neonatal bowel obstruction. *Imperforate anus* is usually evident on physical examination, although in some cases, the perineal fistula often associated with this disorder may have the appearance of an anteriorly displaced anus. *Meconium plug syndrome* is colonic obstruction due to inspissated meconium and mucus. It can occur in association with cystic fibrosis, small left colon syndrome, and Hirschsprung's disease, but is usually an idiopathic phenomenon. Contrast enema confirms the diagnosis and is also usually therapeutic. *Intestinal atresia* or *stenosis* can affect any part of the intestinal tract but most commonly occurs in the ileum or jejunum. X-rays reveal markedly dilated loops of bowel and a "microcolon" is seen on contrast enema. *Small left colon syndrome* typically occurs in infants of diabetic mothers and is also suggested by a characteristic picture on contrast enema. Treatment is supportive, but Hirschsprung's disease needs to be ruled out in these patients as well. *Meconium ileus* is a distal ileal obstruction as a result of inspissated meconium and is associated in nearly all cases with cystic fibrosis. Water-soluble contrast enema is usually diagnostic, showing a microcolon with luminal filling defects in the ileum; it is often therapeutic as well. Other conditions that rarely produce distal bowel obstruction in the newborn include *intestinal duplication cyst, incarcerated hernia,* and *intestinal volvulus.*

Children older than 3 months with constipation will usually be diagnosed with "functional" constipation, although occasionally an older child with constipation will be found to have Hirschsprung's disease. Children with Hirschsprung's disease typically have a history of stooling difficulty since birth, require assistance such as suppositories or enemas to have a bowel movement, and rarely develop encopresis and soiling. In fact, the rectum in patients with Hirschsprung's disease is usually small and empty of stool. Nevertheless, a complete workup, including contrast enema and rectal biopsy, is sometimes necessary to rule out Hirschsprung's disease, even in adolescence or adulthood.

Other less common causes of constipation in young children include *milk protein allergy* and other dietary causes. *Intestinal duplication cysts* and, in particular, *rectal duplication cysts* occasionally manifest in this age-group. Constipation also can be the manifesting symptom in patients with pelvic tumors, such as sacrococcygeal teratoma.

Other forms of intestinal pseudo-obstruction can present in much the same way as Hirschsprung's disease in older patients, but are generally quite rare and typically very difficult to confirm with certainty. *Intestinal neuronal dysplasia* is a somewhat controversial diagnosis that is characterized by hyperganglionosis of the bowel and, to add to the diagnostic uncertainty, can occur in association with Hirschsprung's disease. Chronic intestinal pseudo-obstruction syndromes such as *hollow visceral myopathy* can be confused with Hirschsprung's disease in their early phases, but the progressive nature of these illnesses and the effect on multiple organs eventually distinguishes them. Lastly, *Chagas' disease* is an acquired enteric gangionopathy that causes achalasia but also can affect the colon. It is rare in the United States but is seen with some frequency in Latin America.

DIAGNOSTIC TESTING

The diagnosis of Hirschsprung's disease is usually made on the basis of a contrast enema and a rectal biopsy. In the past, anorectal manometry studies were used as the diagnostic study of choice at some centers. In children older than 2 weeks of age, a balloon inflated in the rectum should cause a reflex relaxation of the internal anal sphincter that is measurable by a pressure transducer positioned in the anus. In children with Hirschsprung's disease, the sphincter does not relax, and the pressure may actually increase in response to rectal balloon inflation.

Contrast enema can support the suspected diagnosis of Hirschsprung's disease, may exclude conditions that can mimic Hirschsprung's disease, and can help to characterize the extent of the disease by demonstrating the location of the transition zone. The enema is usually performed with barium suspension, but the radiologist may prefer to use a water-soluble contrast agent. The classic picture is that of dilated proximal colon that transitions rapidly to a normal- or narrow-caliber rectum (Fig. 12-2). The diameter of the rectum is normally larger than those of the sigmoid and descending colons. When the reverse is true, Hirschsprung's disease should be suspected (Fig. 12-3). This is usually best appreciated radiographically on a lateral view of the rectum. A transition zone may not be appreciated in cases of Hirschsprung's disease in which the entire colon is involved or when the segment is extremely short. Some believe that rectal digital examination performed before the contrast enema can diminish the radiographic findings and lead to a false-negative result, although this has been difficult to confirm. Lastly, a radiograph taken 24 hours after the contrast study that shows incomplete evacuation of barium from the rectum strongly suggests Hirschsprung's disease.

When the contrast enema shows a transition zone, the diagnosis of Hirschsprung's disease must be confirmed before surgical intervention is performed. Likewise, when a contrast enema fails to support the diagnosis despite a strong clinical suspicion, a rectal biopsy should be performed to more definitively rule out the diagnosis. Rectal biopsy is generally performed in one

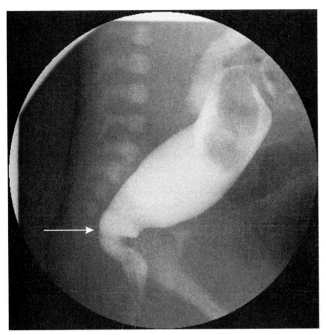

Figure 12-2 Contrast enema in a newborn patient with Hirschsprung's disease. Note the transition zone *(arrow)*, as the more dilated proximal colon tapers to more narrow distal colon at the rectosigmoid junction.

rectum. Suction is applied using a syringe, causing the rectal mucosa and submucosa to be drawn into the lumen. A blade is then activated and a small piece of tissue is harvested. It is important for the biopsy to be performed at least 2 to 3 cm above the dentate line, because the most distal portion of the rectum is normally aganglionic. The procedure is quite safe, although bleeding and bacteremia have been described. Perforations also have been reported but are quite rare. Because of the absence of tactile sensory innervation of the rectum, the procedure is also usually painless.

An adequate suction rectal biopsy specimen must include the submucosa, which is examined using standard histopathologic techniques for the presence of ganglion cells. When ganglion cells are not seen, the diagnostic accuracy of the study is increased by finding hypertrophied nerve trunks (Fig. 12-4). The accuracy of the technique may also be improved by staining for acetylcholinesterase, the level of which is markedly increased in patients with Hirschsprung's disease.

of two ways. In newborns, *suction rectal biopsy* can be performed safely at the bedside and is felt to be quite accurate when adequate submucosa has been obtained. The most commonly used instrument employs a small metal capsule with a side hole that is inserted into the

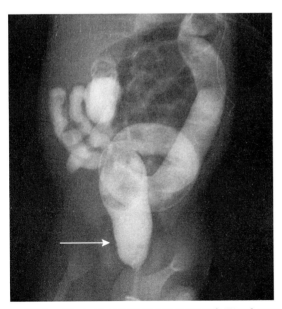

Figure 12-3 Contrast enema in a patient with Hirschsprung's disease. The transition zone is subtle, but the narrow caliber of the rectum *(arrow)* relative to the more proximal sigmoid colon was noted and felt to be suggestive of Hirschsprung's disease. Subsequent rectal biopsy confirmed the diagnosis.

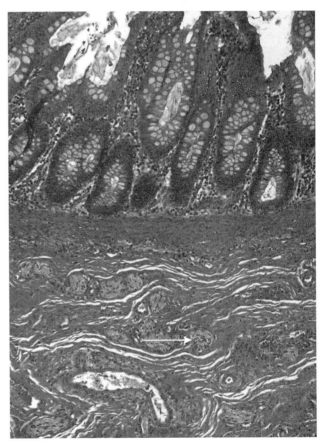

Figure 12-4 *(See also Color Plate 12-4.)* Rectal biopsy of a patient with Hirschsprung's disease. There are no ganglion cells to be found within the myenteric plexus. There are hypertrophied nerves *(arrow)*, however, which serves to confirm the diagnosis of Hirschsprung's disease. (Hematoxylin and eosin stain, × 400.)

Suction rectal biopsy is felt to be very accurate and is the standard approach to the diagnosis of Hirschsprung's disease in most centers. However, in children older than approximately 6 months and in those in whom suction rectal biopsy has been performed but is inconclusive, open rectal biopsy may be necessary. This involves general anesthesia and is performed in the operating room. A full-thickness biopsy is usually performed, and because it provides the opportunity to examine both myenteric and submucosal plexuses for the presence of ganglion cells, it is considered the diagnostic gold standard. It is also very safe and produces very little postoperative discomfort.

TREATMENT

The definitive treatment of Hirschsprung's disease is surgical and includes removal of the aganglionic segment of bowel and replacement with the proximal normally innervated bowel. There are three standard operations, each of which was initially described in the 1950s and 1960s and have similar excellent results (Fig. 12-5). The choice of operation is usually based on the training and experience of the surgeon, but occasionally patient-related issues need to be considered. The first operation was developed by Ovar Swenson in the 1950s and continues to be performed with some frequency. In this operation, the aganglionic bowel is resected full-thickness down to the anus. The aganglionic bowel is pulled down through the pelvis and anastomosed to the anus at the perineum. An internal sphincterotomy was added to the standard operation in the 1960s. Although perhaps less commonly performed than other procedures for Hirschsprung's disease, it continues to have many enthusiastic proponents throughout the world.

The second operation to gain widespread acceptance was described by Bernard Duhamel in 1960 and modified in 1967 by Lester Martin. The Duhamel-Martin operation involves retaining the aganglionic rectum and anastomosing to its posterior aspect the ganglionated bowel that has been pulled through. The anastomosis is usually created in a side-to-side fashion using a gastrointestinal stapling device inserted through the anus, which simultaneously joins the two segments and divides the common wall between them to create a single lumen. The goal of the operation is to retain the normal sensory innervation of the rectum and pelvic organs while the posterior one half of the new rectum provides the motor apparatus needed for proper defecation. This is one of the two most commonly performed operations for Hirschsprung's disease and has had very good results.

The third accepted operation designed to treat Hirschsprung's disease is also probably the one most commonly performed. The endorectal pull-through operation was first described by Soave in 1964 and later modified by Boley. The distal rectal mucosa is stripped, leaving the muscular coat of the rectum intact. The ganglionated bowel is then brought through the muscular cuff and sutured just above the anorectal junction. Thus, the normal bowel is surrounded distally by the muscular coat of the native rectum. There is less pelvic dissection with this operation and therefore theoretically less potential for disruption of pelvic nerves.

Traditionally, all operations for Hirschsprung's disease included an initial diverting colostomy performed just above the transition zone (a "leveling" colostomy), 3 to

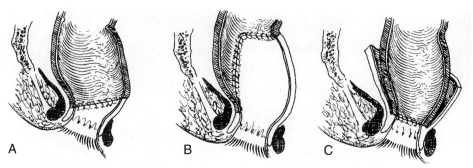

Figure 12-5 The three most popular operations for Hirschsprung's disease. **A,** The Swenson's operation, in which the aganglionic rectum is removed and the normally ganglionated proximal bowel is brought down and sutured at the anus. **B,** The Duhamel-Martin operation, in which the aganglionic rectum is preserved. The normally ganglionated proximal bowel is brought down behind the native rectum and the wall between the two is obliterated with a stapling device to create a single large lumen. **C,** The Soave-Boley operation, in which the mucosa and submucosa of the distal rectum are stripped, preserving a cuff of rectal muscle and, in theory, its sensory and motor innervation; the proximal bowel is brought down within the cuff and sutured to the anus. Traditionally, these operations were performed using a large abdominal incision 6 months after a "leveling" colostomy. Today they are often performed as a primary operation (without prior colostomy), frequently using a minimally invasive approach (laparoscopic and/or transanal). (From Klein MD, Burd RS: Hirschsprung's Disease. In Wyllie R, Hyams J (eds): Pediatric Gastrointestinal Disease: Pathology Diagnosis Management, 2nd ed. Philadelphia, WB Saunders, 1999, pp 489-498).

6 months before definitive surgery. This was felt to be necessary to allow the dilated bowel to return to normal size, and to allow the patient to grow to a size that would make the operation technically easier to perform. More recently, there has been a movement toward primary repair in newborns in whom the diagnosis is made relatively early, before significant bowel dilatation has occurred. This trend has been accompanied by the development of several very good minimally invasive surgical approaches, all of which are modifications of the more standard open operations. For example, a laparoscopic-assisted primary pull-through operation is used with success in some centers. The transanal primary pull-through procedure recently has been popularized with excellent early results. Using this approach, the entire operation is performed through the anus, with no incision placed on the abdomen at all. As with all new surgical techniques, the basic principles of the operation need to be adhered to and the results need to be compared rigorously with those of the standard procedures, which have certainly withstood the test of time.

The operations described above are applicable to most of the 85% of patients with so-called *short-segment* Hirschsprung's disease. *Total colonic aganglionosis* is usually treated with some modification of one of the three principal operations, but the results are generally not as good. *Ultra-short segment Hirschsprung's disease* is a controversial entity in which the disease is purported to involve only the anus and internal sphincter. Diagnostic criteria are not completely agreed on and rectal biopsy is usually normal. Anal manometry may be the only way to make the diagnosis, but it is increasingly difficult to find a center with the equipment and expertise to do the study properly. Treatment is equally controversial and typically involves some combination of a laxative regimen, anal dilatation, and internal sphincterotomy. Older children and the rare adult diagnosed with Hirschsprung's disease pose a challenge given the severe changes associated with chronic colonic dilatation and years of heavy laxative use. These patients almost always require a diverting colostomy for a period of time before definitive repair.

The patient with Hirschsprung's enterocolitis is treated with bowel rest, intravenous hydration, triple antibiotic therapy, and frequent rectal irrigation with normal saline. In the past, mortality from enterocolitis was quite high. Recent data suggest that with proper therapy the mortality should be minimal, but it is not zero. Parents and health care providers need to be educated about the signs and symptoms of enterocolitis to avoid any delay in therapy. Any patient suspected of having enterocolitis should be admitted to the hospital and evaluated carefully. It is far better to overtreat a patient who turns out not to have the disease than to undertreat one who does. The usual signs are abdominal distention, explosive diarrhea, fever, lethargy, and sometimes emesis. A classic finding is that of an explosive bowel movement immediately on removing the examining finger from the anus. There may be blood or mucus in the stool, which is often malodorous. Symptoms may progress to obtundation and shock. Complications also include colonic perforation and overwhelming sepsis. Early symptoms may be confused with garden-variety viral gastroenteritis and therefore require vigilance and a low threshold for aggressive therapy. Treatment continues for 3 to 14 days depending on the severity of the disease and the response to therapy. Prophylactic routine rectal irrigations are used by some surgeons during the first year after operation for Hirschsprung's disease to reduce the incidence of enterocolitis.

The overall results of surgical therapy for Hirschsprung's disease are very good; however, a significant number of patients have a less than satisfactory result. This may be a result of complications, such as recurrent enterocolitis or rectal stricture requiring dilatation, or suboptimal function, including persistent constipation with soiling or frank incontinence. Some complications are clearly related to technical issues (pulling through aganglionic bowel, anastomotic leak or stricture, ischemia of the neorectum) but appear to occur with more-or-less equal frequency regardless of which operation is used. Other complications appear to be related to other as yet undefined factors related to Hirschsprung's disease itself. Parents should be warned that the operation is not always curative and that ongoing problems can occur in this frequently challenging and sometimes frustrating disease.

APPROACH TO THE CASE

This infant has a clinical picture consistent with a bowel obstruction. Standard initial therapy for a bowel obstruction regardless of etiology usually includes bowel rest, nasogastric tube decompression of the stomach, and fluid resuscitation. If fever, lethargy, or other signs of sepsis are present, antibiotics (ampicillin and gentamicin) should be started as well, although some physicians treat empirically with antibiotics in these situations given the high risk of bacterial translocation from the gut and the vulnerability of the newborn to bacteremia. The infant is monitored closely with serial examinations and periodic x-rays, looking especially for signs of sepsis, peritonitis, and bowel perforation. Meanwhile, a pediatric surgeon is consulted and a diagnostic workup is performed.

The workup in this patient includes a barium enema (Fig. 12-6). This is usually an excellent first study because it allows us to rule out other causes of bowel obstruction in a newborn, such as meconium plug syndrome, small left colon syndrome, and meconium ileus, and in many cases is an excellent initial treatment for

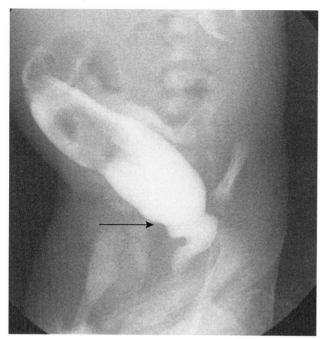

Figure 12-6 Contrast enema for introductory case. There is a transition zone at the rectosigmoid junction *(arrow)*. Rectal biopsy confirmed the diagnosis of Hirschsprung's disease.

these conditions. One should avoid the temptation to request an upper gastrointestinal study in these patients because it is rarely useful as a diagnostic test, it delays definitive treatment, and it can worsen bowel distention, increasing the risk of complications. The contrast enema in this patient is felt to be consistent with Hirschsprung's disease. There is a distinct transition zone from dilated proximal bowel to relatively narrow distal bowel. The transition zone is in the sigmoid colon, which is the most common location. On the lateral view, it is clear that the diameter of the rectum is less than those of the descending and sigmoid colons.

Although the diagnosis is fairly certain at this point, more definitive evidence is required before proceeding with an operation. A suction rectal biopsy is performed at the bedside and an adequate sample of the submucosa is obtained. Acetylcholinesterase staining is positive and despite an exhaustive search through the entire specimen, no ganglion cells are identified. In addition, abundant hypertrophied nerve fibers are seen, enhancing the degree of diagnostic certainty.

With the diagnosis confirmed, discussions begin with the family regarding treatment recommendations, surgical options, and prognosis. Meanwhile, ampicillin and gentamicin are given, and rectal irrigations with normal saline are performed twice daily. If the infant has responded to the initial therapy with significant abdominal decompression and is clinically well, enteral nutrition can be started until the day of surgery. The operation is scheduled at the earliest convenience of the family and the surgeon.

This infant is diagnosed early and responds nicely to initial therapy. He has a relatively short-segment disease and is therefore felt to be an excellent candidate for a primary repair, avoiding a temporary diverting colostomy. A laparoscopic-assisted transanal approach is offered to the family, and they provide informed consent for the operation. The risks of the operation include infection and bleeding, which are uncommon; anastomotic leak, anastomotic stricture, and pelvic abscess, which are rare; and recurrent constipation, fecal incontinence, and injury to pelvic nerves resulting in bladder dysfunction or impotence, which are uncommon and difficult to assess for several years to come.

Before surgery, general anesthesia is induced and the patient is initially placed in a supine position. Laparoscopic access to the abdomen is obtained and the colon is visualized. There is a distinct transition zone near the rectosigmoid junction. A seromuscular biopsy is taken above the transition and sent for immediate pathologic review. The biopsy site is repaired with sutures and the laparoscopic portion of the procedure is concluded. If the transition zone could not be clearly visualized, several biopsies would be taken so as to identify the ganglionated portion of the bowel. Had the aganglionic segment been found to be too long for the operation to be done safely using a transanal approach, the colon would be mobilized as far as was necessary to facilitate the pull-through. This would typically include ligation and division of the inferior mesenteric artery and mobilization of the splenic flexure. Once the colon has been adequately mobilized, the patient is placed in a lithotomy position and an anal retractor is placed into position. The pathologist reports that the biopsy shows normally ganglionated bowel. The rectal mucosa is stripped, preserving a short cuff of muscle wall, and the colon is pulled through the anus by dividing all attachments and blood vessels one by one, until the biopsy site is identified. The colon is divided at this point and anastomosed to the anus.

Postoperatively, the patient does well and is started on feeds on the resumption of normal bowel activity, which typically occurs by the third postoperative day. He will be followed periodically for several years to monitor his bowel habits and to identify potential complications early.

SUMMARY

Hirschsprung's disease is an idiopathic, congenital form of intestinal pseudo-obstruction that affects the rectum and colon, causing severe constipation. Patients also are at risk for enterocolitis, an acute diarrheal illness that can be life-threatening. The disease typically manifests in infancy—the classic presentation is that of a newborn who has not passed meconium in the first 48 hours of life—but it can present at any age. The hallmark of the disease is the absence of ganglion cells in the myenteric plexuses of the rectum. Ganglion cells are derived from the neural crest and form an integral part of the enteric nervous system, where they mediate the relaxation of the bowel wall during peristalsis. Distal to the point where the neural crest cells halted their craniocaudal migration along the bowel, usually in the sigmoid colon, the bowel remains in a state of tonic contraction, resulting in pseudo-obstruction and severe constipation. The diagnosis is confirmed by contrast enema, which typically reveals a dilated colon (megacolon) that tapers down to a narrow-caliber rectum, and by rectal biopsy, which confirms the absence of ganglion cells. The treatment is primarily surgical and involves replacement of the affected bowel with more proximal ganglionated bowel, using one of the three different operations. Some patients require a temporary diverting colostomy before the definitive repair, though there is a current trend toward primary repair in infancy and the use of minimally invasive surgical techniques. The results of treatment are generally very good, but a significant proportion of patients have complications such as recurrent enterocolitis or persistent constipation even after definitive surgical repair. Nevertheless, patients with this interesting and often challenging disease are usually able to enjoy a normal and unrestricted lifestyle.

MAJOR POINTS

Hirschsprung's disease is a congenital disease of unknown etiology. There may be a genetic component in some cases. It occurs with an estimated incidence of 1 in 5000 births.

Associated anomalies occur in approximately 30% of cases, including trisomy 21 and other disorders relating to neural crest differentiation and migration.

Hirschsprung's disease is caused by a lack of ganglion cells within the enteric neural plexuses of the rectum and distal colon.

In 85% of cases, it is the rectum and a small portion of the distal colon that are affected by the disease, although in some cases, the entire colon may be involved.

The disease usually manifests in infancy with failure to pass meconium in the first 48 hours of life and severe constipation, but can manifest at any age.

Patients with Hirschsprung's disease are at risk for a disease process known as enterocolitis, which causes diarrhea, dehydration, and sometimes life-threatening sepsis.

Rectal biopsy and demonstration of the absence of ganglion cells are necessary to confirm a suspected diagnosis of Hirschsprung's disease.

The treatment of Hirschsprung's disease involves one of three operations that have been described to replace or bypass the aganglionic rectum and colon.

A small but significant minority of patients continue to have difficulty with constipation, technical complications, or recurrent enterocolitis even after surgical repair of Hirschsprung's disease.

SUGGESTED READINGS

Badner JA, Sieber WK, Garver KL, Chakravarti A: A genetic study of Hirschsprung disease. Am J Hum Genet 46:568-580, 1990.

Boley SJ: An endorectal pull through operation with primary anastomosis for Hirschsprung's disease. Surge Gynecol Obstet 127:353-357, 1967.

de Oliveira RB, Troncon LE, Dantas RO, Menghelli UG: Gastrointestinal manifestations of Chagas' disease. Am J Gastroenterol 93:884-889, 1998.

Duhamel B: A new operation for the treatment of Hirschsprung's disease. Arch Dis Child 35:38-39, 1960.

Georgeson KE, Cohen RD, Hebra A, et al: Primary laparoscopic-assisted endorectal colon pull-through for Hirschsprung's disease: A new gold standard. Ann Surg 229:678-682, 1999.

Hayakawa K, Hamanaka Y, Suzuki M, et al: Radiological findings in total colon aganglionosis and allied disorders. Radiat Med 21:128-134, 2003.

Hoehner JC, Ein SH, Shandling B, Kim PC: Long-term morbidity in total colonic aganglionosis. J Pediatr Surg 33:961-965, 1998.

Langer JC, Minkes RK, Mazziotti MV, et al: Transanal one-stage Soave procedure for infants with Hirschsprung's disease. J Pediatr Surg 34:148-151, 1999.

Langer JC, Seifert M, Minkes RK: One-stage Soave pull-through for Hirschsprung's disease: A comparison of the transanal and open approaches. J Pediatr Surg 35:820-822, 2000.

Marty TL, Seo T, Matlak ME, et al: Gastrointestinal function after surgical correction of Hirschsprung's disease: Long-term follow-up in 135 patients. J Pediatr Surg 30:655-658, 1995.

Marty TL, Seo T, Sullivan JJ, et al: Rectal irrigations for the prevention of postoperative enterocolitis in Hirschsprung's disease. J Pediatr Surg 30:652-654, 1995.

Nakao M, Suita S, Taguchi T, et al: Y. Fourteen-year experience of acetylcholinesterase staining for rectal mucosal biopsy in neonatal Hirschsprung's disease. J Pediatr Surg 36:1357-1363, 2001.

Proctor ML, Traubici J, Langer JC, et al: Correlation between radiographic transition zone and level of aganglionosis in Hirschsprung's disease: Implications for surgical approach. J Pediatr Surg 38:775-778, 2003.

Rees BI, Azmy A, Nigam M, Lake BD: Complications of rectal suction biopsy. J Pediatr Surg 18:273-275, 1983.

Scharli AF: The practical significance of manometry in pathology of the rectum and anorectum. Prog Pediatr Surg 24:142-154, 1989.

Soave F: A new surgical technique for treatment of Hirschsprung's disease. Surgery 56:1007-1014, 1964.

Stewart DR, von Allmen D: The genetics of Hirschsprung's disease. Gastroenterol Clin North Am 32:819-837, 2003.

Swenson O: Follow-up on 200 patients treated for Hirschsprung's disease during a 10-year period. Ann Surg 146:706-714, 1957.

Teitelbaum DH, Caniano DA, Qualman SJ: The pathophysiology of Hirschsprung's-associated enterocolitis: Importance of histologic correlates. J Pediatr Surg 24:1271-1277, 1989.

Teitelbaum DH, Qualman SJ, Caniano DA: Hirschsprung's disease: Identification of risk factors for enterocolitis. Ann Surg 207:240-244, 1988.

Tomita R, Ikeda T, Fujisaki S, et al: Hirschsprung's disease and its allied disorders in adults: Histological and clinical studies. Hepatogastroenterology 50:1050-1053, 2003.

van Leeuwen K, Teitelbaum DH, Elhalaby EA, Coran AG: Long-term follow-up of redo pull-through procedures for Hirschsprung's disease: Efficacy of the endorectal pull-through. J Pediatr Surg 35:829-833, 2000.

CHAPTER 13

Infectious Diarrhea

MATTHEW R. RILEY
DORSEY BASS

Disease Description
Case Presentation
Epidemiology
Pathophysiology
Differential Diagnosis
Diagnostic Testing
Treatment
    Oral Rehydration Therapy
    Supplemental Therapy
    Antibiotic Therapy
    Public Health
Approach to the Case
Summary
Major Points

DISEASE DESCRIPTION

Infectious diarrhea encompasses a range of clinical syndromes caused by various microbiologic agents, including bacteria, viruses, and parasites. One strict case definition defines diarrhea as the passage of three or more loose stools in a 24-hour period. However, infectious diarrhea may manifest as acute watery diarrhea, dysentery with visible blood in the stool, or persistent diarrhea lasting longer than 14 days.

CASE PRESENTATION

A 7-year-old boy without significant past medical history presents with 3 days of nonbilious emesis and diarrhea. For the first 2 days, he passed two large, loose nonbloody stools per day. On the third day of his illness, his stools became bloody with occasional mucus. He also has had anorexia and numerous episodes of brief epigastric and right lower quadrant pain. He has tolerated only clear liquids, including water, fruit juice, and soda, for the past 2 days. He has been urinating at least four times a day, although his mother states that it appears "dark." No other family members or recent contacts are ill. He lives in an urban area and drinks tap water from the city water system. He eats only home-cooked meals, with the exception of a fast-food hamburger that he ate 4 days ago.

His physical examination is notable for a temperature of 38.3° C, a heart rate of 110, and a blood pressure of 102/66 mm Hg. His mental status is normal. His oral mucous membranes are slightly tacky. He has epigastric and right lower quadrant tenderness without rebound or involuntary guarding. His extremities are warm with brisk capillary refill.

Preliminary bloodwork reveals normal electrolytes, blood urea nitrogen, and creatinine. Complete blood count is normal with the exception of 29% band neutrophils. Erythrocyte sedimentation rate is 24 mm/hour, and stool guaiac is positive.

EPIDEMIOLOGY

Worldwide, approximately 2.5 million children die each year secondary to diarrhea, including 15% of all deaths among children younger than 5 years of age in developing countries. It has been estimated that between 20 and 40 million diarrheal illnesses occur in children younger than the age of 5 years in the United States alone. Only 10% of these episodes require a physician visit and only 1% require hospital admission. Because only a minority of cases of infectious diarrhea require medical attention, data regarding the causes of diarrhea remain unclear. Furthermore, techniques for identifying stool pathogens are limited and cost prohibitive for most cases of uncomplicated and self-limited diarrhea.

Diarrheal illness accounts for only 300 pediatric deaths in the United States yearly, but its social and economic burdens are enormous. Diarrhea accounts for 10% of all pediatric office visits by children younger than 3 years of age, with an associated cost of $0.6 to 1 billion a year.

PATHOPHYSIOLOGY

In a state of health, a balance exists between secretion of water and electrolytes into the gut lumen and absorption into the enterocyte and ultimately the bloodstream. In the small intestine, villus cells are primarily responsible for absorption and crypt cells are primarily responsible for secretion. In the colon, crypt cells secrete a small amount of chloride, and surface cells absorb sodium and water. Normally, this balance favors absorption so that despite relatively high volumes of fluid intake and secretion, the net stool output is small. Multiple molecular transporters and mechanisms are responsible for this balance.

The crypt cells of the small intestine predominantly secrete hydrogen and bicarbonate anions, which allows for passive diffusion of sodium and water into gut lumen. However, this secretion is small compared with the absorption by villus enterocytes. In the villi, the sodium-glucose luminal cotransporter (SGLT-1) transporter couples sodium and glucose absorption, whereas other transporters couple sodium absorption with specific amino acids. A third type of transporter, the Na-hydrogen exchangers (NHEs), exchanges sodium for hydrogen. Sodium is then transported across the basolateral membrane of the enterocyte via Na,K-ATPase. Of note, the integrity of the SGLT-1 transporter during episodes of diarrhea is used to optimize rehydration therapy with fluids containing a balanced ratio of glucose and sodium.

In the colon, the cystic fibrosis transmembrane conductance regulator (CFTCR) likely facilitates chloride and bicarbonate secretion and thus secretion of sodium and water into the colonic lumen. However, a larger amount of sodium absorption, facilitated by the absorption of short-chain fatty acids, results in net absorption of water from the colonic contents.

In disease, one or more mechanisms operate to derange this balance, resulting in a net increase in fluid secretion and thus increased stool output. Increased secretion of anions by crypt cells under the influence of various enterotoxins or derangements in the enteric nervous system can result in secretory diarrhea. Dysfunction of the tight junctions between enterocytes also can allow increased diffusion of water into the gut lumen. Osmotic diarrhea occurs when one or more nutrients fail to be absorbed by the small intestine. These excess particles create an increased osmotic force, causing increased diffusion of water into the stool.

Two additional mechanisms can contribute to the development of diarrhea: inflammation and dysmotility. In cases of invasive intestinal infections, such as those from *Shigella, Salmonella, Yersinia,* and *Campylobacter,* as well as inflammatory bowel disease, inflammation of the small intestinal and colonic mucosa leads to increased stool output. The most common clinical sequela is dysentery, with a small volume of bloody, mucous stools associated with tenesmus, and hypoalbuminemia. Increased intestinal motility can also lead to greater stool output by decreasing the time available for nutrients and water to be absorbed. Causes include thyrotoxicosis, intestinal tumors, and stimulant laxative abuse. Hypomotility, as in pseudo-obstruction and blind loop syndrome, can lead to diarrhea through bacterial overgrowth.

In cases of infectious diarrhea, the exact cause of the imbalance varies depending on the specific pathogen. For example, rotavirus and *Campylobacter jejuni* have a predominant cytopathic effect on enterocytes, resulting in loss of absorptive capacity and increased stool output. Other organisms such as enterotoxigenic *Escherichia coli* and *Vibrio cholerae* increase cyclic nucleotide–mediated secretion through the production of enterotoxins. *Shigella dysenteriae* and *Clostridium difficile* cause cell inflammation and death via cytotoxins. *Giardia lamblia* and enteroadherent *E. coli* may result in malabsorption by adhering to the surface of the villi and directly blocking electrolyte transport. Although any one of these mechanisms may predominate, in most cases of diarrhea, multiple mechanisms are involved.

DIFFERENTIAL DIAGNOSIS

The differential diagnosis of acute diarrhea in children includes both infectious and noninfectious causes. In the case of infectious diarrhea, a wide array of pathogens, including bacteria, viruses, and parasites, can cause similar clinical syndromes (Table 13-1). An understanding of these pathogens and the range of symptoms each can cause is necessary to develop a diagnostic plan. The incidence of the various pathogens is difficult to ascertain, given the current limitations and variations of diagnostic techniques and the lack of methodologically sound epidemiologic studies. In addition, wide variability is present, depending on seasonal and geographic differences. Finally, children with compromised immune systems, secondary to malnutrition, immunodeficiency, or immunosuppressive medications, are susceptible to a broader array of pathogens.

Estimates of the causative agent in cases of acute diarrhea in children are shown in Table 13-2. Of note, no identifiable pathogen is found in approximately 40% of

Table 13-1 Differential Diagnosis of Infectious Diarrhea

Bacterial	Viral	Protozoa
Aeromonas/Plesiomonas	**Nonopportunistic**	**Nonopportunistic**
Bacteroides	Astrovirus	Blastocystis hominis
Campylobacter jejuni	Norwalk virus	Cyclospora cayetanensis
Clostridium difficile	Rotavirus	Entamoeba histolytica
Escherichia coli	Enteric adenovirus	Giardia lamblia
Salmonella	**Opportunistic**	Isospora belli
Shigella	Adenovirus	Cryptosporidium parvum
Staphylococcus aureus	Cytomegalovirus	**Opportunistic**
Vibrio cholerae	Epstein-Barr virus	Cryptosporidium parvum
Yersinia enterocolitica	Human immunodeficiency virus	Microsporida

Table 13-2 Causes of Infectious Diarrhea in Children

Pathogen	Frequency (% of Cases)
None identified	40
Rotavirus	25-40
Calicivirus	10
Adenovirus	4-10
Astrovirus	4-9
Escherichia coli	3-16
Salmonella	3-7
Giardia lamblia	1-15
Campylobacter jejuni	1-8
Cryptosporidium parvum	1-3
Shigella	1-3
Yersinia enterocolitica	1-2
Aeromonas hydrophila	1-2
Entamoeba histolytica	1

cases, using standard laboratory techniques, although the clinical presentation of each pathogen can vary widely. (Table 13-3 categorizes various pathogens by their most common presentations.) Those listed as opportunistic tend to be more common and cause more severe and protracted illness in the immunocompromised. Finally, consideration must always be given to the noninfectious causes of diarrhea that are listed in Table 13-4.

DIAGNOSTIC TESTING

For most cases of uncomplicated acute, watery diarrhea, laboratory examination to seek the causative pathogen is costly and unnecessary. In fact, even when extensive testing is done, a causative agent is found in only 60% to 70% of patients. For hospitalized patients, isolation and contact precautions are recommended to prevent the spread of disease. Testing for specific enteric pathogens may aid in cohorting of patients, if necessary. Rapid testing is available only for rotavirus and C. difficile at most institutions.

However, with dysentery, efforts should be made to identify the causative pathogen. Dysentery is often,

Table 13-3 Common Clinical Presentations of Enteric Pathogens

Acute, Watery Diarrhea	Dysentery	Chronic or Recurrent Diarrhea
Adenovirus	Campylobacter jejuni	Blastocystis hominis
Aeromonas	Clostridium difficile	Cryptosporidium parvum
Astrovirus	Entamoeba histolytica	Cyclospora cayetanensis
Calicivirus	Escherichia coli	Giardia lamblia
Norwalk virus	Plesiomonas	Isospora belli
Rotavirus	Salmonella	
Vibrio cholerae	Shigella	
	Yersinia enterocolitica	

Table 13-4　Noninfectious Causes of Diarrhea
Constipation with encopresis
Carbohydrate malabsorption
Glucose-galactose malabsorption
Lactose intolerance
Laxative abuse
Postinfectious diarrhea
Sucrase-isomaltase deficiency
Fat malabsorption
Cystic fibrosis
Shwachman-Diamond syndrome
Enteropathy
Autoimmune enteropathy
Celiac disease
Crohn's disease
Eosinophilic enteritis
Food allergy
Ulcerative colitis
Structural/anatomic
Lymphangiectasia
Microvillus inclusion disease
Short bowel syndrome
Tufting enteropathy
Motility
Hirschsprung's disease
Pseudo-obstruction
Small bowel bacterial overgrowth
Thyrotoxicosis
"Toddler's diarrhea"
Other
Antibiotic related
Appendicitis
Burns
Immunodeficiency
Radiation enteropathy

Table 13-5　Clinical Clues to Particular Pathogens	
Clinical Feature	**Pathogens**
Daycare attendance	Rotavirus, *Giardia lamblia*, astrovirus
Recent antibiotic use	*Clostridium difficile*
Immunocompromised	Cytomegalovirus (CMV), adenovirus, *Cryptosporidium parvum*
Unpasteurized milk products, exposure to farm animals	*Escherichia coli, Salmonella*
Meningitis, reptile contact	*Salmonella*
Hemolytic anemia, thrombocytopenia	*E. coli O157:H7, Shigella*
Pharyngitis, right lower quadrant pain	*Yersinia enterocolitica*
Dysentery with hepatomegaly or abscess	*Entamoeba histolytica*

although not necessarily, accompanied by crampy abdominal pain, fever, tenesmus, and mucous stools. It is important to note that the presence of melena, blood on the surface of formed stool, or blood detectable only by stool guaiac should not be considered dysentery. Dysentery is most commonly caused by bacterial pathogens that invade the colonic mucosa, causing inflammation and tissue damage. (See Table 13-3 for the various pathogens that can cause dysentery.) Important noninfectious causes include inflammatory bowel disease and enterocolitis.

The choice of diagnostic tests should be guided by each patient's clinical history and presentation. (Clinical clues to particular enteric pathogens are found in Table 13-5.) In addition, some knowledge of the strengths and limitations of common stool tests can help avoid some diagnostic pitfalls (Table 13-6). Figure 13-1 shows an algorithm for the selective use of diagnostic tests. With dysentery, consideration should also be given to evaluating for hemolytic uremic syndrome with blood urea nitrogen, creatinine, and complete blood count.

TREATMENT

Oral Rehydration Therapy

The first step in the management of acute diarrhea is a complete physical assessment. The physical assessment should first focus on establishing the degree of dehydration present (Table 13-7). Although the amount of weight loss can aid in assessing the degree of dehydration, an accurate pre-illness weight is often not available. Thus, the clinician must often rely on other physical signs as well as the reported history of fluid intake and urine output. For infants and toddlers still in diapers, estimates of urine output may be obscured by the presence of watery diarrhea. The presence of tachycardia is often more helpful than blood pressure changes, because many children may not become hypotensive until the onset of cardiovascular collapse. In addition, many of the physical signs outlined in Table 13-7 can be influenced by confounding factors such as room temperature and a child's anxiety during the examination.

Laboratory examinations such as electrolytes, blood urea nitrogen, creatinine, and urinalysis can be helpful in cases in which the physical examination is equivocal or when dehydration of approximately 5% is suspected. However, laboratory testing is usually unnecessary and inaccurate.

Once the degree of dehydration has been established, the proper course of rehydration and ongoing hydration can be established. If severe dehydration is present,

Table 13-6 Laboratory Tests in the Diagnosis of Infectious Diarrhea

Test	Notes
Fecal leukocytes	False-negative results increase if fresh stool samples not examined immediately
Stool guaiac	False-positive results from red meat, vitamin C, non-gastrointestinal bleeding and others; iron does *not* cause false-positive result
Rotavirus EIA	Positive predictive value of positive result affected by wide seasonal variations, of limited use during established outbreaks
Ova and parasites	Three specimens on separate days needed for diagnostic sensitivity >90%, insensitive for *Giardia* and *Cryptococcus*
Giardia EIA	Two samples needed for diagnostic sensitivity >90%
Clostridium difficile toxin assay	Cell culture method has specificity and sensitivity >95%; higher yield for hospital-acquired diarrhea, unhelpful in children <1 year of age
Stool culture	*Escherichia coli* and *Yersinia* require special culture media and may need to be specifically requested; low yield for hospital-acquired diarrhea
Cryptococcus DFA	Cheaper than acid-fast stain
Stool PCR	Most sensitive, not widely available
Entamoeba histolytica Stool EIA	Specificity and sensitivity >95%
Antibodies by IHA	Helpful for those with suspected amebic abscess
CMV, EBV	Serum PCR can provide evidence of disseminated infection, endoscopy with biopsies often needed to confirm diagnosis

CMV, cytomegalovirus; DFA, direct fluorescence antibody; EBV, Epstein-Barr virus; EIA, enzyme immunoassay; IHA, indirect hemagglutination assay; PCR, polymerase chain reaction.

20 mL/kg of normal saline or lactated Ringer's solution should be administered intravenously until perfusion is normalized. The remaining fluid deficit can then be replaced over the next 24 to 48 hours. For children with mild to moderate dehydration, rehydration with 50 to 100 mL/kg of oral rehydration solution (ORS) should be performed over 3 to 4 hours. If the child is unable to tolerate oral liquids, nasogastric administration can be attempted. For patients with no or minimal dehydration, no rehydration therapy is required. Ongoing fluid losses should be replaced in all patients using oral or nasogastric ORS or intravenous fluids, if required. Table 13-8 lists a selection of commercially available products suitable for use as ORS.

Breastfed infants should be allowed to continue breastfeeding during all phases of treatment. Other children should be offered a regular diet after rehydration. Liquids such as sodas and juices should be avoided because they contain excessive amounts of simple carbohydrates and may lead to a secondary osmotic diarrhea. Milk and milk-based formulas should not be limited unless lactose intolerance is clinically evident. In those uncommon cases, lactose-free products such as soy milk or soy-based formulas can be substituted.

Supplemental Therapy

Zinc supplementation with daily doses of two to three times the recommended daily allowance during the first 4 days of a diarrheal illness has been shown to decrease the duration of acute diarrhea and prevent the development of persistent diarrhea in the developing world. Supplementation of vitamin A has been investigated as a preventive therapy, but no protective effect has been shown except in areas with a high prevalence of vitamin A deficiency. The use of antimotility agents is not recommended in children because current data are insufficient to prove any beneficial effects. They are also associated with significant side effects in children, including lethargy, ileus, and coma and may worsen the course of *C. difficile, Shigella, Entamoeba,* and *E. coli* O157:H7 colitis. Bismuth subsalicylate, kaolin-pectin, and fiber are not recommended because of lack of efficacy. Lactobacillus supplementation during diarrheal episodes has been shown only to provide a clinically insignificant decrease in number of stools and diarrhea duration.

Antibiotic Therapy

The use of empiric antibiotics in the treatment of acute diarrhea in children is not recommended. The use of empiric antibiotics should be reserved for the immunocompromised and those with severe life-threatening illnesses. However, antibiotic therapy may be appropriate once a causative pathogen is identified. Indications and recommendations for therapy are shown in Table 13-9.

Public Health

An important element of the care of any patient with infectious diarrhea is the prevention of the spread of the disease to others. Precautions should be taken immediately to isolate hospitalized patients, and specific rigor in

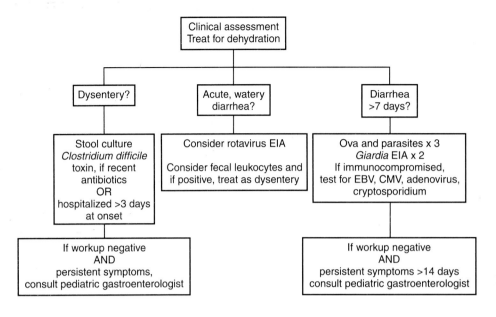

Figure 13-1 Algorithm for diagnosis of infectious diarrhea.

Table 13-7 Physical Assessment for Dehydration

Symptom	Minimal Dehydration	Mild-Moderate Dehydration	Severe Dehydration
Weight	<3% Loss	3%-9% Loss	>9% Loss
Mental status	Alert	Fatigued, restless	Lethargic
Heart rate	Normal	Normal to increased	Increased
Blood pressure	Normal	Normal	Decreased
Mucous membranes	Moist	Dry, tacky	Parched
Capillary refill	Brisk	Prolonged	Prolonged
Extremities	Warm	Cool	Cold, mottled
Urine output	Normal	Decreased	Minimal

Table 13-8 Composition of Commercially Available Electrolyte Solutions

	Sodium (mmol/L)	Chloride (mmol/L)	Potassium (mmol/L)	Base (mmol/L)	Carbohydrate (g/L, Source)	Osmolarity (mOsm/L)
World Health Organization (WHO) Oral rehydration solution (ORS)	75	65	20	30	13.5 glucose	245
Pedialyte (Ross)	45	35	20	30	25 glucose	250
Enfalyte (Mead Johnson)	50	45	25	34	30 rice syrup solids	200
Ceralyte (Cera)	50-90	40-80	20	30	40 long-chain rice solids	220

provider hygiene should be observed. Consideration also should be given to the need for reporting specific infectious pathogens to the local public health department. Although variations in requirements exist in different localities, most nonviral causes of infectious diarrhea are reportable. If doubt exists, providers should contact the local public health department for more information.

APPROACH TO THE CASE

On admission to the hospital, the patient was found to be moderately dehydrated and was given 20 mL/kg of intravenous normal saline. He was allowed to take a regular diet as tolerated, but because of inadequate oral

Table 13-9 Antimicrobial Therapy for Select Causes of Infectious Diarrhea*

Pathogen	Primary Therapy	Alternative	Notes
Blastocystis hominis	Metronidazole 35-50 mg/kg/day ÷ tid × 10 days (max: 2 g/day)	Iodoquinol 30-40 mg/kg/day ÷ tid × 20 days (max: 1.95 g/day) TMP-SMX 6 mg/kg TMP, 30 mg/kg SMX daily × 7 days	Indications for treatment not established
Campylobacter jejuni	Azithromycin 5 mg/kg PO daily × 5-7 days (max: 500 mg/day)	Doxycycline 2-4 mg/kg PO ÷ daily-bid × 5-7 days (max: 200 mg/day)	Early treatment may shorten duration and prevent relapse
Clostridium difficile	Metronidazole 30 mg/kg/day IV/PO ÷ qid × 7-10 days (max: 2 g/day)	Vancomycin 40 mg/kg/day PO ÷ qid × 7-10 days (max: 2 g/day)	Discontinue other antibiotic therapies as soon as possible
Cryptosporidium parvum	Nitazoxanide 12-47 mo: 200 mg ÷ bid × 3 days 4-11 yr: 400 mg ÷ bid × 3 days	Paramomycin 25-35 mg/kg/day PO ÷ bid-qid (max: 3 g/day)	Consider oral IVIG if immunocompromised. Efficacy of antibiotics limited
Cyclospora belli	TMP-SMX 10 mg/kg/day TMP, 50 mg/kg/day SMX ÷ bid × 7-10 days	Ciprofloxacin 25 mg/kg/day ÷ bid × 7 days (max: 1.5 g/day)	Higher doses and longer duration may be needed for immunocompromised patients
Escherichia coli (ETEC or EIEC)	TMP-SMX 12-20 mg TMP/kg ÷ bid-qid × 5-7 days	Azithromycin 5 mg/kg PO daily × 5-7 days (max: 500 mg/day)	Avoid antibiotics for *E. coli* O157:H7 because of risk of HUS
Entamoeba histolytica	Metronidazole 35-50 mg/kg/day ÷ tid × 5-10 days (max: 2 g/day) *and* iodoquinol 30-40 mg/kg/day ÷ tid × 20 days (max: 1.95 g/day) *or* paromomycin 25-35 mg/kg/day PO ÷ bid-qid (max: 3 g/day)	Nitazoxanide 12-47 mo: 200 mg ÷ bid × 3 days 4-11 yr: 400 mg ÷ bid × 3 days	Avoid corticosteroids and antimotility agents Patients with invasive disease require a systemic antibiotic and a luminal amebicide. Use iodoquinol or paromomycin alone for asymptomatic cyst shedders
Giardia lamblia	Metronidazole 15 mg/kg/day ÷ tid × 5 days (max: 2 g/day)	Nitazoxanide 12-47 mo: 200 mg ÷ bid × 3 days 4-11 yr 400 mg ÷ bid × 3 days 12 yr: 1000 mg ÷ bid × 3 days	
Isospora belli	TMP-SMX 10 mg/kg/day TMP, 50 mg/kg/day SMX ÷ bid × 10 days	Ciprofloxacin 25 mg/kg/day ÷ bid × 7 days (max: 1.5 g/day)	Higher doses and longer duration may be needed for immunocompromised.
Salmonella, nontyphoidal	**Amoxicillin, TMP-SMX, cefotaxime, ceftriaxone** based on sensitivities	Ciprofloxacin 25 mg/kg/day ÷ bid × 7 days (max: 1.5 g/day)	Indicated only for those at risk for invasive disease. Treatment may prolong carrier stage
Shigella	**Ampicillin, TMP-SMX** × 5 days based on sensitivities	Ceftriaxone 50-75 mg/kg/day IV/IM daily × 5 days (max: 4 g/day); **ciprofloxacin** 25 mg/kg/day ÷ bid × 5 days (max: 1.5 g/day)	Indicated only for those with severe disease and dysentery, and the immunocompromised. Therapy eradicates organisms in feces and may prevent spread. Avoid antimotility agents
Yersinia enterocolitica	**TMP-SMX, gentamicin, cefotaxime** based on sensitivities	Ciprofloxacin 25 mg/kg/d ÷ bid × 7 days (max: 1.5 g/day)	Indicated only for the immunocompromised

*This chart may contain non–FDA-approved uses of medications.
EIEC, enteroinvasive *E. coli;* ETEC, enterotoxigenic *E. coli;* HUS, hemolytic uremic syndrome; IVIG, intravenous immunoglobulin; TMP-SMX, trimethoprim-sulfamethoxazole.

intake, required supplementation with intravenous D5 ½ normal saline. Stool samples were sent for culture, including *E. coli* and *Yersinia*, ova and parasites, and fecal leukocytes: 2+ neutrophils and 1+ red blood cells were seen on light microscopy.

Because of his right lower quadrant tenderness, fever and bandemia, a computed tomography (CT) scan of the abdomen was obtained. This showed thickening of the cecum and terminal ileum with an unremarkable appendix. After 4 days of continued bloody diarrhea, consultation with a pediatric gastroenterologist was obtained and colonoscopy performed. Biopsies of the colon demonstrated cryptitis and crypt abscesses without architectural distortion, consistent with an acute colitis. Two days later the stool culture became positive for nontyphoidal *Salmonella,* sensitive to ciprofloxacin. The patient was not treated with antibiotics and his symptoms resolved spontaneously over the next 2 days. The county health department was notified of the case, although no definitive source was ever identified.

SUMMARY

Acute diarrhea is a common problem faced by clinicians caring for children. Whereas most cases are likely of viral origin and self limited, the clinician must always be aware of the possibility of other pathogens. For most children, therapy consists of attention to hydration with the use of appropriate oral electrolyte solutions. These solutions not only capitalize on intestinal physiology to maximize fluid absorption but also avoid the creation of a secondary osmotic diarrhea. The presence of bloody diarrhea should increase the clinical suspicion of bacterial pathogens, whereas persistent or recurrent symptoms should prompt a search for parasitic infections. Special consideration should be paid to children with underlying chronic illness, particularly those who are immunocompromised. Although antibiotics may be useful for select pathogens, the empiric use of antibiotics for acute diarrhea in children is not recommended and may lead to increased complications.

MAJOR POINTS

Acute, self-limited watery diarrhea in children is common and requires little, if no, laboratory testing. Treatment should be limited to supportive care, including prevention and treatment of dehydration.

Oral rehydration solutions and the continuation of solid food should be encouraged for most cases of acute infectious diarrhea.

The causative pathogen in all cases of dysentery should be sought with appropriate laboratory tests. Opportunistic pathogens should be sought in cases of diarrhea in immunocompromised children.

Empiric antibiotics should be limited to those with severe systemic disease. Specific antibiotic therapy may be indicated for certain enteric pathogens.

Failure to respond to routine therapy or the development of chronic diarrhea should prompt further evaluation and consideration of referral to a pediatric gastroenterologist.

SUGGESTED READINGS

American Academy of Pediatrics Red Book: 2003 Report of the Committee on Infectious Diseases, 26th ed. Elk Grove Village, Ill, American Academy of Pediatrics, 2003.

Avendano P, Matson DO, Long J, et al: Costs associated with office visits for diarrhea in infants and toddlers. 12:897-902, 1993.

Caeiro JP, Mathewson JJ, Smith MA, et al: Etiology of outpatient pediatric nondysenteric diarrhea: A multicenter study in the United States. 18:94-97, 1999.

Duggan C, Nurko S: "Feeding the gut": The scientific basis for continued enteral nutrition during acute diarrhea. 131: 801-808, 1997.

Glass RI, Lew JF, Gangarosa RE, et al: Estimates of morbidity and mortality rates for diarrheal diseases in American children. 118:S27-S33, 1991.

Grotto I, Mimouni M, Gdalevich M, et al: Vitamin A supplementation and childhood morbidity from diarrhea and respiratory infections: A meta-analysis. 142:297-304, 2003.

King CK, Glass R, Bresee JS, et al: Centers for Disease Control and Prevention. Managing acute gastroenteritis among children: Oral rehydration, maintenance, and nutritional therapy. 52:1-16, 2003.

Strand TA, Chandyo RK, Bahl R, et al: Effectiveness and efficacy of zinc for the treatment of acute diarrhea in young children. 109:898-903, 2002.

Teach SJ, Yates EW, Feld LG: Laboratory predictors of fluid deficit in acutely dehydrated children.[see comment]. 36: 395-400, 1997.

Walker WA: Pediatric Gastrointestinal Disease, 4th ed. New York, BC: Decker, 2004.

Inflammatory Bowel Disease

DOUGLAS JACOBSTEIN

ROBERT BALDASSANO

Disease Description
Epidemiology
Pathophysiology
Clinical Features
Differential Diagnosis
Diagnostic Testing
Treatment
    Nutritional Therapy
    Aminosalicylates
    Corticosteroids
    Antibiotics
    Immunomodulators
        6-Mercaptopurine and Azathioprine
        Methotrexate
        Cyclosporine
        Infliximab
    Surgery
Approach to the Case
Summary
Major Points

DISEASE DESCRIPTION

Inflammatory bowel disease (IBD) represents a spectrum of disorders including ulcerative colitis and Crohn's disease with chronic, idiopathic inflammation of the intestinal tract. Although the specific cause of the disorder is unknown, internal and external environmental factors, genetic predisposition, and an altered immune system all play a role in the development of the disease. Although no cure for IBD currently exists, goals of therapy in pediatrics focus on maintaining long-term remission

CASE PRESENTATION

A 13-year-old female presents with diarrhea, weight loss, and abdominal pain for the past several months. She was previously well until she developed diarrhea. She reports stooling five to eight times per day. Her stools are never formed. Initially there was no blood in her stools, but she notes that over the past few weeks there is some blood mixed with the stool. Her abdominal pain is located in the right lower quadrant and is nonradiating. There have been no fevers. She often feels nauseated but has not vomited. She has lost 10 pounds over the past 3 months. In addition, her mother notes that "she used to be bigger than most of the other girls in her class and now she is one of the smallest." She frequently complains of pain in her right knee. There has been no recent travel and no known sick contacts.

Physical examination reveals a thin, pale female in no acute distress. She is in the 5 to 10 percentile for weight and height. She is anicteric with moist membranes. There are no mouth sores. Lungs are clear; there are no murmurs. Her abdomen is soft with mild tenderness to palpation in the right lower quadrant, and there is no rebound or guarding. Bowel sounds are present. There is no hepatosplenomegaly. Perirectal examination shows two skin tags with no drainage or fistulous tracts. On rectal examination there is a small amount of Hemoccult-positive stool in the rectal vault. Neurologic and musculoskeletal examinations are normal.

EPIDEMIOLOGY

Since the 1930s the incidence of IBD has greatly increased. In the 1950s, ulcerative colitis (UC) was twice as prevalent as Crohn's disease (CD), but recent studies in the United States show that CD has been steadily increasing while ulcerative colitis rates remain more stable. The incidence rate for UC for 10- to 19-year-olds is 2 per 100,000, and the age-specific incidence rate in North America for 10- to 19-year-olds is 3.5 per 100,000 for CD. The incidence of CD has increased in the pediatric age-group. In two population-based surveys, approximately 20% of children and adolescents were less than 10 years of age at diagnosis and 4% presented before 5 years of age. Whereas the overall incidence of CD in females exceeds that of males by 20% to 30%, studies among pediatric populations alone have shown a male predominance. UC appears to affect both sexes equally. There is no simple mendelian genetic mechanism at work in the transmission of IBD, yet multiple familial occurrences are well documented in 15% to 20% of patients. Familial IBD is particularly common with early-onset IBD. For patients diagnosed at younger than age 20 years, 30% had a positive family history. The percentage decreased to 18% for those diagnosed between 20 and 39 years of age, and to 13% among those diagnosed at older than 40 years.

Whites appear to be more commonly affected than nonwhites. CD is also more common among families of middle European origin. It is more common among Jews than non-Jews. Additionally, within the United States, the disease is more common in northern areas than southern areas and urban rather than rural areas. The disease occurs more frequently among patients with Turner's syndrome, Hermansky-Pudlak syndrome, and glycogen storage disease type 1B.

PATHOPHYSIOLOGY

The etiology of inflammatory bowel disease remains unknown. The disease appears to be the result of a combination of antigenic stimulation of an altered immune system in a genetically predisposed individual. The high incidence of disease among first-degree relatives of an affected individual supports the concept of genetic predisposition. The risk of developing CD in monozygotic twins nears 50%, whereas the rate in dizygotic twins is much lower (3.8%). The rate of ulcerative colitis is also higher among monozygotic twins. At diagnosis, there is a 5% to 25% chance of finding inflammatory bowel disease in a first-degree relative of an affected proband, and siblings of a patient with CD are 17 to 35 times more likely to develop CD than the general population. The discovery of the *NOD2/CARD* 15 gene on chromosome 16 further supports the connection between genetics and the environment in the pathophysiology of CD. The gene, which is abnormal in 20% to 30% of pediatric patients with CD, regulates immune responses to bacterial products. Other possible chromosomal susceptibility genes include chromosome 6, which contains the major histocompatability complex and the HLA genes.

The role that infectious agents play in the development of IBD is unclear. To date, no convincing and reproducible evidence has identified a causative organism. Atypical mycobateria were suspected as a possible cause because of the similar pathologic expression of mycobaterial intestinal infection and CD. Other possible bacterial organisms, including *Escherichia coli, Listeria,* and *Streptococcus*, as well as early viral infection with measles have been suggested as stimuli for the disease but none has been identified as the cause. Noninfectious antigenic stimuli, both dietary and environmental, also have been considered as immunotriggers, but to date have not been identified.

Current theories on the development of CD or UC involve a cascade of events that lead to the condition. An antigenic stimulus, either microbial, dietary or environmental, stimulates the active immune system of the intestinal tract. In a normal host this stimulation and subsequent inflammation are self limited and controlled; however, in a genetically predisposed individual, the inflammation is not self limited, and inflammatory mediators are continually produced by activated immune cells, leading to tissue injury and fibrosis. Proinflammatory cytokines including interleukin (IL)-1, IL-6, IL-8, IL-12, and IL-18, as well as tumor necrosis factor-alpha (TNF-α) are found in elevated numbers in affected tissues and serum in patients with CD, and antiinflammatory cytokines such as IL-4 and IL-10 are decreased. These proinflammatory molecules are responsible for the recruitment of inflammatory cells through increased expression of vascular adhesion cell molecules, eosinophil degranulation, induction of nitric oxide synthase in macrophages and neutrophils, and increased collagen production. Inflammatory cell products, including histamine, prostaglandins, and leukotrienes, cause chloride secretion in epithelial cells that contribute to diarrhea.

CLINICAL FEATURES

UC is a diffuse mucosal inflammation limited to the colon; it affects the rectum in approximately 95% of cases, and may extend proximally in a symmetric uninterrupted pattern to involve parts or all of the large intestine. Because UC is a mucosal disease limited to the colon, the most common presenting symptoms are rectal bleeding, diarrhea, and abdominal pain. There are multiple patterns of presentation of UC in the pediatric age-group; 50% to 60% have mild disease. The diarrhea is insidious in onset and later associated with hematochezia. There are no systemic signs of fever, weight loss, or hypoalbuminemia. The disease is usually confined to the distal colon and responds well to therapy. Thirty percent of pediatric patients present with moderate disease characterized by bloody diarrhea, cramps, urgency to defecate, and abdominal tenderness. These patients have associated systemic signs, such as anorexia, weight loss, low-grade fever, and mild anemia. Severe colitis occurs in approximately 10% of patients. This presentation is characterized by more than six bloody stools per day, abdominal tenderness, fever, anemia, leukocytosis, and hypoalbuminemia. Severe hemorrhage, toxic megacolon, and perforation are serious complications in this group of patients. Occasionally, children with UC may have a presentation dominated by extraintestinal manifestations, such as growth failure, arthropathy, skin manifestations, or liver disease. This accounts for less than 5% of the pediatric version of the disease.

Unlike the findings in UC, the intestinal involvement in CD may occur in any portion of the gastrointestinal tract. The presentation is determined primarily by the location and extent of disease involvement. The majority of children have disease involving the terminal ileum (50% to 70%), with more than one half of these patients also having inflammation in varying segments of the colon, usually the ascending colon. Ten percent to 20% of children have isolated colonic disease, and 10% to 15% have diffuse small bowel disease of the more proximal ileum or jejunum. Isolated gastroduodenal disease is uncommon (less than 5% of patients), but there may be endoscopic and histologic evidence of gastroduodenal inflammation in up to 30% to 40% of children with CD. CD involving the small intestine usually presents with evidence of malabsorption including diarrhea, abdominal pain, growth deceleration, weight loss, and anorexia. Initially, these symptoms may be quite subtle, and any one may predominate the clinical picture. The onset of growth failure is usually insidious, and any child or adolescent with persistent alterations in growth should have an appropriate diagnostic evaluation for inflammatory bowel disease. Growth failure may precede the onset of intestinal symptoms by years. There are multiple causes of growth failure in patients with CD, but inadequate nutrient intake is usually present. Anorexia, reduced intake, malabsorption, increased losses, and increased metabolic demands all contribute to poor growth. Small bowel mucosal disease may result in malabsorption of iron, zinc, folate, or vitamin B_{12} deficiency. CD involving the colon may be clinically indistinguishable from UC with symptoms of bloody mucopurulent diarrhea, crampy abdominal pain, and urgency to defecate. Symptoms of painful defecation, bright red rectal bleeding, and perirectal pain may signal perianal disease, which may occur without symptomatic involvement in any other area of the intestinal tract. Perianal involvement includes simple skin tags, fissures, abscesses, and fistulae. The perineum should be inspected in all patients presenting with signs and symptoms of CD, because abnormalities detectable in this region will substantially increase the clinical suspicion of inflammatory bowel disease.

Extraintestinal manifestations can occur in both ulcerative colitis and CD: 25% to 35% of patients with IBD have at least one extraintestinal manifestation. These diseases may be diagnosed before, concurrently with, or after the diagnosis of IBD is made. Extraintestinal manifestations can occur even after colectomy for UC. The presence of extraintestinal manifestations may carry prognostic significance. Patients with UC and extraintestinal manifestations have a significantly higher rate of pouchitis following colectomy and ileoanal anastomosis.

Skin manifestations, which are common in IBD, include erythema nodosum and pyoderma gangrenosum. Erythema nodosum is more common in CD and usually follows the course of the disease. The lesions of erythema nodosum are raised, red, tender nodules that appear primarily on the anterior surfaces of the leg. Pyoderma gangrenosum affects less than 1% of patients with UC and even fewer patients with CD. Pyoderma gangrenosum is often an indolent chronic ulcer that may occur even when the disease is in remission. Aphthous lesions in the mouth are the most common oral manifestation of IBD. This lesion is more common in CD and is commonly associated with skin and joint lesions. Oral lesions appear to parallel intestinal disease in most cases but also may occur before any gastrointestinal symptoms.

Ophthalmologic manifestations occur most frequently, both for CD and UC, when the disease is active. The most common ocular findings are episcleritis and anterior uveitis. The uveitis is usually symptomatic, causing pain or decreased vision. Increased intraocular pressure and cataracts may be seen in children receiving corticosteroid therapy.

Arthritis is the most common extraintestinal manifestation in children and adolescents, occurring in 7% to 25% of pediatric patients. The arthritis is usually transient nondeforming synovitis, asymmetric in distribution and usually involving the large joints of the lower extremities. In adults, the arthritis occurs when the disease is active, but in children the arthritis may occur years before any gastrointestinal symptoms develop. Ankylosing spondylitis occurs in 2% to 6% of patients and is more common in males

Hepatobiliary disease is one of the most common extraintestinal manifestations seen in IBD. It may affect areas from the hepatocytes to the biliary tree, and even extend to the vascular system. As opposed to most other extraintestinal manifestations, hepatobiliary complications may precede the onset of IBD, accompany active disease, or develop after surgical resection of all diseased bowel. Children may first present with liver disease, before any clinical signs of IBD. Abnormal serum aminotransferases are common during the course of IBD in children. Most aminotransferase elevations are transient and appear to relate to medications or disease activity. Persistent aminotransferase elevations (>6 months) should be investigated because the likelihood of serious liver disease is increased. Intrahepatic and extrahepatic manifestations of liver disease occur in children with

IBD. Intrahepatic manifestations include chronic active hepatitis, granulomatous hepatitis, amyloidosis, fatty liver, and pericholangitis. Extrahepatic manifestations include sclerosing cholangitis, and cholelithiasis. Granulomatous hepatitis is rare and is identified by the noncaseating granulomatous lesions on liver biopsy. Pericholangitis could be an early stage of primary sclerosing cholangitis, although few progress to that stage. Sclerosing cholangitis develops in 3.5% of UC pediatric patients and less than 1% of CD pediatric patients. An inexorably progressive disease in adults, it may remain more dormant in children. It is not related to disease activity and may appear years before any gastrointestinal disease develops or even years after a colectomy for UC. Endoscopic retrograde cholangiopancreatography (ERCP) has significantly improved the ability to diagnose this disease in the pediatric population. Cholelithiasis has been described in both UC and CD, but more frequently in CD, especially after ileal resection. Cholesterol and pigment stones occur in patients with IBD.

The urologic manifestations of IBD include nephrolithiasis, hydronephrosis, and enterovesical fistulae. Nephrolithiasis is a common renal complication in pediatrics and occurs in approximately 5% of children with IBD. External compression of the ureter by an inflammatory mass or abscess may lead to hydronephrosis. Enterovesical fistulae, which are more common in boys, may present with recurrent urinary tract infections or pneumaturia.

Thromboembolic disease is an extraintestinal manifestation that occurs in adults as well as children with IBD. It is considered to be the result of a hypercoagulable state that parallels disease activity and is manifested by thrombocytosis, elevated plasma fibrinogen, factor V, factor VIII, and decreased plasma antithrombin III. This may lead to deep vein thrombosis, pulmonary emboli, and neurovascular disease. Vasculitis affecting both the systemic and the cerebral circulation has been described in association with IBD in children. Other extraintestinal manifestations include pancreatitis, fibrosing alveolitis, interstitial pneumonitis, pericarditis, and peripheral neuropathy.

DIFFERENTIAL DIAGNOSIS

Making the diagnosis of IBD is often difficult because of the subtle and varied manner in which it may present. Table 14-1 highlights the lengthy list of diseases that should be considered in the differential diagnosis. Recurrent abdominal pain is a common problem in pediatrics, with 10% of all children complaining of nonspecific periumbilical pain at some time during childhood. Recurrent abdominal pain in children with IBD is generally associated with other problems such as anorexia, growth failure, decreased appetite, diarrhea, or extraintestinal manifestations. Therefore, children with abdominal pain and any of the above problems require a more extensive evaluation for their pain.

Common causes of abdominal pain in children include constipation, functional abdominal pain, lactose intolerance, gastroesophageal reflux, ulcer disease, or urinary tract infection. If the pain is in the right lower quadrant, one must consider appendicitis, lymphoma, intussusception, mesenteric adenitis, Meckel's diverticulum, ovarian cyst, and endometriosis. Causes of abdominal pain associated with rectal bleeding in infancy include Hirschsprung's enterocolitis, intussusception, and allergic colitis. In older children, rectal bleeding may occur in infectious colitis, hemolytic uremic syndrome, Henoch-Schönlein purpura, Meckel's diverticulum, intestinal polyps, hemorrhoids, or anal fissures. Small intestinal lymphoma may manifest with similar clinical and radiographic finding as small intestinal CD. Therefore, it is important to obtain intestinal biopsies at the time of diagnosis.

The differential diagnosis of infectious disease of the gastrointestinal tract mimicking IBD also needs to be considered. *Campylobacter, Yersinia,* and *Aeromonas*

Table 14-1 Differential Diagnosis of Inflammatory Bowel Disease by Symptom

Abdominal pain	Diarrhea
Constipation	Infection
Irritable bowel syndrome	Giardiasis
	Cryptosporidium
Carbohydrate intolerance	Carbohydrate intolerance
	Laxative abuse
Appendicitis	Irritable bowel
Infection	
Mesenteric adenitis	**Bloody diarrhea**
Intussusception	Infection
Lymphoma or other neoplasm	*Clostridium difficile*
	Yersinia enterocolitica
Ovarian cyst	*Campylobacter jejuni*
Peptic disease	*Escherichia coli*
Henoch-Schönlein purpura	*Salmonella*
	Shigella
Diverticulitis	
Rectal bleeding	**Ischemic bowel**
Polyp	Hirschsprung's enterocolitis
Meckel's diverticulum	
Diverticulosis	**Growth delay/weight loss**
Solitary rectal ulcer	Parasitic infection
Fissure	Endocrinopathy
	Anorexia nervosa
Arthritis	Constitutional growth delay
Juvenile rheumatoid arthritis	
Ankylosing spondylitis	
Infection	

can mimic symptoms of IBD. *Clostridium difficile* is an anaerobe that is the causative agent of pseudomembranous enterocolitis. Pseudomembranous enterocolitis has been described following treatment with almost all routine antibiotics used in pediatric practice. Practically speaking, amebiasis is the only parasitic infection in the United States that mimics IBD. This organism is best diagnosed with specific serologic tests that are positive at the time of acute colitis in 90% of patients. Other infectious agents, such as *Cryptosporidium, Giardia,* cytomegalovirus, and *Strongyloides* should be excluded when risk factors exist.

DIAGNOSTIC TESTING

Preliminary workup of suspected IBD should be performed by the primary physician. The importance of the history cannot be overemphasized. History of recent antibiotic intake and family history are important and often overlooked. Abdominal examination is often nonspecific, although a fullness or mass in the right lower quadrant may indicate CD. Rectal examination is important in detecting perianal disease such as fissures or fistulas as well as appraising stool guaiac. A careful assessment of growth and development is an important part of the evaluation of the pediatric patient. Growth abnormalities may be detected by evaluation of several different parameters. These include the measurement of height and weight, including calculations of percent height and weight for age and percent weight for height, measurement of growth velocity, anthropometry to determine body composition, and skeletal bone age to look for delayed bone maturation. The measurement of growth velocity is the most sensitive indicator of growth abnormalities, because a decrease in growth velocity may be seen before the crossing of major percentile lines on standard growth curves.

Laboratory data are also nonspecific. The complete blood cell count may reveal evidence of hypochromic, microcytic anemia, or thrombocytosis. The sedimentation rate is elevated in 90% of patients with CD. The C-reactive protein (CRP) has also recently gained favor as an acute marker of inflammation. Additional testing includes those to assess serum proteins (albumin, transferrin, prealbumin) and micronutrients (folic acid, vitamin B_{12}, serum iron, total iron binding capacity, calcium, magnesium). Antineutrophil cytoplasmic antibody (pANCA) is positive in 19% of patients with CD and 80% of patients with UC. Anti–*Saccharomyces cerevisiae* antibody (ASCA) is positive in 70% of patients with CD. These antibody tests can, at times, help differentiate between UC and CD colitis.

Once infectious causes have been ruled out, it is best for the primary care physician to refer the patient to a pediatric gastroenterologist for further diagnostic evaluation. The next diagnostic study should be flexible colonoscopy with colonic and terminal ileal biopsies as well as esophagogastroduodenoscopy (EGD). The development of flexible small-caliber endoscopes has allowed endoscopic evaluation of pediatric patients of all ages, including infants. Macroscopic findings of aphthous ulcers, cobblestoning, psuedopolyps, erythema, or friability are abnormal and are consistent with IBD. Ulcerative colitis almost always involves the rectum with continuous inflammation, whereas in CD there is rectal sparing and skip lesions. Figure 14-1 shows the representative findings of CD. Microscopically there is evidence of chronic active inflammation with lymphocytes, neutrophils, and/or eosinophils. Often there are crypt abscesses and crypt architectural distortion. Granulomas, although occurring in less than 30% of biopsies, are consistent with CD and do not occur in ulcerative disease. Figure 14-2 shows some of the macroscopic and microscopic findings of ulcerative colitis. A single contrast upper gastrointestinal tract radiologic series with small bowel follow-through studies is then performed to complete the diagnostic workup. Findings of inflammatory bowel disease include nodularity, thickened bowel loops, strictures, ulcers, or fistulas. Figure 14-3 shows narrowing of the terminal ileum consistent with CD. In older children, double contrast radiography (enteroclysis) allows the examination of fine mucosal details to detect early ulceration in the small bowel. Computed tomography and ultrasonography are useful in the assessment of abscesses and fistulae in CD but do not generally play a role in the initial diagnosis.

TREATMENT

The physician or nurse practitioner caring for the pediatric patient with IBD faces many difficult challenges when considering treatment options. Issues including growth, bone development, and sexual maturation should be considered when selecting therapies. General goals for optimizing outcome should achieve the best clinical and laboratory control of disease with the fewest side effects; promote growth through adequate nutrition; and permit the patient to function as normally as possible with consideration for school attendance and participation in activities. Table 14-2 outlines the available therapies for IBD and selected dosing ranges.

Nutritional Therapy

Nutritional therapy in IBD is still underused, although it is gaining wider acceptance. One of the most appealing aspects of nutritional therapy is that it addresses the well-known effects of malnutrition while providing a therapeutic option. Although parental nutrition is tradi-

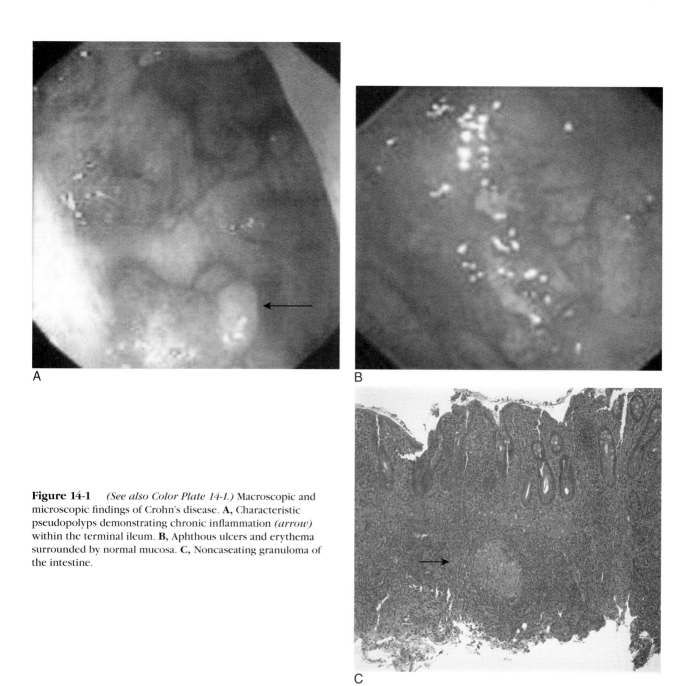

Figure 14-1 *(See also Color Plate 14-1.)* Macroscopic and microscopic findings of Crohn's disease. **A,** Characteristic pseudopolyps demonstrating chronic inflammation *(arrow)* within the terminal ileum. **B,** Aphthous ulcers and erythema surrounded by normal mucosa. **C,** Noncaseating granuloma of the intestine.

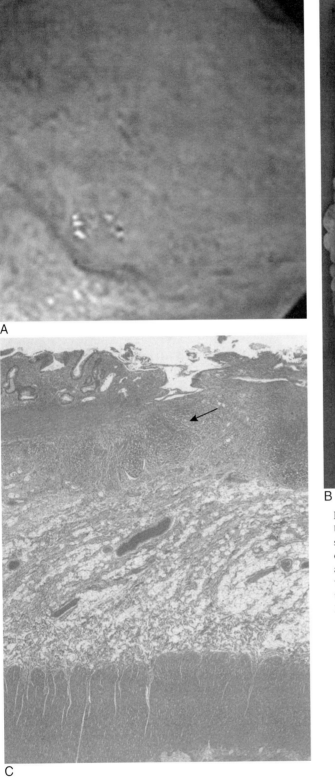
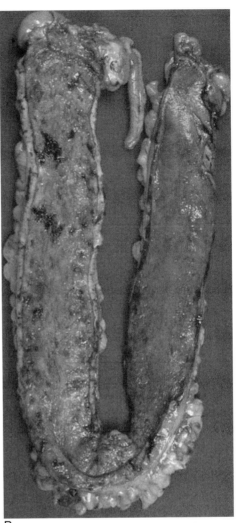

Figure 14-2 *(See also Color Plate 14-2.)* Ulcerative colitis. **A,** Characteristic macroscopic appearance of ulcerative colitis with erythema, continuous irritation, and ulceration. **B,** Colectomy specimen from a patient with ulcerative colitis. **C,** Microscopically there is inflammation located only within the luminal surface.

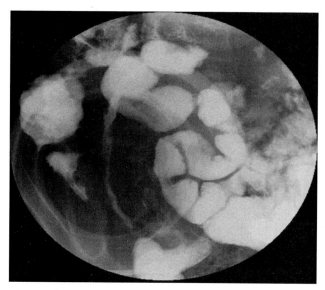

Figure 14-3 Terminal ileal stricture. Upper gastrointestinal series with small bowel follow-through demonstrates a long area of narrowing consistent with a stricture within the terminal ileum.

nutrition represents a more physiologic and safer delivery system. Previous meta-analyses have shown remission rates between 50% and 80% after 4 weeks of exclusive enteral feedings in patients with CD. It should be noted that both TPN and enteral feeding are more effective for CD than for UC, for which these interventions should be reserved for repletion of malnutrition rather than treatment of active disease.

Micronutrient deficiencies are common among patients with IBD despite adequate caloric intake. Practitioners should pay particular attention to the fat-soluble vitamins A, D, and E; selenium, zinc, calcium, folic acid, iron, and vitamin B_{12} also should be monitored. Bone densitometry (DEXA) scans should be obtained, and patients should be monitored for signs of osteopenia and osteoporosis.

tionally reserved for the sickest pediatric patients, enteral nutrition provides needed calories and eliminates dietary antigens that may trigger the immune system.

Perhaps the most basic form of nutritional therapy in IBD is the use of bowel rest and parenteral nutrition. Trials of total parenteral nutrition (TPN) and bowel rest have resulted in clinical remission of CD in adolescents. Response rates as high as 90% have been reported with the use of exclusive TPN, even in steroid-refractory disease. Despite the reported success with TPN, enteral

Aminosalicylates

The aminosalicylates, including sulfasalazine and the newer 5-aminosalicylic acid compounds mesalamine and mesalazine, are first-line drugs with limited anti-inflammatory properties. They are felt to act locally with limited systemic absorption. The primary mechanism of action appears to be the drugs' inhibition of the lipoxygenase pathway of arachidonic acid metabolism. The role for the aminosalicylates has been more clearly established in ulcerative colitis than in CD. Controlled trials have shown proven efficacy in the treatment of mild to moderate ulcerative colitis, whereas the results of their use in CD for both induction and maintenance have been more controversial.

Table 14-2 Pharmacologic Therapy for IBD

	Ulcerative Colitis and Crohn's Disease
Mild disease and remission	Mesalamine (Asacol, Pentasa) 50-100 mg/kg/day divided tid to qid (max: Asacol 4.8 g/day, Pentasa 4 g/day)
	Mesalamine enema (Rowasa) 4 g at bedtime
	Mesalamine suppository (Rowasa) 500 mg at bedtime or bid
	Hydrocortisone enema (Cortenema) daily to bid
	Budesonide enema (Entocort enema 2 g/100 mL daily)
Moderate disease	Metronidazole (Flagyl) 15 mg/kg/day divided tid (max: 1 g/day)*
	Nutritional therapy
	Continue the above therapies with the addition of prednisone, to be tapered depending on clinical remission; 1-2 mg/kg/day, max: 40-60 mg/day
	Budesonide (Entocort) (controlled ileal release) 9 mg daily, may replace prednisone for acute flare*
Refractory disease	Azathioprine (Imuran) 2-2.5 mg/kg/day, daily
	6-Mercaptopurine (Purinethol) 1-1.5 mg/kg/day, daily
	Cyclosporine A (Sandimmune IV or PO) 4-6 mg/kg continuous infusion or bid
	Infliximab (Remicade) 5 mg/kg IV at 0, 2, 6 wk (induction) and then every 8 wk

*For use in the treatment of Crohn's disease only.

Mesalazine appears to be better tolerated than sulfasalazine among children. Nausea and vomiting were more common with sulfasalazine. Other side effects, including pancreatitis, hepatotoxicity, interstitial nephritis, pericarditis, and colitis, have been described with the use of mesalazine. Rash and fever secondary to hypersensitivity can occur and are often linked to the sulfa moiety in sulfasalazine. Because of the limited number of controlled trials among children, dosing guidelines have not clearly been established for the use of the aminosalicylates. There is a trend toward using mesalamine in doses between 50 and 75 mg/kg/day; doses as high as 100 mg/kg/day have been used. Limited availability of liquid preparations for this class of drugs complicates its use among young patients who have difficulty swallowing pills or capsules. For proctitis and distal inflammatory bowel disease, enemas and suppositories are available.

Corticosteroids

Corticosteroids continue to be a mainstay of therapy for acute exacerbations of pediatric IBD. Despite the known long list of side effects, no drug to date has shown a better ability to provide symptomatic relief. Previous studies have shown a 20% to 36% dependency rate among CD patients, and 20% of patients are steroid resistant. There have been no controlled trials using corticosteroids versus placebo among pediatric patients. Previous studies have, however, evaluated enteral nutrition and corticosteroids. Meta-analysis found similar remission rates, close to 85%, among patients using corticosteroids and those treated with enteral nutrition. Recommended dosing for oral corticosteroids is 1 to 2 mg/kg/day to a maximum of 60 mg.

Budesonide, a newer steroid formulation with extensive first-pass hepatic metabolism, has been reported to reduce the unwanted side effects of corticosteroids. Although no placebo-controlled trials have been carried out using this drug in pediatrics, several studies comparing budesonide and prednisolone have been conducted. Although the prednisolone group showed a trend toward being more effective at inducing remission, budesonide demonstrated a better side effect profile, with less adrenal suppression measured by mean cortisol levels and less cosmetic side effects.

Although corticosteroids offer an effective short-term remediation of symptoms for active CD and ulcerative colitis, the side effect profile of this medication prohibits long-term use. Side effects of fluid retention, fat redistribution, hypertension, hyperglycemia, cataracts, and weight gain are well known and appear to be related to dose and duration of therapy. Additionally, bone demineralization and linear growth retardation that also occur with corticosteroid use are more damaging and often more difficult to correct than other unwanted side effects.

Antibiotics

Although bacteria flora have been given a central role in the development of inflammatory bowel disease, the role of antibiotics in the treatment of pediatric inflammatory bowel disease has been studied only on a limited basis. No randomized trials using antibiotics have been published to date. Frequently, the use of antibiotics is reserved for patients with infectious complications of their disease (abscesses or *Clostridium difficile*) and those with significant perirectal involvement.

Side effects such as peripheral neuropathies with the use of metronidazole have been reported in children. Other antibiotics, including the fluoroquinolones, which have demonstrated some efficacy among adult patients with perianal and fistulous CD, have been linked to cartilage damage in laboratory animals.

Immunomodulators

6-Mercaptopurine and Azathioprine

Used for more than 50 years in oncology patients, 6-mecaptopurine (6-MP) and its predrug azathioprine are being used with increasing frequency in pediatric patients with IBD. These medications are converted to 6-thioguanine nucleotides in the liver. This active metabolite then inhibits lymphocyte proliferation by impairing deoxyribonucleic acid (DNA) synthesis. Recent randomized controlled trials have shown significantly shorter duration of steroid use and lower cumulative steroid dose at 6, 12, and 18 months among patients who received 6-MP versus placebo; patients were also maintained in remission longer on 6-MP versus placebo. Dosing of 6-MP should be between 1 and 1.5 mg/kg/day and between 1.5 and 2.5 mg/kg/day for azathioprine.

Given the known side effects of the use of this class of medications, including allergic (pancreatitis, arthralgias, rash, and fever) as well as nonallergic reactions (leukopenia, thrombocytopenia, infection, hepatitis, and malignancy), safety remains a concern when prescribing this drug to pediatric patients. Pediatric studies indicate that side effects occur in 15% to 20% of patients on these medications, and careful monitoring of patients who take azathioprine or 6-MP is required.

Methotrexate

Limited studies have evaluated the use of methotrexate in pediatric IBD, although several adult studies have shown clinical efficacy in inducing and maintaining remission in patients with steroid-dependent and steroid-refractory CD. Recent data in pediatrics suggest that oral methotrexate may be better tolerated and has similar bioavailability to the subcutaneous form.

Side effects include gastrointestinal problems (nausea, anorexia, and diarrhea), headaches, dizziness, fatigue, and mood changes. Additionally, leukopenia, thrombocytopenia, pulmonary toxicity, and opportunistic infections also are possible. Hepatotoxicity, although still a concern, is less common than once believed but still requires careful monitoring.

Cyclosporine

Cyclosporine, developed initially for the prevention of organ rejection, has some role in the treatment of patients with IBD and in particular those patients with refractory, severe ulcerative colitis. Whereas short-term results have been established with cyclosporine, the drug does not appear to alter long-term outcomes. To date, no controlled trials have been conducted using cyclosporine in refractory ulcerative colitis.

Significant side effects are known to occur with the use of cyclosporine. No studies regarding its use in pediatric IBD patients have been done, but side effects including paresthesias, hypertrichosis, renal damage, hypertension, and hepatotoxicity are well described in adult studies.

Infliximab

Infliximab, a humanized, chimeric, monoclonal anti–TNF-α antibody, represents the first biologic agent approved for use in children with IBD. Indications for use include patients with CD that is refractory to corticosteroids and immunomodulators as well as those patients with significant perianal disease or fistulas. Infliximab also has been used with some limited success in pediatric patients with ulcerative colitis. Typical initial dosing is 5 mg/kg given intravenously. Dosing schedules involve the administration of three initial doses given at weeks 0, 2, and 6. Repeat doses are then given every 8 to 12 weeks, provided the patient demonstrated an initial response.

Side effects of the medication, including opportunistic infections such as tuberculosis and herpes zoster, lupus, serum sickness, and malignancies (although rare), have been reported. More common side effects from the medication are infusion reactions. Believed to occur in about 6% of patients who receive infliximab, well-documented reactions include diaphoresis, shortness of breath, blood pressure changes, and tachycardia. Recent studies in pediatrics have focused on the role that human antichimeric antibodies (HACA) play in infusion reactions and efficacy of the medication. The concomitant use of an immunomodulator is believed to provide some protection against the formation of antibodies and thus reduce infusion reactions and promote drug efficacy.

Surgery

Surgical indications in inflammatory bowel disease include uncontrollable bleeding, intractability of disease despite appropriate medical management, perforation, obstruction/stricture, abscess formation, or carcinoma. Although surgery for CD may provide the patient with short-term improvements in disease activity to allow for catch-up growth and progression to puberty, research has shown that disease is likely to recur in almost 50% of patients within 2 to 5 years. Patients who are referred for surgery should understand this and expect to remain on medical therapies in the postoperative period to help delay or prevent recurrence.

Although disease returns in almost 50% of Crohn's patients following surgery, patients with ulcerative colitis fare much better following surgical resection. Colectomy with the creation of an ileoanal pouch is curative for most patients with UC and should be considered for those patients with disease that is unresponsive to medical therapies.

APPROACH TO THE CASE

The patient exhibits some of the clear hallmarks of the presentation of IBD. She has ongoing symptoms of weight loss, abdominal pain, diarrhea, and hematochezia. Physical examination findings of right lower quadrant abdominal pain without rebound or guarding and perirectal skin tags also are suggestive of IBD. The patient should have blood chemistries, a complete blood count, and inflammatory markers including erythrocyte sedimentation rate and CRP measured. Additionally, an infectious process should be ruled out with stool cultures. It is likely that this patient will require upper and lower endoscopies as well as a radiographic study using oral contrast.

SUMMARY

IBD represents a spectrum of disorders involving chronic inflammation of the intestinal tract. Although the classic triad of diarrhea, abdominal pain, and weight loss can be seen, the presentation may be more indolent, and diligence among practitioners is required. Laboratory studies including hypoalbuminemia, anemia, and elevation of inflammatory markers (CRP or erythrocyte sedimentation rate [ESR]) are suggestive of the diagnosis; however, ultimately the diagnosis is made based on radiographic and/or endoscopic findings. Presently, no cure exists for IBD. Medications are aimed at minimizing symptoms and maximizing the growth potential for children with the disease.

MAJOR POINTS

The incidence of IBD continues to rise and is more prevalent in developed nations than in Third World countries.

The specific pathophysiology of IBD is unknown. The disease is believed to be due to an interplay of environmental factors and immunoregulatory factors in a genetically predisposed individual.

UC causes diffuse mucosal inflammation limited to the colon, whereas CD can occur anywhere within the gastrointestinal tract.

Patients with UC commonly present with rectal bleeding, abdominal pain, and diarrhea.

The presentation of CD is more varied and depends on the location of the disease within the intestinal tract.

The classic triad of abdominal pain, diarrhea, and weight loss occurs in only 30% of patients diagnosed with CD.

Extraintestinal manifestations of IBD are common and can include skin findings, arthralgias/arthritis, fever, nephrolithiasis, ophthalmologic disorders, hematologic problems, and hepatobiliary disease.

Gastrointestinal infections can mimic symptoms of IBD and should be ruled out before making a diagnosis.

The findings of hypoalbuminemia, microcytic anemia, or an elevation of the CRP or ESR are suggestive but not diagnostic of IBD.

The gold standard for diagnosis is based on classic microscopic findings of chronic inflammation on endoscopic biopsies.

Radiographic studies including upper GI with small bowel follow-through, abdominal computed tomography (CT) scans, and magnetic resonance imaging (MRI) are useful adjunctive tests when making the diagnosis.

General goals for selecting therapeutics should focus on achieving the best clinical and laboratory control of disease with the fewest side effects; promote growth through adequate nutrition; and permit the patient to function as normally as possible with consideration for school attendance and participation in activities.

SUGGESTED READINGS

Baldassano RN, Piccoli DA: Inflammatory bowel disease in pediatric and adolescent patients. Gastroenterol Clin North Am 28:445-445, 1999.

Escher JC, Taminiau JAJM, Nieuwenhuis EES, et al: Treatment of inflammatory bowel disease in childhood: Best available evidence. Inflamm Bowel Dis 9:34-58, 2003.

Griffiths AM: Inflammatory bowel disease. Nutrition 14: 788-791, 1998.

Griffiths AM, Ohlsson A, Sherman PM, et al: Meta-analysis of enteral nutrition as a primary treatment of active Crohn's disease. Gastroenterology 108:1056-1067, 1995.

Hendrickson BA, Gokhale R, Cho JH: Clinical aspects and pathophysiology of inflammatory bowel disease. Clin Micro Rev 15:79-94, 2002.

Hyams JS: Crohn's disease in children. Pediatr Clin North Am 43:255-277, 1996.

Hyams JS: Extraintestinal manifestations of inflammatory bowel disease in children. J Pediatr Gastroenterol Nutr 19: 7-21, 1994.

Kirschner BS: Differences in the management of inflammatory bowel disease in children and adolescents compared to adults. Neth J Med 53:S13-S18, 1998.

Kirschner, BS: Growth and development in chronic inflammatory bowel disease. Acta Paediatrica Scand Suppl 366:98-104, 1990.

Mamula P, Markowitz JE, Baldassano RN: Clinical features and natural history of pediatric inflammatory bowel diseases. In Sartor RB, Sanborn WJ (eds): Kirsner's Inflammatory Bowel Diseases. Philadelphia, Saunders, 2004.

Mamula P, Markowitz JE, Baldassano RN: Inflammatory bowel disease in early childhood and adolescence: Special considerations. Gastroenterol Clin North Am 32:967-995, 2003.

Markowitz J, Grancher K, Kohn N, et al: A multicenter trial of 6-mercaptopurine and prednisone in children with newly diagnosed Crohn's disease. Gastroenterology 119:895-899, 2000.

Podolsky DK: Inflammatory bowel disease. N Engl J Med 347:417-429, 2002.

Seidman E, LeLeiko N, Ament M, et al: Nutritional issues in pediatric inflammatory bowel disease. J Pediatr Gastroenterol Nutr 12:424-438, 1991.

Intussusception

JANICE A. KELLY

Disease Description
Case Presentation
Epidemiology
Pathophysiology
Differential Diagnosis
Diagnostic Testing
Treatment
Approach to the Case
Summary
Major Points

DISEASE DESCRIPTION

Intussusception occurs when a portion of the digestive tract becomes telescoped into the adjacent bowel segment. The intussuscipiens (the receiving loop) contains the folded intussusceptum (the donor loop), which has two components—the entering limb and the returning limb.

CASE PRESENTATION

A 10-month-old female is referred to the emergency department for abdominal pain, vomiting, and bloody stools. Physical examination was unremarkable except for currant-jelly stools on rectal examination and intermittent lethargy. On further questioning, the parents mentioned that the child had one prior episode of similar symptoms, at 8 months of age, which seemed to resolve after 6 hours.

EPIDEMIOLOGY

Intestinal intussusception is the most common abdominal emergency in children less than 2 years of age, and is the second most common cause of intestinal obstruction after pyloric stenosis. Most cases (approximately 90%) begin near the ileocecal valve. The incidence rate for intussusception for children younger than 24 months of age has been described as 33 per 100,000. Approximately 76% of cases are in children less than 12 months of age. Although not confined to children, the peak incidence of intussusception is between 4 and 14 months of age, when most cases are idiopathic, although benign lymphoid hyperplasia may act as a lead point. In older children, a pathologic lead point, such as a Meckel's diverticulum, may be found. A male predominance is described in a ratio of 3:2.

The duration between onset of symptoms and medical examination averaged 21 hours in one study. Irritability, vomiting, and bloody stools were the most common presenting signs or symptoms. The triad of vomiting, bloody stools, and abdominal mass was present in only 20 of 86 children (23%) in one series. Peritonitis, with shock, was detected in 1 out of 95 children, who also had necrosis of the intestine at surgery. Initial diagnosis was based on clinical findings in 42% of children, ultrasound in 31%, and radiography in 22%. The most common site was ileocolic, regardless of age at presentation. Recurrence was the only complication noted in one series for the children whose intussusception was resolved by enema, and it occurred more frequently in these cases than in cases resolved by surgery.

PATHOPHYSIOLOGY

Idiopathic childhood intussusception is considered to result from hyperplasia of lymphoid tissue (Peyer's patches) in the distal ileum. An identifiable lead point or pathologic lead point in an intussusception has been reported to occur in 1.5% to 12% of children with intussusception. A higher number of lead points is found in young infants and children older than 3 years of age.

Intussusception is an invagination of the bowel lumen with the invaginated portion (the intussusceptum) passing distally into the ensheathing outer portion (the intussuscipiens) via peristalsis. There are four types: ileocolic, ileo-ileocolic, colo-colic, and ileo-ileal. The majority of intussusceptions are ileocolic, and the intussusception is usually found along the course of the ascending colon. However, during reduction, the intussusceptum may be encountered as far distal as the sigmoid.

Intussusception causes compression of the intramural and mesenteric veins, leading to edema and hemorrhage in the bowel wall. Eventually, arterial inflow is impaired and ischemia and infarction follow. This precipitates the typical lower gastrointestinal (GI) bleeding, or currant-jelly stool, which is believed to be a mixture of blood, stool, and mucoid exudates.

The typical presentation is an infant who is drawing his or her legs up to the abdomen with bouts of colicky pain, with associated vomiting, pallor, poor perfusion, and passage of currant-jelly stool. These bouts are separated by periods of apathy. These features are typical but are present in only perhaps 30% to 60% of patients. Up to 20% of infants have no obvious pain. An abdominal mass, described as sausage-like, may be present on examination.

DIFFERENTIAL DIAGNOSIS

Most cases are labeled idiopathic because there is no obvious predisposing lesion or lead point. Some cases may be secondary to hypertrophied Peyer's patches in the ileal region, secondary to presumed viral infections, most often enteric adenovirus, that act as lead points. Other specific causes are listed in Table 15-1. Lead points are more common in older children.

Table 15-1 Specific Causes of Intussusception

Intestinal lymphoid hyperplasia	Ventriculoperitoneal shunt
Intramural hematoma	Meckel's diverticulum
Cystic fibrosis (inspissated stool)	Hemangioma
	Parasites
Lymphoma or other neoplasm	Adhesions
	Postsurgical
Henoch-Schönlein purpura	
Polyps (Peutz-Jeghers syndrome, juvenile polyps)	
Hemolytic uremic syndrome	

DIAGNOSTIC TESTING

Plain x-rays are not required. Ultrasound has been suggested as a screening test, but its sensitivity and specificity are unclear. On ultrasound, the intussusception in transverse section has a hypoechoic outer ring and a hyperechoic center, which is known as the target or doughnut sign. The hypoechoic layer represents the edematous bowel, whereas the echoic center represents the mucosa and trapped intraluminal contents. Multiple layers represent an ileo-ileocolic lesion (Fig. 15-1). Currently, a contrast (air or radiopaque) enema under fluoroscopy is the accepted diagnostic test. This should be performed whenever the diagnosis is suspected. A contrast enema is performed to confirm the diagnosis, and to attempt a nonoperative reduction by hydrostatic pressure via a barium column or air pressure (Figs. 15-2 and 15-3). The absolute contraindications to attempted nonoperative reduction are clinical signs of peritonitis or pneumoperitoneum on plain x-ray or fluoroscopy. Some clinicians feel pneumatic reduction is quicker, cleaner, and perhaps safer if perforation were to occur.

TREATMENT

Nonoperative reduction is the treatment of preference. A plain abdominal x-ray must be done first to check for signs of free air, perforation, or intestinal infarction before any attempts at reduction. Patients will require fluid resuscitation and careful monitoring for development of third spacing of fluid, shock, and sepsis.

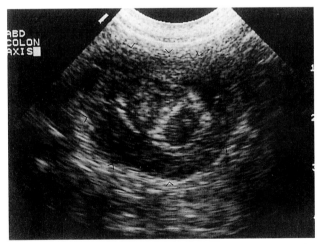

Figure 15-1 Transabdominal ultrasound shows target-like (*arrowheads*) appearance of intussusception. (Photo courtesy of Altschuler SM, Liacouras CA (eds): Clinical Pediatric Gastroenterology, Philadelphia, Churchill Livingstone, 1998, p 473, with permission.)

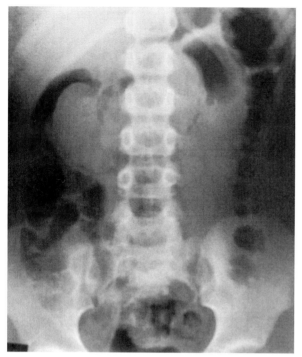

Figure 15-2 Abdominal x-ray shows an intussusception in the right upper quadrant; distal colonic gas defines the intussusceptum. (Photo courtesy of Altschuler SM, Liacouras CA (eds): Clinical Pediatric Gastroenterology, Philadelphia, Churchill Livingstone, 1998, p 536, with permission.)

Air or barium may be used as a contrast agent, with success rates approaching 70% with experienced radiologists. Fluoroscopic monitoring of reduction is favored, but hydrostatic reduction using water or water-soluble contrast agent and ultrasound is sometimes used. Confirmation of reduction is witnessed by the presence of contrast or air in the small bowel. Sometimes this doesn't occur if the ileocecal valve is edematous. However, by itself, this finding is not an indication for surgery. This situation should prompt continued observation of the patient. A successful reduction is evidenced by recovery and absence of pain. If symptoms persist, a repeat attempt at reduction may be successful.

Intussusception reduction is painful, and should be performed with adequate analgesia. For cases of repeated bouts of intussusception, or clinically symptomatic, persistent intussusception that has failed attempts at reduction, surgical exploration is required to relieve the intussusception and isolate any potential lead point.

APPROACH TO THE CASE

The second episode prompted a barium enema, which showed a midtransverse ileocolic intussusception, which was reduced by an air enema. The barium

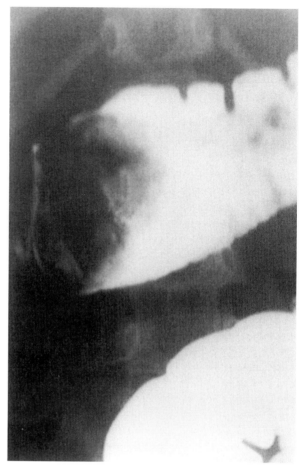

Figure 15-3 Barium enema shows intussusception (indenting the column of contrast) in the transverse colon. (Photo courtesy of Altschuler SM, Liacouras CA (eds): Clinical Pediatric Gastroenterology, Philadelphia, Churchill Livingstone, 1998, p 473, with permission.)

enema revealed multiple, small, round filing defects along the right transverse colon and ascending colonic areas consistent with lymphoid hyperplasia.

All patients with suspected intussusception should have an assessment of vital signs and overall clinical status. These patients are at risk for third spacing and shock. Intravenous access should be obtained, and intravenous hydration begun. The patient should be clinically reassessed periodically, especially before any attempts at reduction of the intussusception to ensure that their clinical condition has not deteriorated. This patient was in a typical age group for intussusception, and had typical presenting features, as well.

Because the patient appeared clinically stable, a barium enema was performed to assess for a lead point, and more important, as a possible therapeutic procedure. The radiographic findings were consistent with lymphoid hyperplasia, the most typical cause for intussusception. Because the procedure was well tolerated and was able to reduce the intussusception, surgery was not required. Some physicians might argue the need for exploratory surgery to rule out a lead point, but because lymphoid hyperplasia is the most common etiology, a conservative course could also be argued.

After a discussion about the treatment options, the parents elected to start a tapering course of steroids. A repeat barium enema 2 months later showed a marked decrease in lymphoid hyperplasia. No further episodes were noted over a 2-year follow-up period.

SUMMARY

Intussusception is the most common abdominal emergency in children younger than 2 years of age. Symptoms include vomiting, waves of abdominal pain, bloody stools, altered mental status, and in some cases, a shock-like state. The majority of cases occur in children younger than 12 months of age. Barium or air enema is most commonly used to attempt to reduce the intussusception. The vast majority of cases do not have a pathologic lead point as a cause, with the most common etiology being benign lymphoid hyperplasia. A small number have recurrent bouts of intussusception. If barium enema fails to reduce the intussusception in a symptomatic patient, surgery is indicated.

MAJOR POINTS

Intussusception is the most common abdominal emergency in children younger than 2 years of age.
Of all cases, 76% occur in children younger than 12 months of age.
There is a 3:2 male predominance.
The classic symptoms are vomiting, abdominal pain, and bloody stools.
Some cases can be associated with shock.
Diagnostic tests include a barium or air contrast enema.
Evidence of intestinal perforation or infarction is an absolute contraindication to a barium or air enema.
The majority of cases can be reduced by barium or air enema.
Cases that fail to reduce by enema, and remain symptomatic, require surgery.
Patients can have recurrent episodes of intussusception (10% of cases); this is more likely to occur in patients who had a barium or air reduction, rather than a surgical correction.
Only about 10% of cases have an actual pathologic lead point as a cause for their intussusception.
The vast majority of cases result from benign lymphoid hyperplasia.

SUGGESTED READINGS

Carty H: Paediatric emergencies: Non-traumatic abdominal emergencies. Emerg Radiol 12:2835-2848, 2002.

del-Pozo G, Albillos JC, Tejedor D, et al: Intussusception in children: Current concepts in diagnosis and enema reduction. Radiographics 19:299-319, 1999.

Harty M, Meyer, J: Plain abdominal radiography. In Altschuler S, Liacouras C (eds): Clinical Pediatric Gastroenterology. Philadelphia, Churchill Livingstone, 1998, p 535.

Jones R, Schirmer B: Intestinal obstruction, pseudo-obstruction, and ileus. In Sleisenger M, Fordtran JS (eds): Gastrointestinal and Liver Disease: Pathophysiology, Diagnosis, and Management. Philadelphia, WB Saunders, 1989, p 372.

Navarro O, Dugougeat F, Kornecki, A, et al: The impact of imaging in the management of intussusception owing to pathologic lead points in children. Pediatr Radiol 30:594-603, 2000.

O'Ryan M, Luccro Y, Pena A, et al: Two year review of intestinal intussusception in six large public hospitals of Santiago, Chile. Pediatr Infect Dis J 22:717-721, 2003.

Shteyer E, Koplewitz BZ, Gross E, et al: Medical treatment of recurrent intussusception associated with intestinal lymphoid hyperplasia. Pediatrics 3:682-685, 2003.

Stringer, D: Radiography: Contrast studies. In Walker WA, Durie P (eds): Pediatric Gastrointestinal Disease: Pathophysiology, Diagnosis, Management, vol 2, 2nd ed. St. Louis, Mosby-Year Book, 1996, pp 1703-1705.

Snyder J: The Surgical Abdomen. In Walker, Goulet (eds): Pediatric Gastroenterology, 4th ed. Philadelphia, BC Decker, 1989, p 609.

Lactose Intolerance

RAMAN SREEDHARAN

JOHN TUNG

Disease Description
Case Presentation
Epidemiology
Pathophysiology
Differential Diagnosis
Diagnostic Testing
    Lactose Breath Test
    Stool pH and Reducing Sugars
    Disaccharidases
Treatment
Approach to the Case
Summary
Major Points

DISEASE DESCRIPTION

Lactose intolerance occurs when the ability of the gastrointestinal (GI) tract to digest lactose is impaired. Lactose is a disaccharide sugar found in milk and is produced exclusively by the mammary glands of mammals. The digestion of lactose depends on the small intestinal brush border enzyme lactase-phlorizin hydrolase (lactase). Low levels of lactase enzyme result in indigestion of the lactose sugar. The undigested lactose increases the osmotic force in the bowel lumen and is fermented by the intestinal flora in the colon. The effects of the increased osmotic force and the products of fermentation of lactose together produce the symptoms of lactose intolerance, which are bloating, diarrhea, flatulence, and cramping.

CASE PRESENTATION

An 11-year-old African American boy presents with complaints of recurrent abdominal pain of 6 months' duration. His mother is unsure when the symptoms started but feels that the symptoms are getting worse. She states that the pain is episodic in nature and lasts 15 minutes to 1 hour. The pain is described as "cramps" throughout the abdomen. Sometimes there is relief on defecation. There is no history of constipation, although at times the stools are loose with flatulence. He complains of "feeling full," with belching. There is no history of vomiting or weight loss and his appetite has been normal. Even though he has a preference for nonvegetarian food, according to his mother his diet is well balanced and includes vegetables, fruits, and milk.

The past medical history is only significant for a broken arm at 6 years of age. There are no allergies. He is currently not on any medications. All the immunizations are up to date.

Physical examination reveals normal vital signs. Height is at the 50th percentile and the weight is at the 75th percentile. Gastrointestinal system examination reveals a nondistended abdomen that is soft and nontender with no palpable masses. The bowel sounds are normal. Rectal examination is normal and the occult blood negative. Examinations of the other systems also are within normal limits.

EPIDEMIOLOGY

Lactose intolerance is found in a variety of settings. There are approximately 50 million people in North America afflicted with lactose intolerance. Lactose intolerance can be found in the following:

1. *Congenital lactase deficiency:* In this rare condition, the expression of lactase is congenitally very low or absent. This condition is extremely rare and is inherited in an autosomal recessive manner, which manifests in the neonatal period with the symptoms of diarrhea and malabsorption. Because the neonate relies primarily on milk intake, this condition is potentially

lethal. Timely diagnosis and lactose-free formula are lifesaving.

2. *Primary lactase deficiency (adult type hypolactasia)* (Table 16-1).

Primary lactase deficiency is most commonly seen after 5 years of age and is genetically predetermined. However, the decline in the lactase levels starts only after the weaning suckling transition is well past, usually after 5 years of age. In this situation, the child is no longer reliant solely on milk for nutrition, thus this is not a lethal condition. The loss of lactase occurs in a mosaic pattern, as the expression of the lactase-phlorizin hydrolase protein is lost in some enterocytes and not others. Studies have shown that loss of lactase-phlorizin hydrolase is not due to the cessation of milk intake but is regulated at the transcriptional level.

As the loss increases, the phenotypic expression of lactose intolerance is seen. This loss is more marked in some races, especially in African American and Asian children. In these children, lactase levels falls to as low as 5% to 10% of the levels present at birth. In most adults there is still some expression of this protein and a limited ability to absorb lactose. Because the condition of lactose intolerance is present in the majority of humans, we should consider the condition of lactose intolerance to be normal. The cultural-historical hypothesis implies that some humans from dairy-predominant cultures have evolved mutations that allow the persistence of the lactase-phlorizin hydrolase protein into adulthood. This trait is believed to be inherited in an autosomal dominant fashion. Some ethnic groups have adapted to lactose intolerance by removal of lactose from milk. Some African tribes consume fermented yogurt, called *Nono,* and many people in India eat yogurt; in both these foods, the fermentation process reduces the lactose content in milk.

3. *Secondary or acquired lactase deficiency:* The enzyme lactase-phlorizin hydrolase is expressed on the enterocyte at the tips of the microvilli of small intestinal mucosa. If there is significant injury to a large surface area of the small intestinal mucosa, it can lead to secondary lactase deficiency by reducing enterocyte lactase expression. Causes for mucosal injury leading to secondary lactase deficiency include gastroenteritis, parasitic infestation, radiation enteritis, drug-induced enteritis, celiac disease, Crohn's disease, and bacterial overgrowth.

On recovery, it takes about 3 days for the premature enterocytes to migrate from the crypts and differentiate into mature enterocytes that express lactase-phlorizin hydrolase at the brush border of the villi. In conditions in which there is rapid intestinal transit, there will be inadequate time for lactase-phlorizin hydrolase to hydrolyze the lactose sugar, resulting in lactose intolerance.

PATHOPHYSIOLOGY

Regardless of the type or nature of the deficiency, the pathophysiology leading to the symptoms in lactose intolerance is the same. The nonhydrolyzed lactose increases the osmotic pressure in the small intestine, thereby drawing water into the lumen. This stimulates the peristalsis and shortens the transit time, which further impairs absorption. The effects are manifested as bloating, cramps, pain, and borborygmi. Lactose that reaches the colon is fermented by the intestinal flora, producing gas (hydrogen, carbon dioxide, and methane) and short-chain fatty acids (acetate, butyrate, and propionate). The effect of this is distention of the bowel and acidity that stimulates peristalsis in the colon. These events manifest as bloating, flatulence, cramps, pain, and diarrhea. The increased osmotic effect due to undigested lactose draws water into the bowel, and the increased peristalsis decreases transit time and absorption, leading to diarrhea.

There is a wide variability in the presentation of symptoms among individuals with lactose intolerance. This depends on a number of factors including lactose intake, lactase activity, gastric emptying, intestinal motility, other foods that influence the bowel content and motility, and the intestinal flora. Many individuals with lactose intolerance will cope with all the symptoms without complaint but present with abdominal distention, cramping, and pain. Always consider lactose intolerance in children who present with recurrent abdominal pain. The intestinal microflora can be different among different individuals; hence the degree of fermentation of lactose is variable, leading to a spectrum of manifestations. People with

Table 16-1 Incidence of Lactose Intolerance in Adults of Different Ethnicities

Ethnic Group	% Intolerant
African black	97-100
Dravidian Indian	9-100
Mediterranean	6-90
North/Central India	25-50
Middle European	10-20
Asian	90-100
Mexican	70-80
Jewish	60-80
Northwest India	3-15
Northern European	1-5
North American Indian	8-90
South American Indian	70-90
African American	7-75
North American white	7-15
Pakistan	3-15

Adapted from Breath Tests & Gastroenterology, QuinTron Instrument Company, 1998, Milwaukee, WI, USA.

inherent slow motility of the bowel and prolonged transit time probably may have more time for absorption and may have less severe symptoms.

DIFFERENTIAL DIAGNOSIS (Table 16-2)

Symptoms of bloating, belching, cramps, pain, flatulence, and diarrhea can be seen in different combinations in a variety of disorders. A detailed history is essential for making a clinical diagnosis. The physical examination primarily helps to eliminate other diagnoses because there are no specific physical findings that will give the diagnosis of lactose intolerance.

DIAGNOSTIC TESTING

Lactose Breath Test (Figs. 16-1, 16-2, and 16-3)

Definitive diagnosis of lactose intolerance is made by breath hydrogen test. This is a safe and noninvasive test. The patient is fasted and a lactose load (2 g/kg to a maximum of 50 g) is fed orally. End-expired air is collected every 15 minutes for the next 2 to 3 hours, and the hydrogen concentration in each sample is measured and plotted on a graph. A peak hydrogen level of 20 parts per million (ppm) above the baseline is considered a positive test.

Bacterial fermentation of carbohydrate substrate in the colon produces hydrogen that increases in the expired gas after a test dose of lactose is given to the patient. H_2 is found in the breath of normal nonfasting children after a carbohydrate meal. In normal people, it is estimated that 8% to 10% of carbohydrates from bread and 22% red lentil beans will enter the colon. To ensure a successful test, patients must fast for at least 12 hours the night before the study.

The basal fasting breath H_2 in normal subjects is usually less than 10 ppm, although in some studies values of up to 40 ppm have been found to be normal. The fi-

Table 16-2	Differential Diagnosis of Lactose Intolerance

Celiac disease
Tropical sprue
Irritable bowel syndrome
Parasitic infestations
Food allergy
Viral infections
Bacterial infections
Pancreatic insufficiency
Laxative abuse
Whipple's disease
Sucrase-isomaltase deficiency
Excessive juice intake

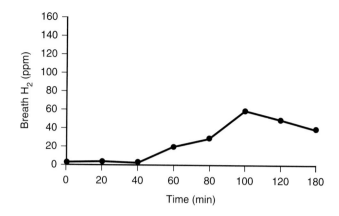

Figure 16-1 Lactose intolerance breath testing.

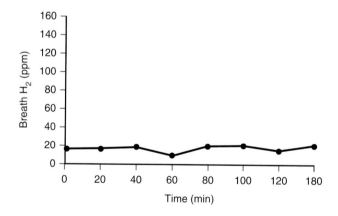

Figure 16-2 Elevated basal breath hydrogen as a result of carbohydrate loading the night before testing.

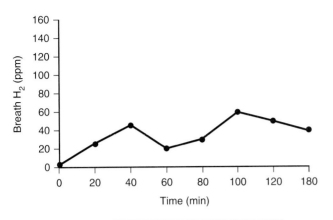

Time (min)	Breath H$_2$ (ppm)
0	3
20	25
40	45
60	20
80	30
100	60
120	50
180	40

Figure 16-3 Double peak as a result of small bowel bacterial overgrowth.

Component Value	Flag	Low	Units Stat
Lactase activity	2.5	15.5	uMol/min/g protein
Maltase activity	230.9	101.1	uMol/min/g protein
Sucrase activity	82.8	25.8	uMol/min/g protein
Palatinase activity	17.6	7.9	uMol/min/g protein
Glucoamylase activity	11.6	8.8	uMol/min/g protein

Figure 16-4 Disaccharidase analysis, which shows lactase-phlorizin hydrolase deficiency.

ber content in the diet may also contribute to differences, as seen in Indians in Asia who have a higher fiber content in their diets (basal H$_2$ mean of 21 ppm) compared with Asian Indians who have migrated to the United States (mean 12 ppm). Younger children who have a higher colonization of bacteria may have higher fasting breath H$_2$ levels with a higher interindividual variation than older children

Our advice to our patients is to have a 12-hour fast, following a diet that is not rich in fiber and slowly digested foods the day before. We also exclude patients who have had recent antibiotic treatment, which can alter the bowel flora. Excessive bacterial colonization of the small intestine can give rise to an early peak in breath hydrogen in addition to a later peak when the lactose reaches the colon.

There are some instances of false-negative tests. Recent antibiotic treatment alters the bowel flora and may alter the test. Also, decreased intestinal motility, decreased transit time, bacterial overgrowth, smoking, and crying can affect the test results.

The addition of methane measurement appears to increase the sensitivity of breath testing because bacteria metabolizes carbohydrates to produce acids, water, and gases. Gases produced include carbon dioxide (CO$_2$) and hydrogen (H$_2$). Some patients with lactose malabsorption do not produce H$_2$ but will generate CH$_4$ instead and such patients will be detected if the testing also measures methane in addition to hydrogen. Some breath-testing equipment such as the QuinTron Microlyzer (QuinTron Instrument Company, Milwaukee, WI) Model P can also measure methane output, whereas others will measure only breath hydrogen.

Stool pH and Reducing Sugars

These tests are indirect tests for lactose intolerance and are not specific.

Disaccharidases (Fig. 16-4)

Direct estimation of lactase levels from jejunal biopsy specimens obtained by endoscopy or capsule biopsy is an invasive method for making the diagnosis. Biopsy specimens from the duodenum may not be very reliable because the lactase activity can be patchy in the duodenum.

The lactose tolerance test, which measures blood glucose levels before and after a lactose diet, requires a fasted patient to have basal fasting blood sugar as a baseline; a slight increase in blood glucose is an indirect indicator of lactase activity. This test requires the monosaccharide transport system to be functioning (lactase splits lactose into the monosaccharides glucose and galactose), and any irregularity with this can affect the test and give an abnormal test result.

TREATMENT

Milk is an important source of nutrients, especially calcium, in an American diet. The Recommended Dietary Allowance (RDA) for calcium for pregnant women and nursing mothers is 1200 to 1500 mg/day; for men, 1000 mg/day; for adolescents and young adults 1200 to 1500 mg/day; and for postmenopausal women 1000 to 1500 mg per day. Adequate calcium intake should be ensured in lactose-intolerant patients. Yogurt is an excellent source of calcium for many lactose-intolerant people because the fermentation process reduces the lactose in the milk.

Commercially available lactase (LactAid, Lactase) changes the lactose to glucose and galactose. It is a yeast-derived β-D-galactosidase in a glycerol carrier; four or five drops are added to a quart of milk. After 24 hours, 70% of the lactose is converted to glucose and galactose. Using 10 drops reduces the lactose by more than 90%, but this results in an increase in sweetness because of increased monosaccharides.

APPROACH TO THE CASE

Detailed history taking is the key to the diagnosis. A high index of suspicion is essential. Ethnic background and age can be clues. History of symptoms in temporal relation to food items containing lactose is a pointer to the diagnosis—targeted questioning while history taking is essential. The symptoms, even though severe at times, are not life threatening (outside the neonatal period and very young age). Weight loss is usually not present. Physical examination should be thorough so that other causes for the pain with physical findings can be eliminated. A history suggestive of lactose intolerance with no history of weight loss and a normal physical examination is usually the picture in an uncomplicated case of lactose intolerance.

SUMMARY

Lactose intolerance is a widespread problem seen across different ethnic populations in varying proportions. The inability to digest lactose sugar found in milk and milk products does not pose a serious threat to health outside the neonatal period. The diagnosis of lactose intolerance can be established by noninvasive tests. Although there is no cure, the disease can be easily controlled by a lactose-free diet or by taking lactase supplements.

MAJOR POINTS

- Lactose is a sugar solely produced by the mammary glands of mammals and is found in milk and milk products.
- Lactose is hydrolyzed by the brush border enzyme lactase into the monosaccharides glucose and galactose, which are absorbed by intestinal transport mechanisms.
- Low levels of lactase in the intestinal brush border lead to lactose malabsorption.
- The unabsorbed lactose exerts osmotic effect, drawing water into the intestine, producing distention and increased peristalsis. The unabsorbed lactose is fermented by the microflora in the colon, producing fatty acids, gas, and bowel distention.
- Genetic late-onset lactose intolerance is seen worldwide and the frequency is variable in different ethnic populations.
- Congenital lactase deficiency is extremely rare.
- Secondary lactose intolerance occurs as result of mucosal injury to the intestinal mucosa or due to quick transit time in the jejunum.
- The best test for the diagnosis of lactose intolerance is the lactose breath hydrogen test.
- The treatment of lactose intolerance is by avoiding lactose in the diet or by taking lactase enzyme supplements with lactose-containing food.

SUGGESTED READINGS

Arola H, Koivula T, Jokela H, et al: Comparison of indirect diagnostic methods for hypolactasia. Scand J Gastroenterol 23:351-357, 1988.

Banai J, Szanto I, Nagy I, Kun M: Measurement and demonstration of lactase and sucrase activities in jejunal mucosa. Am J Gastroenterol 85:157-160, 1990.

Buller HA, Rings EH, Montgomery RK, Grand RJ: Clinical aspects of lactose intolerance in children and adults. Scand J Gastroenterol Suppl 188:73-80, 1991.

Chao CK, Sibley E: PCR-RFLP genotyping assay for a lactase persistence polymorphism upstream of the lactase-phlorizin hydrolase gene. Genet Test 8:190-193, 2004.

Chaussain M, Kheddari K, Roche R, et al: Abdominal pain in children caused by lactose intolerance: Prospective use of the hydrogen breath test. Presse Med 23:881-885, 1994.

Cierna I, Cernak A, Krajcirova M, Leskova L: Lactose intolerance in the differential diagnosis of abdominal pain in children. Cesk Pediatr 48:651-653, 1993.

Cochet B, Griessen M, Balant L, et al: Diagnosis of lactase deficiency with the expired hydrogen (H_2) test. Schweiz Med Wochenschr 111:192-193, 1981.

Dahlqvist A: Assay of intestinal disaccharidases. Enzymol Biol Clin (Basel) 11:52-66, 1970.

de Vrese M, Stegelmann A, Richter B, et al: Probiotics: Compensation for lactase insufficiency. Am J Clin Nutr 73(2 Suppl):421S-429S, 2001.

Gremse DA, Greer AS, Vacik J, DiPalma JA: Abdominal pain associated with lactose ingestion in children with lactose intolerance. Clin Pediatr (Phila) 42:341-345, 2003.

Jarvela I, Sabri EN, Kokkonen J, et al: Assignment of the locus for congenital lactase deficiency to 2q21, in the vicinity of but separate from the lactase-phlorizin hydrolase gene. Am J Hum Genet 63:1078-1085, 1998.

Kolars JC, Levitt MD, Aouji M, Savaiano DA: Yogurt: An autodigesting source of lactose. N Engl J Med 310:1-3, 1984.

Lerebours E, N'Djitoyap NC, Lavoine A, et al: Yogurt and fermented-then-pasteurized milk: Effects of short-term and long-term ingestion on lactose absorption and mucosal lactase activity in lactase-deficient subjects. Am J Clin Nutr 49:823-827, 1989.

Levitt MD, Kolars JC, Savaiano DA: Carbohydrate malabsorption and intestinal gas production. Neth J Med 27:258-261, 1984.

Mobassaleh M, Montgomery RK, Biller JA, Grand RJ: Development of carbohydrate absorption in the fetus and neonate. Pediatrics 75:160-166, 1985.

Montgomery RK, Buller HA, Rings EH, Grand RJ: Lactose intolerance and the genetic regulation of intestinal lactase-phlorizin hydrolase. FASEB J 5:2824-2832, 1991.

Naim HY: Molecular and cellular aspects and regulation of intestinal lactase-phlorizin hydrolase. Histol Histopathol 16:553-561, 2001.

Patel YT, Minocha A: Lactose intolerance: Diagnosis and management. Compr Ther 26:246-250, 2000.

Saarela T, Simila S, Koivisto M: Hypercalcemia and nephrocalcinosis in patients with congenital lactase deficiency. J Pediatr 127:920-923, 1995.

Scrimshaw NS, Murray E: Lactose tolerance and milk consumption: Myths and realities. Arch Latinoam Nutr 38:543-567, 1988.

Scrimshaw NS, Murray EB: The acceptability of milk and milk products in populations with a high prevalence of lactose intolerance. Am J Clin Nutr 48(4 Suppl):1079-1159, 1988.

Shaw AD, Davies GJ: Lactose intolerance: Problems in diagnosis and treatment. J Clin Gastroenterol 28:208-216, 1999.

Sieber R, Stransky M, de Vrese M: Lactose intolerance and consumption of milk and milk products. Z Ernahrungswiss 36:375-393, 1997.

Sinden AA, Sutphen JL: Dietary treatment of lactose intolerance in infants and children. J Am Diet Assoc 91:1567-1571, 1991.

Srinivasan R, Minocha, A: When to suspect lactose intolerance: Symptomatic, ethnic, and laboratory clues. Postgrad Med 104:109-123, 1998.

Stallings VA, Oddleifson NW, Negrini BY, et al: Bone mineral content and dietary calcium intake in children prescribed a low-lactose diet. J Pediatr Gastroenterol Nutr 18:440-445, 1994.

Suarez FL, Savaiano DA, Levitt MD: A comparison of symptoms after the consumption of milk or lactose-hydrolyzed milk by people with self-reported severe lactose intolerance. N Engl J Med 333:1-4, 1995.

Suarez FL, Savaiano DA, Levitt MD: Review article: The treatment of lactose intolerance. Aliment Pharmacol Ther 9:589-597, 1995.

Swagerty DL Jr, Walling AD, Klein RM: Lactose intolerance. Am Fam Physician 65:1845-1850, 2002.

Tamm A: Management of lactose intolerance. Scand J Gastroenterol Suppl 202:55-63, 1994.

Vesa TH, Marteau P, Korpela R: Lactose intolerance. J Am Coll Nutr 19(2 Suppl):165S-175S, 2000.

Webster RB, DiPalma JA, Gremse DA: Lactose maldigestion and recurrent abdominal pain in children. Dig Dis Sci 40:1506-1510, 1995.

Malrotation and Volvulus

VINCENT BIANK

MICHAEL C. STEPHENS*

Disease Description
Case Presentation
Epidemiology
Pathophysiology
Differential Diagnosis
Diagnostic Testing
Treatment
Approach to the Case
Summary
Major Points

DISEASE DESCRIPTION

Intestinal malrotation or "bad rotation" of the intestine refers to the improper positioning of the intestines within the abdominal cavity. However, this abnormal position in itself does not cause problems. Instead, the abnormal position and fixation allow the intestines to twist or volvulize, possibly resulting in obstruction, or in severe cases of volvulus, death.

CASE PRESENTATION

A 2-week-old term male is brought to the primary care physician's office for routine checkup and weight check following delivery. His mother states that the patient has had good urine output, but has only had or three bowel movements since being discharged from the hospital. She recalls the patient had daily bowel movements while in the nursery and feels his stooling pattern has diminished since coming home. The patient is exclusively breastfed and nurses every 2 to 3 hours for 10 to 15 minutes. He frequently "spits up" after eating. The mother states that the patient has otherwise behaved the same as her two previous children and was wondering if she should be concerned.

More careful questioning reveals that the "spitting up" is forceful and that the patient's emesis is intermittently dark green. The few stools passed since discharge appeared "tarry." The mother has brought the most recent stool to be examined.

His weight is 300 g below his birthweight of 3.2 kg. The remainder of the physical examination is normal. Specifically, the abdomen is soft, nontender, and nondistended without appreciable masses, and bowel sounds are present. The stool is dark black and positive for occult blood.

EPIDEMIOLOGY

The reported incidence of malrotation ranges from 1 in 500 to 1 in 6000 live births. The true incidence is difficult to determine because many patients with malrotation may remain asymptomatic through adulthood. Males are more commonly affected than females with reports as high as a 2:1 predominance. The majority of cases present in the first year of life, with 60% to 90% of cases in the first month of life.

Malrotation is commonly associated with anomalies of the abdominal wall (i.e., gastroschisis or omphalocele) and diaphragmatic hernia. Varied gastrointestinal anomalies also have been associated with malrotation, including intestinal atresia, Meckel's diverticulum, intussusception, Hirschsprung's disease, persistent cloaca, and anomalies of the extrahepatic biliary system.

---

*The authors wish to thank John Sty, M.D., Chief and Clinical Professor of Radiology, Children's Hospital of Wisconsin, for graciously providing the radiographic images.

PATHOPHYSIOLOGY

Malrotation is the result of a failure of one of two events in the embryonic development of the intestine. During the second month of gestation, the midgut undergoes tremendous elongation, eventually outgrowing the abdominal cavity. It extrudes into the umbilical cord for further development. During the third month of gestation, the intestine returns to the abdominal cavity. At this time, both the duodenojejunal junction and the cecum undergo a 270° counterclockwise rotation around the superior mesenteric vessels. This rotation is followed by fixation of the duodenojejunal junction at the ligament of Treitz and the cecum to the right lower quadrant of the abdominal cavity. The normal midgut is therefore affixed via a broad base extending from the ligament of Treitz in the left upper quadrant to the cecum in the lower right quadrant of the abdominal wall. Failure of either of these two processes (rotation or fixation) results in a narrow mesenteric base, making the midgut susceptible to volvulus around the superior mesenteric vessel axis. Volvulus about this axis leads to intestinal ischemia. In malrotation, peritoneal (Ladd) bands connecting the displaced cecum to the abdominal wall may stretch across the duodenum or small bowel, creating another source of obstruction.

Malrotation can be classified into nonrotation, incomplete rotation or reverse rotation depending on the degree of rotation and the direction (Fig. 17-1). Nonrotation, the most common form, is an early form of arrested rotation resulting in the small bowel on the right and the cecum on the left of the superior mesenteric axis. Incomplete rotation, a later form of arrested rotation, results in the duodenojejunal junction partially rotating around the superior mesenteric axis and the cecum in the left upper quadrant. Reversed rotation is a very rare form of malrotation that results from the midgut rotating in a clockwise rather than counterclockwise direction. The result is that the duodenum is anterior to the superior mesenteric artery and the transverse colon is posterior.

DIFFERENTIAL DIAGNOSIS

The manifesting symptoms of malrotation with volvulus may range from chronic intermittent vomiting to overt obstruction with bilious vomiting. Therefore, the differential diagnosis is quite extensive. The clinician must narrow this diagnosis with a careful history and a thorough physical examination. A directed differential for vomiting is listed in Table 17-1.

DIAGNOSTIC TESTING

Despite the frequently emergent nature by which malrotation with volvulus manifests, diagnosis can be challenging. This is because contrast studies demonstrate only the position of the intestine, not the fixation. One must infer based on the position whether adequate fixation exists. Numerous reports have documented malrotation with volvulus in the presence of a normally positioned duodenum, or more commonly, a normally positioned cecum. Although malrotation is most commonly detected through upper gastrointestinal (UGI) contrast series, evaluation of both the upper and lower intestinal tracts may be necessary if the diagnosis is in doubt or if clinical symptoms demand additional workup.

In evaluating a patient with suspected malrotation with volvulus, plain x-ray is commonly the first examination. Findings range from normal to a gasless abdomen.

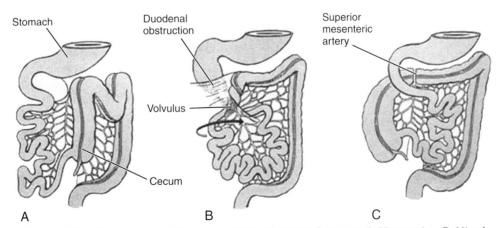

Figure 17-1 Illustrations of different anomalies of intestinal rotation. **A**, Nonrotation. **B**, Mixed rotation wavith volvulus. **C**, Reversed rotation. (From Moore K, Persaud T: The Developing Human: Clinically Oriented Embryology. Philadelphia, Saunders, 1993, p 254.)

Table 17-1 Differential Diagnosis of Vomiting			
Infant	Choledochal cyst	Crohn's disease	*Neurologic*
Anatomic	Adrenal hyperplasia	Ulcerative colitis	Hydrocephalus with shunt
Pyloric stenosis	Ureteropelvic obstruction	Ménétrier's disease	dysfunction
Malrotation	Overfeeding	Chronic granulomatous	Concussion
Duplication	**Child**	disease	Subdural hematoma
Duodenal web/sling	*Infectious*	*Anatomic*	Subarachnoid hemorrhage
Meconium ileus	Gastroenteritis	Inguinal hernia	Intracranial neoplasm
Congenital atresia or	Infectious colitis	Malrotation with volvulus	Reye's syndrome
stenosis	Parasitic infections	Intussusception	Migraine headaches
Tracheoesophageal fistula	*Helicobacter pylori* gastritis	Duodenal hematoma	Epilepsy
Hirschsprung's disease	Hepatitis	Ovarian or testicular torsion	Pseudotumor cerebri
Pseudo-obstruction	Giardiasis	*Miscellaneous*	Abdominal migraine
Metabolic	Pneumonia	Pancreatitis	Mucosal injuries
Organic acidemias	Meningitis	Renal stones	Peptic ulcer or duodenitis
Fatty acid oxidation defects	Streptococcal pharyngitis	Hydrometocolpos	Celiac disease
Amino acidemias	Acute or chronic sinusitis	Toxic ingestion	Crohn's disease
Urea cycle defects	Pyelonephritis	Lead poisoning	Ulcerative colitis
Storage diseases	Appendicitis	**Adolescent**	GERD
Mitochondriopathies	*Neurologic*	*Infectious*	*Anatomic*
Infectious	Hydrocephalus with shunt	Gastroenteritis	Malrotation with volvulus
Meningitis	dysfunction	Infectious colitis	SMA syndrome
Pyelonephritis	Concussion	Acute or chronic sinusitis	Surgical adhesions
Pneumonia	Subdural hematoma	Streptococcal pharyngitis	Duodenal hematoma
Gastroenteritis	Subarachnoid hemorrhage	Parasitic infection	Inguinal hernia
Otitis media	Intracranial neoplasm	*H. pylori* gastritis	Ovarian or testicular
Neurologic	Reye's syndrome	Giardiasis	torsion
Subdural hematoma	Migraine headaches	Hepatitis	*Miscellaneous*
Hydrocephalus	Epilepsy	Meningitis	Toxic ingestion
Arnold-Chiari malformation	Mucosal injuries	Pneumonia	Psychogenic vomiting
Miscellaneous	Peptic ulcer or duodenitis	Appendicitis	Bulimia
Bezoar	Gastroesophageal reflux	Pyelonephritis	Cyclic vomiting
Cow's milk or soy protein	disease (GERD)	Pelvic inflammatory	
sensitivity	Celiac disease	disease	

Nonspecific but rapid and inexpensive multiview abdominal radiographs can help the clinician assess the degree of obstruction and determine if surgical intervention should proceed without further diagnostic tests. Contrast studies remain the diagnostic method of choice. Review of the literature favors performing a UGI contrast study. Although an abnormally located cecum is suggestive of malrotation, this finding on contrast enema is not specific to malrotation with volvulus. However, a misplaced duodenum found by UGI is more suggestive of malrotation.

Figure 17-2 shows the common UGI findings in malrotation. In analyzing the UGI examination, one is specifically looking for positioning of the duodenojejunal junction, which, in classic malrotation, will lie to the right of midline. Other diagnostic signs may include a spiral or corkscrew appearance of the second or third portion of the duodenum or the proximal jejunum lying on the right side of midline. Despite the ease with which classic malrotation may be identified, current recommendations suggest that if clinical symptoms persist, regardless of a negative UGI examination, a barium enema should be performed.

TREATMENT

Initial management includes rapid intervention to stabilize fluid and metabolic disturbances until an accurate diagnosis can be made. Rapid diagnosis and prompt surgical intervention are the keys to avoiding disastrous complications. The initial surgical step is to reduce any volvulized segment of bowel and determine the viability of the segment. Following this inspection, a Ladd procedure is performed. Since its description in the early 1930s, the Ladd procedure consists of lysing any existing Ladd bands and repositioning both the small and large intestines. The duodenum will subsequently lie to the right of midline and the cecum will lie in the left lower quadrant, therefore providing a broad mesenteric base. More recent debate had been whether to perform an appendectomy at the time of procedure, because the appendix will reside in the left lower quadrant and therefore may pose a diagnostic dilemma if appendicitis were to ensue following the Ladd procedure. If necrotic bowel is present, and the remaining segments are viable and of adequate length, the non-viable bowel should be resected and either a primary or secondary anastomosis be conducted. Additionally, if

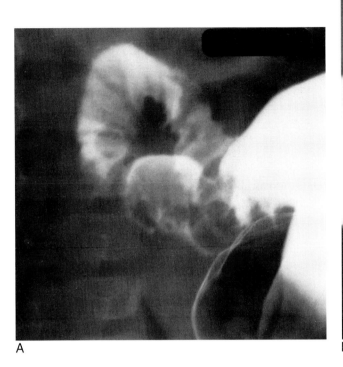
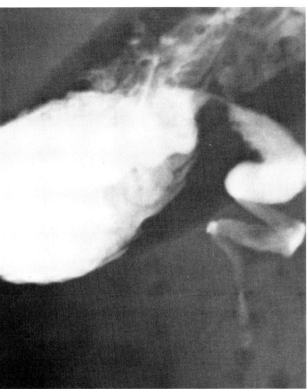
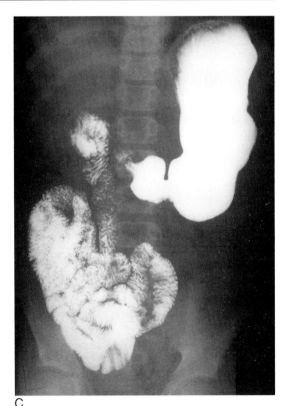

Figure 17-2. Upper gastrointestinal series in the evaluation of malrotation. **A,** Normal anatomy with incidental duodenal ulceration. **B,** Malrotation with volvulus; classic corkscrew appearance of second and third portions of duodenum. **C,** Nonrotation, with the entire small intestine located in the right abdomen.

the volvulized segment is of questionable viability, a second-look procedure should be done. A second-look procedure consists of reducing the segment of volvulized bowel then re-examining the segment after a period of time (usually 24 to 48 hours) in order to better determine the viability of the volvulized segment.

The mortality rate for midgut volvulus has remained between 3% and 10% for decades. This reflects the fact that outcome is primarily related to early diagnosis and prompt intervention rather than technical advances in management. Complications include recurrent volvulus, adhesive bowel obstruction, and "short-gut syndrome" after resection of a large ischemic segment of bowel and the attendant morbidity and mortality of chronic dependence on parenteral nutrition. Because of these devastating complications, prompt elective Ladd procedure is required even in the asymptomatic patient.

APPROACH TO THE CASE

The classic manifesting symptom of malrotation with volvulus is bilious vomiting. Although vomiting is by far the most common manifesting symptom, it is not always bilious. Bilious vomiting may be the manifesting symptom in as little as 20% of cases. Other manifesting symptoms include abdominal distention, colicky abdominal pain, diarrhea, constipation, or melanotic stools. The presentation of malrotation may be less dramatic, with occasional vomiting and abdominal pain or failure to thrive. Because the severity of symptoms is not a reliable predictor of malrotation, one should maintain a low threshold to investigate for anatomic problems such as malrotation in the child with idiopathic vomiting. In more severe cases in which volvulus has created significant intestinal ischemia, manifesting symptoms may include overwhelming sepsis, abdominal ascites, or cardiorespiratory decompensation.

The symptoms presented in this case warrant investigation for malrotation or other anatomic intestinal abnormalities. The differential diagnosis also includes infection (i.e., necrotizing enterocolitis, gastroenteritis, or infectious colitis) and allergy (i.e., cow's milk or soy allergy) in addition to mechanical causes (i.e., malrotation, intussusception, intestinal duplication, duodenal webs or slings). A UGI series should be ordered early in the evaluation of this patient to ensure rapid referral for prompt surgical intervention. Early intervention remains the key to avoiding devastating outcomes in malrotation.

SUMMARY

Malrotation with volvulus remains a common pediatric disease process with catastrophic consequences. Subsequently, prompt evaluation should be considered in any newborn presenting with vomiting. Malrotation with volvulus is a congenital disorder that results from either improper rotation or fixation of the intestine. The result is a narrow mesenteric base on which the bowel may twist and subsequently cut off its own blood supply. The incidence ranges from 1 in 500 to 1 in 6000 births. However, individuals may go a lifetime without symptoms. The classic presentation is that of a neonate with bilious vomiting, although bilious vomiting is not always present. Older individuals may present with poor weight gain and occasional nonbilious vomiting. Malrotation with volvulus is commonly identified by UGI contrast study, although if the result is negative and symptoms remain suspicious, barium enema is recommended. On diagnosis, emergent surgical intervention is mandated. The Ladd procedure remains the surgical correction since its description in the early 1930s. Despite advancements in medical and surgical technology, mortality has remained fairly unchanged primarily because of the devastating consequences of total midgut volvulus. Subsequently, incidental findings of malrotation should be surgically corrected regardless of symptomatology.

MAJOR POINTS

Vomiting in an infant can be a sign of malrotation and intermittent volvulus, and a low threshold of tolerance should be held for further investigation to rule out this life-threatening disorder.

Malrotation is a congenital disorder resulting from either improper rotation or fixation of the intestine.

Malrotation is common; the incidence ranges from 1 in 500 to 1 in 6000 births.

Classic symptoms include bilious vomiting in the neonate, although the absence of bilious vomiting does not rule out malrotation.

Older individuals may go a lifetime without symptoms and present with only intermittent nonbilious vomiting or poor weight gain.

UGI series is a useful test to diagnose malrotation.

If UGI contrast study is negative, but symptoms are highly suspicious, barium enema should be considered.

Once diagnosed, emergent surgical intervention is mandated.

Mortality remains unchanged despite the advances in medical and surgical technology due to the devastating consequences of midgut volvulus, implying there should be a low threshold to investigate for malrotation.

Due to the devastating consequences, the incidental finding of malrotation should lead to surgical revision regardless of symptomatology.

SUGGESTED READINGS

Azizkhan R, Frykman P: Anomalies of intestinal rotation. In Rudolph C, Rudolph A, Hostetter M, et al (eds): Rudolph's Pediatrics, New York, McGraw-Hill, 2003, pp 1400-1402.

Ford EG, Senac MO Jr, Srikanth MS, Weitzman JJ: Malrotation of the intestine in children. Ann Surg 215:172-178, 1992.

Long FR, Kramer SS, Markowitz RI, Taylor GE: Radiographic patterns of intestinal malrotation in children. Radiographics 16:547-556, 1996.

Long FR, Kramer SS, Markowitz RI, et al: Intestinal malrotation in children: Tutorial on radiographic diagnosis in difficult cases. Radiology 198:775-780, 1996.

Millar AJ, Rode H, Cywes S: Malrotation and volvulus in infancy and childhood. Semin Pediatr Surg 12:229-236, 2003.

Moore K, Persaud T: The Developing Human: Clinically Oriented Embryology, Philadelphia, Saunders, 1993, pp 237-264.

Phillip J: Abdominal surgical emergencies. In Pediatric Gastrointestinal Disease: Pathophysiology, Diagnosis, and Management, Philadelphia, Saunders, 1999.

Rescorla FJ, Shedd FJ, Grosfeld JL, et al: Anomalies of intestinal rotation in childhood: Analysis of 447 cases. Surgery 108:710-715, 1990.

Torres AM, Ziegler MM: Malrotation of the intestine. World J Surg 17:326-331, 1993.

Wesson D, Haddok G: Congenital anomalies. In Walker W, Durie P, Hamilton, J, et al (eds): Pediatric Gastrointestinal Disease: Pathophysiology, Diagnosis, and Management, Hamilton, Ontario, BC Decker, 2000, pp 424-434.

Wesson D, Haddok G: The surgical abdomen. In Walker W, Durie P, Hamilton, J, et al (eds): Pediatric Gastrointestinal Disease: Pathophysiology, Diagnosis, and Management, Hamilton, Ontario, BC Decker, 2000, pp 235-249.

Wyllie R: Intestinal atresia, stenosis, and malrotation. In Behrman R, Kliegman R, Jensons H (eds): Nelson's Textbook of Pediatrics. Philadelphia, Saunders, 2004, pp 1232-1236.

CHAPTER 18

Meckel's Diverticulum

EDISIO SEMEAO

Disease Description
Case Presentation
Epidemiology
Clinical Features and Pathophysiology
Differential Diagnosis and Diagnostic Testing
Treatment
Approach to the Case
Summary
Major Points

DISEASE DESCRIPTION

Meckel's diverticulum (MD) is the most common congenital abnormality of the gastrointestinal tract. It occurs in approximately 2% of the population. In pediatric patients the most common clinical presentation is with painless rectal bleeding. Other symptoms that may be described include recurrent abdominal pain, abdominal distention, and nausea and/or vomiting.

CASE PRESENTATION

A 4½-year-old boy was admitted to the gastroenterology service after a second visit to an emergency department (ED) with complaints of rectal bleeding. The first visit was 2 weeks prior to the admission with the complaint of 2 days of blood per rectum. It happened several times per day and was not associated with any discomfort or diarrhea. Evaluation in the ED revealed normal vital signs and an examination revealed a questionable anal fissure. The patient was discharged to home with constipation precautions.

Two weeks later the patient returned to the ED with continued symptoms of rectal bleeding. After the initial visit, the bleeding seemed to resolve for several days, but then returned, with the patient seeing blood for the past 3 days on a regular basis. The patient did not complain of pain and had normal bowel movements with no straining. The patient denied fevers, history of trauma, and vomiting. Evaluation in the ED showed a blood pressure of 90/65 mm Hg and a pulse rate of 105 beats/minute. The abdominal examination was unremarkable and the external rectal examination was normal with no evidence of an external fissure. The stool was guaiac positive with gross blood.

EPIDEMIOLOGY

Meckel's diverticulum was first described by Johann Meckel in 1809. This abnormality results from the incomplete obliteration of the fetal omphalomesenteric-vitelline duct between the seventh and eighth weeks of gestation. The vitelline duct communicates with the yolk sac and involutes as the placenta replaces the yolk sac as the source of fetal nutrition. Failure of this process results in various anomalies of which MD accounts for 90% of the vitelline duct anomalies. It is a true diverticulum, containing all three layers of the bowel wall; its vascular supply comes from a remnant of the vitelline artery, a terminal branch of the superior mesenteric artery. MD is usually located on the antimesenteric border and is usually between 2 and 4 cm in length. Approximately 50% of diverticula contain ectopic tissue, with gastric tissue accounting for 60% to 85%. Pancreatic tissue accounts for 5% to 16%, and other less common tissue types include colonic and duodenal.

MD tends to be more common in males, with a ratio of males to females of 3:2; also, males have more symptomatic diverticula. MD has been associated with several other congenital anomalies that include cardiac malformations, anorectal atresia, exophthalmos, cleft palate, annular pancreas, and some central nervous system malformations.

CLINICAL FEATURES AND PATHOPHYSIOLOGY

Although the presence of MD is 2% in the population, the rarity of this anomaly in clinical practice is that only 4% to 6.5% of patients with MD are symptomatic. The majority of symptomatic MD contains ectopic tissue. In children, the most common presentation is with painless rectal bleeding, which may range from occult blood to frank bright red blood and hemodynamic instability. The bleeding is believed to occur due to the highly acidic secretions of the gastric tissue on the adjacent tissues, which may cause ulcerations that lead to bleeding. Similarly, the alkaline secretions of the pancreatic tissue may also cause ulcerations and lead to bleeding.

Intestinal obstruction is another complication that arises from MD. It is the most common type of presentation in adults and can occur in up to 40% of pediatric patients. This results from intussusception, in which the MD serves as a lead point, inflammation, omphalomesenteric bands, or adhesions. The clinical symptoms in this setting include recurrent abdominal pain, abdominal distention, nausea, and vomiting.

Another common presentation for symptomatic MD is inflammation or diverticulitis, which can occur in 12% to 40% of cases. Patients often present with signs and symptoms consistent with appendicitis, and the diagnosis is made at the time of surgical exploration. In a subset of this group, the diverticulum may perforate from infarction or ulceration and lead to a more acute and toxic presentation. Malignancies also have been reported in association with MD. These are present within the diverticulum and can cause obstructive symptoms or can be found incidentally. Sarcomas are the most common, followed by carcinoids and adenocarcinomas.

DIFFERENTIAL DIAGNOSIS AND DIAGNOSTIC TESTING

The diagnosis of symptomatic MD is difficult to make and requires a high index of suspicion. This diagnosis should be considered in any patient with recurrent unexplained abdominal pain, nausea and vomiting, or rectal bleeding. Table 18-1 lists a variety of common problems that can mimic the presentation of MD.

Physical examination findings are variable and depend on the type of presenting complications. In children with rectal bleeding, the examination is usually

Table 18-1 Differential Diagnosis for Meckel's Diverticulum

Appendicitis	Rectal fissure
Polyps	Intestinal duplication
Intussusception	Arteriovenous malformation
Malrotation/volvulus	Colonic diverticulitis
Allergic proctitis	Hirschsprung's enterocolitis
Infectious colitis	Peptic ulcer disease
Lymphonodular hyperplasia	

benign except for a positive rectal examination and usually low blood pressure and tachycardia. Patients with obstructive symptoms may have abdominal distention and tenderness and hyperactive bowel sounds. Patients with an inflammatory (diverticulitis) type of presentation will have similar findings as in appendicitis, with the possibility of peritoneal signs in cases of perforation.

The diagnosis cannot be made with laboratory evaluation or plain x-ray. Laboratory analysis may be helpful to determine the degree of bleeding with a hemoglobin count and a coagulation profile to rule out an underlying bleeding disorder. Plain x-rays may show evidence of obstruction, but are not diagnostic of MD. Contrast studies such as upper gastrointestinal series with small bowel follow-through or enterocolysis studies are limited in value because the layers of barium in the bowel can obscure the diverticulum. A computed tomography (CT) scan and ultrasound are often nonspecific in the diagnosis of MD but can be helpful in looking for other causes of presenting symptoms. Endoscopy and colonoscopy are not sensitive for the diagnosis of MD, but can be helpful in identifying other causes that may explain symptoms. Angiography may not be helpful because the vascular supply is usually normal.

The most useful method for the diagnosis of MD is with a Meckel's scan, technetium-99m pertechnetate scan. This technique, however, depends on the presence of ectopic gastric mucosa in the MD in order to have uptake of the isotope by the gastric mucosa. Because not all diverticula contain gastric mucosa, this scan may not be of value in all situations. However, because complications such as bleeding are usually (90%) associated with ectopic gastric tissue, this test may be diagnostic in many symptomatic cases. In children, the scan has a sensitivity and specificity of 85% and 95%, respectively, but in adults these values fall to 62.5% and 9%, respectively. Because this scan is dependent on the presence of ectopic gastric tissue, a number of factors can lead to a false-positive or a false-negative scan (Table 18-2).

The accuracy of the scan can be enhanced by the use of a variety of pharmacologic agents. Pentagastrin can

Table 18-2 Conditions That Can Lead to a Misinterpretation of a Meckel's Scan	
False Positive	**False Negative**
Ectopic gastric mucosa (localized in other segments of the gastrointestinal tract, duplication)	**Lack of adequate or absent gastric mucosa**
Focal small bowel pathology (intussusception, volvulus, appendicitis, Crohn's disease, abdominal abscess)	**Impaired vascular supply** (intussusception or obstruction that causes compression of vascular supply and does not allow tracer to reach mucosa)
Neoplasm (leiomyosarcoma, carcinoid, hemangioma, arteriovenous [AV] malformation, uterine fibroids, small bowel lymphoma)	**Brisk bleeding** (dilution of tracer and inadequate focal uptake)
Genitourinary tract (external pelvis, vesicoureteral reflux, ectopic kidney)	**Technique** (pharmacologic agents can enhance study, pentagastrin; can lead to wash-out by increasing peristalsis, overlying organs such as bladder or kidney; atropine; insufficient isotope)
Uterine "blush" (uterine pooling of blood)	

increase uptake of technetium in the gastric mucosa and cimetidine inhibits the intraluminal release of technetium, which allows for a higher concentration of isotope in the mucosa. Glucagon also can be used to decrease peristalsis and thus decrease washout of the isotope. In situations in which the Meckel's scan is nondiagnostic or in patients with nonbleeding symptoms but with a high index of suspicion for MD, laparoscopy has been shown to be effective and have less morbidity than an exploratory laparotomy.

TREATMENT

The treatment for MD that is symptomatic and identified is surgical removal. This can be done either with simple diverticulectomy, or in cases in which the adjunct ileum is damaged or further evidence of ectopic tissue, a limited resection may be required. The bigger dilemma is what the approach is when an MD is found incidentally and the patient is asymptomatic. Previous research has indicated that the morbidity for diverticulectomy is approximately 9% and that because the risk of developing symptoms during a lifetime was 4%, these diverticula should be left in place. More recent work has shown a much lower morbidity (2%) associated with the removal of the diverticulum, and thus some researchers have advocated removal of the diverticulum that is found incidentally. The development of new techniques such as laparoscopy and stapling devices has aided in decreasing the morbidity and mortality in this procedure.

Several series have compared features of symptomatic with asymptomatic diverticula to see if there are characteristics that would help in deciding the approach to asymptomatic MD. Several have been identified, which significantly increases the risk of developing complications from a MD that is asymptomatic. These include age, younger patients (less than 8 to 10 years of age), longer diverticulum (>2 cm), and a narrower base (<2 cm in diameter); all were associated with increased risk of developing symptoms later in life.

APPROACH TO THE CASE

Laboratory evaluation was remarkable for a hemoglobin level of 10.2 g/dL with normal electrolytes, albumin, transaminases, and clotting studies. The abdominal x-ray was normal. The patient was admitted and given intravenous fluids. Stool studies were obtained for infectious evaluation. In the next 24 hours, the rectal bleeding continued with no other symptoms and the hemoglobin dropped to 8.6 g/dL. The infectious workup remained negative and a colonoscopy was performed to the region of the cecum and revealed no gross colonic abnormality. Biopsies were obtained. The bleeding persisted and a Meckel's scan using technetium-99m pertechnetate was performed to exclude MD. A trace of isotope was noted in the right side of the abdomen (Fig. 18-1) and a tentative diagnosis of MD was made. The patient was then taken to the operating room for a diagnostic laparoscopy that revealed an MD (Fig. 18-2), which was removed by the surgeon.

SUMMARY

Meckel's diverticulum is the most common congenital abnormality of the gastrointestinal tract. However, only a small percentage cause clinical symptoms, and thus the clinician needs to have a high degree of

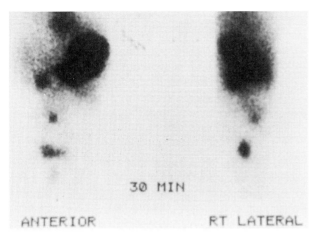

Figure 18-1 Meckel's scan. Following premedication with pentagastrin, an abnormal focus was seen above the bladder and to the right of the midline.

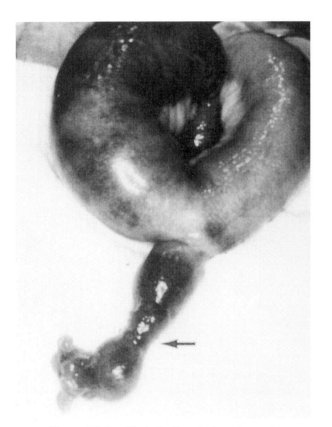

Figure 18-2 Meckel's diverticulum *(arrow)*.

suspicion in order to make a prompt and accurate diagnosis. The most common symptoms include rectal bleeding in children and obstructive symptoms in adults. Patients may also present with inflammatory changes that mimic diverticulitis. Most MD that presents with symptoms has ectopic tissue, with gastric and pancreatic tissues being the most common. A Meckel's scan is the most efficient, least invasive test in making the diagnosis. However, the limitation is the need for the presence of ectopic gastric tissue in the diverticulum. The treatment of choice for symptomatic MD is surgical removal. Although there is still some disagreement about the treatment for asymptomatic MD found incidentally, the development of minimally invasive laparoscopy and new stapling techniques have made the removal of even these diverticula more straightforward.

MAJOR POINTS

MD is the most common congenital anomaly of the gastrointestinal tract, occurring in approximately 2% of the general population.

Approximately 50% have ectopic tissue, with gastric tissue the most common. Pancreatic, colonic, and duodenal tissues also may be present in the diverticulum.

The clinician needs a high degree of suspicion in order to make a prompt and accurate diagnosis.

In children, the most common presenting symptom is painless rectal bleeding. Other complications of MD include intestinal obstruction, which can cause abdominal pain, distention, and nausea and vomiting. Inflammation or diverticulitis also accounts for a large number of complications and can mimic the symptoms of appendicitis.

Factors that lead to symptoms and complications with MD include the presence of ectopic tissue, young age, long diverticulum, and narrow-based diverticulum.

A Meckel's scan is the most useful noninvasive test in diagnosing an MD. It is limited by the need for the presence of ectopic gastric tissue to take up the isotope, technetium-99m pertechnetate. In cases in which there is no gastric tissue but significant symptoms, the clinician needs to exclude other diagnoses, and if a high degree of suspicion for MD exists, laparoscopy has become the modality of choice to further evaluate for MD.

The treatment of choice for symptomatic MD is surgical removal. Incidentally found diverticula, especially in younger patients (pediatric age-group) or with higher risk features are now recommended to be removed. The development of newer surgical techniques (laparoscopy, stapling devices) has made the morbidity of the procedure lower than the lifetime risk of developing complications from an MD left in place.

SUGGESTED READINGS

Artigas V, Calabuig R, Badra F, et al: Meckel's diverticulum: Value of ectopic tissue. Am J Surg 151:631-634, 1986.

Bani-Hani K, Shatnawi N: Meckel's diverticulum: Comparison of incidental and symptomatic cases. World J Surg 28:917-920, 2004.

Chao H, Kong M, Chen J, et al: Sonographic features related to volvulus in neonatal intestinal malrotation. J Ultrasound Med 19:371-376, 2000.

Cooney D, Duszynski D, Camboa E, et al: The abdominal technetium scan (a decade of experience). J Pediatr Surg 17:611-619, 1982.

Cullen J, Kelly K, Moir C, et al: Surgical management of Meckel's diverticulum: An epidemiological, population-based study. Ann Surg 220:564-568, 1994.

Daneman A, Lobo E, Alton D, Shuckett B: The value of sonography, CT and air enema for detection of complicated Meckel diverticulum in children with non-specific clinical presentation. Pediatr Radiol 28:928-932, 1998.

DiGiacomo J, Cottone F: Surgical treatment of Meckel's diverticulum. South Med J 86:671-675, 1993.

Heyman S: Nuclear medicine. In Altschuler S, Liacouras C (eds): Clinical Pediatric Gastroenterology. Philadelphia, Churchill Livingstone, 1998, p 501, figure 67-5.

Hollands C, Hoffman M: Congenital anomalies of the intestine. In Altschuler S, Liacouras C (eds): Clinical Pediatric Gastroenterology. Philadelphia, Churchill Livingstone, 1998, p 159, figure 21-5.

Leijonmarck C, Bonman-Sandelin K, Frisell J, Raf L: Meckel's diverticulum in the adult. Br J Surg 73:146-149, 1986.

Mackey W, Dineen P: A fifty year experience with Meckel's diverticulum. Surg Gynecol Obstet 156:56-64, 1983.

Martin J, Conner P, Charles K: Meckel's diverticulum. Am Fam Physician 61:1037-1042, 1044, 2000.

McCollough M, Sharieff G: Abdominal surgical emergencies in infants and young children. Emerg Med Clin N Am 21:909-935, 2003.

Mendelson K, Bailey B, Balint T, Pofahl W: Meckel's diverticulum: Review and surgical management. Curr Surg 58:455-457, 2001.

Miele V, DeCicco M, Andreoli C, et al: US and CT findings in congenital Meckel diverticulum. Radiol Med 101:230-234, 2001.

Onen A, Cidem M, Ozturk H, et al: When to resect and when not to resect an asymptomatic Meckel's diverticulum: An ongoing challenge. Pediatr Surg Int 19:57-61, 2003.

Sfakianakis G, Conway J: Detection of ectopic gastric mucosa in Meckel's diverticulum and in other aberrations by scintigraphy: I. Pathophysiology and 10-year clinical experience. J Nucl Med 22:647-655, 1981.

Shalabi R, Soliman S, Fawy M, Samaha A: Laparoscopic management of Meckel's diverticulum in children. J Pediatr Surg 40:562-567, 2005.

Simms M, Corkery, J: Meckel's diverticulum: Its association with congenital malformations and the significance of atypical morphology. Br J Surg 67:216-219, 1980.

Soltero M, Bill A: The natural history of Meckel's diverticulum and its relation to incidental removal: A study of 202 cases of diseased Meckel's diverticulum found in King County, Washington, over a fifteen year period. Am J Surg 132:168-173, 1976.

Turgeon D, Barrett J: Meckel's diverticulum. Am J Gastroenterol 85:777-781, 1990.

Wahchouchy E, Marano A, Etienne J, Fingerhut A: Meckel's diverticulum. J Am Coll Surg 192:658-662, 2001.

Williams R: Management of Meckel's diverticulum. Br J Surg 68:477-480, 1981.

Yau K, Siu W, Lau B, et al: Laparoscopy-assisted surgical management of obscure gastrointestinal bleeding secondary to Meckel's diverticulum in a pediatric patient: Case report and review of the literature. Surg Laparosc Endosc Percutan Tech 15:374-377, 2005.

CHAPTER 19

Necrotizing Enterocolitis

MICHAEL POSENCHEG

GILBERTO PEREIRA

Disease Description
Case Presentation
Epidemiology
Pathophysiology
Differential Diagnosis
Diagnostic Testing
Treatment
Approach to the Case
Summary
Major Points

DISEASE DESCRIPTION

Necrotizing enterocolitis (NEC) is a potentially devastating inflammatory process causing ischemia and necrosis of the intestinal tract of the newborn (and particularly the premature) infant. The absolute etiology remains elusive; however, there are two features almost universally associated with NEC: prematurity and feeding. NEC is the most common intestinal emergency in the preterm infant.

CASE PRESENTATION

An 18-day-old former 28-week gestation, 1100-g male infant was born to a 27-year-old $G_2 P_1$ mother. Her prenatal course was significant for premature labor at 27 and 4/7 weeks gestation, for which she was administered betamethasone and magnesium sulfate. Her prenatal laboratory tests were remarkable for blood type O+, antibody screen negative, rubella immune, hepatitis B Ag negative, and rapid plasma reagin (RPR) nonreactive. She denied any substance use or abuse and had a negative toxicology screen. Despite tocolytic effort, her infant was born via spontaneous vaginal delivery after 48 hours of steroids. The infant's Apgar scores were 7 at 1 minute and 8 at 5 minutes and he received continuous positive airway pressure (CPAP) in the delivery room for increased work of breathing. Umbilical venous and arterial lines were placed, and the infant was transferred to the neonatal intensive care unit (NICU) for further evaluation. His initial arterial blood gas (ABG) was 7.28/56/85/23/-1 and he remained on CPAP of 5 and 30% FIO_2. Ampicillin and gentamicin were started and continued for 48 hours after blood cultures were sent from the newly placed umbilical catheters. He had no cardiovascular instability, and did not require inotropic support.

Over the next 4 days the infant was weaned from CPAP to oxygen by nasal cannula, and his umbilical arterial line was removed. On day 5 of life enteral nutrition was initiated with standard preterm formula, 20 kcal/ounce, at 20 mL/kg via nasogastric tube. A 7-day feed advance was initiated after initial tolerance of feedings at a rate of 20 mL/kg/day until a full volume of 150 mL/kg/day was reached. His umbilical venous line was removed on day 12 of life when the infant reached full feeding volume. On day 17 of life the baby developed abdominal distention, heme-positive stools, and bilious gastric residuals. At this point, his feedings were held and intravenous fluids were initiated. His laboratory evaluation included a blood culture, complete blood count, electrolytes, and arterial blood gas, and ampicillin and gentamicin were started. This evaluation was significant for a white blood cell count of 3.5K, a platelet count of 95K, and a significant metabolic acidosis as demonstrated on his ABG—7.15/35/80/7/-17. Abdominal x-rays in two views were obtained and demonstrated dilated intestinal loops, bowel wall thickening, and pneumatosis intestinalis throughout the abdomen.

Over the next 6 hours, with further distention of the abdomen, the infant suffered from multiple episodes of apnea and bradycardia, leading to respiratory failure requiring intubation and mechanical ventilation. Follow-up x-rays demonstrated free air under the diaphragm, and he concurrently developed significant hypotension requiring dopamine at a dose of 20 µg/kg/minute and epinephrine at 0.05 µg/kg/minute. A peripheral arterial line was placed for blood pressure monitoring and blood sampling. Hydrocortisone was added for blood pressure support and metronidazole (Flagyl) was added to enhance antimicrobial coverage. He developed abdominal wall erythema and severe distention, requiring significant increases in ventilatory support. Subsequently, he was taken to the operating room for an exploratory laparotomy, where it was determined that the infant had 20 cm of necrotic intestine, which was resected. After returning from the operating room, he had persistent acidosis and hypotension that was unresponsive to bicarbonate administration and increasing inotropic support. The infant expired by the following morning despite prolonged resuscitative efforts.

EPIDEMIOLOGY

The incidence of NEC ranges from 1% of all NICU admissions to up to 10% in the very low birthweight category of preterm infants. The relation between incidence and gestational age is inversely correlated, with the most premature infant at greatest risk. The age at onset of this disease is also inversely correlated, with the most premature infants acquiring NEC at an older age than more mature infants. Stoll and colleagues report a mean age at diagnosis of 20.2 days for infants 30 weeks' gestation or less, 13.8 days for 31- to 33-week-gestation infants, and 5.4 days for 34 weeks or greater. Additionally, greater than 90% of babies diagnosed with NEC have been enterally fed. Additional factors associated with the development of NEC include the presence of a patent ductus arteriosus, use of umbilical arterial catheters, and the administration of indomethacin alone or in conjunction with postnatal steroids. The common thread among these factors is the relation to mesenteric blood flow and gut ischemia. However, only prematurity and enteral nutrition have consistently been associated with NEC in this population.

Full-term infants are not immune to this disorder because they make up nearly 10% of all cases; however, most full-term infants who acquire NEC have additional risk factors associated with this disease that differ from their premature counterparts. Risk factors in the full-term group include congenital heart disease, polycythemia, maternal cocaine use, hypothyroidism, small for gestational age (SGA), birth asphyxia, gastroschisis, and history of exchange transfusion. The age at onset in full-term infants is also much younger than premature infants. Wiswell and colleagues report a median age at onset of 2 days in 43 full-term infants with NEC. Furthermore, a recent publication suggests a possible role of birth by cesarean section as a risk factor for NEC in full-term infants.

A number of short- and long-term complications are related to NEC. In the short-term, infants may experience general feeding intolerance as well as intestinal obstruction from stricture and adhesion formation. Long-term complications are related to the amount of bowel affected by the initial insult. In the most severe cases, especially when more than 50% of the intestine is resected, short gut syndrome may result with subsequent malabsorption of nutrients and reliance on intravenous nutrition for survival. Ultimately, this may progress to total parenteral nutrition (TPN) cholestasis, and subsequent liver failure. At this time, transplantation of intestine with or without an associated liver transplant is being performed at a select few centers in the United States with some success.

The mortality rate associated with NEC is dependent on birthweight, with an overall mortality rate of 10% to 44% in infants weighing less than 1500 g and 0% to 20% in infants weighing more than 2500 g.

PATHOPHYSIOLOGY

Although the absolute pathogenesis of NEC remains elusive, there have been many investigations identifying risk factors and their relative contributions to the development of this disorder. The only two risk factors that have been consistently associated with NEC are prematurity and enteral feeding. However, multiple studies have demonstrated inflammation, loss of integrity of the intestinal mucosa, and presumed subsequent bacterial translocation as other features in the overall pathogenesis.

Prematurity is the most consistent risk factor associated with NEC because the incidence of NEC increases with decreasing gestational age. It is hypothesized that immaturity of the mucosal barrier of the intestine, including dysregulation of splanchnic blood flow, may be primarily responsible for the increased susceptibility in this population. This mucosal barrier may be more susceptible to inflammation-mediated injury inducing apoptotic cell death, resulting in loss of integrity and subsequent bacterial translocation.

Feeding the preterm infant has been an area of much investigation for many years, because more than 90% of infants who develop NEC have been enterally fed. Researchers have evaluated the time of initiation of feedings, type of feeding (formula vs. breast milk), method of feeding (continuous vs. bolus), and rate of advancement of feeding as they pertain to the development of NEC.

With respect to time of initiation of feeding, method of feeding, and rate of advancement, Cochrane meta-analysis reviews are done on each of these topics, demonstrating no difference in the incidence of NEC. However, there is some evidence that breast milk may be protective for preterm infants. Factors believed to be present in human milk that may confer this protective effect include immunoglobulins (specifically IgA), platelet-activating factor (PAF)-acetylhydrolase, IL-10, and epidermal growth factor.

New evidence has emerged with respect to the timing of advancement of feedings that may offer improved outcomes. Berseth and associates have demonstrated in a randomized controlled trial that maintaining preterm infants on 20 mL/kg/day (minimal feeding group) for 10 days before advancing feeding volumes confers an advantage over advancing feeding by 20 mL/kg/day (advancing feeding group) to a maximum of 140 mL/kg/day over a 7-day period. In their single-center study, the minimal feeding group had an incidence of NEC of 1.4% versus 10% in the advancing feeding group, and the study was halted prematurely due to the significant difference between the groups. This evidence, if confirmed, may alter future feeding practices of preterm infants.

Inflammation plays a major role in the pathogenesis of NEC. A number of inflammatory mediators have been associated with the development of NEC including platelet-activating factor (PAF), inducible nitric oxide synthase (iNOS), tumor necrosis factor-alpha (TNF-α), interferon-gamma (IFN-γ), and interleukin-8 (IL-8). Specifically, according to Ford and coworkers, increased levels of iNOS and 3-nitrotyrosine, a combined marker of oxidative and nitrative stress, have been co-localized with evidence of apoptosis in the intestinal mucosa of infants with NEC compared with infants undergoing bowel resection for other indications. Caplan and Jilling have demonstrated that increased PAF levels are found in both the serum and stool of infants with NEC when compared with controls and that PAF is a potent inducer of apoptosis in intestinal cells. This information supports the hypothesis that inflammation induces cellular injury and death by apoptosis, causing a breakdown in the mucosal barrier, and potential subsequent bacterial translocation resulting in further bowel injury.

DIFFERENTIAL DIAGNOSIS

The differential diagnosis that includes NEC is a differential diagnosis of intestinal obstruction in a newborn, the most common presenting symptoms of NEC.

The differential diagnosis of intestinal obstruction and/or perforation in a neonate includes the following:
Necrotizing enterocolitis
Feeding intolerance
Septic ileus
Malrotation with volvulus
Hirschsprung's disease
Intestinal atresias (jejunal, ileal)
Meconium plug
Meconium ileus
Spontaneous intestinal perforation

DIAGNOSTIC TESTING

Unfortunately, there is no good diagnostic test for NEC. If there is clinical suspicion that the infant's symptoms are more exaggerated than would be expected from feeding intolerance, including abdominal distention, increased gastric residuals, bilious emesis, gross blood in the stool or abdominal erythema, an initial evaluation is instituted. This is especially true if these symptoms of feeding intolerance are combined with systemic signs and symptoms such as apnea, bradycardia, lethargy, and temperature instability. The initial evaluation includes a complete blood count with differential to determine the presence of leukopenia and thrombocytopenia specifically, an arterial blood gas to evaluate for metabolic or respiratory acidosis, a blood culture to document infection, and an abdominal radiograph to evaluate the intestinal gas pattern (presence of ileus) as well as findings more suggestive of NEC including pneumatosis intestinalis, portal venous gas, and, at the extreme, pneumoperitoneum (Figs. 19-1 and 19-2). When infants are x-rayed, they are often supine, and pneumoperitoneum may manifest as a football sign—free air that collects in the middle of the abdomen with displacement of the falciform ligament. Obtaining a left lateral decubitus view of the abdomen helps to differentiate questionable cases of pneumoperitoneum as the air layers over the liver edge, making it easier to appreciate. It is crucial that these x-rays are followed serially to evaluate for progression of disease.

In 1978, Bell and coworkers developed staging criteria for the categorization of the severity of NEC that were subsequently revised in 1986 by Kleigman and Walsh. These criteria are listed in Table 19-1.

TREATMENT

The medical management of NEC is primarily supportive. At the suggestion of disease, infants should be made nothing per mouth (NPO) and a Replogle or Salem sump orogastric tube should be placed under low continuous suction to decompress the abdomen. Infants may require mechanical ventilation because of respiratory failure secondary to abdominal competition. Hypotension is managed with vasoconstrictors, inotropic

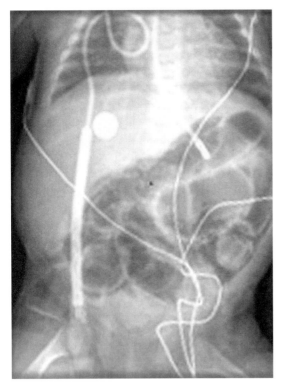

Figure 19-1 X-ray of the abdomen demonstrating generalized abdominal distension, bowel wall thickening and pneumatosis intestinalis, consistent with stage IIA NEC.

agents, and steroids. Broad antibiotic coverage is initiated, usually with ampicillin or vancomycin, and gentamicin. In the setting of portal venous gas or pneumoperitoneum, many experts advocate the addition of anaerobic coverage with metronidazole. Metabolic acidosis also may develop and is treated with base administration (either bicarbonate or tromethamine [THAM] in the setting of hypercarbia).

The duration of therapy is an area of controversy. Most experts advocate for treatment with antibiotics and NPO duration of at least 10 to 14 days for stage II or greater NEC. Once portal venous gas is present, surgical management should be considered. Additional indications for operative care include pneumoperitoneum, abdominal wall erythema, or continued clinical deterioration despite optimal medical management. Two surgical options currently are being used: open laparotomy and percutaneous drainage. To date, there is no evidence-based guideline for the optimal operative procedure because much of the current evidence has significant selection bias. The choice of which procedure to perform is surgeon and institution based; there also is a bias for smaller infants (<1000 g) to undergo percutaneous drainage; however, their outcomes are expected to be worse on the basis of birthweight and gestational age alone. A recently published multicentered, randomized clinical trial by Moss and colleagues found no apparent difference in the short-term outcomes of survival to 90 postoperative days, dependence on total parenteral nutrition, or length of stay, regardless of surgical approach. These results should be taken with caution, as the outcomes of infants eligible, but not enrolled, in the trial were superior to those of the enrolled infants. Further studies should also include neurodevelopmental outcome as a major focus.

A number of experimental therapies aimed at the prevention of NEC hold some promise. Breast milk has been found to be associated with a decreased incidence of NEC and in attempting to determine the mechanism, researchers have evaluated enteral administration of immunoglobulins. A Cochrane Database of Systematic Reviews meta-analysis on the topic did not find a beneficial effect on the combined use of IgG and IgA, but there are no studies examining IgA alone, which may hold more promise. Separately, it has been demonstrated in both mouse and piglet models that the intravenous or enteral administration of L-arginine, the precursor of nitric oxide production that may help to regulate mesenteric blood flow, has been protective for the development of NEC. To date, there has been only one small study examining this effect in preterm infants. This study demonstrated a decrease in the incidence in NEC with the enteral administration of L-arginine, but the difference was mostly attributable to the decrease in stage I NEC, a more difficult and subtle diagnosis to make. Further investigation in a large multicentered, randomized controlled trial is needed to evaluate the effect on stages II and III NEC.

APPROACH TO THE CASE

The case detailed is not an uncommon one in the NICU. Infants who present with NEC often have an unremarkable hospital course until the presentation of symptoms. The timing of the symptoms also is not uncommon, with infants of a more premature gestational age presenting later (1 month or later) and infants closer to term presenting earlier (in the first week). This infant presented in an abrupt fashion with the onset of bilious gastric aspirates, abdominal distention, and heme-positive stool, which was quickly followed by clinical deterioration and the need for both respiratory and cardiovascular support. NEC may also present in a more insidious fashion, with the slow development of feeding intolerance over days to one week, eventually developing radiographic findings to corroborate the clinical picture. Neonatologists have been investigating ways to determine which baby has or will develop NEC in this more insidious presentation. One common clinical parameter that is followed is the volume of gastric residuals. Cobb and associates demonstrated the gastric residuals of greater than 40% of the previous feeding volume was associated with the diagnosis of NEC.

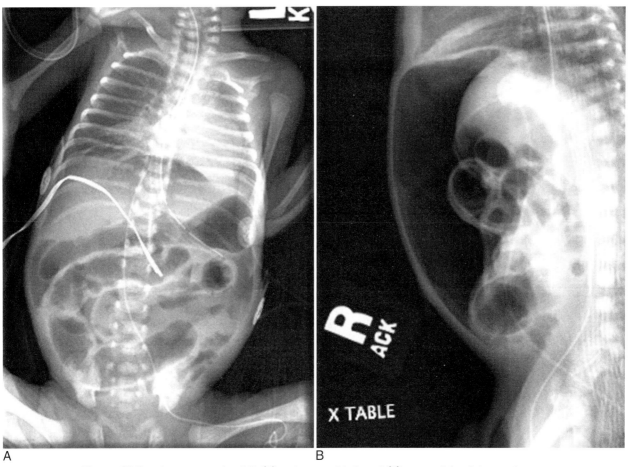

Figure 19-2 Anteroposterior (AP) **(A)** and cross-table lateral **(B)** x-rays of the abdomen demonstrating the presence of dilated intestinal loops and pneumoperitoneum, consistent with stage IIIB NEC.

Table 19-1 Bell's Staging Criteria for Categorization of the Severity of NEC

Stage	Systemic Signs	Intestinal Signs	Radiographic Signs
I: suspected NEC	Apnea, bradycardia, temperature instability	Increased gastric residuals, abdominal distention, occult blood in stool	Normal or mild ileus
IIA: mild NEC	Apnea, bradycardia, temperature instability	Abdominal distention ± tenderness, absent bowel sounds, grossly bloody stools	Ileus, dilated bowel loops with focal pneumatosis intestinalis
IIB: moderate NEC	Mild acidosis and thrombocytopenia	Abdominal wall edema and tenderness ± palpable mass	Extensive pneumatosis intestinalis, early ascites, ± portal venous gas
IIIA: advanced NEC	Respiratory and metabolic acidosis, mechanical ventilation, oliguria, disseminated vascular coagulation (DIC)	Worsening wall edema and erythema with induration	Prominent ascites, persistent bowel loop, no free air
IIIB: advanced NEC	Vital sign and laboratory evidence of deterioration, shock	Evidence of perforation	Pneumoperitoneum

Bell MJ, Ternberg JL, Feigin RD, et al: Neonatal necrotizing enterocolitis: Therapeutic decisions based upon clinical staging. Ann Surg 187:1-7, 1978.
Revised by Walsh M, Kliegman RM: Necrotizing enterocolitis: Treatment based on staging criteria. Pediatr Clin North Am 33:179-201, 1986.

The eventual outcome of this case also is not uncommon, especially with infants that have an abrupt clinical deterioration. It is essential that practitioners have a keen eye for this diagnosis and initiate supportive therapy quickly. Early involvement of pediatric surgery also will allow for a timely intervention, if necessary. Nevertheless, even when the diagnosis is made quickly and therapy initiated, the severe morbidity and mortality associated with NEC may not be avoidable.

SUMMARY

NEC is a devastating inflammatory gastrointestinal disorder of newborn infants. Its incidence is inversely correlated with gestational age and birthweight and is associated with the institution of enteral feeding. There are significant mortality and long-term morbidity, making NEC a significant problem for the newborn infant. Its pathophysiology is multifactorial, but includes a premature mucosal barrier in the gut, the institution of enteral nutrition, mucosal ischemia, an intense inflammatory response, and bacterial translocation. There is no diagnostic test for NEC, so the diagnosis is made on a combination of systemic and abdominal signs and symptoms and radiographic findings. Treatment is mainly supportive with respiratory and cardiovascular support, abdominal decompression, bowel rest, base administration, antibiotic use, and, in severe cases, surgical intervention. Experimental therapies to prevent NEC are being evaluated and include the enteral administration of IgA and L-arginine.

SUGGESTED READINGS

Amer MD, Hedlund E, Rochester J, et al: Platelet-activating factor concentration in the stool of human newborns: Effects of enteral feeding and neonatal necrotizing enterocolitis. Biol Neonate 85:159-166, 2004.

Bell MJ, Ternberg JL, Feigin RD, et al: Neonatal necrotizing enterocolitis: Therapeutic decisions based upon clinical staging. Ann Surg 187:1-7, 1978.

Berseth CL, Bisquera JA, Paje VU: Prolonging small feeding volumes early in life decreases the incidence of necrotizing enterocolitis in very low birth weight infants. Pediatrics, 111:529-534, 2003.

Caplan M, Jilling T: The pathophysiology of necrotizing enterocolitis. NeoReviews. 2:e103-e110, 2001.

Cobb BA, Carlo WA, Ambalavanan N: Gastric residuals and their relationship to necrotizing enterocolitis in very low birth weight infants. Pediatrics 113:50-53, 2004.

Dimmitt R, Moss R: Clinical management of necrotizing enterocolitis. NeoReviews 2:e110-e117, 2001.

MAJOR POINTS

- NEC is the most common intestinal emergency in preterm infants.
- The most consistent risk factors for the development of NEC include prematurity and enteral feeding; more than 90% of infants with NEC have been fed.
- The incidence and age at onset of NEC are inversely correlated with gestational age.
- Full-term infants are not immune to NEC and have unique risk factors.
- NEC is associated with significant short- and long-term morbidity as well as up to 50% mortality in the most premature infants.
- Human breast milk may offer protection against the development of NEC.
- Practitioners should consider maintaining preterm infants on 20 mL/kg/day of enteral nutrition for 10 days before starting the advancement of feeding.
- The pathophysiology of NEC most certainly involves factors related to the immaturity of the preterm infant intestine, multiple inflammatory mediators such as PAF and iNOS, and the induction of apoptosis of the intestinal epithelium, leading to mucosal breakdown and bacterial translocation.
- The clinical presentation of NEC includes increased gastric residuals, bilious emesis, grossly bloody or heme-positive stools, abdominal distention, apnea, bradycardia, lethargy, and temperature instability. These may be confused with general feeding intolerance, a more common occurrence in the preterm infant.
- The differential diagnosis of NEC includes other diseases that result in intestinal obstruction or perforation, such as atresias, volvulus, septic ileus, Hirschsprung's disease, and spontaneous intestinal perforation.
- There is no diagnostic test specific for NEC; therefore, the diagnosis is based on a combination of clinical and radiographic criteria.
- Treatment is primarily supportive, including bowel rest, antibiotics, mechanical ventilation, blood pressure and acid-base management, and surgical intervention when indicated.
- Potential therapies for the prevention of NEC include enteral administration of IgA and L-arginine.

Ford H, Watkins S, Reblock K, et al: The role of inflammatory cytokines and nitric oxide in the pathogenesis of necrotizing enterocolitis. J Pediatr Surg 32:275-282, 1997.

Kennedy KA, Tyson JE, Chamnanvanikij S: Early versus delayed initiation of progressive enteral feedings for parenterally fed low birth weight or preterm infants. Cochrane Neonatal Group. Cochrane Database Syst Rev 2004.

Kennedy KA, Tyson JE, Chamnanvanikij S: Rapid versus slow rate of advancement of feeding for promoting growth and preventing necrotizing enterocolitis in parenterally fed low birth weight infants. Cochrane Neonatal Group. Cochrane Database Syst Rev, 2004.

Maayan-Metzger A, Itzchak A, Mazkereth R, et al: Necrotizing enterocolitis in full-term infants: Case-control study and review of the literature. J Perinatol 24:494-499, 2004.

Moss RL, Dimmitt RA, Barnhart DC, et al: Laparotomy versus peritoneal drainage for necrotizing enterocolitis and perforation. N Engl J Med 354:2225-2234, 2006.

Sato T, Oldham K: Abdominal drain placement versus laparotomy for necrotizing enterocolitis with perforation. Clin Perinatol 31:577-589, 2004.

Stoll B: Epidemiology of necrotizing enterocolitis. Clin Perinatol 21:205-218, 1994.

Stoll BJ, Kanto WP, Glass RI, et al: Epidemiology of necrotizing enterocolitis: A case-control study. J Pediatr 96:447, 1980.

Walsh M, Kliegman RM: Necrotizing enterocolitis: Treatment based on staging criteria. Pediatr Clin North Am 33:179-201, 1986.

Wiswell TE, Robertson CF, Jones TA, et al: Necrotizing enterocolitis in full-term infants: A case-control study. Am J Dis Child 142:532, 1988.

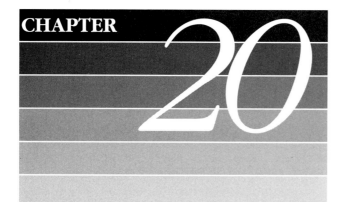

Parasitic Infections

ROSALYN DIAZ
ASIM MAQBOOL

Disease Description
Case Presentation
Epidemiology
Most Common Parasitic Infections in Children
    Protozoan Flagellates
        Giardia lamblia
    Amebic
        Entamoeba hystolytica
        Dientamoeba fragilis
        Blastocystis hominis
        Cryptosporidium Species
        Cyclospora cayetanensis
    Nematodes (Roundworm)
        Strongyloides stercoralis
        Ascaris lumbricoides
        Trichuris trichuria (Whipworm)
        Enterobius vermicularis (Pinworm)
        Necator americanus (Hookworm)
    Blood Flukes
        Schistosoma Species
Approach to the Case
Summary
Major Points

DISEASE DESCRIPTION

Parasites are organisms that live in or on a host at the expense of the host. Parasitic infections are prevalent worldwide but more common in developing countries. Nevertheless, children are traveling internationally more than ever; therefore, health professionals in industrialized nations need to be aware of the presentation and treatment of these diseases as well.

CASE PRESENTATION

A 3-year-old boy presents with abdominal pain, poor appetite, decrease in energy, and significant decline in growth velocity over the preceding 6 months. The abdominal pain is poorly localized, but mostly periumbilical, and vague but occasionally severe. Pain is not associated with meals, diarrhea, constipation, or vomiting. His parents report occasional unrelated low-grade fever. On further inquiry he is found to eat dirt, paper, and sometimes flakes from wall paint. The past medical history is remarkable for recurrent episodes of diarrhea and upper respiratory tract infections. Parents describe occasional whistling sounds from the chest. The boy was born full term after an uneventful home delivery; birthweight was 2.8 kg. He was the fourth child in a lower socioeconomic class family. He was partially immunized. He was almost exclusively breastfed for the first 6 months of life, but weaning was started late and food habits were erratic.

On physical examination, his vital signs are stable. He appears pale, well hydrated, but small for his age. Both height and weight are in the 10th percentile. Head, eyes, ears, nose, and throat (HEENT) examination is remarkable for poor oral hygiene but no obvious lead lines on his gums. Lungs are clear to auscultation. Heart auscultation reveals a regular rate and rhythm without a murmur appreciated. Abdomen is protuberant, but soft, depressible, not tender, and without organomegaly. There is no clubbing, edema, or rash. The remainder of the systemic examination is within normal limits.

EPIDEMIOLOGY

Intestinal parasites infect millions of people worldwide, especially in developing countries where potable water is not as available and/or sanitation is poor.

Human behavior is often implicated for the persistence of parasitic disease. The most common form of intestinal parasitic infection is asymptomatic carrier state. Asymptomatic geohelminthic intestinal carrier states, and subclinical infections may exist for years, even following migration from endemic areas. Symptoms presented by the patient will depend in part on the competency of the host's immune system, the degree of malnutrition (which in itself may be exacerbated by the infection), environmental load, and exposure history. Increased morbidity is observed when parasitic infections coexist with malnutrition and immunodeficiency, underlining the need for consideration of these infections in the diagnoses.

Typically these infections may manifest with gastrointestinal symptoms such as abdominal pain and diarrhea, anemia, and blood in the stool, often with obstructive symptoms, anemia, or poor growth and delayed development. Given the seriousness and the implications that growth failure can have in children, and the interval of time during essential periods of growth to reverse trends in declining growth velocity, it is important to suspect parasitic infections in the appropriate clinical context, pursue appropriate and adequate testing, and promptly institute therapy.

MOST COMMON PARASITIC INFECTIONS IN CHILDREN

Protozoan Flagellates

Giardia lamblia
Epidemiology

The most common cause of parasitic enteritis in the United States is *Giardia*, which causes diarrhea in all age-groups around the world. It is also among the more common parasites associated with traveler's diarrhea, and a higher incidence is noted among immigrants to developed countries, as well as in individuals living in crowded conditions, including orphanages and prisons. Children are more typically affected. In developed countries the prevalence of *Giardia* is as low as 2% to 5%, versus up to 30% in developing areas.

Giardiasis is associated with diarrheal outbreaks stemming from contaminated water supplies. *Giardia* is resistant to chlorination and can be found in rivers, swimming pools, lakes, and beaches. Cysts have been discovered in chlorinated municipal water supplies, and in animal reservoirs such as beavers and muskrats; infections are frequently reported in campers and hikers drinking from contaminated streams. Fecal to oral transmission is an additional risk factor.

Life Cycle/Transmission

Giardia is one of the four common species of intestinal flagellates. It is a protozoan, single-celled parasite that exists in two forms, a motile trophozoite and cyst, with the latter form causing infection (Fig. 20-1). Transmitted by fecally contaminated water or food, and direct person-to-person contact, only 10 to 100 microorganisms are needed to cause infection and symptoms. Cysts multiply in the duodenum and jejunum of the human host. They reside in close approximation to the mucosa, may penetrate into the secretory mucosa, and have been isolated in the gallbladder and biliary system as well. A sucking disk located on the antral portion of the ventral surface facilitates anchorage to the mucosa, akin to a sucking disk producing mechanical tissue irritation.

Clinical Presentation

Early in life, infants and young children are usually symptomatic and develop diarrhea, vomiting, and anorexia. Symptoms may range from mild diarrhea and flatulent crampy abdominal pain and epigastric pain with tenderness to a full-blown malabsorptive state with steatorrhea. Severe giardiasis may be accompanied by hypoporteinemia, hypogammaglobinemia, and folic acid and fat-soluble vitamin deficiencies.

Older children and adults are usually asymptomatic. After ingestion of cysts, the incubation period before diarrhea starts is usually 3 to 40 days. Chronic diarrhea and malabsorption may lead to failure to thrive. Giardiasis may coexist with a chronic disease called Whipple's disease, which is a rare disorder caused by the bacterium *Tropheryma whippelii*. This disease is characterized by diarrhea, arthralgias, abdominal pain, and malabsorption.

Diagnosis

Giardia cysts and trophozoites can be found in stool microscopy, as well as duodenal fluid and mucosal biopsy (Fig. 20-2). It may take 10 to 36 days of infection before patient presents with symptoms or before organism may be detected. Excretion patterns vary from high (with parasites present in nearly all stool samples), to intermittent and low—on the order of 40% of stool specimens, necessitating multiple stool specimens to increase diagnostic yield. Usually, three stool samples taken on different days are required to make the diagnosis. Diagnosis alternatively can be made by identifying trophozoites in duodenal fluid aspirates obtained by endoscopy, intubation, the string test, and on biopsy. Enzyme immunoassays (EIAs) are used commercially for detection of *Giardia* in stools. The sensitivity and specificity of an EIA have been reported anywhere from 88% to 98% and 87% to 100%, respectively.

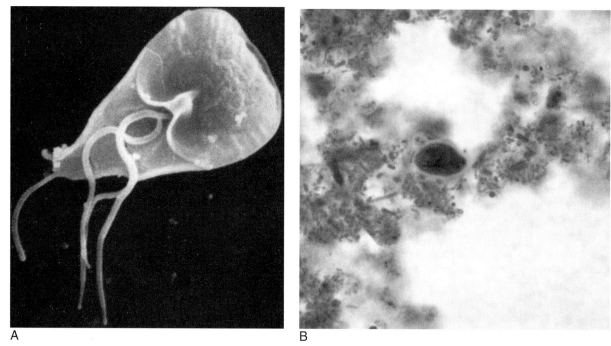

Figure 20-1 *(See also Color Plate 20-1.)* **A,** Scanning electron microscopy of *Giardia lamblia* showing its flagella. **B,** Trichrome stain revealing cystic form of *Giardia* (in blue in center). (**A,** From the Public Health Image Library from the Centers for Disease Control and Prevention [CDC] website, http://phil.cdc.gov [provider CDC/Janice Carr]; **B,** from the Public Health Image Library from the CDC website, http://phil.cdc.gov [provider CDC/DPDx /Melanie Moser].)

Treatment

Spontaneous eradication has been reported, as have chronic infections, with the latter more common in younger children. Drugs of choice are metronidazole, nitazoxanide, and tinidazole. Other alternatives are paromomycin, furazolidone, and quinacrine.

Prevention

Contamination with *Giardia* may be prevented by the use of clean water supplies; the organism is able to withstand filtration and chlorination. For hikers with portable water purification systems, iodine solutions are effective.

Amebic

Entamoeba histolytica

E. histolytica, of the intestinal amebae, is a common large intestinal parasite in humans and primates, with the majority of cases asymptomatic.

Epidemiology

E. histolytica occurs in between 1% and 5% of the world's population. Prevalence rates are highest in areas of crowding, poor sanitation, and in particular, in the tropics. Cysts are usually ingested from contaminated water; in the tropics, contaminated vegetables and food also may serve as cyst sources. Asymptomatic cyst carriers are the major source of contamination, and have been linked to epidemic outbreaks when sewage leaks into the water supply, and under poor sanitation and hygiene (such as in prisons and orphanages). High-carbohydrate, low-protein diets in these environments may increase the risk of amebic dysentery.

Life Cycle

E. histolytica primarily inhabits the colon. Trophozoites induce the pathologic changes. The trophozoites live in the lumen and may invade colonic crypts, feed on erythrocytes, coalesce, and form shallow ulcers. Chronic infections may occur in the terminal ileum and cecum, and may lead to obstruction. An ameboma (inflammatory, tumor-like mass) also may form on the intestinal wall and lead to obstruction. The sigmoid colon and rectum are common sites for recurrence of infection.

Deeper penetration into the intestinal wall with perforation has been reported. Invasion into the vascular system may lead to amebic dysentery. If the organisms penetrate the capillaries, the infection may disseminate through the bloodstream to the liver (primarily) as well as to other organs (lung and brain), where abscess may form. Enteric amebae may be expelled in liquid or semiformed stools in the trophozoite form. If motility is impaired, the amebae may differentiate into four nucleated,

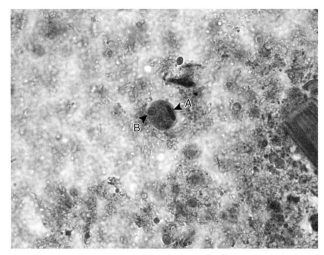

Figure 20-3 *(See also Color Plate 20-3.) Entamoeba histolytica.* Notice in this trichrome stain the cystic form of *Entamoeba* with a body (A) and well-demarcated nucleus (B). (From the Public Health Image Library from the Centers for Disease Control and Prevention (CDC) website, http://phil.cdc.gov [provider CDC/DPDx /Melanie Moser].)

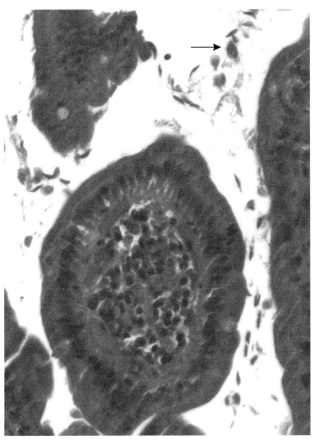

Figure 20-2 *(See also Color Plate 20-2.)* Light microscopy of *Giardia (arrow)* in a duodenal biopsy.

resistant cyst stages. *E. histolytica* cysts are not produced in the tissues. Eight small trophozoites are generated from each infected cyst.

Clinical Presentation

Symptoms depend on the site involved and extent of colonic lesions, if any. Symptoms may develop in as little as 4 days to as late as one year after exposure, or in mild cases, never. In less acute disease, symptoms appear and progress gradually with days to weeks of cramps, abdominal discomfort, anorexia, weight loss, and malaise that may progress to diarrhea, increased abdominal cramping and pain, and nausea. Liquid stools with flecks of blood, mucus, and trophozoites may be observed in this stage. Significant abdominal tenderness, fulminant dysentery, and dehydration occur with progression or with more severe cases, with obstruction and perforation possible. Extraintestinal symptoms are the result of primarily hematogenous spread (although lung abscesses can occur from extension of liver abscesses). Amebic hepatitis or abscesses are the most common extraintestinal manifestation, occurring in less than 5% of cases. These abscesses are commonly nonsupperative, progressive, and destructive but lack wall formation. The contents are necrotic, usually devoid of bacteria, with active amebae confined to the margins. In more than 50% of cases of amebic hepatic abscesses, there is no preceding indication of intestinal disease.

Diagnosis

Coproscopic diagnoses are made on fresh and warm stool for examination for trophozoites; immediately fixed in sodium acetate acetic acid formalin (SAF) solution or in polyvinyl alcohol, and examined microscopically (Fig. 20-3). A single stool sample examination has a yield of 50% to 60%, with higher sensitivity in the range of 95% by successive stool specimen evaluation over 3 successive days. Saline purges have been used to detect cysts and trophozoites. Formed feces can be examined for the presence of cysts. Endoscopic scrapings also can be examined. Stool cultures may also be employed. A newer polymerase chain reaction (PCR) is used to differentiate *E. histolytica* from *Entamoeba dispar.* Coproantigen can be detected in stool by enzyme-linked immunosorbent assay (ELISA) based on monoclonal antibodies. Liver abscess aspirates have the highest yield from the edges, not the center, which is most likely necrotic and debris ridden. Serologic assays are very sensitive (>95%) and aid in differentiation between *E. histolytica* and *E. dispar.*

Treatment

Asymptomatic amebiasis can be treated with dioxanide furoate, paromomycin, or metronidazole. Amebic dysentery, liver abscesses, and amebomas should be treated with metronidazole. Alternatives are nitroimidazoles, ornidazole, or tinidazole.

Prevention
Travelers to endemic areas should drink filtered, boiled water and avoid fresh prepeeled fruits, vegetables, and salads and uncooked foods. There is no current chemoprophylaxis.

Dientamoeba fragilis
Epidemiology
D. fragilis is an unflagellated protozoan that infects the large intestine of humans worldwide. Most commonly it is a binucleated trophozoite, but nuclear variations occur, and between one and four nuclei can be seen per organism. Prevalence in developed countries, including the United States, is reported to be between 2% and 4%; rates as high as 69% have been reported in areas with poor hygiene, crowded living conditions, in Native American populations, and in childcare facilities. The most common age at presentation is 5 to 10 years old; infections have been reported in all age-groups.

Life Cycle/Transmission
No cystic form of *Dientamoeba* has been identified and its cycle is not completely known. This organism is believed to be transmitted via the fecal–oral route and, given its common concomitant presentation with *Enterobius vermicularis*, it has been postulated that *Dientamoeba* infects humans via pinworm eggs.

Clinical Presentation
Abdominal pain and diarrhea are the most common symptoms presented by children infected with *Dientamoeba*. Mucus may be seen in the stool; blood is rarely present. Diarrhea may last for a couple of weeks, and it is not uncommon to have abdominal pain for 1 or 2 months. Other symptoms such as nausea, vomiting, weight loss, fatigue headache, and bloating are seen less frequently.

Diagnosis
Diagnosis is made by microscopically visualizing trophozoites in fresh stool (Fig. 20-4). Multiple permanently stained samples, using trichrome or hematoxylin, should be examined in order to accurately make the diagnosis.

Treatment
Symptomatic patients have been treated effectively with iodoquinol, paromomycin, or tetracycline.

Blastocystis hominis
Epidemiology
The classification of *Blastocystis* has been controversial as well as its clinical significance. It is currently classified as a protozoan with three stages: vacuolar, granular, and ameboid. It is present worldwide, with a reported prevalence of 33% to 54%, but in the United States it has been seen in 1% to 20% of stools tested in laboratories for ova and parasites. It is usually present in the cecum and proximal colon.

Life Cycle/Transmission
Its transmission is believed to be fecal–oral, but is not well described. The entire life cycle of this organism has not been completely elucidated. The thick-walled cysts are believed to be transmitted via the fecal–oral route, whereas the thin-walled cysts are believed to multiply in the intestinal tract of animals.

Clinical Presentation
The clinical significance of detecting *Blastocystis* in the stool is controversial, given that it frequently presents as an asymptomatic state in an unsuspecting host. Infections related to *Blastocystis* infections present with bloating, nausea, abdominal pain, flatulence, diarrhea and constipation, and perianal pruritus. Untreated, the organism may survive in the intestine from weeks to years.

Diagnosis
Although the diagnosis can be made by detecting the cyst-like form in stool by wet mount or trichrome, some prefer the former technique (Fig. 20-5). At least three specimens should be examined to confirm the diagnosis, avoid confusion of debris with the organism, and to be certain that no other organism is present.

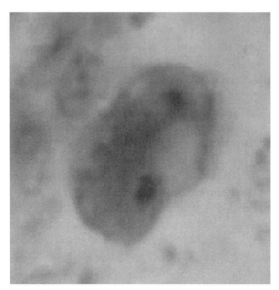

Figure 20-4 *(See also Color Plate 20-4.) Dientamoeba fragilis.* Trichrome stain of a binucleated trophozoite. (From the Public Health Image Library from the Centers for Disease Control and Prevention [CDC] website, http://phil.cdc.gov [provider CDC].)

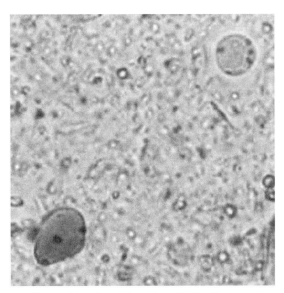

Figure 20-5 *(See also Color Plate 20-5.) Blastocystis hominis.* Iodine stain of the cyst-like form of *Blastocystis*. (From the Public Health Image Library from the Centers for Disease Control and Prevention [CDC] website, http://phil.cdc.gov [provider CDC].)

Treatment

In those cases in which gastrointestinal symptoms are present with positive detection of *Blastocystis*, and in the absence of any other readily identifiable bacteria or virus that may produce similar symptoms, treatment with metronidazole or iodoquinol is reported to be effective.

Cryptosporidium Species
Epidemiology

Cryptosporidium is a worldwide, intracellular protozoan found in fish, birds, reptiles, mammals, and humans. Many species have been described that infect humans, but *Crytosporidium parvum* and *Crytosporidium hominis* are the two most common. Infections are seen mostly in immunocompromised patients, especially those with human immunodeficiency virus (HIV), typically presenting with intractable diarrhea. Residents of endemic areas (tropical developing areas), children in daycares, and international travelers also are at risk. *Cryptosporidium* is found worldwide, but outbreaks such as that which occurred in Milwaukee in 1993 have been described in healthy immunocompetent individuals.

Life Cycle/Transmission

The organism resides in the small and large intestines, as well as in the respiratory epithelia. It is spread by fecally contaminated food and water and direct person-to-person contact. The precise mechanism by which this parasite causes diarrhea is not well known, but adherence of the organism to epithelial cells is believed to contribute to its pathogenesis. Typically, *Cryptosporidium* resides in the stomach and intestines, and, in particular, the ileum.

Clinical Presentation

It presents as profuse watery, self-limited (most cases; immunocompetent hosts) to intractable diarrhea (in immunocompromised individuals, the young and elderly), fever, nausea, anorexia, abdominal discomfort, and vomiting, which usually follow an incubation period of 1 to 7 days in an immunocompetent host.

Diagnosis

Cryptosporidium oocytes can be detected in feces using immunofluorescence microscopy with good yield. Acid-fast staining also is used, as well as enzyme immunoassays.

Treatment

Cryptosporidiosis usually has an uncomplicated course in immunocompetent children, in whom disease resolves in 10 to 14 days without requiring therapy other than rehydration. On the other hand, immunocompromised patients are usually treated with the drug of choice, which is nitazoxanide. There is no effective specific treatment with HIV other than aggressive treatment for HIV. HIV patients on highly active antiretroviral therapy (HAART) have parasite numbers that are reduced to clinically insignificant levels while the patient is on this therapy.

Cyclospora cayetanensis
Epidemiology

C. cayetanensis is present worldwide but the prevalence is higher in Peru, Nepal, and Haiti.

Life Cycle/Transmission

Oocysts passed in stool become infective after they undergo sporulation in the environment. Oocysts, ingested in fresh produce and water, release sporozoites in the small bowel, which then invade the epithelium.

Clinical Presentation

Diarrhea, abdominal pain, anorexia, and fever among other symptoms, usually start after 1 week of incubation. Diarrhea may last up to 3 months.

Diagnosis

Examination of stool under light microscope allows for identification of oocysts.

Treatment

Infection with this protozoan is usually self limited in immunocompetent patients, but requires therapy with trimethoprim-sulfamethoxazole in immunocompromised hosts.

Nematodes (Roundworm)

Strongyloides stercoralis

Epidemiology

This roundworm's geographic distribution includes the tropics, subtropics, and the southern Unites States.

Life Cycle/Transmission

Strongyloides goes through two cycles: the free-living cycle, in which the larvae undergo different stages outside of the human host; and the parasitic cycle. Larvae penetrate the skin, causing a local skin reaction. After penetrating the skin, they migrate via lymphatics and venules to the alveoli, presenting 1 week later with respiratory symptoms. The larvae continue traveling through the respiratory tract until they are swallowed. Once in the small intestine, they mature to adults, and 2 weeks later diarrhea begins. The organism invades the small bowel mucosa, specifically duodenum and jejunum, causing enteritis and eosinophilia.

Clinical Presentation

Although often asymptomatic, healthy children may present with mild diarrhea and abdominal discomfort. Immunosuppressed or malnourished patients may present with a more serious infection characterized by sepsis, shock, and pulmonary and neurologic disease, which may be fatal. Dissemination of the infection may occur in patients receiving steroids or immunosuppressant therapies.

Diagnosis

Larvae may be detected microscopically in stool, duodenal fluid or jejunal biopsy. In patients with disseminated disease, sputum also may be positive. Special techniques of concentration and culture should be done in order to detect the larvae in stool samples. Serum antibodies, which are positive in up to 80% of patients, also should be done.

Treatment

Albendazole is the drug of choice. Other alternatives include ivermectin and thiabendazole.

Ascaris lumbricoides

Epidemiology

Ascariasis is one of the most common human parasitic infections, and the most common helminthic human infection. It is found worldwide, but it is more prevalent in developing areas with poor sanitation. Highest prevalence rates are in Southeast Asia, Africa, and Latin America. Eggs are ingested by contact with contaminated foods, soil, and drinking water. Children bear the brunt of both prevalence and intensity of infections in endemic areas.

Life Cycle/Transmission

Ascariasis is transmitted by ingestion of larvae in soil and by eating raw fruits and vegetables. The eggs become infective when fertilized (Fig. 20-6). Larvae then hatch, and can mature in the lumen of the small intestine, where they penetrate the intestinal wall and migrate into the reticuloendothelial system to the liver, lungs, and eventually into the alveoli. Tracheopharyngeal migration to the gastrointestinal tract occurs when the adult worm differentiates and matures. The sexually mature female worm can produce more than 100,000 eggs per day, usually shed in the feces. Eggs remain viable in moist soil for years, but are very sensitive to desiccation. The average life span of these parasites is approximately one year to 18 months.

Clinical Presentation

Nausea, anorexia, vomiting, and passage of adult worms may accompany colicky epigastric pain. Children and adults with significant infections may present with intestinal obstruction. Usually, infections are asymptomatic. Subclinical infections in children may be associated with anemia and poor growth. In addition to growth failure, *Ascaris* infection may cause malabsorption of fat and protein. Infrequently, pancreatitis, bile duct obstruction, and appendicitis may complicate the disease (worm migration).

During the lung phase of the cycle, children may present with cough, hemoptysis, dyspnea, wheezing, fever, and eosinophilia. Hemorrhages and inflammatory infiltrations may occur with a characteristic diffuse mottling in the peribronchial area appreciable radiographically on plain x-rays (Löffler's syndrome).

Diagnosis

Ascaris may be seen in microscopic examination of concentrated stool or in wet mount if heavy infection. During the pulmonary phase, it also may be found on sputum or gastric aspirate. Occasionally, adult worms may be passed in the stool or come out through the mouth or nose. Migrating ascarid larvae have been identified by serologic antibody (IgE) testing.

Treatment

Drugs of choice for the treatment of ascariasis are albendazole, mebendazole, ivermectin, and pyrantel pamoate. Drug therapies during the migratory stages of the infection are not effective; subsequent treatment 2 to 3 weeks after the initial treatment regimen is therefore indicated. In cases of intestinal obstruction, drugs plus intestinal suction are common

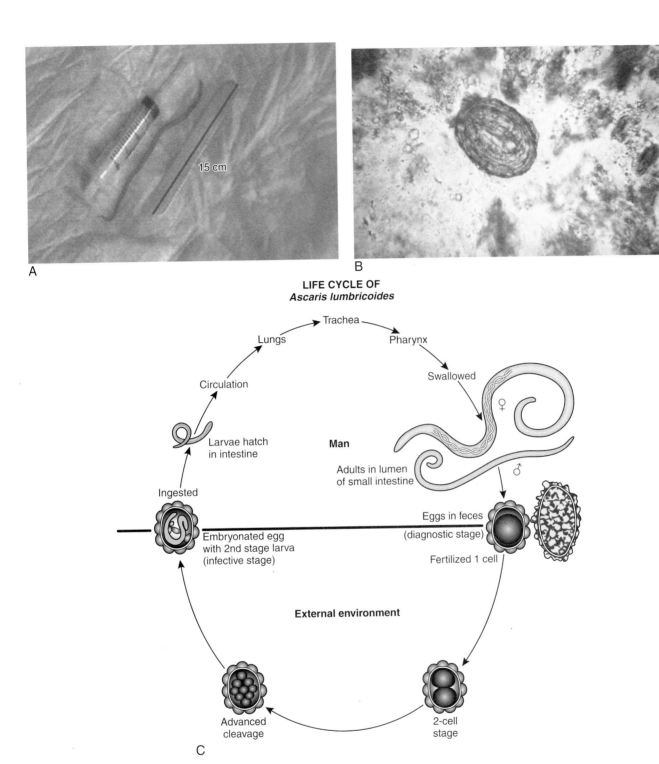

Figure 20-6 *(See also Color Plate 20-6.)* **A,** Adult ascaris male. **B,** Fertilized ascaris egg. **C,** Life cycle of ascaris. (**A,** From Batyraliev T: Pulmonary edema associated with *Ascaris lumbricoides* in a patient with mild mitral stenosis: A case report. Eur J Gen Med 1:43-45, 2004; **B,** from the Public Health Image Library from the Centers for Disease Control and Prevention [CDC] website, http://phil.cdc.gov [provider CDC]; **C,** from Public Health Image Library from the CDC website, http://phil.cdc.gov [provider CDC].)

measures; occasionally surgery is required. Endoscopic removal of bile and pancreatic obstruction is indicated in select cases.

Prevention

Improved, appropriate sewage disposal, sanitation and hygiene about food preparation, regular screening, and appropriate therapy are indicated in endemic areas.

Trichuris trichuria (Whipworm)
Epidemiology

Worldwide distributed, it is most common in the tropics and in regions with high rates of poor sanitation, and where human feces are used as fertilizer. In the United States, infections are most commonly seen in the southeastern states, and in immigrants.

Life Cycle/Transmission

Infection is acquired by the ingestion of embryonated eggs, which require 10 days outside of the human host to reach the infective stage. Typically, the outside shell is digested in the small intestine, where the larvae transiently reside, and subsequently pass to the cecum. In the cecum, they permanently attach to the mucosa. Whipworm can be present all the way to the rectum; each worm is typically 3 to 5 cm long (Fig. 20-7).

Clinical Presentation

Light worm burdens are usually asymptomatic, whereas heavier manifestations can present with abdominal pain, distention, and mucoid to bloody diarrhea, accompanied by tenesmus, weight loss, and weakness; anemia, nutritional deficiencies, growth restriction, and rectal prolapse (secondary to edema) may occur in children with heavy infection. Appendicitis precipitated by obstruction of the lumen by worms has been reported.

Treatment

Albendazole is the drug of choice, administered for a total of 3 days. Repeat pharmacologic therapy may be required because the treatment is not very efficacious. Oral mebendazole is an alternative.

Enterobius vermicularis (Pinworm)
Epidemiology

The pinworm is the most common helminth of industrialized nations and temperate climates. The pediatric population in particular is prone to infection, as are situations of crowding.

Life Cycle/Transmission

The eggs may survive for days in dry dust and can become airborne. Mature eggs are ingested by the host, usually by hand contamination. The eggs hatch in the duodenum, and the larvae develop to maturity in the small intestine, proceed to the large intestine, and reside there, growing up to 13 mm long (females). Gravid females migrate out of the anus and lay their eggs on the perineum, from where pruritus may reinfect the host by means of oral transmission. The eggs can survive for weeks outside the human host, and can remain in unwashed clothing. Alternative routes of reinfection of the host are by the hatched worms re-entering the rectum from the anus and perineum, and back into the colon; the eggs are fully infective within a few hours of being deposited (Fig. 20-8).

Clinical Presentation

Most infections are believed to be asymptomatic. Perianal pruritus is most often reported; migration to the vagina may occur in females, producing local irritation. Attachment of adult worms to the intestinal wall may produce inflammation. Pinworms are not uncom-

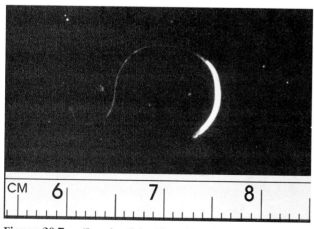

Figure 20-7 *(See also Color Plate 20-7.) Trichuris.* This adult whipworm measures approximately 4 cm in length. (From the Public Health Image Library from the Centers for Disease Control and Prevention [CDC] website, http://phil.cdc.gov [provider CDC/Dr. Mae Melvin].)

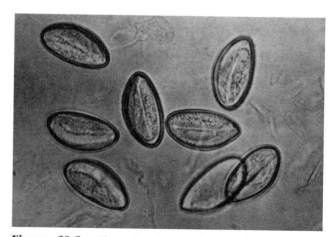

Figure 20-8 *(See also Color Plate 20-8.) Enterobius.* Picture shows pinworm eggs caught on cellulose tape. (From the Public Health Image Library from the Centers for Disease Control and Prevention [CDC] website, http://phil.cdc.gov [provider CDC].)

monly recovered from the appendix during appendectomy, but it is unclear if these are incidental findings or causative agents.

Diagnosis
Recovery of eggs from the perineum in children with pruritus ani can be made by direct observation/examination of the perianal area, as well as by the application of double-sided tape to trap the eggs when they are deposited

Treatment
Tapwater enemas for reducing worm burden have been used. A single oral dose of albendazole followed 2 weeks later by an additional dose is recommended. Pyrantel pamoate may be used in a similar fashion. Empiric treatment of all family members should be considered.

Necator americanus (Hookworm)
Epidemiology
This is the only hookworm found in North and South America, and is native to sub-Saharan Africa and India. Soil contamination by feces and lack of shoes facilitate infection through the skin. Adequate rainfall and loose soil in mostly the tropics and subtropics (and some extension into temperate zones) facilitate infection and survival. Pica can be observed, usually in response to the iron deficiency anemia of the initial infection, increasing the risk for reinfection, and for coinfection with other soil-based parasites.

Life Cycle/Transmission
Eggs in moist soil hatch within 1 to 2 days, where they grow and develop into infective larvae over the subsequent week. These infective larvae do not feed until they infect a host, and can survive for up to 14 days without nourishment. They reside in the upper layers of the soil, and when in contact with the host's skin, can penetrate and enter the host. From the subcutaneous tissue, they enter the venules, are transported to the lungs and enter the alveoli, migrate up the trachea, are swallowed, and enter the small intestine, where maturation occurs, feeding on blood from the host tissue. Mature hookworms mate, and eggs are passed through the stool. *N. americanus* may survive for more than a decade.

Clinical Presentation
Skin penetration by the larvae may produce a significant allergic reaction. Pulmonary symptoms are usually absent. Gastrointestinal symptoms include abdominal discomfort and diarrhea, flatulence, and epigastric pain. Eosinophilia may be present and progressive, and anemia may develop if iron intake is insufficient. Hypoproteinemia and severe anemia can occur with chronic infections.

Treatment
A single oral dose of albendazole is recommended, with mebendazole as the alternative (3-day dosing regimen). Pyrantel pamoate also is effective. Ferrous sulfate therapy coincident to deworming and continuing after treatment is completed should be entertained for anemic patients.

Blood Flukes
Schistosoma Species
Epidemiology
Schistosoma japonicum, Schistosoma mansoni, and *Schistosoma haematobium* are the three species known to most commonly infect humans. They are found in the Caribbean, South America, Africa, and the Middle East. In fact, there are reports of this disease in Africa as early as 3200 BC. Most of the infected humans are asymptomatic, but in some cases the disease can have serious consequences. Rodents are a reservoir in endemic areas, as are domesticated animals. Humans are the only important host for *S. haematobium*. Water snails play roles in contamination of water sources, as intermediate hosts.

Life Cycle/Transmission
Schistosomiasis is transmitted by ingestion of water contaminated with urine *(S. haematobium)* or of feces containing eggs (Fig. 20-9). These worms are dioecious (the sexes are separate). Eggs are produced in the veins from where they penetrate to the small intestine and/or bladder, and they are eliminated in the urine and stools. Eggs in the water hatch and infect snails, an intermediate host that then produces cercariae. Infection follows exposure to contaminated water, by direct skin penetration by the cercariae, to invade the circulatory system. Once penetration has occurred, morphologic changes in the worm occur (such as a loss of the forked tail and glands that facilitated penetration), and it transforms from an aerobic to anaerobic metabolism. The immature fluke, after residing in the subcutaneous tissues for about 2 days invades the circulatory system, first to the lungs and subsequently to the hepatic sinusoidal tissue. In the liver, growth and maturation occur. After approximately 2 weeks, the maturing worms migrate against blood flow into the portal system to the mesenteric or vesicular vasculature. The final location for *S. mansoni* is in the smaller tributaries of the inferior mesenteric vein, in the lower colonic region. *S. japonicum* worms come to reside in the superior mesenteric vein branches in proximity to the small intestine; subsequent invasion of the inferior mesenteries and caval system may occur. *S. haematobium* migrate to the vesical plexus, including prostatic and uterine plexi. Heavy egg infestations and infections with *S. haemotobium* are associated with increased risk of bladder carcinogenesis.

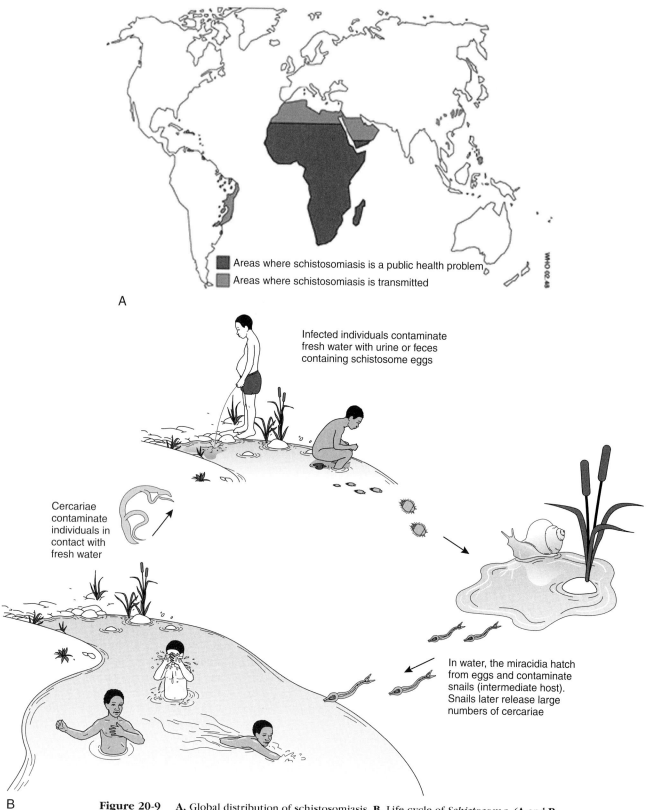

Figure 20-9 **A,** Global distribution of schistosomiasis. **B,** Life cycle of *Schistosoma*. (**A** and **B,** from the World Health Organization website, www.who.int/en.)

Clinical Presentation

Many infections are asymptomatic. Symptoms depend on the organ(s) affected and by the organism causing the infection. The adult worms laying eggs in the mesenteric vasculature trigger the acute stage of the disease, which can last for 1 to 3 months. Egg extrusion subsequently from the bladder wall (*S. haematobium*) may retrigger some of the symptoms seen with the acute symptom presentation and an accompanying hematuria. Infections may cause fever, eosinophilia, localized erythema and pruritus (at the site of penetration), gastrointestinal symptoms (colitis, abdominal pain), acute hepatitis, hepatosplenomegaly (*S. mansoni* and *S. japonicum*), and portal hypertension as well as hepatic and pulmonary cirrhosis and central nervous system symptoms (cerebral granulomatous disease with *S. japonicum;* transverse myletis with *S. mansoni*). Hemoptysis may occur in the pulmonary stages of migration (most with *S. haematobium*). Intestinal disease, usually confined to the colon, occurs with *S. mansoni* and *S. japonicum,* with a granulomatous picture, polyposis, diarrhea, bloody stools, and a protein-losing enteropathy; strictures may occur. Chronic schistosomiasis is related to egg emboli released into the circulation.

Diagnosis

Diagnosis is made by detecting eggs in feces, urine, or duodenal aspirate.

Treatment

Praziquantel is the drug of choice; multiple doses are more effective than single dose treatment. Both periportal fibrosis and bladder wall thickening respond to treatment. The most effective treatment is against the adult worms—treatment during immature forms may actually exacerbate symptoms. Oxamniquine may be used as an alternative when patients don't respond to praziquantel.

Prevention

Prevention includes control in intermediate hosts, elimination of snails from endemic water sources, sanitation, and hygiene measures to prevent contamination; vaccines are in development (Table 20-1).

APPROACH TO THE CASE

The approach to a patient who presents with abdominal pain, poor appetite, and poor growth has to include an evaluation for parasitic infections. In this case, other diagnoses to be considered are failure to thrive, anemia, malnutrition, and lead poisoning, among others. Workup should include evaluation of diet, complete blood count, stool ova and parasites, lead levels, urinalysis, and, given patient's location and incidence of tuberculosis, a Mantoux test. This boy's hemoglobin was 9.0 g/dL, mean corpuscular volume (MCV) 70, mean corpuscular hemoglobin (MCH) 25, mean corpuscular hemoglobin concentration (MCHC) 30, all consistent with hypochromic microcytic anemia. White blood cell (WBC) count was 6500, with a differential of 45% polymorphonuclear cells, 51% lymphocytes, and 4% eosinophils, which is not considered significant eosinophilia. Lead level, urinalysis, and Mantoux test were negative. Stool examination revealed the presence of *A. lumbricoides.* Nutrition evaluation revealed significant deficiencies of all food groups. Besides nutritional and general health advice, he was placed on mebendazole 100 mg twice a day for 3 days, along with ferrous sulfate 6 mg/kg/day divided in three doses for 2 months. Other children in the family were also given mebendazole therapy for presumed infection. Follow-up 1 month later revealed improvement in his general health as well as eating habits. Hemoglobin increased to 10 g/dL. Plans included follow-ups of growth, development, and nutritional status with the pediatrician and iron supplementation.

SUMMARY

Parasitic infections vary geographically, with incidence not confined to traditionally endemic areas in the modern era of globalization and immigration. The recognition of clinical symptoms, diagnosis, appropriate treatment, and surveillance for comorbidities and complications as well as sequelae are relevant to the modern practice of medicine.

MAJOR POINTS

Parasitic infections are prevalent worldwide.
Most commonly, parasitic infections present as an asymptomatic carrier state.
Symptoms vary depending on the mode of infection and host's immune system, among other things.
They usually infect the human host through the mouth or skin.
Significant morbidity may be associated with these infections, especially in the immunocompromised host.
Early detection and treatment are necessary to prevent serious sequelae.

Table 20-1 Other Common Intestinal Parasitic Infections

Parasite	Epidemiology	Transmission/Life Cycle	Location	Symptoms	Diagnosis	Treatment
Protozoan						
Dientamoeba fragilis (amoeba)	Institutionalized populations; homosexual men	Egg transmission suspected	Colonic mucosal crypts; do not invade tissue	Diarrhea, abdominal pain, occasional bloody/mucoid stools, fever, flatulence, fatigue	Binucleated; stained trophozoites in the fresh stool samples fixed with polyvinyl alcohol	Iodoquinol; tetracycline; paromomycin for drug-resistant strains
Balantidium coli (ciliate)	Institutionalized populations; worldwide outbreaks	Fecal-oral; cyst passed in feces; trophozoites in large intestine; mucosal invasion can occur and simulate amebic dysentery. Swine serve as hosts/occasional transmission to humans	Colon, cecum, terminal ileum	Mild colitis, diarrhea; extension to liver, pulmonary system and, urogenital tract possible	Stool; cysts stained with iodine	Oxytetracycline; iodoquinol
Isospora belli (sporozoa)	Developing world; common presentation of HIV/AIDS	Matures in the small intestine	Small intestinal epithelial cell parasite	Usually asymptomatic and self limited; range from mild gastrointestinal (GI) distress cramps, pain, malaise, fever, weakness, weight loss to severe dysentery; eosinophilia; malabsorption	Stool oocyte recovery; duodenal string test	Trimethoprim-sulfamethoxazole for 3 weeks (immunocompromised patients)

Microsporidia	Present in most invertebrates. Mostly in HIV/AIDS patients; coinfection with *Cryptosporidium* common	Primarily by ingestion and inhalation of spores	Obligate intracellular intestinal epithelium	GI: diarrhea, wasting, abdominal pain, nausea, malabsorption; cholangitis	Spores in feces, bile, other GI secretions; organisms in intestinal biopsy Giemsa stains, periodic acid–Schiff positive	Albendazole; may not clear infection
Cestodes *Diphyllobothrium latum* (fish tapeworm)	Worldwide; northern temperate climates; freshwater fish improperly cooked, prepared, pickled	Eggs in contaminated fresh water eaten by two intermediate hosts prior to human transmission	Two intermediate hosts required for life cycle Eggs passed in feces develop in fresh water; embryo eaten by copepod where larva develops; copepod eaten by fish; larva then develops into plerocercoid, ingested by humans; develops into adult worm in the small intestine	Usually asymptomatic; when in proximal jejunum, vitamin B_{12} deficiency and anemia, akin to/ complicating pernicious anemia in genetically susceptible populations	Eggs or worms in stool Worms can grow to several meters in length	Praziquantel for all three species; single dose usually effective Niclosamide is the alternative
Taenia saginata	Taiwan, Korea, China, the Philippines, Malaysia, Indonesia	Eggs are found in feces, infecting raw or undercooked meats (pork)	Small intestine Intermediate hosts include cattle, goats, monkeys, wild boars, pigs	Mild GI complaints and only rarely causes appendicitis, pancreatitis, or cholangitis	Microscopic examination of eggs and proglottids in feces	Praziquantel or niclosamide

Table 20-1 Other Common Intestinal Parasitic Infections—Cont'd

Parasite	Epidemiology	Transmission/Life Cycle	Location	Symptoms	Diagnosis	Treatment
Taenia solium	Latin America, Africa, India, Southeast Asia, China, the Slavic countries	Eggs are found in feces, infecting raw or undercooked meats (pork)	Small intestine. The pig is the intermediate host; eggs once hatched migrate to the duodenum, where they penetrate the intestinal wall. Adult worms can be several meters in length	Adult worm causes mild GI complaints; moderate eosinophilia. Larval infection may cause cysticercosis (epilepsy, retinitis, uveitis, conjunctivitis)	Microscopic examination of eggs and proglottids in feces; perianal tape test also useful. Calcifications may be seen on x-rays. Biopsy of skin nodules	Praziquantel or niclosamide
Nematodes						
Ancylostoma duodenale (Old World hookworm)	Europe, the Mediterranean, South America (west coast), India, China	Eggs are transmitted in the stool and infect humans through skin penetration	Migrate through the heart, lungs, into the small intestine (see *Necator americanus*).	Iron deficiency anemia, skin eruption (ground itch) and cardiac, GI and lung symptoms	Microscopic inspection of eggs in the stool	In endemic areas, it is often not treated, but in the U.S. it is treated with albendazole, mebendazole, levamisole, or pyrantel pamoate; oral iron
Anisakis spp.	North America (herring, salmon, mackerel); also cod, halibut, Pacific red snapper, sardines, squid; Japan and the Netherlands, with infections from sushi, smoked, pickled fish	Transmitted by infected fish consumption	Marine mammal parasites. Eggs passed in mammal feces hatch and free-swimming larvae ingested by crustaceans; crustaceans eaten by fish and squid; migration to muscle tissues, eaten by other fish and squid and transmitted; fish and squid maintain larvae infective to humans and marine mammals; humans become infected from undercooked seafood	Transient cases mostly in North America. Gastric invasion, intestinal tract invasion; abrupt onset 1 to 5 days following ingestion; abdominal pain, nausea, emesis, diarrhea, peritonitis, adynamic ileus, perforation possible; eosinophilic infiltrates	Endoscopic worm removal from the stomach; gastric filling defect on upper GI series; worms in emesis	Transient cases: no treatment required. GI form: EGD/surgery required/curative with removal. Albendazole twice daily for 3 weeks or more may be required

Trichinella spiralis	Follows dietary patterns and sanitation; highest rates in China; also in the United States, Spain, France, Italy, Slavic countries	Parasite of carnivorous animals; undercooked pork/meat with larvae present; rats and swine are reservoirs (fed refuse)	Ingestion of undercooked pork with larvae; larvae are encysted in skeletal muscle. When ingested, adult worms enter wall of small intestine; penetrate wall, enter bloodstream and are carried to muscle where they encyst	Intestinal symptoms usually minor; if present, nonspecific gastroenteritis picture. Eosinophilia, leukocytosis, hyper-IgE; myositis prominent; subungual splinter hemorrhages; meningoencephalitis possible/CVA and CNS symptoms possible	Serologic tests Skeletal muscle biopsy	Mebendazole three times daily for 3 to 10 days Albendazole for 8 to 14 days is an alternative Corticosteroids in symptomatic/toxicity cases

AIDS, acquired immunodeficiency syndrome; CNS, central nervous system; CVA, cardiovascular accident; EGD, esophagogastroduodenoscopy; HIV, human immunodeficiency virus; IgE, immunoglubulin E.

SUGGESTED READINGS

Abramowicz M: Drugs for parasitic infections. Med Lett 1-12, 2004.

Ali IK, Zaki M, Clark CG: Use of PCR amplification of tRNA gene-linked short tandem repeats for genotyping *Entamoeba histolytica*. J Clin Microbiol 43:5842-5847, 2005.

Amadi B, Kelly P, Mwiya M, et al: Intestinal and systemic infection, HIV, and mortality in Zambian children with persistent diarrhea and malnutrition. J Pediatr Gastroenterol Nutr 32:550-554, 2001.

Aziz H, Beck CE, Lux MF, Hudson MJ: A comparison study of different methods used in the detection of *Giardia lamblia*. Clin Lab Sci 14:150-154, 2001.

Calderaro A, Gorrini C, Bommezzadri S, et al: *Entamoeba histolytica* and *Entamoeba dispar:* Comparison of two PCR assays for diagnosis in a non-endemic setting. Trans R Soc Trop Med Hyg 100:450-457, 2006.

Centers for Disease Control and Prevention (CDC) website: www.dpd.cdc.gov.

Christie JD, Crouse D, Kelada AS, et al: Patterns of *Schistosoma haematobium* egg distribution in the human lower urinary tract. III. Cancerous lower urinary tracts. Am J Trop Med Hyg 35:759-764, 1986.

Crompton DWT, Nesheim MC: Nutritional impact of intestinal helminthiasis during the human life cycle. Annu Rev Nutr 22:35-59, 2002.

Eisenberg JN, Seto EY, Colford JM Jr, et al: An analysis of the Milwaukee cryptosporidiosis outbreak based on a dynamic model of the infection process. Epidemiology 9:255-263, 1998.

Farthing MJ: Immune response–mediated pathology in human intestinal parasitic infection. Parasite Immunol 25:247-257, 2003.

Fenollar F, Lepidi H, Gerolami R, et al: Whipple disease associated with giardiasis. J Infect Dis 188:828-834, 2003.

Gendrel D, Treluyer JM, Richard-Lenoble D: Parasitic diarrhea in normal and malnourished children. Fundam Clin Pharmacol 17:189-197, 2003.

Hodder SL, Mahmoud AA, Sorenson K, et al: Predisposition to urinary tract epithelial metaplasia in *Schistosoma haematobium* infection. Am J Trop Med Hyg 63:133-138, 2000.

Jong E: Intestinal parasites. Prim Care Clin Office Pract 29:857-877, 2002.

Macpherson CN: Human behaviour and the epidemiology of parasitic zoonoses. Int J Parasitol 35:1319-1331, 2005.

Moon TD, Oberhelman RA: Antiparasitic therapy in children. Pediatr Clin North Am 52:917-948, viii, 2005.

O'Ryan M, Prado V, Pickering L: A millennium update on pediatric diarrheal illness in the developing world. Semin Pediatr Infect Dis 16:125-136, 2005.

Petri WA: Pathogenesis of amebiasis. Curr Opin Microbiol 5:443-447, 2002.

Podewils LJ, Mintz ED, Nataro JP, Parashar UD: Acute, infectious diarrhea among children in developing countries. Semin Pediatr Infect Dis 15:155-168, 2004.

Ruffer MA: Note on the presence of *Bilharzia haematobia* in Egyptian mummies of the twentieth dynasty (1250-1000 BC). BMJ I:16, 1910.

Scott ME, Koski KG: Zinc deficiency impairs immune responses against parasitic nematode infections at intestinal and systemic sites. J Nutr 130:1412S-1420S, 2000.

Weinstock JV, Summers R, Elliott DE: Helminths and harmony. Gut 53:7-9, 2004.

Zardi EM, Picardi A, Afeltra A: Treatment of cryptosporidiosis in immunocompromised hosts. Chemotherapy 51:193-196, 2005.

CHAPTER 21

Perianal Anomalies

GREGORZ TELEGA

Disease Description
Case Presentation
Epidemiology
Pathophysiology
Definitions
Differential Diagnosis
Diagnostic Testing
Treatment
Approach to the Case
Summary
Major Points

DISEASE DESCRIPTION

Perianal diseases in children are common and encompass a broad spectrum of pathologic processes, including congenital anomalies, fissures, fistulae, abscesses, hemorrhoids, rectal prolapse, and pilonidal sinus. Most of perianal pathology is related to local disease, but the clinician should be aware of the fact that some perianal pathology can be associated with sequences of congenital anomalies or with systemic illnesses such as inflammatory bowel disease.

CASE PRESENTATION

A 15-year-old female presented with tenesmus and perianal pain. The patient has been symptomatic for the past 3 weeks. Pain with defecation is present daily, and she passes three or four bowel movements per day. Stools are formed, are small with no visible blood, and have no mucus. The patient has a sensation of incomplete defecation. A trial of mineral oil did not improve symptoms. On review of symptoms the patient reports fatigue ("I am not so good at sports anymore"). There is no abdominal pain and no weight loss. The patient does not have menarche yet. All other systems have been reviewed and are normal. The past medical history shows no medical problems, and the family history shows no chronic disorders.

On physical examination, the patient is active and alert. Findings are as follows: weight—42.2 kg (5th percentile), height—146 cm (<5th percentile), heart rate—74, respiratory rate—16, blood pressure—95/60 mm Hg. Head, eyes, ears, nose, and throat (HEENT): oral mucosa moist, tympanic membranes pale, mobile with insufflations; no oral ulcers. Neck: supple, no goiter. Chest: no retractions, no dullness on percussion, lungs clear to auscultation. Breasts—Tanner II. Abdomen: soft, not distended, not tender, no hepatosplenomegaly, no masses; bowel sounds present. Musculoskeletal: short stature; joints—full range of motion, no swelling, and no erythema. Skin: no rash, adequate subcutaneous fat. Genital: no anatomic abnormalities, intact hymen, and pubic hair: Tanner II. Neurologic examination: intact cranial nerves, symmetric muscle tone, symmetric deep tendon reflexes, normal gait, normal speech, and normal cognitive skills. Rectal examination: an indurated, tender area with erythema is present on the posterior aspect of the anus. Patient refused digital examination due to fear of pain.

EPIDEMIOLOGY

Anorectal anomalies (imperforate anus) occur in approximately 1 in 2500 live births. Cloacal exstrophy is very rare, and its prevalence is probably less than 1 in 200,000 or 1 in 400,000 live births, slightly more frequent in males. Up to 15% of children with Crohn's disease will present with perianal abscesses or fistulae.

PATHOPHYSIOLOGY

The anus, as the rest of the gastrointestinal (GI) tract, has two major muscular layers: the muscularis externa and the muscularis mucosae. The rectum differs from the colon by its lack of taeniae. In their place is a complete layer of longitudinal muscle fibers. Mucosal folds known as the valves of Houston are characteristic anatomic features of the rectum; the distal third of the rectum is devoid of peritoneum, and the proximal segment of rectum has peritoneum on its anterior wall. The anal canal is defined as a portion of bowel that passes through the levator ani muscles and opens onto the anal verge. The external and internal sphincter muscles function as a continence mechanism.

The main events in the embryologic development of the anorectal area include cloaca formation at approximately 21 days' gestation and separation of an anterior urogenital cavity and a posterior anorectal cavity by 6 weeks of gestation. Disruption of this process results in a variety of congenital anomalies.

Cloacal exstrophy is a major defect of the abdominal wall; patients will present with a combination of omphalocele, a bladder exstrophy, and anal atresia. The corpora of the penis or clitoris can be found on separated pubic bones. Other malformations can be present. Assignment of gender may be difficult and should be postponed until the patient's evaluation is complete.

Anal atresia is an anomaly in which there is no anal opening within the ring of external anal sphincter. The abnormally located opening is usually in the midline within the urethra, scrotum, or perineum in males or within the vagina, vulva, or perineum in females.

Duplication cysts are attached to the alimentary canal; they have a muscle layer and an epithelial lining.

About 60% of infants with anorectal anomalies will have other congenital defects, including genitourinary, cardiac, gastrointestinal, or vertebral anomalies, known as the VACTERL (vertebral, anorectal, cardiac, tracheoesophageal, renal, limb) sequence. Johanson-Blizzard syndrome is associated with morphologic abnormalities: congenital aplasia of the alae nasi, ectodermal scalp defects, imperforate anus, and pancreatic insufficiency.

DEFINITIONS

Perirectal abscess is one of the most common disorders of the perianal area. A perirectal abscess is a localized pus collection in the perirectal tissues. Abscesses can be classified according to their location in relation to the levator ani and eternal anal sphincter. Abscesses in the perianal location are the most common, followed by abscesses in ischioanal, intersphincteric, and supralevator locations. Perirectal abscesses usually arise from the crypts between columns of Morgagni; cryptitis can evolve into a perianal abscess. Abscesses can lead to formation of the fistulas. Perirectal abscesses or fistulas can be a presentation of systemic diseases like Crohn's disease, diabetes and chronic granulomatous disease, neutropenia, leukemia, and human immunodeficiency virus (HIV), as well as side effects from the use of immunosuppression. Of children with Crohn's disease, 15% will present with perianal abscesses or fistulae.

Perianal infections are common in infants in diapers. Usually there is no specific inciting event, but occasionally there is an accompanying diaper rash. In these cases, infection may be the result of an inward spread from the skin. *Candida albicans* and group A β-hemolytic streptococci are common organisms that cause infections in the diaper area.

Anal fissure is a tear of the anoderm (the skin of the anal canal). The tear is commonly linear. Simple tears usually heal within 1 or 2 days without scarring. Chronic fissure usually develops as a consequence of infection of the simple tear. Resolution of chronic fissures leads to formation of a skin tag. Chronic fissures and skin tags can be associated with Crohn's disease.

Hemorrhoids are varices of perirectal venous plexus. They are classified into two types: external and internal. External hemorrhoids involve the skin of the anus, and their nerve supply is derived from the skin. As a result, external hemorrhoids are associated with acute pain when infected or thrombosed. Internal hemorrhoids are located under the rectal mucosa; they usually present with hematochezia. Chronic constipation and excessive straining are implicated in the development of hemorrhoids. Internal hemorrhoids may also be associated with portal hypertension.

Rectal prolapse is more common in boys than in girls. The condition is usually self limited. Usually prolapse is associated with a history of prolonged straining at defecation. Rectal prolapse may also be associated with an acute diarrheal episode, cystic fibrosis, or a neurologic or anatomic anomaly. Children with unexplained or recurrent rectal prolapse should have a sweat chloride test to rule out cystic fibrosis.

Pilonidal abscess is an abscess in the sacrococcygeal region in the midline, which is often accompanied by draining sinus tracts. A pilonidal sinus usually begins at the site of an ingrown hair follicle. It usually is located 1 or 2 inches above the anus.

DIFFERENTIAL DIAGNOSIS

The differential diagnosis for perirectal induration and tenesmus can be found in Table 21-1.

Table 21-1 Most Common Disorders of Perianal Area

Disease	Presentation
Perirectal abscess	Perirectal induration, perirectal fistula, mucopurulent drainage, tenesmus, constipation, perirectal tenderness, low-grade fevers, pelvic pain
External hemorrhoids	Induration within anal opening, tender when clot or inflammation forms within the varix, common cause of bleeding with the blood on the surface of stool or on toilet paper
Crohn's perianal disease	Single or multiple abscesses and fistulas in perianal area. Usually associated with other symptoms of bowel inflammation (diarrhea, blood in the stool, abdominal pain, early satiety), malnutrition (weight loss, failure to thrive, short stature, delayed puberty) or systemic inflammation (low-grade fevers, joint pain, fatigue)
Anal fissure	Linear fissure, indurated only when infected. Pain with defecation. Bleeding with blood on the surface of stool or on toilet paper
Rectal prolapse	Prolapse usually occurs after defecation or straining. Induration is circular present within anal opening, prolapsed mucosa can be swollen and erythematous; tenesmus can be present,
Pilonidal abscess	Persistent pain in the sacrococcygeal region accompanied by a boil located in the midline just above the anus. Often results in a chronic pilonidal sinus

The early sign of perianal abscess is an indurated, tender area in the perianal area. Erythema can be present, although it is not universal. Inspection of the perianal area and digital rectal examinations identify the abscess in the majority of patients. Constant crying or irritability that is worse with diaper changing can suggest perirectal abscess. Rupture of abscess can lead to formation of a fistula, and to persistent drainage. With perirectal abscess or fistula, one must always consider associated diseases, particularly in older children.

DIAGNOSTIC TESTING

Proper examination of the anus, perineal area, and rectum will detect many obvious causes of lower GI bleeding, rectal pain, or tenesmus. Without proper examination, the clinician often ends up performing unnecessary tests. Anorectal anomalies are usually detected during routine newborn examination. An anogenital index can be calculated by dividing the distance from the vagina or scrotum to the anus, by the distance from the vagina or scrotum to the coccyx. The normal anogenital index in females is 0.39 ± 0.09, whereas 0.56 ± 0.2 is normal for males.

The lower back should be examined for evidence of sacral agenesis. Neurologic examination of the lower extremities should be performed to exclude spinal cord lesions. When congenital anorectal anomalies are detected, active investigation for associated anomalies should be initiated. Ultrasonography of the kidneys and spinal cord, echocardiography, echocardiography karyotyping should be considered.

Simple, nonrecurrent perianal abscess in infants and young children may be treated surgically without additional tests. Investigation of the perianal abscess in older children should include review of the growth chart and sexual maturation. A complete blood count (CBC), chemistry panel, and erythrocyte sedimentation rate (ESR) should be tested to screen for diabetes or irritable bowel disease (IBD). If "red flags" like failure to thrive, delayed puberty, anemia, or hypoalbuminemia are present, further evaluation with colonoscopy, esophagogastroduodenoscopy and upper-GI barium study with small bowel follow-through should be considered. If surgical fistulectomy is contemplated, pelvic magnetic resonance imaging (MRI) should be considered to define anatomy of rectal fistulas.

TREATMENT

The goal of initial management of imperforate anus is relief of the distal bowel obstruction and protection of the anal sphincter mechanism. Usually, the surgeon creates a colostomy and in a second stage, performs definitive reconstruction. Only low lesions with the anomaly distal to the anal sphincter are amenable to one-stage reconstructive procedures without diverting a colostomy. Most anorectal anomalies are amenable to reconstruction via a posterior sagittal approach. Laparotomy is often required in girls with cloacal anomaly and boys with rectovesical fistula. Superb surgical technique is necessary to optimize the long-term outcome. Children with "high" malformations tend to have a worse outcome, with higher rates of fecal incontinence. Constipation occurs frequently even in children with "low" lesions.

Treatment of simple uncomplicated rectal abscesses includes surgical drainage and systemic antibiotics if necessary. Abscesses with draining fistula should be drained, but if the fistula persists, a fistulectomy should be considered. Precise imaging of fistulas in relationship to rectal structures increases safety of the procedure. Abscesses and fistulas associated with systemic disease should be approached in the context of the specific disease. For example in Crohn's disease 6-mercaptopurine (MP) and azathioprine in combination with antibiotics (metronidazole, ciprofloxacin) can be tried. Recently anti–tumor necrosis factor (TNF) chimeric antibody (infliximab) has been shown to be effective in the treatment of fistulizing Crohn's disease.

APPROACH TO THE CASE

Presence of systemic symptoms like fatigue, short stature, delayed puberty in combination with local complaints (tenesmus, perianal induration), suggests Crohn's disease. Initial laboratory workup should include CBC, chemistry panel, and ESR (or C-reactive protein [CRP]). The clinician should take into account the history, physical examination, and laboratory workup to estimate the likelihood of Crohn's disease. A high index of suspicion should be applied because Crohn's disease can present with subtle nonspecific symptoms. If Crohn's disease is suspected, referral should be made to a pediatric gastroenterologist for further evaluation. Diagnosis of Crohn's disease is made by endoscopy (colonoscopy in combination with esophagogastroduodenoscopy) and histologic evaluation of colonic and intestinal mucosa.

The diagnosis is based on the presence of chronic inflammation involving the small intestine or chronic granulomatous inflammation of any segment of gastrointestinal (GI) tract. The presence of abscesses, fistulas, skip lesions, rectal sparing, transmural inflammation supports a diagnosis of Crohn's disease. Cases of chronic colitis without diagnostic features of Crohn's disease but not following the classic pattern of ulcerative colitis are classified as indeterminate colitis. Once diagnosis is established, gastroenterologists may choose to define the extent of the disease and investigate potential complications. Upper GI with small bowel follow-through can be done to investigate the small bowel not accessible to endoscopy. This study can also be used if small bowel stenosis or fistulas are suspected. Limitation of the barium study is poor visualization of the small bowel mucosa. If investigation of small bowel mucosa is necessary, enteroclysis or capsule endoscopy can be performed. When intra-abdominal abscess is suspected, abdominal and pelvic computed tomography (CT) scanning with oral and IV contrast should be performed. In some cases of colitis (including Crohn's colitis) sclerosing cholangitis can be present. Endoscopic retrograde cholangiogram is the study of choice for a diagnosis of sclerosing cholangitis.

Once the diagnosis of Crohn's disease is established, therapy is based on immunomodulatory agents; 5-aminosalicylic acid components (sulfasalazine and mesalamine) are not effective in modifying the long-term course of the disease. In mild cases of Crohn's disease oral or local 5-aminosalicylic acid (5-ASA) compounds can be used for symptomatic improvement. Azathioprine or 6-mercaptopurine (6-MP) can modify the course of the disease, decrease frequency of relapses, and decrease their severity. Steroids are effective in treating acute exacerbations of Crohn's disease, but they do not alter the course of the disease and are associated with significant side effects. Steroids are not effective in the treatment of perianal Crohn's disease. Antibiotics (metronidazole or ciprofloxacin) have been used with success in some cases, but no randomized controlled trial has been done to support this claim. Side effects of therapy (peripheral neuropathy) are common with metronidazole. Infliximab is a chimeric anti-TNF antibody. This medication is available as an IV infusion and is effective in treating Crohn's disease, with reported response rates close to 70%. Infliximab has been successful in treating fistulizing and perianal Crohn's disease, but the response rate for perianal disease is only 46%.

SUMMARY

Examination of the perianal area is an important part of a physical examination. Main categories of disorders include congenital anatomic anomalies (anal atresia, cloacal exstrophy, duplication cyst) and inflammatory disorders (perirectal abscess, rectal fistula, pilonidal abscess, perianal Crohn's disease).

MAJOR POINTS

Examination of the perianal area is an important part of the physical examination.

Without a proper examination, a clinician often performs unnecessary tests.

About 60% of infants with anorectal anomalies will have other congenital defects including genitourinary, cardiac, gastrointestinal, or vertebral anomalies.

Infants crying or irritability that is worse with diaper changing can suggest perirectal abscess.

Simple, nonrecurrent perianal abscesses in infants and young children may be treated surgically without additional tests.

Perirectal abscesses or fistulas can be a presentation of systemic disease; a clinician should investigate for presence of "red flags."

Chronic fissures and skin tags can be associated with Crohn's disease.

Children with unexplained or recurrent rectal prolapse should have a sweat chloride test to rule out cystic fibrosis.

Pilonidal abscess is located in the sacrococcygeal region in the midline and is often accompanied by draining sinus tracts.

SUGGESTED READINGS

Bar-Maor JA, Eitan A: Determination of the normal position of the anus (with reference to idiopathic constipation). J Pediatr Gastroenterol Nutr 6:559-561, 1987.

Festen C, van Harten H: Perianal abscess and fistula-in-ano in infants. J Pediatr Surg 33:711-713, 1998.

Forrester MB, Merz RD: Descriptive epidemiology of anal atresia in Hawaii, 1986-1999. Teratology 66 Suppl S12-S16, 2002.

Jeshion WC, Larsen KL, Jawad AF, et al: Azathioprine and 6-mercaptopurine for the treatment of perianal Crohn's disease in children. J Clin Gastroenterol 30:294-298, 2000.

Langer JC: Abdominal wall defects. World J Surg 27:117-124, 2003.

Lichtenstein GR: Treatment of fistulizing Crohn's disease. Gastroenterology 119:1132-1147, 2000.

Markowitz J, Daum F, Aiges H, et al: Perianal disease in children and adolescents with Crohn's disease. Gastroenterology 86:829-833, 1984.

Pena A, Hong A: Advances in the management of anorectal malformations. Am J Surg 180:370-376, 2000.

Pena A: Surgical management of anoectal malformations: A unified concept. Pediatr Surg Int 3:82-93, 1988.

Present DH, Rutgeerts P, Targan S, et al: Infliximab for the treatment of fistulas in patients with Crohn's disease. N Engl J Med 340:1398-1405, 1999.

Schouten WR, Briel JW, Auwerda JJ, et al: Anal fissure: New concepts in pathogenesis and treatment. Scand J Gastroenterol 31(Suppl 218):78-81, 1996.

Siafakas C, Vottler TP, Andersen JM: Rectal prolapse in pediatrics. Clin Pediatr (Phila) 38:63-72, 1999.

Singh B, Mortensen NJ McC, Jewell DP, George B: Perianal Crohn's disease. Br J Surg 91:801-814, 2004.

Soffer SZ, Rosen NG, Hong AR, et al: Cloacal exstrophy: A unified management plan. J Pediatr Surg 35:932-937, 2000.

CHAPTER 22

Polyps and Polyposis Syndromes

MEI-LUN WANG

ANIL RUSTGI

Disease Description
Case Presentation
Clinical Presentation
Polyp Classification and Histology
    Harmartomatous Polyps
        Juvenile Polyps
        Juvenile Polyposis Syndrome
        Cowden Syndrome and Bannayan-Riley-Ruvalcaba
            Syndrome
        Peutz-Jeghers Syndrome
    Familial Adenomatous Polyposis
Principles of Genetic Screening
Summary
Major Points

DISEASE DESCRIPTION

Although the vast majority of childhood polyps are benign, a small subset is found in the setting of inherited predisposition that may increase the risk of colorectal cancer or other neoplasms. This chapter reviews the classification of polyps in children, including an overview of major polyposis syndromes (Table 22-1). Clinical management and indications for screening colonoscopy are reviewed and principles of genetic testing and counseling are discussed.

CASE PRESENTATION

A 4-year-old boy presents to the clinic with a 3-month history of intermittent hematochezia. He has daily, soft, formed bowel movements, in which there is occasionally bright red blood. At the onset of the symptoms, his pediatrician started him on a stool softener. Although the stools are now softer, intermittent bright red rectal bleed-

ing persists. The patient does not have abdominal pain, and his appetite is normal. The review of systems is negative for fevers, chills, nausea, or vomiting. He is not on any medications. His past medical history, family history, and social history are all unremarkable. On physical examination, he is at the 75th percentile for height and the 50th percentile for weight. His abdomen is soft and nontender without organomegaly or masses. The rectal examination is notable for soft brown stool in the rectal vault that is heme positive. There are no perianal skin tags or fissures. The patient's hemoglobin, platelet count, prothrombin time/International Normalized Ratio (PT/INR), and partial thromboplastin time (PTT) are all within normal limits. At colonoscopy, two pedunculated polyps are found in the rectosigmoid colon.

CLINICAL PRESENTATION

Most childhood polyps are asymptomatic, and are found incidentally at colonoscopy. However, gastrointestinal polyps can manifest as rectal bleeding, abdominal pain, or rarely, intestinal obstruction. The differential diagnosis of rectal bleeding is outlined in Table 22-2. Visible rectal bleeding can result from trauma from the passage of stool. The surface of a polyp may also ulcerate and bleed as it outgrows its own blood supply. A polyp may also serve as a lead point for intussusception, resulting in colicky abdominal pain or obstructive symptoms.

POLYP CLASSIFICATION AND HISTOLOGY

Visually, polyps are described as pedunculated or sessile. Pedunculated polyps are mushroom-like lesions that are attached to the intestinal mucosa by a stalk. Sessile polyps are flat, elevated lesions that are attached to the mucosa by a broad base.

Table 22-1 Polyposis Syndromes in Children					
	Age at Presentation	Gene Mutation	Polyp Histology	Cancer Risk	Benign Extraintestinal Manifestations
Juvenile polyposis syndrome (JPS)	1st to 2nd decade	SMAD4 BMPR1A	Hamartoma	Colon Stomach Duodenum	None
Peutz-Jeghers syndrome (PJS)	1st decade	STK11/LKB1	Hamartoma	Colon Breast Testes Ovary Pancreas Lung	Mucocutaneous pigmentation Polyps in sinuses, bronchi, bladder
Bannayan-Riley-Ruvalcaba syndrome (BRRS)/Cowden syndrome (CS)	2nd to 3rd decade	PTEN	Hamartoma Adenoma Ganglioneuroma Lipoma	Breast Thyroid	Macrocephaly Mucocutaneous pigmentation Uterine abnormalities Thyroid disease
Familial adenomatous polyposis (FAP)	2nd decade	*APC*	Adenoma	Colon (100%) Hepatoblastoma Medulloblastoma Glioblastoma multiforme Thyroid Adrenal	Osteomas Epidermoid cysts Congenital hypertrophy of retinal pigment epithelium (CHRPE) Desmoid

Most pediatric polyps are either hamartomas or adenomas. Rarely, lipomas or neuromas are found in the intestinal tract in children. Hamartomatous polyps, also referred to as inflammatory polyps, tend to be pedunculated. Grossly, these polyps may appear ulcerated and friable. Histologically, the majority of hamartomatous polyps are characterized by an expanded lamina propria, dilated mucin-filled cystic glands, and an infiltration of inflammatory cells (Fig. 22-1). Hamartomas are not malignant, and rarely have dysplastic features. In contrast, adenomatous polyps are dysplastic lesions with malignant potential. Grossly, adenomas tend to have lobulated surfaces as a result of uneven growth. Histologically, adenomas have irregular nuclei with increased mitotic figures (Fig. 22-2). Foci of intestinal epithelial proliferation expand into zones of normally nonproliferating epithelium. As the rate of cell proliferation increases, polypoid lesions develop; thus the larger the adenoma, the greater the risk for malignant transformation.

Harmartomatous Polyps

Juvenile Polyps

The most frequently encountered intestinal polyps in the pediatric population are juvenile polyps, which occur with an estimated frequency of 1:50 to 1:100 in children ages 1 to 18. Juvenile polyps occur with greatest frequency in the first decade of life, with a peak incidence between 2 and 5 years. Juvenile polyps in the first 12 months of life are exceedingly rare. Although symptoms such as abdominal pain and iron deficiency anemia can occur in up to one third of patients, the majority of patients present with only painless rectal bleeding. At colonoscopy, 50% of patients with juvenile polyps have more than one polyp: 53% of juvenile polyps are found in the rectosigmoid colon, and the remainder are found at approximately equal distribution throughout the remainder of the colon (16% ascending, 16% transverse, and 13% descending

Table 22-2 Differential Diagnosis of Rectal Bleeding in Children
Infectious diarrhea
Anal fissures
Polyps
Inflammatory bowel disease
Meckel's diverticulum
Allergic enteropathy
Intussusception
Henoch-Schönlein purpura
Vascular lesions

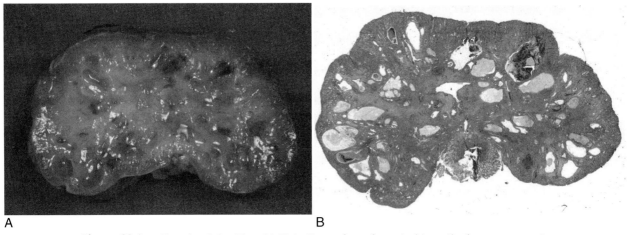

Figure 22-1 *(See also Color Plate 22-1.)* **A,** Cut surface of a typical juvenile (hamartomatous) polyp. **B,** Hematoxylin and eosin–stained hamartomatous polyp with dilated mucin-filled cystic glands and inflammatory infiltrate. (Courtesy Eduardo D. Ruchelli, MD, Children's Hospital of Philadelphia.)

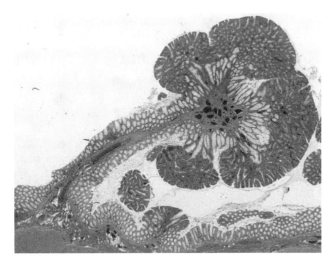

Figure 22-2 *(See also Color Plate 22-2.)* Hematoxylin and eosin–stained adenoma, with a multilobulated surface (×100). (Courtesy Eduardo D. Ruchelli, MD, Children's Hospital of Philadelphia.)

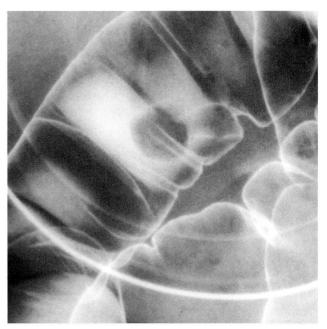

Figure 22-3 Isolated juvenile polyp (hamartoma). Spot radiograph from double-contrast barium enema shows a 1-cm pedunculated polyp in the sigmoid region. The head of the polyp is manifested as a translucent filling defect in the barium pool; the stalk of the polyp as two parallel barium-etched lines. (Courtesy Stephen E. Rubesin, MD, Hospital of the University of Pennsylvania.)

colon). The radiographic appearance of a solitary juvenile polyp is depicted in Figure 22-3.

The risk for neoplasia in patients with juvenile polyps is extremely low; in fact, there have been only eight cases in the literature of neoplasia in the setting of typical juvenile polyps. Juvenile polyps should be endoscopically removed, even if found incidentally on colonoscopy. Removal of solitary polyps followed by histologic confirmation is usually sufficient, and endoscopic surveillance is not necessary unless there is a relevant family history or if the symptoms recur.

Juvenile Polyposis Syndrome

Juvenile polyposis syndrome (JPS) is a rare syndrome characterized by multiple hamartomatous polyps within the gastrointestinal tract, albeit with a proclivity in the colon. Transmitted in an autosomal dominant fashion, the condition has a mean age of presentation at 9 years, although many cases of JPS present in the second or third decade of life. Like solitary juvenile polyps, JPS can present with rectal bleeding, abdominal pain, and anemia. More unusual presentations of JPS include prolapse of the polyp or rectum, diarrhea, or a protein-losing enteropathy.

JPS can be subdivided into three categories based on the clinical presentation and polyp location. JPS of infancy is extremely rare, with affected individuals presenting in the first year of life with bloody diarrhea, failure to thrive, and protein-losing enteropathy. Death occurs by the end of the first year of life. In juvenile polyposis coli (JPC), polyps are restricted to the colon and rectum (Fig. 22-4). The mean age at presentation in JPC ranges from age 5 to 15 years. In generalized JPS, any site from the stomach to the rectum can be affected, with the total number of polyps ranging from 10 and 200. Affected patients with generalized JPS tend to present at a younger age (<5 years) than patients with JPC.

The development for JPS has recently been linked to mutations of the transforming growth factor-beta (TGF-β) superfamily. TGF-β functions as a growth inhibitor in the intestinal epithelium by initiating cell cycle arrest. In certain individuals with JPS, a mutation in Smad4, a key signaling molecule in the TGF-β pathway, interrupts growth inhibitory signaling by TGF-β, resulting in unopposed epithelial growth and polyp formation. Mutations in Smad4 are currently believed to be responsible for approximately 25% of JPS cases. Mutations of another member of the TGF-β superfamily, bone morphogenetic protein receptor 1A (BMPR1A), disrupt signaling through the Smad4 pathway, also resulting in unopposed epithelial growth. Identification of JPS genotype may have implications on specific JPS phenotypes. For example, whereas Smad4 mutation–positive cases are associated with generalized JPS, Smad4 mutation–negative cases are more likely to have JPC.

In contrast to patients with typical juvenile polyps, patients with JPS are at increased risk for the development of gastrointestinal neoplasia. Approximately 50% of JPS patients develop colon cancer, based on studies of affected JPS families. Studies of adult patients with JPS have shown that the risk of developing colorectal carcinoma increases from 15% at age 35, to up to 68% at age 60. In a retrospective study of 57 patients with JPS who developed colon cancer, the mean age of cancer diagnosis was 38 years. Malignancies of the small intestine and stomach have also been described in adults with JPS.

Given the implications for surveillance and outcome, it is important to distinguish between the diagnoses of typical juvenile polyps and JPS. However, current controversy exists regarding the number of polyps that must be found to raise suspicion for JPS. Retrospective reviews of JPS suggest that patients with as few as three juvenile polyps should be undergo genetic screening for Smad4 and PTEN mutations. Other diagnostic criteria for JPS include the finding of any number of juvenile polyps in the gastrointestinal tract in any patient with a family history of JPS. Screening recommendations for JPS and other polyposis syndromes are outlined in Table 22-3.

Cowden Syndrome and Bannayan-Riley-Ruvalcaba Syndrome

A subset of patients with JPS likely includes cases of Cowden syndrome (CS) and Bannayan-Riley-Ruvalcaba syndrome (BRRS). Both are rare autosomal dominant disorders characterized by gastrointestinal hamartomas in the setting of a wide range of phenotypic abnormalities. The extraintestinal signs and symptoms of these disorders may be subtle, underscoring the importance of a detailed family history and physical examination.

Affected individuals with CS have mucocutaneous lesions including acral keratoses, oral papillomas, and facial trichilemmomas (90% to 100%). CS is also characterized by the finding of hamartomas in multiple sites, including the intestine, breast, thyroid gland, oral gland, oral mucosa, and brain. Gastrointestinal polyps are found in 40% to 60% of CS patients, and may be typical juvenile polyps, lipomas, ganglioneuromas, or adenomas. Pediatric CS patients may present with progressive macrocephaly with normal ventricle size in the first 2 years of life. All patients with CS are primarily at increased risk for the development of thyroid (10%) and breast cancer (50%). The risk for cancer of the intestinal

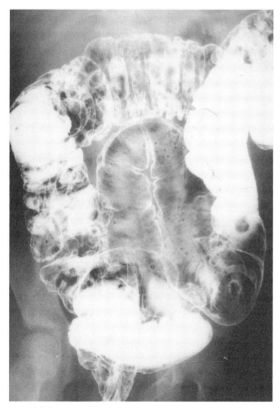

Figure 22-4 Juvenile polyposis syndrome (hamartomas). Overhead view from double-contrast barium enema shows innumerable polyps throughout the colon, varying from 0.2 to 1.3 cm in size. (Courtesy Igor Laufer, MD, Hospital of the University of Pennsylvania.)

Table 22-3	Surveillance Recommendations
Juvenile polyposis syndrome (JPS)	Colonoscopy at onset of symptoms or early in second decade, every 1 to 3 years depending on number of polyps found
	Upper endoscopy every 3 years
Peutz-Jeghers syndrome (PJS)	Colonoscopy at onset of symptoms or in midteens, every 1 to 2 years
	Upper endoscopy every 1 to 2 years, from age 10 years
	Abdominal ultrasound every 1 to 2 years, from age 30 years
	Annual hemoglobin
	Small bowel series every 2 to 3 years from age 10 years
	Mammography every 2 to 3 years from age 25 years
	Annual testicular examination from age 10 years
Bannayan-Riley-Ruvalcaba syndrome (BRRS)/Cowden syndrome (CS)	Annual thyroid examination, starting in 2nd decade of life
	Annual breast examination
	Annual mammography from age 30 years
Familial adenomatous syndrome (FAP)	Annual colonoscopy, from ages 10 to 12 years
	Upper endoscopy every 1 to 3 years from 20 to 25 years
	Head computed tomography (CT) (in affected Turcot families)
	Annual hepatic ultrasound and alpha-fetoprotein during first decade of life

tract is low, although patients with adenomatous polyps are at increased risk for gastrointestinal malignancy.

Criteria for BRRS include intestinal hamartomas, subcutaneous and/or visceral lipomas, hemangiomas, macular pigmentation of the genitalia, and a range of neurologic findings including macrocephaly with normal ventricle size, developmental delay, hypotonia, and seizures. In contrast to CS, the development of neoplasia in affected organs has not been reported.

Germline mutations in the protein-tyrosine phosphatase and tensin homolog (PTEN) gene account for up to 80% of cases of both CS and BRRS. Mutations in PTEN affect embryonic development, cell cycle regulation, apoptosis, and tumor formation.

Peutz-Jeghers Syndrome

Peutz-Jeghers syndrome (PJS) is a hamartomatous polyposis syndrome, which is inherited in an autosomal dominant fashion. This disorder is characterized by the presence of mucocutaneous pigmentation, including hyperpigmented lesions of the lips, buccal mucosa, areas around the eyes and nostrils, and perianal region. Hyperpigmented lesions of the hands and feet may be found at presentation, but often abate in adolescence. Pigmented macules range from blue to black, and often develop during infancy in affected individuals. Gastrointestinal polyps are found in the small intestine (70% to 90%), colon (50%), and less commonly in the stomach. Polyps may also be found at extraintestinal sites, including the sinuses and bronchi. Patients with PJS may present with rectal bleeding, abdominal pain, or even intussusception due to polypoid lead points.

Histologically, intestinal polyps in PJS are distinguished from juvenile polyps and other hamartomatous polyps by the presence of "arborizing" smooth muscle within the stalk and head of the polyp, surrounded by otherwise normal-appearing intestinal mucosa (Fig. 22-5). The malignant potential of intestinal lesions is low, but affected individuals (48%) develop cancer in other organs such as the breast, pancreas, ovaries, testes, or uterus. Malignancies of the lung and cervix have also been described.

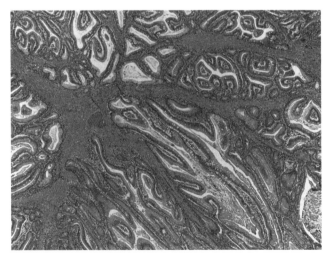

Figure 22-5 *(See also Color Plate 22-5.)* Hematoxylin and eosin–stained section of Peutz-Jeghers polyp. Note the appearance of "arborizing" smooth muscle within the polyp, which distinguishes these polyps from typical hamartomatous polyps. (Courtesy Eduardo D. Ruchelli, MD, Children's Hospital of Philadelphia.)

Germline mutations in the *STK11/LKB1* tumor suppressor gene are found in approximately 70% of patients with PJS, and screening for these mutations is commercially available. The mutated gene encodes a serine-threonine kinase, and is located on chromosome 19p13.3. Once mutations have been identified, first-degree relatives should undergo screening for mutations. Individuals with known mutations should have endoscopic surveillance (upper and lower endoscopy) every 1 to 2 years, starting at age 10 years. Extraintestinal screening by abdominal ultrasound, breast, and pelvic/testicular examinations should begin in the second or third decade of life.

Familial Adenomatous Polyposis

Familial adenomatous polyposis (FAP) is the most common polyposis syndrome with an underlying genetic basis. Occurring with an estimated frequency between 1:17,000 and 1:5000, FAP is inherited in an autosomal dominant fashion. Patients with FAP typically present in the second decade of life, with an average age of 16 years. Polyps are found in most affected individuals by age 35. Adenomatous polyps can be found throughout the gastrointestinal tract, but are most commonly distributed in the colon and rectum (Figs. 22-6 and 22-7). In the small intestine, polyps are found most frequently in the duodenum, where affected individuals are at increased risk for the development of duodenal and periampullary carcinomas. Nearly 100% of patients with FAP will develop gastrointestinal cancer by the fifth decade of life.

Mutations in the *APC* gene are responsible for the development of FAP, and more than 400 *APC* mutations have been identified to date. *APC* is a tumor-suppressor gene that has been mapped to chromosome 5q21. This gene encodes a cytoplasmic protein that binds and regulates the degradation of β-catenin, a protein whose target genes are associated with cellular proliferation. *APC* mutations thus lead to tumor development through the accumulation and unregulated activity of β-catenin.

Patients with FAP typically have extraintestinal manifestations, including benign epidermal growths, including osteomas of the mandible and occipital bones, dental abnormalities, epidermoid cysts, congenital hypertrophy of the retinal pigment epithelium (CHRPE), and desmoid tumors. Turcot syndrome, which is considered to be a phenotypic variant of FAP, includes FAP in the setting of central nervous system tumors. Medulloblastoma is the most common type of central nervous system (CNS) tumor in Turcot syndrome, although glioblastoma multiforme also has been reported.

Of particular concern in pediatric patients is the known association of FAP and hepatoblastoma. Studies of children with both hepatoblastoma and FAP demonstrate not only that the development of this rare, rapidly progressive liver tumor often occurs before age 5, but also that the development of hepatoblastoma in FAP kindreds is associated with germline *APC* mutation in the 5′ end of the gene. It is estimated that the risk of the development of hepatoblastoma in children born to a parent with FAP is 1.6%, with a relative risk 850 times higher than that of the general population; thus, annual alpha-fetoprotein (AFP) analysis and liver ultrasound have been recommended by some investigators for at-risk children starting between 0 and 5 years of age.

Because of the inevitable risk for colorectal carcinoma in FAP, early diagnosis and genetic screening are essential. Genetic testing in first-degree relatives should be performed in FAP family members by ages 10 to 12 years, and can be completed using commercially available protein truncation assays or by deoxyribonucleic acid (DNA) sequencing in peripheral blood lymphocyte DNA. Carriers should undergo flexible sigmoidoscopy every 1 to 2 years until adenomas are found, at which point annual colonoscopies should be performed. Older individuals, however, should undergo a full colonoscopy in light of the greater risk for advanced polyposis. Family members without identified *APC* mutations are believed to have a cancer risk equivalent to that of the general population. The finding of colonic adenomas is an indication for additional screening via upper gastrointestinal endocsopy every 1 to 2 years. A side-viewing endoscope should be used in order to better view the ampulla.

Prophylactic total colectomy should be performed once adenomas are identified. Given the psychological ramifications of colectomy in childhood, colectomy should be postponed until after high school, if possible. In such cases, annual colonoscopy is recommended. Colectomy should be strongly considered in cases of

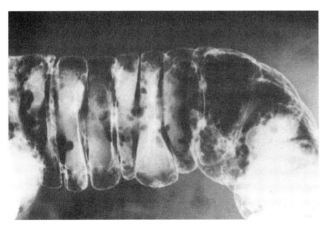

Figure 22-6 Familial adenomatous polyposis syndrome. Spot radiograph of ascending colon shows numerous polyps manifested as 4- to 6-mm radiolucent filling defects in the barium pool or ovoid barium-etched lines. (From Rubesin SE, Laufer I: Tumors of the colon. In Levine MS, Rubesin SE, Laufer I (eds): Double Contrast Gastrointestinal Radiology, 3rd ed. Philadelphia, WB Saunders, 2000, pp 357-416, Figure 12-91B.)

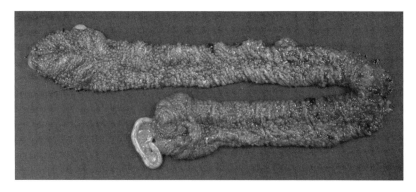

Figure 22-7 *(See also Color Plate 22-7.)* Familial adenomatous polyposis coli. Cut surface of resected specimen demonstrates the presence of polyps throughout the colon. (Courtesy Eduardo D. Ruchelli, MD, Children's Hospital of Philadelphia.)

large adenomas (5 mm or larger) or multiple adenomas (100 or more), regardless of patient age. In the upper gastrointestinal tract, transesophageal ultrasound is indicated if ampullary polyps are found by upper endoscopy. Ampullectomy should be performed once the presence of adenomas is confirmed. In cases of high-grade dysplasia, the Whipple procedure is indicated.

PRINCIPLES OF GENETIC SCREENING

Inherited polyposis syndromes together constitute about 3% to 5% of all colon cancers, underscoring the need for comprehensive genetic testing in at-risk patients and family members of affected patients. In this regard, genetic testing should be performed in order to (1) confirm the diagnosis of an inherited polyposis syndrome or (2) determine the carrier status of a family member of a patient with a known mutation. All genetic screening should be performed knowing that the lack of a known mutation in an affected patient does not rule out the diagnosis. Subsequent genetic screening of family members in these situations is therefore much more difficult, mandating a greater reliance on medical history and clinical judgment. When mutations are identified in index cases, however, subsequent testing of other family members for the presence or absence of the same mutations is highly accurate. In the arena of genetic testing, it is imperative that all studies are performed at designated centers with genetic counseling expertise.

SUMMARY

The management of gastrointestinal polyps in children presents multiple challenges to the practitioner, in clinical decision-making and in the ramifications of genetic screening. Our understanding of the genetic basis for the development of inherited polyposis syndromes has increased dramatically in the past decade. It is clear that discoveries in this area will continue to benefit patients and their families, through more comprehensive genetic screening and clinical applications.

MAJOR POINTS

- Gastrointestinal polyps are a common cause of rectal bleeding in childhood.
- In children, the majority of gastrointestinal polyps are either hamartomas or adenomas.
- Hamartomas are not malignant, and rarely have dysplastic features. Adenomatous polyps are dysplastic lesions with malignant potential. The larger the adenoma, the greater the risk for malignant transformation.
- Uncomplicated juvenile polyps have no malignant potential, and manifest between the ages of 2 and 5 years.
- Patients with 3 or more juvenile polyps should be screened for Smad4 mutations associated with JPS. Patients with JPS may have up to a 50% risk of gastrointestinal cancer.
- A subset of patients with JPS includes cases of Cowden syndrome and Bannayan-Riley-Ruvalcaba syndrome. Affected patients have multiple extraintestinal manifestations including macrocephaly and an increased risk for the development of breast and thyroid cancers.
- Individuals with Peutz-Jeghers syndrome have gastrointestinal hamartomatous polyps in the setting of mucocutaneous pigmentation. This syndrome is associated with increased risk for extraintestinal malignancies including the breast, testes, and uterus.
- FAP, the most common genetic polyposis syndrome, is caused by mutations in the *APC* gene. The risk for intestinal cancer is 100%. Because of the known association between FAP and hepatoblastoma, children of affected patients with FAP should undergo early screening.
- Genetic testing for most polyposis syndromes is widely available, and should be used in the context of a thorough clinical evaluation and family history.

SUGGESTED READINGS

Coburn MC, Pricolo VE, DeLuca FG, et al: Malignant potential in intestinal juvenile polyposis syndromes. Ann Surg Oncol 2:386-391, 1995.

Corredor J, Wambach J, Barnard J: Gastrointestinal polyps in children: Advances in molecular genetics, diagnosis, and management. J Pediatr 138:621-628, 2001.

Cynamon HA, Milov DE, Andres JM: Diagnosis and management of colonic polyps in children. J Pediatr 114:593-596, 1989.

Eng C, Ji H: Molecular classification of the inherited hamartoma polyposis syndromes: Clearing the muddied waters (see comment). Am J Hum Genet 62:1020-1022, 1998.

Erdman SH, Barnard JA: Gastrointestinal polyps and polyposis syndromes in children. Curr Opin Pediatr 14:576-582, 2002.

Fearnhead NS, Britton MP, Bodmer WF: The ABC of APC. Hum Mol Genet 10:721-733, 2001.

Friedl W, Kruse R, Uhlhaas S, et al: Frequent 4-bp deletion in exon 9 of the SMAD4/MADH4 gene in familial juvenile polyposis patients. Genes Chromosomes Cancer 25:403-406, 1999.

Giardiello FM, Offerhaus JG: Phenotype and cancer risk of various polyposis syndromes. Eur J Cancer 31A:1085-1087, 1995.

Giardiello FM, Hamilton SR, Kern SE, et al: Colorectal neoplasia in juvenile polyposis or juvenile polyps. Arch Dis Child 66:971-975, 1991.

Giardiello FM, Petersen GM, Brensinger JD, et al: Hepatoblastoma and APC gene mutation in familial adenomatous polyposis (see comment). Gut 39:867-869, 1996.

Giardiello FM, Welsh SB, Hamilton SR, et al: Increased risk of cancer in the Peutz-Jeghers syndrome. N Engl J Med 316:1511-1514, 1987.

Giardiello FM, Brensinger, JD, Petersen GM: AGA technical review on hereditary colorectal cancer and genetic testing. Gastroenterology 121:198-213, 2001.

Gorlin RJ, Cohen MM JR, Condon LM, et al: Bannayan-Riley-Ruvalcaba syndrome. Am J Med Genet 44:307-314, 1992.

Groden J, Thliveris A, Samowitz W, et al: Identification and characterization of the familial adenomatous polyposis coli gene. Cell 66:589-600, 1991.

Hanssen AM, Fryns JP: Cowden syndrome. J Med Genet 32:117-119, 1995.

Hemminki A, Markie D, Tomlinson I, et al: A serine/threonine kinase gene defective in Peutz-Jeghers syndrome. Nature 391:184-187, 1998.

Howe JR, Roth S, Ringold JC, et al: Mutations in the SMAD4/DPC4 gene in juvenile polyposis (see comment). Science 280:1086-1088, 1986.

Howe JR, Mitros FA, Summers RW: The risk of gastrointestinal carcinoma in familial juvenile polyposis. Ann Surg Oncol 5:751-756, 1998.

Hyer W, Beveridge I, Domizio P, et al: Clinical management and genetics of gastrointestinal polyps in children. J Pediatr Gastroenterol Nutr 31:469-479, 2000.

Jass JR, Williams CB, Bussey HJ, et al: Juvenile polyposis—A precancerous condition. Histopathology 13:619-630, 1988.

Jenne DE, Reimann H, Nezu J, et al: Peutz-Jeghers syndrome is caused by mutations in a novel serine threonine kinase. Nat Genet 18:38-43, 1998.

King JE, Dozois RR, Lindor NM, et al: Care of patients and their families with familial adenomatous polyposis. Mayo Clin Proc 75:57-67, 2000.

Marsh DJ, Dahia PL, Zheng Z, et al: Germline mutations in PTEN are present in Bannayan-Zonana syndrome. Nat Genet 16:333-334, 1997.

Marsh DJ, Dahia PL, Caron S, et al: Germline PTEN mutations in Cowden syndrome-like families. J Med Genet 35:881-885, 1998.

Mestre JR: The changing pattern of juvenile polyps. Am J Gastroenterol 81:312-314, 1986.

Offerhaus GJ, Giardiello FM, Krush AJ, et al: The risk of upper gastrointestinal cancer in familial adenomatous polyposis (see comment). Gastroenterology 102:1980-1982, 1992.

Powell SM, Petersen GM, Krush AJ, et al: Molecular diagnosis of familial adenomatous polyposis (see comment). N Engl J Med 329:1982-1987, 1993.

Ray JE, Heald RJ, Chiram: Growing up with juvenile gastrointestinal polyposis: Report of a case. Dis Colon Rectum 14:375-378, 1971.

Rubesin SE, Laufer I: Tumors of the colon. In Levine MS, Rubesin SE, Laufer I (eds): Double Contrast Gastrointestinal Radiology, 3rd ed. Philadelphia, WB Saunders, 2000, pp 357-416, Figure 12-91B.

Rustgi AK: Hereditary gastrointestinal polyposis and nonpolyposis syndromes (see comment). N Engl J Med 331:1694-1702, 1994.

Sachatello CR, Hahn IL, Carrington CB: Juvenile gastrointestinal polyposis in a female infant: Report of a case and review of the literature of a recently recognized syndrome. Surgery 75:107-114, 1974.

Sachatello CR, Pickren JW, Grace Jr JT: Generalized juvenile gastrointestinal polyposis. A hereditary syndrome. Gastroenterology 58:699-708, 1970.

Waite KA, Eng C: Protean PTEN: Form and function. Am J Hum Genet 70:829-844, 2002.

Woodford-Richens K, Bevan S, Churchman M, et al: Analysis of genetic and phenotypic heterogeneity in juvenile polyposis. Gut 46:656-660, 2000.

CHAPTER 23

Chronic Intestinal Pseudo-Obstruction

LEONEL RODRIGUEZ
ALEJANDRO FLORES

Disease Description
Case Presentation
Epidemiology
Pathophysiology
Diagnosis
   Kidney, Ureter, and Bladder
   Barium Studies
   Ultrasound
   Esophageal Manometry
   Antroduodenal Manometry
   Colonic Manometry
   Anorectal Manometry
   Sphincter of Oddi Manometry
   Electrogastrography
   Full-Thickness Biopsy
   Metabolic Screen
Treatment
   Nutrition
   Small Bowel Bacterial Overgrowth
   Medical Therapy
      Prokinetics
      Antiemetics
      Antibiotics
      Surgery
      Pyloric Botox Injection
      Gastric Pacing
      Intestinal Transplantation
Outcome
Approach to the Case
Summary
Major Points

DISEASE DESCRIPTION

Chronic intestinal pseudo-obstruction (CIPO) is a severe and disabling disorder characterized by episodes of continuous symptoms and signs of bowel obstruction in the absence of a fixed lumen-occluding lesion. The presence of radiologic features of obstruction were initially included in the diagnostic features, but they are not always present and their absence should not rule out CIPO; histologic and manometric findings are more reliable and reproducible. CIPO is the end of the spectrum that includes irritable bowel syndrome and non-ulcer dyspepsia.

CASE PRESENTATION

A female presented at the age of 3 months with symptoms of gastroesophageal (GE) reflux (vomiting), hypotonia, and failure to thrive. On initial evaluation, upper gastrointestinal (UGI) series were done and showed GE reflux but normal anatomy; abdominal ultrasound was normal, UGI endoscopy was performed and showed no esophagitis and mild duodenal atrophy, and a pH probe study showed no GE reflux. She was initially on oral (PO) feedings, and after few months of failure to thrive, she underwent a gastrostomy placement for supplementation. A metabolic evaluation including serum amino acids and urine organic acids showed normal results; also, cystic fibrosis and glycogen storage disease were ruled out.

EPIDEMIOLOGY

The majority of patients present with symptoms during the first year of life, (43% in the first month) on occasion in a transient form in the premature newborn, and in some instances can carry a high morbidity even in term newborns. Abdominal distention is the most common sign, it can be present soon after birth, usually associated with bilious vomiting, and beyond the neonatal period with episodic vomiting and constipation. The presence of megacystis at birth should alert the physician to underlying CIPO. The most common signs

Table 23-1 Epidemiologic Data of CIPO							
	No.	Family History	Urologic Involvement	Myopathy	Neuropathy	Mixed or Nondiagnostic	TPN Dependent	Died
United States	85	1	35	32 (A)	48 (A)	5 (A)	53(62)	22(27)
United Kingdom	44	11	16	16 (13A/16H)	22 (14A/22H)	6 (3A/6H)	32(73)	14(32)
United Kingdom 2	20			13 (H)	4 (3H/1AD)	3 (H)	8(40)	2(10)
Spain	16	N/A	7	N/A	N/A	N/A	3(19)	3(19)
France 1	22	4	N/A	8 (H)	13 (H)	N/A	11(50)	5(23)
France 2	105	N/A	N/A	17	58	24	39(37)	11(10)
Brazil	7	2	5	2	1	4	2(29)	3(43)
Argentina	4	N/A	0	4	0	0	4(100)	N/A
Total	303	18	63	92(30)	146(48)	42(14)	152(50)	60(20)

AD, antroduodenal manometry; CIPO, chronic intestinal pseudo-obstruction; H, histology; N/A, not applicable; TPN, total parenteral nutrition.

and symptoms in decreasing frequency are abdominal distention, vomiting, constipation, abdominal pain, poor weight gain, and diarrhea. Family history is significant in up to 29% (Table 23-1).

Among the associated anomalies, urologic involvement is significantly present in 3% to 71%, is more frequently seen in the myopathic type, and is associated with increased risk to develop urinary tract infections (UTIs). Another well-defined association is malrotation: partial or full in 88% patients who had intestinal dysmotility, similar to neuropathic CIPO, after surgical correction of malrotation. In a study of 23 patients with CIPO, hypogammaglobulinemia was found in 78% (78% of those required intravenous immune globulin), autonomic dysfunction in 43%, recurrent hypoglycemia in 39%, asthma in 39%, cholecystitis in 30%, low serum carnitine level in 26%, urinary dysfunction in 26%, pancreatitis in 22%, behavioral problems in 22%, myopathy in 9%, idiopathic thrombocytopenia in 8%, velopharyngeal insufficiency in 4%, oculocutaneous albinism in 4%, Pierre Robin syndrome in 4%, and protein C deficiency in 4%. Biliary tract motility is also affected in children, which could explain the increased incidence of cholelithiasis in these patients not solely from total parenteral nutrition (TPN). Recently, an association with autoimmune hepatitis in a case of leiomyositis with CIPO has been reported.

PATHOPHYSIOLOGY

During fasting, the antrum and the small intestine show a motility pattern known as migrating motor complex (MMC), described initially in animals and later further characterized in humans. This MMC is generated at the intracellular level as a "slow wave" of electrical activity. The MMC is composed of three phases: phase I is characterized by motor quiescence, phase II (the longest) shows irregular and intermittent phasic contractions, and phase III shows regular and rhythmic contractions that progress from the antrum to the ileum. The MMC is shorter in children and its duration increases with age. After a meal, the MMC stops and the intestine shows contractions of larger duration and amplitude.

This rhythmic enteric activity is generated by the enteric nervous system (ENS), a role that has been elucidated recently. Increasing evidence of abnormalities of the ENS by mechanisms such as inflammation, degeneration, or autoimmune responses may explain the resulting intestinal dysmotility. ENS is composed of the interstitial cell of Cajal (ICC), neurons, and glial cells. The ICCs are believed to act as the pacemaker (slow wave generation) of the GI tract. These ICCs have been the focus of extensive research oriented to their detection and localization on the GI tract in motility disorders. The proto-oncogene c-kit encodes a transmembrane tyrosine kinase receptor c-kit that is critical for the development of the ICCs and has become the marker for the identification of these cells in tissues. Recently, this network of ICCs has been found to be abnormal in children and adults with CIPO, and a delayed maturation of ICCs was observed in a transient form of CIPO in neonates. ICCs were absent in CIPO patients when compared with adult controls, mechanical obstruction, and other motility disorders as well as Crohn's disease and colorectal cancer. ICCs from deep muscular plexus (DMP) and intermuscular ICCs were absent in a newborn with CIPO. Another important marker for dysmotility is nitric oxide synthase (NOS), which is known to mediate relaxation in sphincters in the GI tract. NOS-containing ganglionic cells were found increased in patients with CIPO. NOS also was found increased and c-kit was found decreased in Japanese children with CIPO. Another possible mechanism of ENS dysfunction is inflammation, probably secondary to autoimmune responses from either paraneoplastic syndromes (small cell lung carcinoma) or infections (*Trypanosoma cruzi,* Epstein-Barr virus [EBV], and cytomegalovirus [CMV]).

CIPO can be classified as primary and secondary. The primary CIPO includes the visceral neuropathies and myopathies, which can be sporadic or familial; both types are described in children as well as adults. Among the secondary causes of CIPO, infectious etiologies can induce an autoimmune inflammatory response against the ENS and the smooth muscle. A commonly unrecognized group of patients with secondary CIPO are the mitochondrial disorders, which can affect the GI tract as well as the liver, cardiovascular system (CVS), and central nervous system (CNS). More common causes of CIPO in adults are infiltrative diseases and collagen vascular disorders, probably because they are more common in adults and it takes time for the damage to the ENS and the smooth muscle to develop and produce symptoms. The most common causes of CIPO are depicted in Table 23-2.

DIAGNOSIS

Patients with symptoms suggestive of CIPO should be extensively evaluated for other conditions emulating pseudo-obstruction, especially mechanical obstruction, pain-associated disability syndrome (PADS), pediatric condition falsification, Munchausen syndrome by proxy, and rarely Kawasaki disease and SMA syndrome. The diagnosis of CIPO is clinical and includes a thorough medical interview and physical examination, and careful review of the diagnostic tests to exclude these conditions to avoid unnecessary invasive testing and treatment. Also important is a metabolic screening to rule out important disorders of metabolism associated with CIPO. The following are the most commonly performed diagnostic studies and their clinical usefulness.

Kidney, Ureter, and Bladder

A kidney, ureter, and bladder (KUB) usually shows dilated loops of bowel with air-fluid levels and no stricture (Fig. 23-1). In rare instances it may show pneumoperitoneum and/or pneumatosis intestinalis. KUB can be normal in some patients, so GI series are important to exclude mechanical obstruction. Severe bowel dilatation is more commonly seen with a myopathic type of CIPO.

Barium Studies

UGI and small bowel series are indicated to rule out anatomic obstruction and malrotation. Barium enema is used to rule out Hirschsprung's disease and megacystis microcolon intestinal hypoperistalsis syndrome (MMIHS) in patients suffering also from constipation. Gastric emptying scintigraphy assesses solid and liquid gastric emptying.

Ultrasound

Antenatal ultrasound can verify the presence of megacystis, and possibly midgut malrotation. Postnatal it can be used for urologic involvement and to rule out pyloric stenosis and possibly malrotation by the "whirlpool sign" (wrapping of the superior mesenteric vein and bowel loops around the superior mesenteric artery).

Esophageal Manometry

Esophageal manometry is useful when antroduodenal manometry (AD) is not available, and is abnormal in the majority of adult patients showing aperistalsis. It is especially important in visceral neuropathies in children, showing low amplitude, low duration, and/or simultaneous waves, although presence of these abnormalities is not as constant as in adults with CIPO, suggesting that esophageal involvement is a late development.

Antroduodenal Manometry

Always abnormal in CIPO, a normal AD manometry excludes CIPO. Because the majority of centers use water perfusion systems, it is recommended to use isotonic solutions like Pedialyte instead of water to avoid water intoxication. AD manometry includes a recording of a fasting period followed first by stimulation of antral contractions by erythromycin, which also helps to prevent the antral inhibition from octreotide used later for the intestine stimulation. In CIPO, the AD manometry aids not only to confirm abnormal upper GI motility but also differentiate between neuropathic and myopathic subtypes. A normal AD manometry in the suitable clinical setting should raise the concern of pediatric falsification disorder, Munchausen syndrome by proxy, or PADS. Typical manometric findings in CIPO include antral hypomotility; in the neuropathic variety, the typical findings include absence of MMC during fasting and phase III-like activity during feeding. In the myopathic variety, the typical findings include low amplitude or absent contractions. Also, the absence of MMC is associated with need for total parenteral nutrition (TPN) and its presence with good response to jejunal feedings. The presence of waves that are simulta-

Table 23-2 Etiology of Pseudo-Obstruction by Age-Group

Primary
Visceral neuropathy
Sporadic or familial
Visceral myopathy
Sporadic or familial
Secondary
Infant
Cytomegalovirus (CMV)
Neurologic
Stenosis of the aqueduct of Sylvius
Neuromuscular
Myotonic dystrophy (Steinert's)
Mitochondrial diseases
OXPHOS defects
Myopathy (complex 1 deficiency)
SOX10 mutation
Mitochondrial NeuroGastroIntestinal Encephalopathy (MNGIE)
Pearson marrow-pancreas syndrome
Infiltrative
Lipoblastomatosis
Autoimmune
Idiopathic myositis
Toxic insult
Fetal alcohol syndrome
Other
Megacystis-microcolon-intestinal hypoperistalsis syndrome
Children
Epstein-Barr virus (EBV)
Metabolic
Hypokalemia
Collagen vascular disorders
Juvenile rheumatoid arthritis
Dermatomyositis
Systemic lupus erythematosus (SLE)
Systemic sclerosis
Neuromuscular
Myotonic dystrophy
Oculopharyngodistal myopathy
Duchenne's disease
Werdnig-Hoffmann disease
Type IV Waardenburg syndrome
Mitochondrial disorders
Peripheral neuropathy with hypomyelination, and deafness related to a SOX10 mutation
MNGIE
Pearson marrow-pancreas syndrome
Familial mitochondrial intestinal pseudo-obstruction and neurogenic bladder
Vasculitis
Kawasaki disease
Neurologic
Neurofibromatosis
Autoimmune
Macrophagic myofasciitis from vaccination
Autoimmune enteric leiomyositis
Inflammation
Celiac disease
Paraneoplastic
Ganglioneuroblastoma
Toxic insult
Chemotherapy agents

Adults
Infectious
Chagas' disease
Clostridium difficile
EBV, CMV, varicella-zoster virus (VZV)
Celiac disease
Metabolic
Hypokalemia
Endocrine
Hypothyroidism
Hypoparathyroidism
Diabetes (mitochondrial A32436 mutation)
Maternally inherited diabetes and deafness (MIDD)
Collagen vascular disorders
SLE
SLE with presence of autoantibodies against proliferating cell nuclear antigen (PCNA)
Rheumatoid arthritis
Scleroderma
Neuromuscular
Myasthenia gravis
Thymoma
Polymyositis
Sjögren's disease
Myotonic dystrophy
Desmin myopathy
Infiltrative disorders
Intestinal endometriosis
Amyloidosis
Primary
Dialysis
Rheumatoid arthritis
Multiple myeloma
RS3PE syndrome and multiple myeloma
Neurologic
Friedreich's ataxia
Pheochromocytoma
Neurofibromatosis
Dysautonomia
Spinal muscular atrophy
Mitochondrial myopathy, encephalopathy, lactic acidosis and stroke-like episodes (MELAS)
MNGIE
Autoimmune
Small cell lung cancer (anti-Hu antibody)
Toxic insult
Neuroleptic malignant syndrome (amitriptyline and lithium carbonate)
Radiotherapy
Haloperidol + benztropine
Chemotherapy agents: vinca alkaloids, cytarabine, Fludarabine
Morphine
Baclofen
Diltiazem
Charcoal and sorbitol (theophylline intoxication)
Amitriptyline
Verapamil
Heroin
Alcohol
Amanita
Other
Angioedema
Macroglobulinemia
Hereditary coproporphyria

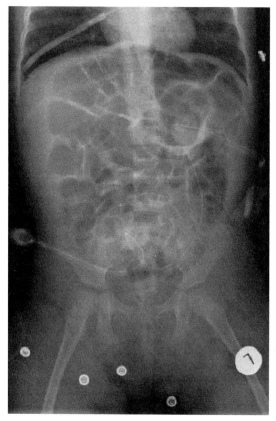

Figure 23-1 Kidney, ureter, and bladder (KUB).

neous and/or of long duration should raise concern for a missed mechanical obstruction. When a patient has a jejunostomy, the manometry catheter can be placed via the stoma and a jejunal manometry performed (Fig. 23-2).

Colonic Manometry

Abnormal in the majority of patients, the neuropathic type shows abnormal basal activity and absence of high amplitude peristaltic contractions (HAPC) and gastrocolic response; the myopathic type shows low amplitude peristaltic contractions or no contractions. When constipation was evaluated in CIPO, 75% had no HAPC and no significant gastrocolic response (Fig. 23-3).

Anorectal Manometry

Normal in almost all patients with CIPO, anorectal manometry has no significant clinical usefulness unless indicated for defecation disorders like internal anal sphincter achalasia.

Sphincter of Oddi Manometry

Dilatation of the common hepatic duct has been recognized in CIPO for some time, suggesting sphincter of Oddi (SO) increased pressure, but the only case report of SO manometry in adults showed SO low basal pressure and low amplitude phasic contractions. In the only pediatric case report of biliary motility in CIPO, gallbladder wall motility was impaired. Further studies are needed to support these findings and to help to elucidate the increased incidence of pancreatitis and intermittent elevation of pancreatic enzymes in CIPO.

Electrogastrography

Electrogastrography (EGG) is a noninvasive method to evaluate the myoelectrical activity of the stomach. Although the consensus is that EGG does not substitute AD manometry as a diagnostic tool, growing evidence supports its use as an adjunct in the evaluation of CIPO. In one study, CIPO patients showed an abnormal dominant frequency, dominant power, and postprandial bradygastria significantly different than controls; another study showed 63% of CIPO patients with abnormal EGG, showing no dominant frequency, also gastric dysrhythmias have been observed in 72% to 93% of CIPO patients.

Full-Thickness Biopsy

Full-thickness biopsy should be performed only when a surgical operation is planned, and if possible from both dilated and undilated segments. An experienced pathologist should interpret the specimen. In neuropathies the histologic changes consist of aganglionosis, neuronal intranuclear inclusions and apoptosis, neural degeneration, intestinal neuronal dysplasia, hypoganglionosis, hyperganglionosis, neuronal hyperplasia and ganglioneuromas, mitochondrial dysfunction, neurotransmitter diseases, ICC network abnormalities, and autoimmune inflammatory neuropathies. Identification of the last one may be particularly important because immunosuppressive therapy may be of benefit. In myopathies, the histologic changes include inflammation, fibrosis and atrophy of the outer longitudinal smooth muscle layer, abnormalities in intestinal muscle layering and intrinsic myocyte defects, and/or changes in the extracellular matrix. Changes specific for mitochondrial myopathies include smooth muscle cells with bulbous protrusions filled with lateralized mitochondria.

Metabolic Screen

It is important to include a complete metabolic evaluation consisting of serum amino acids, urine organic acids, serum lactate, serum pyruvate, electrolytes, liver function tests (LFTs), and thyroid function tests (TFTs) to rule out a disorder of metabolism like mitochondrial disorders, hypothyroidism, or hypokalemia (Fig. 23-4).

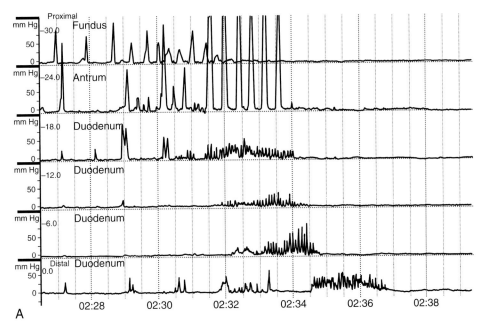

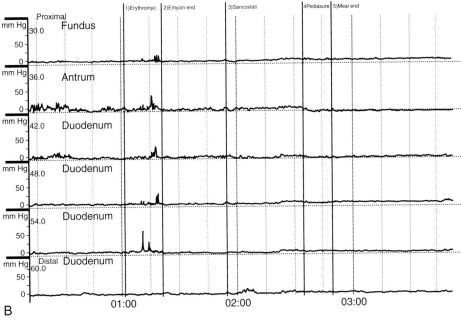

Figure 23-2 Antroduodenal manometry (AD). **A,** Normal AD manometry. **B,** Abnormal AD manometry.

TREATMENT

Treatment for idiopathic CIPO is supportive, not curative. In the evaluation it is very important to exclude secondary causes of CIPO that could improve with the appropriate treatment. A multidisciplinary team should be involved in the management in patients with CIPO, including a nutritionist, psychologist, metabolism specialist, urologist, and a social worker (Fig. 23-5). Nutritional support is the mainstay of treatment in CIPO. Treatment of the complications from CIPO can be very difficult, especially for bacterial overgrowth and central catheter-related sepsis.

Nutrition

Nutritional support is imperative. A trial of enteral feedings is always warranted. Enteral route is preferred over parenteral, especially before puberty because regular pubertal growth is achieved in only 25% of children on cycled nocturnal TPN. Even in cases of TPN dependency, it is imperative to ascertain some enteral nutrition; the amount needed to prevent complications is not known.

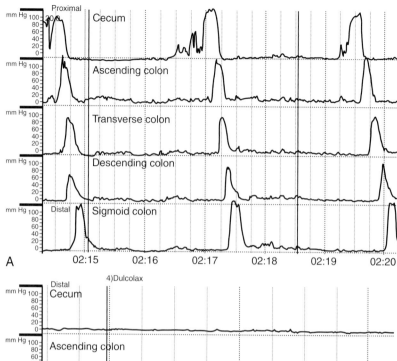
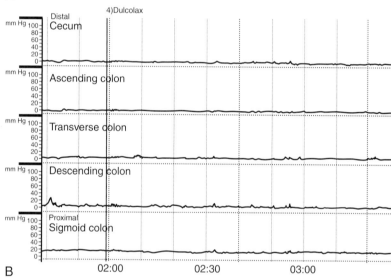

Figure 23-3 Colonic manometry. **A,** Normal colonic manometry. **B,** Abnormal colonic manometry.

Enteral feedings may be attempted via a gastrostomy (G) tube as much as possible, and jejunostomy (J) feedings may be required when G feedings are not tolerated. The institution of home parenteral nutrition has proved to be safe and has slightly higher survival rates compared with chronic dialysis programs. The age at the start of home parenteral nutrition and the degree of enteral independence are important prognostic factors in the survival rates in irreversible intestinal failure (IF).

Small Bowel Bacterial Overgrowth

One of the mechanisms to control small bowel bacterial overgrowth (SBBO) is motility, especially the phase III MMC. Common symptoms include diarrhea, weight loss, and macrocytic anemia. Therapy includes treatment of the underlying cause when possible; replacement of nutritional deficits including vitamins and antibiotics, and a role for probiotics is being explored.

Medical Therapy

The following are the most useful medications in treating patients with CIPO.

Prokinetics
Erythromycin (EES)
Effective inducing antral motility and intestinal phase III MMC in children with chronic GI functional symptoms, the higher the dose the more likely it is to obtain a clinical response but it is also more likely to have side effects. EES may be of benefit for gastroparesis but not for intestinal dysmotility, and when given orally may be

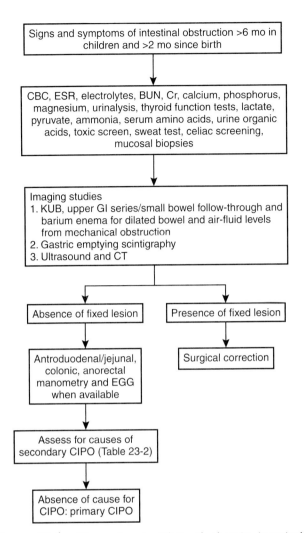

Figure 23-4 Diagnostic algorithm of chronic intestinal pseudo-obstruction (CIPO). BUN, blood urea nitrogen; CBC, complete blood count; Cr, creatinine; CT, computed tomography; EGG, electrogastrography; ESR, erythrocyte sedimentation rate; GI, gastrointestinal; KUB, kidney, ureter, and bladder.

more effective in males with the myopathic variety not taking opiates for pain. Better results are achieved when used in combination with octreotide because inhibition of antral hypomotility is blocked.

Metoclopramide
The most commonly used prokinetic, metoclopramide's use is limited because of the associated CNS side effects. Although useful for delayed gastric emptying, it has little if any effect on small bowel motility.

Domperidone
Domperidone is an alternative for patients who experience side effects from metoclopramide and/or show no response. As with metoclopramide, it is useful for the delayed gastric emptying component.

Octreotide
An impaired somatostatin response after feeding in CIPO has been reported. When used subcutaneously it induces phase III of the MMC but decreases antral motility during AD manometry. This effect can be blocked with EES. In clinical practice it has not shown significant benefit except in adults with scleroderma-induced CIPO.

Tegaserod
A partial and selective 5-HT4 receptor agonist, tegaserod has stimulatory effects on the GI tract and is approved for adults with irritable bowel syndrome (IBS) with constipation and refractory constipation. Recently, it has shown prokinetic effects in gastroparesis and dyspepsia. Only one report of a child receiving tegaserod for CIPO showed immediate response by tolerating enteral feedings, and TPN was discontinued. In the authors' experience tegaserod has been helpful only in a select group of patients, especially in those with associated colonic dysmotility with constipation.

Antiemetics
Ondansetron
Probably the most potent antiemetic, ondansetron may be indicated for severe nausea that does not respond to prokinetics.

Antibiotics
Central catheter (CC)-related infections require treatment with antibiotics and at times the removal of the catheter. Neutropenia and lack of antibiotic prophylaxis prior to CC placement were found to be associated with a higher rate of early infection. Screening culture of central lines does not detect the majority of infections in patients on home TPN. An alternative is the delivery of antibiotics locked within the lumen of the catheter or flushing the catheter with a combination of vancomycin, heparin, and ciprofloxacin. Antibiotic management for SBBO ranges from treatment of every bout of SBBO to cycling antibiotics, the latter associated with antibiotic resistance.

Surgery
Surgical resections are not indicated in the management of CIPO.

Gastrostomy
Used primarily for venting the upper GI tract, gastrostomy usually is not useful for feeding purposes.

Jejunostomy
Jejunostomy may be used for feedings, but is not suitable for venting.

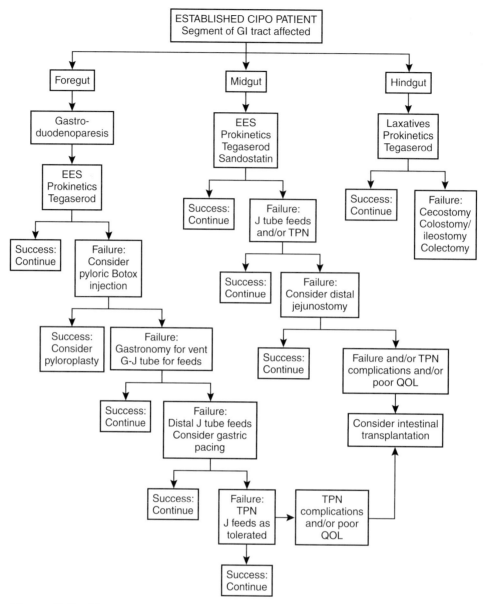

Figure 23-5 Treatment algorithm of chronic intestinal pseudo-obstruction (CIPO). EES, erythromycin; GI, gastrointestinal; G-J gastrojejunostomy; J, jejunostomy; QOL, quality of life; TPN, total parenteral nutrition.

Pyloric Botox Injection

Reported to be effective in improving gastric emptying and symptoms in adults with idiopathic gastroparesis, pyloroplasty can be considered if Botox is successful.

Gastric Pacing

Gastric pacing improves symptoms of gastroparesis in adults but effects of gastric emptying are not consistent.

Intestinal Transplantation

Intestinal transplantation (IT) is now considered the only potential curative treatment for life-threatening intestinal failure (IF). IF can be defined as the inability of the native GI tract to provide nutritional autonomy. An early and extensive evaluation is recommended, as well as attempts to wean TPN to establish the irremediable nature of irreversible IF for the correct use and timing of IT. IT is indicated for irreversible IF, mainly for complications related to TPN (recurrent central venous infections, liver failure, and loss of central venous access) and poor quality of life. Survival rates are not as good as other solid organ transplantations, but outcomes have improved with new immunosuppressive therapies like sirolimus, and the results are promising. In the three largest series of long-term follow-up after liver–small bowel transplantation for CIPO from three different centers in the United States, one center reported 8 patients received six small bowel and three liver–small bowel transplants; the median survival graft was 15 months, two casualties and two rejections in 1 patient, the 5 survivors with full enteral nutrition. The second center showed very similar numbers: of 8 children transplanted 6 had rejection (1 died) and 3 died within 4 years after transplantation; all 5 survivors tolerate full enteral feedings. The third center (the most recent) reported 16 patients (divided in two periods according to different immunosuppressive agents) showed survival rates of 1 and 2 years for periods one and two of 57% and 43% and 89% and 78%, respectively; none of the long-term survivors is on TPN and all tolerate enteral feedings. A group in Italy reported a 1-year patient and graft survival of 83% and 67% from 6 patients after a mean follow-up of 25 months. Quality of life and self-esteem are essential in these patients; one study reported that the perception of physical and psychosocial functioning on transplant recipients was not different from controls.

OUTCOME

The neuropathic type carries a better prognosis than the myopathic type and is the most common type in children, possibly because myopathic is more likely to be secondary to GI involvement from systemic diseases that not only are more common in adults but also take a long time to develop. Most of the patients with CIPO will require some source of enteral or parenteral nutrition during their lives, and a significant number will eventually depend on it.

Quality of life is an important outcome that needs further investigation. A telephone interview questionnaire showed that CIPO patients had less freedom from pain and more depression and anxiety than controls and juvenile rheumatoid arthritis (JRA) patients; also, parents of CIPO patients required more time to care for their child and had poorer emotional status than parents of healthy controls and JRA patients. The prognosis is poor in primary CIPO, with most of the patients requiring enteral or parenteral nutrition, and a significant number will die from TPN-related complications. In the secondary forms the prognosis depends on the etiology. Most patients with CIPO will require some source of enteral or parenteral nutrition and a majority will eventually depend on it, although this could change with the emergence of small bowel transplantation. Mortality in pediatric CIPO ranges in most studies from 10% to 43%.

The clinical presentation of CIPO during adulthood can be quite different, with vague abdominal pain followed by vomiting and constipation as main symptoms (most have CIPO secondary to another condition). The prognosis is very similar, with many having multiple surgical interventions during their lifetime. A minority tolerated oral nutrition, and most have tried multiple prokinetics with partial success.

APPROACH TO THE CASE

Our patient did well until a few weeks before her second birthday when she developed gastroparesis (clinical and delayed gastric emptying by scintigraphy) and required multiple prokinetics without success. She then underwent a muscle biopsy that confirmed complex I mitochondrial disorder. She did not tolerate the gastrostomy tube feedings anymore, so a gastrojejunostomy tube was placed, which she initially tolerated. An AD was performed to delineate the motility pattern and findings were consistent with neuropathy. She then underwent a jejunostomy tube placement and initially tolerated jejunostomy tube feedings, until tolerance limited enteral nutrition and TPN was initiated. The gastrostomy tube has been used since then only for venting. She has been unable to tolerate more than 5 to 10 mL/day of jejunostomy tube feedings since then (now 5 years old) and she has had six CVL infections (five bacterial and one fungal) with subsequent sepsis. She also has had thrombosis of the neck veins (on enoxaparin [Lovenox]) and at present she has liver disease with coagulopathy (low factor IX) probably related to TPN that requires multiple infusions with fresh frozen plasma and cryoprecipitate. Despite these complications that impair her quality of life significantly, causing her to spend most of her life in the hospital, she is neurologically intact. She is awaiting liver–small bowel transplantation.

SUMMARY

CIPO is a disorder that includes a group of symptoms that resemble mechanical obstruction without a fixed lesion. The diagnosis of CIPO is evolving, as new etiologies are being discovered and characterized (mitochondrial disorders) and few cases should remain as primary. The treatment is supportive and is based on nutritional support. Enteral is the preferred route, and TPN should be used when enteral cannot be tolerated. Drug treatment is suboptimal. Intestinal transplantation should be considered in patients with intestinal failure and TPN complications and/or poor quality of life. CIPO should be an area of extensive investigation because in many cases the etiology is still unknown and the treatment is only supportive. Intestinal transplantation may evolve into the curative treatment, but experience and more studies are required.

MAJOR POINTS

Always rule out mechanical obstruction, pediatric falsification, Munchausen syndrome by proxy, and PADS before further invasive treatment.

Recent advances in diagnostic testing have caused a decrease in the number of primary CIPO as new etiologies (mitochondrial disorders) emerge.

AD manometry is always abnormal in CIPO.

Full-thickness biopsies are performed only when a surgical procedure is indicated.

Nutritional support is the mainstay of treatment in CIPO.

Enteral feedings are always preferred over TPN.

Surgical intervention has a limited role in the management of CIPO.

Intestinal transplantation may develop into the optimal treatment for irreversible intestinal failure.

SUGGESTED READINGS

Devane SP, Coombes R, Smith VV, et al: Persistent gastrointestinal symptoms after correction of malrotation. Arch Dis Child 67:218-221, 1992.

Di Lorenzo C, Flores AF, Tomomasa T, et al: Effect of erythromycin on antroduodenal motility in children with chronic functional gastrointestinal symptoms. Dig Dis Sci 39:1399-1404, 1994.

Di Lorenzo C, Lucanto C, Flores AF, et al: Effect of octreotide on gastrointestinal motility in children with functional gastrointestinal symptoms. J Pediatr Gastroenterol Nutr 27:508-512, 1998.

Emmanuel AV, Shand AG, Kamm MA: Erythromycin for the treatment of chronic intestinal pseudo-obstruction: Description of six cases with a positive response. Aliment Pharmacol Ther 19:687-694, 2004.

Goulet O, Jobert-Giraud A, Michel JL, et al: Chronic intestinal pseudo-obstruction syndrome in pediatric patients. Eur J Pediatr Surg 9:83-89, 1999.

Heneyke S, Smith VV, Spitz L, et al: Chronic intestinal pseudo-obstruction: Treatment and long term follow up of 44 patients. Arch Dis Child 81:21-27, 1999.

Lapointe SP, Rivet C, Goulet O, et al: Urological manifestations associated with chronic intestinal pseudo-obstructions in children. J Urol 168:1768-1770, 2002.

Lux G, Katschinski M, Ludwig S, et al: The effect of cisapride and metoclopramide on human digestive and interdigestive antroduodenal motility. Scand J Gastroenterol 29:1105-1110, 1994.

Mousa H, Hyman PE, Cocjin J, et al: Long-term outcome of congenital intestinal pseudoobstruction. Dig Dis Sci 47:2298-2305, 2002.

Peracchi M, Basilisco G, Bareggi B, et al: Plasma somatostatin levels in patients with chronic idiopathic intestinal pseudo-obstruction. Am J Gastroenterol 92:1884-1886, 1997.

Quigley EM: Chronic intestinal pseudo-obstruction. Curr Treat Options Gastroenterol 2:239-250, 1999.

Rudolph CD, Hyman PE, Altschuler SM, et al: Diagnosis and treatment of chronic intestinal pseudo-obstruction in children: Report of consensus workshop. J Pediatr Gastroenterol Nutr 24:102-112, 1997.

Schwankovsky L, Mousa H, Rowhani A, et al: Quality of life outcomes in congenital chronic intestinal pseudo-obstruction. Dig Dis Sci 47:1965-1968, 2002.

Shimotake T, Iwai N, Yanagihara J, et al: Biliary tract complications in patients with hypoganglionosis and chronic idiopathic intestinal pseudoobstruction syndrome. J Pediatr Surg 28:189-192, 1993.

Soykan I, Sarosiek I, McCallum RW: The effect of chronic oral domperidone therapy on gastrointestinal symptoms, gastric emptying, and quality of life in patients with gastroparesis. Am J Gastroenterol 92:976-980, 1997.

Tack J, Vos R, Janssens J, et al: Influence of tegaserod on proximal gastric tone and on the perception of gastric distension. Aliment Pharmacol Ther 18:1031-1037, 2003.

Vantini I, Benini L, Bonfante F, et al: Survival rate and prognostic factors in patients with intestinal failure. Dig Liver Dis 36:46-55, 2004.

Vargas JH, Sachs P, Ament ME: Chronic intestinal pseudo-obstruction syndrome in pediatrics: Results of a national survey by members of the North American Society of Pediatric Gastroenterology and Nutrition. J Pediatr Gastroenterol Nutr 7:323-332, 1988.

Verne GN, Eaker EY, Hardy E, et al: Effect of octreotide and erythromycin on idiopathic and scleroderma-associated intestinal pseudoobstruction. Dig Dis Sci 40:1892-1890, 1995.

CHAPTER 24

Short Bowel Syndrome

MARIA MASCARENHAS
MATTHEW J. RYAN

Disease Description
Case Presentation
Epidemiology
Pathophysiology
Diagnostic Testing
Treatment
   Medical Management of Short Bowel Syndrome
      Nutrition (Enteral and Parenteral)
   Treatment of Complications
   Surgical Management of Short Bowel Syndrome
   Other
Approach to the Case
Summary
Major Points

DISEASE DESCRIPTION

Short bowel syndrome (SBS) refers to malabsorption in the presence of a shortened intestine. Typically, this occurs in patients who have undergone a significant resection of their intestine. Functional SBS occurs when malabsorption is present with normal intestinal length; its causes include intestinal pseudo-obstruction, refractory sprue, radiation enteritis, and congenital villous atrophy. Complications of SBS include profuse, watery diarrhea; disruptions in fluid balance; weight loss; and nutritional deficiencies.

CASE PRESENTATION

The patient is a 6-month-old female who is a former 24-week preemie. She developed necrotizing enterocolitis and required resection of her ileum, ileocecal valve, and all but 20 to 30 cm of her colon. She required parenteral nutrition, cycled over 16 hours through a Broviac catheter. She took Pregestimil 20 kcal/ounce by mouth: 45 mL every 3 hours, with 0.5 mL of MCT oil added to every ounce of Pregestimil. She had four or five bowel movements daily with moderate water loss. She had wet burps after feeds, but no emesis. Her birthweight was 620 g, with a weight today of 3 kg (<5th percentile). Her parents became concerned about her watery stools and her small size. They wanted to know if there was any better way to increase calories through her gut without worsening her bowel movements.

EPIDEMIOLOGY

The incidence and frequency of short bowel syndrome in children are dependent on the underlying disorder. Although surgical resection due to inflammatory bowel disease may be the predominant cause of SBS in adults, the vast majority of pediatric cases are in premature infants with surgical resection due to necrotizing enterocolitis. Malrotation resulting in intestinal volvulus is another common cause of SBS. Functional SBS occurs when malabsorption is present with normal intestinal length; causes include intestinal pseudo-obstruction, refractory sprue, radiation enteritis, and congenital villous atrophy (Fig. 24-1).

PATHOPHYSIOLOGY

In the term neonate, the small bowel is estimated to be 250 cm and the colon 40 cm. The jejunum, ileum, and colon can double in length during the last trimester. Therefore, premature babies born at 28 weeks already have one half the small bowel as a term neonate. The

Acquired
NEC
Crohn's
Volvulus
Hirschsprung's
Tumors
Radiation

Congenital
Gastroschisis
Atresia

Figure 24-1 Causes of short bowel syndrome. NEC, necrotizing enterocolitis.

adult small intestine ranges from 400 to 700 cm, divided into the duodenum (approximately 30 cm), the jejunum (160 to 200 cm), and ileum (160 to 200 cm).

The adult distal intestinal tract is responsible for absorbing 2 to 3 L of ingested food and water on a daily basis. It also resorbs the 7 to 9 L of fluid secreted by the intestines each day. Protein, fat, and carbohydrate absorption occurs throughout the duodenum, jejunum, and ileum. The duodenum is responsible for the absorption of iron, carbohydrates, and electrolytes. Bile acids mix with the fats to form chylomicrons and allow for fat absorption in the ileum. In the jejunum, electrolytes, carbohydrates, trace elements, folate, fat-soluble vitamins, and water get absorbed. The ileum absorbs fats, bile salts, water, and vitamin B_{12}. Overall, the small bowel absorbs greater than 95% of ingested fat and protein. Carbohydrates are absorbed with an efficiency of between 8% and 98% (Fig. 24-2). To appreciate the physiology of SBS, it is important to understand that not all parts of the gut are created equally. Villous height, motility, absorptive capacity, and transporters all vary depending on the region of bowel being examined. The jejunum has long villi, a large absorptive surface area, high concentrations of enzymes and carrier proteins, and large tight junctions allowing for the passage of larger molecules. In contrast, the ileum has short villi, small tight junctions, less absorptive capacity, and increased lymphoid tissue. The ileum is the site of production for peptide YY and enteroglucagon. Peptide YY is responsible for a phenomenon known as the "ileal brake" and controls the rate of gastric emptying. The ileum also absorbs bile acids and vitamin B_{12} through site-specific receptors.

The severity of SBS symptoms depends a great deal on the presence or absence of the ileocecal valve. The ileocecal valve prevents the reflux of colonic bacteria into the small intestine and also controls the emptying of fluids and nutrients into the colon. After bowel resection, healing of the gut occurs through a process known as intestinal adaptation. Adaptation refers to the process in which the bowel changes functionally to meet nutritional needs in spite of the reduced surface area available for absorption. The first step in adaptation is mucosal hyperplasia. The hyperplasia includes increased crypt number and lengthening of villi, leading to an increase in absorptive surface area.

Stomach
1. Intrinsic factor binds to vitamin B_{12}
2. Pepsin aids in protein digestion
3. Mechanical digestion

Duodenum
1. Bile mixes to help form chylomicrons
2. Lipase aids in fat digestion
3. Amylase and protease aid in protein digestion
4. Brush border enzymes break down carbohydrates
5. Iron absorbed
6. Calcium, magnesium, and zinc absorption

Jejunum
1. Absorption of trace elements
2. Folate absorbed
3. Free fatty acids and fat-soluble vitamins absorbed
4. Moderate amount of water absorbed
5. Calcium and mineral absorption
6. Mono- and disaccharide absorption

Ileum
1. Bile salts absorbed
2. Intrinsic factor absorbed
3. Vitamin B_{12} absorbed
4. Water absorbed
5. Fat absorbed

Colon
1. Remainder of water resorbed
2. Minimal electrolyte absorption
3. Short-chain fatty acids

Figure 24-2 Functions of bowel segments.

The increased surface area also results slightly from intestinal lengthening, but much more from the increased villous height and luminal diameter. Another step in intestinal adaptation is changing the function of the enterocytes (functional adaptation). It should be noted that the increased cell number does not translate into increased nutrient transporters or the production of proper digestive enzymes.

Very little adaptation occurs until enteral feeding resumes again, stressing the importance of resuming enteral feeds. Nutrients are believed to stimulate adaptation include long- and short-chain fatty acids, omega-3 fatty acids, fiber, and glutamine. Long-chain fats tend to be more trophic than medium-chain triglycerides. Long-chain fats rapidly reduce starvation-induced mucosal atrophy compared with high-carbohydrate and high-protein diets. Arachidonic acid is an omega-3 fatty acid shown to be a major stimulant for adaptation through prostaglandins. Glutamine has received a lot of attention recently—it may work through several mechanisms to enhance adaptation and has been shown to reduce bacterial translocation as well as prevent mucosal atrophy. Unfortunately, even though studies suggest IV glutamine may have some trophic effects, oral glutamine produces minimal intestinal hyperplasia.

Stomach
- Upper GI
- Endoscopy

Duodenum
- Upper GI
- Upper endoscopy
- Intestinal disaccharidases
- Duodenal aspirate for culture
- Lactose breath test

Jejunum
- Upper GI with small bowel follow-through
- DEXA (assessment of nutrient absorption)

Ileum
- Upper GI with small bowel follow-through
- Vitamin levels

Colon
- Colonoscopy
- Barium enema
- Gastric emptying study

Figure 24-3 Imaging and diagnostic tools. DEXA, dual-energy x-ray absorptiometry; GI, gastrointestinal.

DIAGNOSTIC TESTING

An important initial step in evaluating the patient with SBS is to determine exactly how many centimeters of intestine remain, what type of intestine it is (jejunum, ileum, or colon), and whether the ileocecal valve is present. Valuable imaging studies include upper gastrointestinal (UGI) with small bowel follow-through and barium enema. These two imaging modalities can give a rough estimate of the entire length of the bowel from mouth to anus and an idea about transit time (Fig. 24-3). Initially, electrolyte and mineral levels (calcium, magnesium, and phosphorus) should be monitored frequently. Subsequently, regular assessment of fat-soluble and specific water-soluble (folic acid and vitamin B_{12}) vitamins and trace minerals (zinc, iron) is essential for proper management of the patient with SBS. Additional testing depends on symptoms and the clinical course of the individual patient. Our patient had weekly labwork initially until she was on a stable regimen, then twice a month labwork for the first several months after going home on TPN. With time, labwork were changed to a monthly schedule (see Fig. 24-3).

TREATMENT

Treatment of the patient with SBS consists of normalizing fluid and electrolyte status, maintaining normal growth, and preventing complications of SBS. The goal of therapy is to maintain the patient so that bowel adaptation and growth occur and the patient can be weaned off nutrition intervention measures (parenteral nutrition [PN], tube feeds, and so on). Complications of SBS include fluid, electrolyte, vitamin, and mineral abnormalities; feeding intolerance; dysmotility; gastric ulcers; cholelithiasis; bacterial overgrowth; and malnutrition.

Medical Management of Short Bowel Syndrome

Nutrition (Enteral and Parenteral)

After initial surgery, PN is started to provide nutritional support and to give the bowel time to heal. When the ileus resolves, trophic feeds are started at a slow continuous rate. Continuous feeds tend to be tolerated better than bolus feeds initially. After a sufficient rate of continuous feeding has been achieved, the patient is transitioned to bolus feedings. This should be done before discharge to allow for a more manageable home regimen and a more natural feeding schedule. If bolus feeds are not tolerated, continuous feeds can be arranged at home. Choice of initial formula should be based on age of the patient and the amount and location of the intestine resected. In infants, if maternal breast milk is available, it is the preferred type of nutrition. Patients who do not tolerate maternal breast milk or partially hydrolyzed formulas are often tried on amino acid–based formulas with good success.

If the patient cannot be completely weaned off PN, then the PN should be cycled to allow time off from the continuous infusion as well as improved lifestyles for the patient and family. Cycling the PN (administering PN over less than 24 hours per day) may also spare the liver from PN-related damage. A long course on PN can lead to a nonreversible cholestasis that can progress to liver failure. Cycling times can range from 12 to 20 hours depending on age, liver status, presence of hypoglycemia, convenience, and hydration status. Calorie and nitrogen requirements in infants fall with time, so frequent weight/height and blood urea nitrogen (BUN) monitoring is necessary to prevent overfeeding. Care must be taken to avoid underhydration and metabolic acidosis, which could have adverse effects on renal function and bone resorption, respectively (Fig. 24-4).

Treatment of Complications

Long-term complications include gastric ulcers, cholelithiasis, and bacterial overgrowth. Proton pump inhibitors and H_2 blockers are used to reduce gastric hypersecretion that occurs in patients with SBS. Hypersecretion typically resolves about 3 months after the initial surgery,

> Parenteral nutrition
> • Lasts the first 1-4 weeks
> • Components — carbohydrates, lipids, protein, fluid, electrolytes, vitamins, minerals, and trace elements
>
> Enteral nutrition
> • Adaptation occurs more rapidly in patients receiving enteral nutrition
> • Start with a continuous infusion to gain better caloric control, and less emesis and constantly saturate the intestine. This may be best managed initially with NG or G-tube feeding.
> • Withhold enteral feeding only if stool losses increase by more than 50% or the stool becomes significantly positive for reducing substances (>0.5%)
>
> Introduction of solids
> • Start with high-protein, starchy foods before introducing carbohydrates
> • BRAT diet and Pedialyte. Oral feedings will be mainly for preservation of oral skills rather than nutrition initially

Figure 24-4 Nutritional management. BRAT, bananas, rice, apples, toast; G, gastrostomy; NG, nasogastric.

> Initial
> • CBC
> • Complete metabolic panel (CMP)
> • Magnesium
> • Phosphorus
> • Triglycerides
> • Cholesterol
> • γ-glutamyl-transferase (GGT)
> • Prealbumin
>
> Daily
> • Basic metabolic panel
> • Calcium
> • Magnesium
> • Phosphorus
> • Triglycerides
>
> Weekly
> • CMP
> • Calcium
> • Magnesium
> • Phosphorus
> • Triglycerides
> • Cholesterol
> • Prealbumin
> • Hepatic function panel
> • GGT
>
> Monthly
> • CBC
> • Serum iron
> • Total iron binding capacity (TIBC)
> • Ferritin
> • Reticulocyte count
>
> Every 3-6 months
> • Serum selenium
> • Manganese
> • Zinc
> • Molybdenum
> • Copper
> • Ceruloplasmin
> • Vitamin A
> • Vitamin 25-D hydroxy
> • PIVKII

Figure 24-5 Laboratory protocol. CBC, complete blood count; CMP, complete metabolic panel.

and the acid blockade can be discontinued. Loperamide can be used to help slow bowel transit and increase time for absorption. It is important to frequently monitor levels of zinc, fat-soluble vitamins, water-soluble vitamins, hemoglobin, and electrolytes (Figure 24-5 shows a suggested regimen for monitoring laboratory evaluation).

Gallbladder stones form due to disruption of the enterohepatic circulation of bile salts. Cholesterol secretion is increased as the liver tries to keep up with the intestinal bile losses. The increased proportion of hydrophobic bile salts creates a more lithogenic bile. In patients who have had extensive ileal resection, increased oxalate absorption by the colon occurs because of the increased concentration of bile acids in the colon. The rising oxalate level leads to the formation of oxalate renal stones. This can be treated with a low-oxalate diet (exclusion of cocoa, peanut products, collards, soybeans, citrus drinks, fruits from the diet) and cholestyramine to bind bile salts.

Bacterial overgrowth is an easily treatable cause of diarrhea and bloating associated with SBS that often gets overlooked. With the loss of the ileocecal valve and disrupted motility of the bowel, colonic bacteria are able to overgrow into the small intestine. Determination of bacterial overgrowth can be done through breath hydrogen measurements or aspiration of duodenal fluid and culture. Long-term effects of bacterial overgrowth can include mucosal inflammation leading to steatorrhea, D-lactic acidosis, and vitamin B_{12} deficiency. Alternating courses of broad-spectrum antibiotics are used. Treatment with a probiotic such as *Lactobacillus* GG may help prevent bacterial overgrowth by populating the bowel with "good" bacteria.

Surgical Management of Short Bowel Syndrome

The goal of the initial operation is to save as much bowel as possible. Often the patient is left with an ostomy. The appropriate length of time from initial surgery to the time of re-anastomosis depends on the recovery of the patient and the length of bowel remaining. Patients with high jejunostomies often present unique challenges with respect to fluid and electrolyte management. In some centers, stool output from the proximal jejunum is fed into the distal jejunum to help minimize fluid and electrolyte shifts. The timing of re-anastomosis usually depends on the weight of the infant. A weight of 3 kg is often a goal, and infants usually require a combination of enteral and PN to achieve this goal. Patients with persistent feeding intolerance, fluid and electrolyte shifts, acidosis and carbohydrate malabsorption may require re-anastomosis sooner than anticipated because of their feeding intolerance. Complications from ostomies can include prolapse, stenosis, bleeding, and skin breakdown/infection. A comprehensive approach with the family, pediatrician, gastroenterologist, and surgeon works best to treat these complications. Every attempt is made to close an ostomy before discharge. If this is not possible, the presence of an ostomy should not limit or restrict the patient's activity at home in any way.

Stricture formation is a complication that occurs at the anastomotic site some time after surgery. This usually presents with symptoms of partial or complete small bowel obstruction: feeding intolerance, vomiting, constipation, abdominal obstruction, bleeding, and bacterial overgrowth. Treatment consists of resection of the stricture. Surgical techniques have been developed for bowel lengthening as an option to help get children off PN. The Bianchi procedure involves transecting the bowel longitudinally to create a bowel segment twice the length but one half the diameter. This can be performed only on bowel that is dilated. A newer procedure called serial transverse enteroplasty (STEP procedure) has been developed. This involves stapling the bowel in alternating and opposite directions, then separating the bowel to create a zigzagging luminal pattern, resulting in increased intestinal length.

Patients who are unlikely to wean off PN or who have minimal adaptation of their bowel may be candidates for small bowel transplantation. This can be performed either as an isolated small bowel transplant or in combination with a liver transplant. Unfortunately, liver failure can occur as a result of long-term TPN use. Patients who develop liver failure may be candidates for a dual small bowel/liver transplant. Complications of transplant can include sepsis, rejection, and lymphoproliferative disease.

Other

Recent research has focused on trying to aid the remaining bowel in growing and adaptation through dietary supplementation or new medications. Growth hormone and glucagon-like peptide are two agents currently on trial. Growth hormone seems to enhance small bowel growth in rats and mice. Few data are available on the effects of growth hormone in human bowel. Glucagon-like peptides are secreted from the GI tract after a meal. These peptides regulate nutrient absorption through motility and transport mechanisms.

APPROACH TO THE CASE

This was a typical presentation of SBS. These infants and children need to be followed closely and monitored for weight gain, diarrhea, vitamin deficiencies, cholestasis (depending on how long they remain on PN), feeding aversion, and electrolyte imbalance. The patient showed good weight gain from birth but did not demonstrate adequate catch-up growth. She could benefit from nasogastric feeds in order to increase nutrient intake and improve absorption with the use of continuous feeds. With tube feeds it would be important to control the rate of nutrient intake so as to not worsen the diarrhea. Loperamide should be added to the regimen to help slow motility. The patient's diarrhea may be a result of malabsorption of bile salts given the fact that she has lost her terminal ileum. Cholestyramine could be helpful because it binds bile acids that get reabsorbed in the ileum. By binding the bile salts, the osmotic load delivered to the short remaining colon is decreased.

She was started on continuous overnight nasogastric feeds with oral feeds during the day so she would not lose her oral motor skills. Loperamide was started to decrease motility, and a proton pump inhibitor was prescribed for gastric hypersecretion. She tolerated tube feeds and her diarrhea improved. Ultimately, at the age of 2 years, she was weaned off PN and at age 5 years was weaned off enteral feeds.

SUMMARY

SBS commonly occurs in neonates due to necrotizing enterocolitis. With the judicious use of PN and enteral feeds, these infants can be supported until sufficient intestinal adaptation occurs. Careful monitoring is important. Prompt treatment of complications will result in decreased mortality and morbidity. Bowel-lengthening procedures and intestinal transplantation are useful in those patients who cannot be successfully transitioned to enteral feeds.

> **MAJOR POINTS**
>
> The presence of the ileocecal valve is critical in determining outcome. Prognosis is improved and patients can tolerate larger resections if the ileocecal valve is present.
>
> The site of the intestinal resection will guide the practitioner as to what nutrient abnormalities to expect. Each section of bowel is responsible for the absorption of different nutrients.
>
> Frequent complications include bacterial overgrowth, diarrhea, liver disease, cholelithiasis, gastric ulcers, and poor growth.
>
> Newer surgical techniques (STEP procedure) are being used for bowel lengthening. Small bowel transplantation remains an option. Consultation with a transplant center should be done early in the course of the disease to determine the best options available for each patient.

SUGGESTED READINGS

Ana Abad-Sinden JS: Nutritional management of pediatric short bowel syndrome. Pract Gastroenterol 12:28-48, 2003.

Borkowski S: Pediatric stomas, tubes and appliances. Pediatr Clin North Am 45:1419-1435, 1998.

Jeejeebhoy KN: Short bowel syndrome: A nutritional and medical approach. CMAJ 166:1297-1302, 2002.

Kaufman S: Personal communication (2005). Children's Hospital of Philadelphia.

Kim HB, Fauza D, et al: Serial transverse enteroplasty (STEP): A novel bowel lengthening procedure. J Pediatr Surg 38:425-429, 2003.

Vanderhoof JA: Short-Bowel Syndrome and Intestinal Adaptation. Hamilton, Ontario, BC Decker, 2004.

Vanderhoof JA, Langnas AN: Short-bowel syndrome in children and adults. Gastroenterology 113: 1767-1778, 1997.

Warner BW, Vanderhoof JA, et al: What's new in the management of short gut syndrome in children. J Am Coll Surg 190:725-736, 2000.

Small Bowel Bacterial Overgrowth

TIMOTHY A.S. SENTONGO

Disease Description
Case Presentation
Epidemiology
Pathophysiology
    Normal Bowel Flora
    Diarrhea and Malnutrition
    Anemia
    D-Lactic Acidosis
    Hepatobiliary Inflammation
Diagnostic Testing
Treatment
    Medical Therapy
    Dietary Treatment
    Probiotic Therapy
    Surgery
Approach to the Case
Summary
Major Points

DISEASE DESCRIPTION

Small bowel bacterial overgrowth (SBBO) syndrome, also referred to as contaminated small bowel syndrome and blind loop syndrome, refers to the clinical signs and symptoms that arise secondary to excessive growth of bacterial organisms in the proximal intestine. The proximal small bowel is normally colonized by commensal microbes similar to oral flora in counts equal to or less than 105/mL. Patients with SBBO have bacterial counts in excess of 105/mL of proximal bowel luminal contents comprising mostly colonic-type flora. The clinical presentation ranges from asymptomatic to anemia, hepatic dysfunction, abdominal pain, gaseous discomfort, diarrhea, recurring pseudo-obstruction symptoms, carbohydrate intolerance, metabolic acidosis, malabsorption, and impaired growth.

CASE PRESENTATION

A 2-year-old toddler with short gut (gastroschisis) and partial parenteral nutrition (PN) dependency is brought to the local emergency department because of recurring episodes of unexplained lethargy. The lethargy is mostly after meals, generally worsens as the day progresses and tends to improve early in the morning after receiving the overnight PN infusion. The patient also has a history of chronic abdominal distention and frequent bowel movements that are attributed to the short gut syndrome. There is no history of abdominal pain, vomiting, fever, intercurrent illness, new medications, or trauma. During the month prior to presentation, oral feeding had increased and the PN was being weaned. Laboratory evaluation showed hemoglobin (Hgb) 9.8 g/dL; mean corpuscular volume (MCV) 91 fl/L; platelets 161 thousand; white blood cells 5.1 K; blood urea nitrogen (BUN) 9 mg/dL; creatinine 0.2 mg/dL; glucose 94 mg/dL; ammonia 33 mg/dL; sodium (Na) 139 mEq/dL; potassium (K) 3.9 mEq/dL; chloride (Cl) 103 mEq/dL; bicarbonate (HCO_3), 12 mEq/dL, respectively. Albumin 3.5 g/dL; bilirubin 2 mg/dL; alanine aminotransferase (ALT) 71 IU/L; aspartate transaminase (AST) 83 IU/L; alkaline (ALK) 105 IU/L; D-lactic acid 0.5 mEq/L.

EPIDEMIOLOGY

Generally, clinical symptoms of SBBO are uncommon in healthy individuals without a predisposing risk factor. Bacterial overgrowth diagnosed on the basis of increased breath hydrogen measurements was found in

15.6% of asymptomatic adults older than 61 years, 27% of rural children ages 5 years or younger in the tropics, and up to 34% of children ages 2 years or younger with chronic abdominal pain, diarrhea, and fetid stool. Recurring symptoms of SBBO suggest an underlying premorbid disease associated with impaired intestinal motility, immune dysfunction, and malnutrition. Therefore, the prevalence of recurring SBBO mirrors the incidence of the premorbid disorders that increase the risk for SBBO (Table 25-1).

PATHOPHYSIOLOGY

Normal Bowel Flora

The intestinal microbial flora are composed of more than 400 species of bacterial organisms that under normal circumstances cause no ill effects to their host. These organisms, also referred to as commensals (colonizing and deriving benefit without causing injury) or endogenous microflora become established during early childhood and persist throughout life with relatively little change. Interaction between environmental influences, host characteristics, and microbial properties determines whether exposure to a microbe results in mere colonization or infection and pathogenicity. There is a transition from principally aerobic organisms in the proximal bowel to predominantly facultative aerobes, anaerobes, and strict anaerobes in the distal small bowel and distal colon. The predominant aerobic commensals include *Lactobacillus*, *Enterococcus*, enteric organisms, *Corynbacterium*, *Streptococcus*, and *Staphylococcus* bacteria. Among the anaerobic bacteria, *Bacteroides* and *Bifidobacterium* account for 30% and 25% of the total counts, respectively.

The number of bacterial organisms also vary considerably along the human gastrointestinal (GI) tract; increasing from less than 10^4/mL in the stomach and proximal small intestine to 10^6 to 10^7/mL in the ileocecal region, and 10^{11} to 10^{12}/g of fecal matter in the colon. Approximately 60% of fecal mass consists of bacteria. The scarcity of bacteria in the proximal gastrointestinal tract is partly from the bacteriostatic effects of saliva, gastric acid, bile, and pancreatic secretions. The phasic propulsive peristaltic movements prevent stable colonization of bacteria in the small intestine, and an intact ileocecal valve impedes proximal migration of microorganisms from the colon. Mucosal barrier function, intestinal secretions, surface secretory immunoglobulin A (IgA), and cell-mediated immune function also play important roles in controlling intestinal flora. Therefore, the risk factors for SBBO are impaired intestinal motility, significant intestinal resection, loss of functional ileocecal valve, malnutrition, geriatric patients, and impaired immune function. Disruption of any one of these factors affects the balance between the normal gut protective mechanisms and bacterial contamination, proliferation, and pathogenicity in the proximal bowel. The symptoms of SBBO are listed in Table 25-2.

Diarrhea and Malnutrition

The proximal bowel is a specialized region for nutrient digestion and assimilation. Overgrowth of bacteria in the proximal small bowel is associated with intestinal inflammation, increased intestinal secretion, and disruption of nutrient digestion, resulting in diarrhea and malabsorption. Excess bacteria in the proximal bowel deconjugate bile salts and form free bile acids that rapidly get absorbed, which depletes the luminal bile concentration and impairs adequate micelle formation, resulting in maldigestion of dietary

Table 25-1 Risk Factors for Short Bowel Bacterial Overgrowth

Anatomic abnormalities of the gut (congenital and acquired)
Congenital intestinal obstruction (jejunoileal webs/atresias, gastroschisis, omphalocele)
Acquired perinatal obstruction (necrotizing enterocolitis [NEC], midgut volvulus, ischemia)
Intestinal strictures and obstruction, e.g., Crohn's disease
Duodenal or jejunal diverticulosis
Gastrointestinal fistulas
Disorders of intestinal motility
Intestinal pseudo-obstruction
Scleroderma
Degeneration of the myenteric plexus
Diabetic autonomic neuropathy
Postoperative problems
Afferent loop stasis
Intestinal adhesions
Gastroenterostomy
Postoperative blind loops
Enteroenterostomy
Continent ileostomy
After colectomy or jejunoileal bypass
Without demonstrable anatomic defect
Temporary monosaccharide malabsorption
Childhood malnutrition
Tropical sprue
Malabsorption in the elderly
Cholangitis
Cirrhosis
Immune deficiency states
Hypochlorhydria

From Gracey M: The contaminated small bowel syndrome. Am J Clin Nutr 32:2324-2343, 1979, Table 1.

Table 25-2	Symptoms of Short Bowel Bacterial Overgrowth
Symptoms	Abdominal pain, gaseous discomfort/distention
	Chronic diarrhea
	Poor growth
	Occult gastrointestinal bleeding
	Functional intestinal obstruction
	Encephalopathy
Clinical findings	Anemia: iron, folate, and vitamin B_{12} deficiencies
	Steatorrhea
	Protein losing enteropathy
	Metabolic acidosis
	Cholestasis, elevated transaminases
Radiographic findings	Dysmotility, gastroparesis, delayed transit
	Dilated bowel, strictures
	Pneumatosis

fat, steatorrhea, and diarrhea. Furthermore, malabsorbed free bile acids exert a carthartic effect on the colon and may contribute to the patchy enteropathic lesions associated with SBBO. The by-products from bacterial isolates in patients with bacterial overgrowth also inhibit intestinal dissacharidase activity, resulting in incomplete digestion and malabsorption of disaccharide sugars. Dumping of these osmotically active and easily fermentable sugars into the distal bowel and colon may result in increased flatulence and osmotic diarrhea.

Anemia

The mechanisms of anemia in patients with SBBO include malnutrition, micronutrient malabsorption, competitive bacterial assimilation of nutrients, and increased losses secondary to SBBO-associated enteropathy. A clinical presentation of iron deficiency and microcytic anemia may develop secondary to iron malabsorption and chronic occult GI bleeding from SBBO-associated bowel inflammation and enteropathy. Vitamin B_{12} and folate deficiencies causing macrocytic anemia may result from competitive assimilation of the vitamins by excessive growth of enteric bacteria. Vitamin B_{12} deficiency also may present atypically without obvious macrocytosis but instead as easy bruisability, progressive neuropsychiatric changes with serum vitamin B_{12} level in the low-normal range. Delay in diagnosis increases the risk for irreversible neurologic injury. Confirmation of metabolic stress from vitamin B_{12} deficiency is made by measuring the serum concentration of methylmalonic acid, which is significantly increased when there is tissue depletion of vitamin B_{12}. Management of vitamin B_{12} deficiency from terminal ileum resection requires lifetime replacement therapy with vitamin B_{12}. Onset of a refractory normocytic anemia in patients with short gut or SBBO should prompt suspicion of multiple micronutrient deficiencies including iron, vitamin B_{12}, folate, and copper.

D-Lactic Acidosis

D-Lactic acid is an optical isomer of L-lactic acid, which is produced endogenously during anaerobic glycolysis. D-Lactic acid is exogenously produced in the GI tract by bacterial fermentation of luminal carbohydrates. *Lactobacillus acidophilus* and *Lactobacillus fermentatum* are normal intestinal flora that produce D-and L-lactic acid from easily fermentable carbohydrates. D-Lactic acid is systemically absorbed, and excessive production may overwhelm normal metabolism, resulting in accumulation, metabolic acidosis, hyperventilation, and onset of encephalopathy-like symptoms in the human host. Serum D-lactic acid is not detected by routine assays for L-lactic acid. This is measured using specialized assays only available at designated reference laboratories. Therefore, the supportive biochemical findings for D-lactic acidosis are metabolic acidosis with an increased anion gap yet normal serum L-lactic acid concentration.

Hepatobiliary Inflammation

Bacterial endotoxin and cell wall components cause canalicular and hepatocellular inflammation. Peptidoglycan polysaccharides are bacterial cell wall polymers with potent inflammatory and immunoregulatory properties. Systemic uptake of peptidoglycan polysaccharides derived from gut bacteria is associated with hepatic inflammation in experimental animals with SBBO. Bacterial culture-negative hepatic injury in association with elevated serum antipeptidoglycan antibodies significantly correlates with increased bacterial counts in the small intestine. The hepatobiliary injury may be preventable by pretreatment with antibiotic therapy using metronidazole.

DIAGNOSTIC TESTING

The gold standard for diagnosis of SBBO is a duodenal aspirate and culture yielding bacterial counts in excess of 105/mL of proximal bowel luminal contents. Appropriate specimen handling and processing are critical because survival and growth of anaerobic bacteria are retarded in atmospheric oxygen. Nonetheless, obtaining a duodenal aspirate and culture is impractical in most patients during routine clinical care. Therefore, alternative noninvasive indirect tests, with reasonably good specificity, albeit lower sensitivity, have been developed (Table 25-3). The ^{14}C-bile acid and ^{14}C-xylose tests are based on bacterial deconjugation of the radiolabeled bile acids and metabolism of labeled xylose, respectively, liberating 14-labeled CO_2 that gets rapidly absorbed and eliminated in expired breath. The detection of the 14-labeled CO_2 in exhaled breath indicates active deconjugation and metabolism of xylose in the proximal bowel, suggesting a high luminal concentration of bacteria. However, use of radioactive markers is to be avoided in children; therefore, these tests have no application in pediatrics. Alternative use of stable isotopes is possible; however, widespread use is prevented by the prohibitive costs associated with analysis.

Hydrogen (and or methane) breath tests are safe, inexpensive, and are the most commonly used tests to diagnose SBBO in children. The physiologic basis for measuring change in breath hydrogen and/or methane is that intermediary metabolism in mammals does not generate hydrogen or methane. Therefore, an increased fasting level of breath hydrogen has a high specificity for active fermentation by enteric bacteria. Likewise, a significant rise in breath hydrogen following administration of a carbohydrate meal indicates a source exogenous to the host, for example, enteric bacteria residing in the host. Glucose is a simple sugar that normally gets rapidly and entirely absorbed in the proximal bowel without requirement for digestion. Therefore, a significant rise in breath hydrogen after administration of a glucose meal suggests excess bacterial contamination of the proximal bowel or rapid transit into the distal bowel and colon.

Determination that the rise in breath hydrogen is from overgrowth of bacteria in the proximal bowel and not merely rapid transit into the colon can be made by using the Lactulose breath hydrogen test. Lactulose is a nondigestible and nonabsorbable disaccharide, which when orally administered results in two measurable peaks in increased breath hydrogen in patients with SBBO. The initial peak is from fermentation of the lactulose by bacteria in the proximal bowel and the second peak is from fermentation by bacteria in the distal bowel and colon. Other supportive tests include upper GI series x-ray used to detect anatomic risk factors predisposing to the development of SBBO, such as strictures, dilated bowel, and enteric fistulas.

TREATMENT

It is uncommon, though not impossible, to develop SBBO as a primary disorder without predisposing risk factors. Recurring symptoms of SBBO should prompt a careful history and evaluation for the common predisposing risk factors listed in Table 25-1. Definitive therapy for recurring SBBO symptoms requires correction of the predisposing risk factors; however, this is often not possible or practical during routine clinical care. Treatment of SBBO can be categorized under (1) antibiotic therapy and prophylaxis, (2) dietary approaches, (3) probiotics, and (4) corrective or palliative surgery of the intestinal anatomic abnormalities leading to stasis or microbial proliferation.

Medical Therapy

This is the most common approach for controlling symptoms of SBBO. A wide variety of antibiotic regimens have been used for the treatment of SBBO. However, safe and efficacious antibiotic therapy is based on the fundamental understanding that (1) the bacterial pathogens responsible for SBBO symptoms are usually

Table 25-3 Tests for Bacterial Overgrowth

Test	Simplicity	Sensitivity	Specificity	Safety
Culture	Poor	Excellent*	Excellent	Good
Urinary indicant	Good	Poor	Poor	Excellent
Jejunal fatty acids	Poor	Fair	Excellent	Good
Jejunal bile acids	Poor	Fair	Excellent	Good
Fasting breath H_2	Excellent	Poor	Good	Excellent
^{14}C-bile acid BT	Excellent	Fair	Poor	Good
^{14}C-xylose BT	Excellent	Excellent	Excellent	Excellent
Lactulose-H_2 BT	Excellent	Fair	Fair-good	Excellent
Glucose-H_2 BT	Excellent	Good	Fair-good	Excellent

*Appropriate microbial specimen handling, anaerobic chambers, and quantitative culture techniques are required.
BT, breath test.
From Toskes PP, Kumar A: Enteric bacterial flora and bacterial overgrowth syndrome. In Feldman M, Scharschmidt BF, Sleisenger MH (eds): Sleisenger & Fordtran's Gastrointestinal and Liver Disease: Pathophysiology, Diagnosis, Management, 6th ed. Philadelphia, WB Saunders, 1998, pp 1523-1535.

part normal endogenous anaerobic and facultative anaerobic colonic flora that have migrated proximally from the distal bowel and colon; (2) antibiotic therapy only suppresses but cannot completely eradicate endogenous bacterial flora; and (3) chronic injudicious use of antibiotics disrupts and suppresses the normal balance of endogenous flora, promotes antibiotic resistance, and increases the risk for developing *Clostridium difficile,* yeast, and other opportunistic enteric and systemic infections.

There are no adequate clinical trials that have identified preferred or most effective antimicrobial agents, duration of therapy, or appropriate management of recurrences. Therefore, it is important that an initial positive SBBO diagnosis is made before subsequent empiric and/or cyclic antibiotic therapy in patients with recurring symptoms. Antibiotics with poor activity against enteric anaerobes or oral aminoglycosides should be avoided. The commonly used antibiotics are metronidazole (bacteroides and anaerobic coverage), trimethoprim-sulfamethoxazole (broad spectrum), and rifaximin (anaerobic coverage and nonabsorbable). When significant intestinal inflammation is present, as evidenced by occult bleeding and inflammatory changes on intestinal biopsy, therapy with sulfasalazine and corticosteroids may be used concurrently with antibiotics.

Dietary Treatment

Dietary modification is most beneficial for patients with recurring episodes of D-lactic acidosis. Decreased or controlled dietary intake of carbohydrates affects the luminal substrate available for fermentation by the enteric bacteria, resulting in lower serum D-lactate levels. Bacteria lack the enzyme capacity for digestion of complex carbohydrates. Therefore, the dietary carbohydrate composition should mostly consist of complex sugars. These are also fermented at much slower rates and, compared with simple sugars, associated with less production of lactic acid. Supportive maintenance therapy with oral alkalizing agents such as citrate and bicarbonate is helpful to buffer the metabolic acidosis in patients with chronic or recurring D-lactic acidosis. Other nutritional manipulations in patients with SBBO include supplementation with iron, folate, vitamin B_{12}, and other micronutrients.

Probiotic Therapy

Probiotics are dietary supplements that contain one or more cultures of living organisms that play a beneficial role in "improving" the host's endogenous microflora. Probiotic organisms alter intestinal microbial flora and intestinal permeability, stimulate the nonimmunologic gut defense barrier and mucosal IgA responses, and influence the balance between pro- and antiinflammatory cytokines; however, these effects vary with the different probiotics. Probiotic therapy has been helpful in reducing symptoms of diarrhea and D-lactic acidosis in patients with short bowel syndrome. More studies are required to define the benefits and applications of probiotic therapy in several disease disorders, including SBBO.

Surgery

Surgery is normally considered when severe symptoms recur, such as functional intestinal obstruction despite adequate medical therapy (antibiotics and diet). Surgical correction of anatomic anomalies leading to stasis and proliferation of bacteria can be immediately corrective of recurring SBBO symptoms. The anatomic abnormalities predisposing to SBBO include adhesions, strictures, dilated bowel, fistulas, and diverticula.

APPROACH TO THE CASE

What is the likely cause of the presenting symptoms? The initial evaluation of a child with lethargy involves a history, physical examination, and laboratory assessment to identify common causes of lethargy and altered mental status. The differential diagnosis includes hypoglycemia, intoxication, encephalopathy, trauma, infection, poisoning, and seizures. The labs show significant metabolic acidosis with a normal serum lactate. Metabolic acidosis may manifest with lethargy and encephalopathy. When associated with a normal anion gap [Na − (Cl + HCO_3) ≤12] the etiology of metabolic acidosis is increased bicarbonate losses that may be secondary to renal or excessive gastrointestinal losses, for example, renal tubular acidosis, severe diarrhea, and high output ileostomies. Metabolic acidosis with an increased anion gap suggests increased serum concentrations of an organic acid. In the setting of short gut syndrome, this is commonly D-lactic acid produced exogenously by fermentation of dietary carbohydrates by enteric bacteria. Megaloblastic anemia may develop secondary to malabsorption or competitive assimilation of vitamin B_{12} or folic acid by luminal bacteria in patients with SBBO. The other risk factors for vitamin B_{12} deficiency in children are impaired absorption due to surgical or functional loss of the terminal ileum and infestation by *Diphyllobothrium latum* (fish tapeworm).

Our patient was evaluated with a glucose breath test that detected a high fasting breath hydrogen followed by a significant rise in breath hydrogen after the glucose load. He had an upper GI small bowel follow-through series x-ray that revealed stasis and a significantly dilated small bowel (Fig. 25-1). The metabolic acidosis was corrected with IV hydration and therapy with bicarbonate replacements. Breath hydrogen testing after administration of oral glucose showed a rise in breath hydrogen greater than 20 parts per million (ppm). The SBBO was treated with oral metronidazole for 2 weeks and therapy repeated for 1 week every other week. The serum vitamin B_{12} level was within normal range, at 332 pg/mL (normal range 200 to 1000 pg/mL); however, with an increased serum methylmalonic acid concentration of 10.9 μmol/L (normal <0.4 μmol/L). The secondary methylmalonic acidemia was indicative of physiologic and metabolic stress from decreased vitamin B_{12} availability, despite being within low-normal serum levels. Vitamin B_{12} deficiency was corrected using intramuscular vitamin B_{12} replacements.

SUMMARY

SBBO is a common, though not frequently recognized, condition characterized by symptoms that develop secondary to excessive growth of bacteria in the proximal small intestine. The clinical presentation is protean, ranging from asymptomatic to primarily gastrointestinal symptoms, malnutrition, metabolic acidosis, and encephalopathy. Those at greatest risk are children with malnutrition, short gut, anatomic abnormalities of the gastrointestinal tract, impaired intestinal motility, and immunodeficiency. A high index of suspicion in at-risk individuals is necessary for early detection, diagnosis, and appropriate management. The case demonstrates the presentation and a management approach that addresses SBBO and its associated complications. The definitive therapy in patients with recurring symptoms is correction of the predisposing factor; otherwise, management is mostly supportive therapy.

MAJOR POINTS

- These symptoms should prompt evaluation for SBBO in children: chronic diarrhea or anemia, unexplained lethargy, confusion, and excessive flatulence.
- The risk factors for developing SBBO include malnutrition, short gut, GI surgery, immunodeficiency, and severe GI motility disorders.
- The following diagnostic tests should be considered for a child with symptoms suggestive of SBBO: duodenal aspiration for bacterial cell count and culture and hydrogen breath tests.
- Treatment strategies for children with recurring SBBO consist of appropriate antibiotic therapy (prophylaxis); changes in diet; probiotics; and corrective surgery of intestinal anatomic abnormalities.

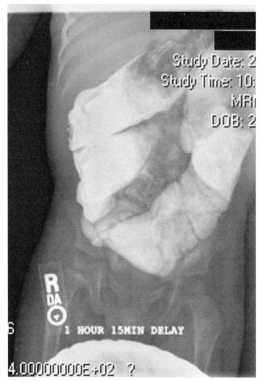

Figure 25-1 Upper gastrointestinal series x-ray demonstrating stasis and significantly dilated bowel.

SUGGESTED READINGS

Bongaerts GP, Tolboom JJ, Naber AH, et al: Role of bacteria in the pathogenesis of short bowel syndrome-associated lactic acidemia. Microb Pathog 22:285-293, 1997.

Chelminsky G, Blanchard S, Sivit C, et al: Pneumatosis intestinalis and diarrhea in a child following renal transplantation. Pediatr Transpl 7:236-239, 2003.

de Boissieu D, Chaussain M, Badoual J, et al: Small-bowel bacterial overgrowth in children with chronic diarrhea, abdominal pain or both. J Pediatr 128:203-207, 1996.

Di Stefano M, Malservisi S, Veneto G, et al: Rifaximin versus chlortetracycline in the short-term treatment of small intestinal bacterial overgrowth. Aliment Pharmacol Ther 14:551-55, 2000.

Gracey M: The contaminated small bowel syndrome: Pathogenesis, diagnosis, and treatment. Am J Clin Nutr 32:234-243, 1979.

Greg CR, Toskes PP: Enteric bacterial flora and bacterial overgrowth syndrome. In Feldman M, Scharschmidt BF, Sleisenger MH (eds): Sleisenger & Fordtran's Gastrointestinal and Liver Disease: Pathophysiology, Diagnosis, Management, 7th ed. Philadelphia, WB Saunders, 2003, pp 1783-1793.

Guarner F, Malagelada JR: Gut flora in health and disease. Lancet 361:512-519, 2003.

Heikens GT, Schofield WN, Dawson S: The Kingston project. II. The effects of high energy supplement and metronidazole on malnourished children rehabilitated in the community: Anthropometry. Euro J Clin Nutr 47:160-173, 1993.

Kaufman SS, Loseke CA, Lupo JV, et al: Influence of bacterial overgrowth and intestinal inflammation on duration of parenteral nutrition in children with short bowel syndrome. J Pediatr 131:356-361, 1997.

Keshavarzian A, Isaacs P, McColl I, Sladen GE: Idiopathic intestinal pseudo-obstruction and contaminated small bowel syndrome: Treatment with metronidazole, ileostomy and indomethacin. Am J Gastroenterol 78:562-565, 1983.

Kocoshis SA, Schletewitz K, Lovelace G, et al: Duodenal bile acids among children: Keto derivatives and aerobic small bowel bacterial overgrowth. J Pediatr Gastroenterol Nutr, 6:686-696, 1987.

Lichtman SN, Keku J, Schwab JH, Sartor RB: Evidence of peptidoglycan absorption in rats with experimental small bowel bacterial overgrowth. Infect Immun 59:555-562, 1991.

Lichtman SN, Okuruwa EE, Keku J, et al: Degradation of endogenous bacterial cell wall polymers by the muralytic enzyme mutanolysin prevents hepatobiliary injury in genetically susceptible rats with experimental intestinal bacterial overgrowth. JCI 90:1313-1322, 1992.

Mayne AJ, Handy DJ, Preece MA, et al: Dietary management of D-lactic acidosis in short bowel syndrome. Arch Dis Child 65:229-231, 1990.

Parlesak A, Klein B, Schecher K, et al: Prevalence of small bowel bacterial overgrowth and its association with nutrition intake in nonhospitalized older adults. J Am Geriatr Soc 51:768-773, 2003.

Pereira SP, Khin-Muang-U, Bolin TD, et al: A pattern of breath hydrogen excretion suggesting small bowel bacterial overgrowth in Burmese village children. J Pediatr Gastroenterol Nutr 13:32-38, 1991.

Perlmutter D, Boyle JT, Campos JM, et al: D-lactic acidosis in children: An unusual metabolic complication of small bowel resection. J Pediatr 102:234-238, 1983.

Piccoli DA: Breath testing. In Altschuler SM, Liacouras CA (eds): Clinical Pediatric Gastroenterology. Philadelphia, Churchill Livingstone, 1998, pp 567-574

Ramakrishnan T, Toskes : Beneficial effects of fasting and low carbohydrate diet in D-lactic acidosis associated with short-bowel syndrome. J Parenter Enteral Nutr 9:361-363, 1985.

Salminen S, Bouley C, Boutron-Ruault MC, et al: Functional food science and gastrointestinal physiology and function. British J Nutr 80(Suppl 1):S147-S171, 1998.

Schwobel M, Hirsig J, Illi O, Battig U: The influence of small bowel contamination on the pathogenesis of bowel obstruction. Prog Pediatr Surg 24:165-172, 1989.

Stephen AM, Cummings JH: The microbial contribution to human fecal mass. J Med Microbiol 13:45-56, 1980.

Toskes PP, Kumar A: Enteric bacterial flora and bacterial overgrowth syndrome. In Feldman M, Scharschmidt BF, Sleisenger MH (eds): Sleisenger & Fordtran's Gastrointestinal and Liver Disease: Pathophysiology, Diagnosis, Management, 6th ed. Philadelphia, WB Saunders, 1998, pp 1523-1535.

Vanderhoof JA: Probiotics and intestinal inflammatory disorders in infants and children. J Pediatr Gastroenterol Nutr 30(Suppl 2):S34-S38, 2000.

Vanderhoof JA, Young RJ, Murray N, Kaufman SS: Treatment strategies for small bowel bacterial overgrowth in short bowel syndrome. J Pediatr Gastroenterol Nutr 27:155-160, 1998.

Walshe K, Healy MJ, Speekenbrink AB, et al: Effects of enteric anaerobic bacterial culture supernatant and deoxycholate on intestinal calcium absorption and dissacharidase activity. Gut 31:770-776, 1990.

Weir DG, Scott JM: Vitamin B_{12} cobalamin. In Shils ME, Olson JA, Shike M, Ross CA (eds): Modern Nutrition in Health and Disease, 9th ed. Philadelphia, Williams & Wilkins, 1999, pp 447-458.

HEPATIC DISORDERS

PART 2

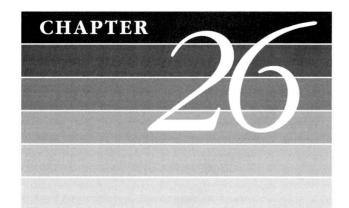

Alagille Syndrome

BINITA M. KAMATH
DAVID A. PICCOLI

Disease Description
Case Presentation
Epidemiology
Pathophysiology
Differential Diagnosis
Diagnostic Testing
Treatment
Approach to the Case
Summary
Major Points

DISEASE DESCRIPTION

Alagille syndrome (AGS) is a highly variable autosomal dominant multisystem disorder involving predominantly the liver, heart, eyes, face, and skeleton. The main clinical manifestations of AGS are cholestasis, characterized by bile duct paucity on liver biopsy; congenital cardiac defects, primarily involving the pulmonary arteries; posterior embryotoxon in the eye; typical facial features; and butterfly vertebrae. Renal and central nervous system abnormalities also are described.

CASE PRESENTATION

The patient is a 7-week-old boy who presented with persistent jaundice. He is the product of an unremarkable delivery and pregnancy and the parents were nonconsanguineous. Of note, the paternal aunt had a repair of tetralogy of Fallot in childhood. There is no family history of liver disease. The patient is feeding well and has pale stools by history.

On physical examination the patient's weight and length are at the 10th percentile. He has scleral icterus, and a small and pointy chin. Cardiovascular examination reveals normal heart sounds and a systolic murmur that radiates to the axillae. Abdominal examination is notable for 3 cm hepatomegaly but no splenomegaly. Laboratory evaluation reveals a conjugated hyperbilirubinemia with total bilirubin 13.0 mg/dL and conjugated fraction of 9.4 mg/dL. His serum aminotransferases are elevated with an alanine aminotransferase of 198 U/L and aspartate aminotransferase of 165 U/L. The γ-glutamyl-transferase (GGT) is markedly elevated at 996 U/L.

EPIDEMIOLOGY

One of the hallmark features of AGS is highly variable expressivitiy, making estimates of prevalence difficult. The advent of molecular screening has widened the spectrum of clinical phenotypes associated with mutations in *Jagged1* (*JAG1*), the disease gene in AGS, and has identified individuals with subclinical features who do not meet classic criteria for the syndrome. The prevalence of classic AGS has been reported as 1 in 100,000 live births, although this is most likely an underestimate because these patients were ascertained based solely on the finding of neonatal liver disease. The prevalence of *JAG1* mutation associated disease is likely to be greater still.

PATHOPHYSIOLOGY

AGS is a developmental disorder predominantly caused by mutations in *JAG1*, located on chromosome 20. To date, more than 400 AGS probands have been studied molecularly, and *JAG1* mutations have been demonstrated in 94%. Total gene deletions have been identified in 5% to 7% of these patients. Approximately 50% of these patients have protein truncating mutations. *JAG1* mutations have been found to be de novo in 5% to 70% of cases. Recently, Notch2 mutations have been identified in a minority of AGS patients without *JAG1* mutations. These individuals appear to have a prominent renal phenotype.

The majority of symptomatic patients with AGS present in the first year of life with a conjugated hyperbilirubinemia in the neonatal period. The magnitude of the hyperbilirubinemia is minor compared with the degree of cholestasis. Cholestasis manifests with pruritus, which is among the most severe in any chronic liver disease. It is rarely present before 3 to 5 months of age, but is seen in nearly all children by the third year of life even in those who are anicteric. The presence of severe cholestasis results in the formation of xanthomas, characteristically on the extensor surfaces of the fingers, the palmar creases, popliteal fossa, buttocks, and the inguinal region. The lesions persist throughout childhood but may gradually disappear after 10 years of age. Hepatomegaly is common in infancy, and although splenomegaly is unusual early in the course of the disease, it is eventually found in up to 70% of patients. Synthetic liver failure is extremely uncommon in the first year of life, nevertheless, progression to cirrhosis and hepatic failure, is recognized in approximately 20% of AGS patients.

Liver biopsy in patients with AGS classically shows intrahepatic bile duct paucity (Fig. 26-1), although the diagnostic histopathologic lesion of duct paucity is progressive and may not be evident in the newborn period. Depending on when a biopsy is performed, there may be a broad range of histologic findings, including portal fibrosis, and rarely, bile duct proliferation.

Congenital heart disease is present in 81% to 100% of individuals with AGS (see Fig. 26-1). The pulmonary vasculature (pulmonary valve, artery and/or its branches) is most commonly involved, with peripheral pulmonic stenosis being the most prevalent. Intracardiac lesions are seen in 24%. The most frequent complex cardiac malformation seen in these patients is tetralogy of Fallot (TOF) (7% to 10%). Cardiac disease accounts for nearly all the early mortality in AGS. Furthermore, cardiovascular disease contributes significantly to the morbidity of the disorder, and has been implicated in the increased post-transplantation mortality seen in some series.

The hepatic and cardiac disease described account for most of the morbidity and mortality in AGS. The remaining three cardinal features of AGS, namely facial features, skeletal (usually butterfly vertebrae), and eye abnormalities (typically posterior embryotoxon) are of little significance

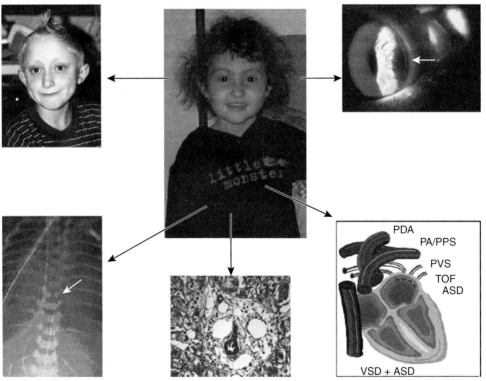

Figure 26-1 *(See also Color Plate 26-1.)* Clinical manifestations of Alagille syndrome. Clockwise upper right and central panels: facial features; posterior embryotoxon; common cardiac anomalies; liver biopsy showing bile duct paucity; butterfly vertebrae on thoracic x-ray. ASD, atrial septal defect; PA/PPS, pulmonary atresia/peripheral pulmonary stenosis; PVS, pulmonary valve stenosis; TOF, tetralogy of Fallot; VSD, ventricular septal defect.

but are relevant for diagnostic purposes (see "Diagnostic Testing" later). The constellation of facial features seen in AGS patients includes a prominent forehead, deep-set eyes with moderate hypertelorism, pointed chin, and saddle or straight nose with a bulbous tip. The combination of these features gives the face a triangular appearance (see Fig. 26-1).

Intracranial bleeding is becoming increasingly recognized as a significant cause of morbidity and mortality in AGS, with occurrences as high as 16%. Additional reports have noted the association of various vascular malformations with AGS including renovascular anomalies and moyamoya syndrome. This may indicate that there is an underlying "vasculopathy" present in some individuals with *JAG1* mutations.

Severe growth retardation is seen in 50% to 87% of patients. It is particularly evident in the first 4 years of life. Malnutrition due to malabsorption is a major factor in this failure to thrive, and chronic wasting is severe in AGS. There appear to be limitations in linear growth even when protein-calorie malnutrition is not evident.

Renal anomalies, although clinically diverse, have been reported in 2% to 74% of AGS patients and as such should be considered an important clinical manifestation of AGS. Reported renal abnormalities have included structural anomalies, such as solitary kidney and ectopic kidney; metabolic kidney disease, in particular, renal tubular acidosis; and renal vascular disease (arterial stenosis), that may result in systemic hypertension.

DIFFERENTIAL DIAGNOSIS

Many other forms of cholestatic liver disease (biliary atresia, cystic fibrosis) may present with conjugated hyperbilirubinemia in the neonatal period (Table 26-1). AGS is most easily confused with extrahepatic disorders such as biliary atresia and metabolic disorders with elevated GGT. AGS is often misdiagnosed as biliary atresia because of the overlap of biochemical, scintiscan, and cholangiographic features. The pattern of histologic involvement of the ducts is significantly different, however, and biopsy must be a routine component of the evaluation. In biliary atresia, bile duct proliferation is the typical histologic lesion, and paucity is extremely rare at diagnosis, whereas in AGS, proliferation is rare, and paucity is nearly always present by 6 months of age. Because the evaluation commonly occurs in the first 2 months of life, the histologic findings may be nondiagnostic, and operative or endoscopic cholangiography is required.

AGS must also be distinguished from other syndromes in which right-sided cardiac defects and vertebral anomalies coexist, such as Noonan syndrome and chromosome 22q11 deletion.

Table 26-1 Differential Diagnosis of Cholestasis in Infancy

Bile duct obstruction	Biliary atresia
	Choledochal cyst
	Alagille syndrome
	Sclerosing cholangitis
	Congenital hepatic fibrosis
	Inspissated bile
Neonatal hepatitis	Viral—cytomegalovirus (CMV), herpes, rubella, adenovirus, hepatitis B
	Bacterial—sepsis, urinary tract infection, listeriosis
	Parasitic—toxoplasmosis
	Idiopathic
Cholestasis syndromes	Progressive familial intrahepatic cholestasis
	Type 1/FIC-1 associated disease (Byler, BRIC)
	Type 2/BSEP
	Type 3/MDR3 deficiency
	Dubin-Johnson syndrome
	Rotor
Metabolic disorders	α_1-Antitrypsin deficiency
	Hypothyroidism
	Cystic fibrosis
	Tyrosinemia
	Galactosemia
	Storage disorders
	Bile acid synthetic disorders
Toxic	Drugs
	Parenteral nutrition

BRIC, benign recurrent intercurrent cholestasis; BSEP, bile salt export pump deficiency; MDR-3, multi-drug resistance gene 3 deficiency.

DIAGNOSTIC TESTING

The diagnosis of AGS in patients with neonatal cholestasis requires a careful physical examination and a thorough biochemical and radiologic evaluation. AGS is most easily confused with extrahepatic disorders such as biliary atresia. Laboratory findings in AGS most commonly include elevations of serum bile acids, conjugated bilirubin, alkaline phosphatase, cholesterol, and γ-glutamyl-transpeptidase indicative of a defect in biliary excretion. Less frequently elevations of serum aminotransferases and triglycerides may be present. Hypercholesterolemia and triglyceridemia may be profound in severe cholestasis. Excretion of nuclear tracer into the duodenum (hepatobiliary scintigraphy) can be helpful to eliminate biliary atresia from consideration; however, nonexcretion is common in AGS as well. The initial noninvasive testing should be followed by a liver biopsy. Liver biopsy classically shows intrahepatic bile duct paucity (see Fig. 26-1), although the diagnostic histopathologic lesion of paucity is progressive and may not be evident in the newborn period. In one large series, bile duct paucity was only evident in 60% of infants younger than 6 months, but present in 95% of older patients.

Evaluation of the facies is an important part of the diagnostic testing for AGS (see Fig. 26-1). The facial features are characteristic although they are dynamic with adult facial features and quite different from those seen in infancy and childhood. Because the facial features are one of the most penetrant features of AGS, they are a valuable diagnostic tool and should be evaluated by a dysmorphologist or a gastroenterologist familiar with the syndrome.

The presence of a murmur in a child with cholestasis should prompt a cardiologic evaluation. The absence or presence of peripheral pulmonary stenosis should be specifically evaluated for because it may be missed on routine echocardiography. Posterior embryotoxon (a prominent centrally positioned Schwalbe's ring) (see Fig. 26-1), visualized by slit-lamp examination, has been reported in up to 89% of patients and is therefore important diagnostically although it is of no consequence for visual acuity. Posterior embryotoxon also occurs in the general population with a frequency of 8% to 15%; therefore, its value as a diagnostic tool is limited. The most common skeletal abnormality in AGS is butterfly vertebrae (see Fig. 26-1). Butterfly vertebrae are usually asymptomatic radiologic findings and can be detected on plain x-rays of the thoracic vertebrae. The frequency of butterfly vertebrae ranges from 2% to 87% in reported cases of AGS.

The diagnosis of AGS is largely based on this clinical testing. Molecular testing for deletions of or mutations within *JAG1* is a useful adjunct for diagnosis in atypical cases or in individuals with subtle manifestations. Fluorescent in situ hybridization (FISH) detects deletions in 5% to 7% of cases of AGS and mutational analysis can now identify mutations in approximately 90% of clinically diagnosed individuals. Mutational analysis is available from commercial companies and on a research basis. The diagnosis of AGS remains largely a clinical one.

TREATMENT

Patients with Alagille syndrome present significant management challenges (Table 26-2). Cholestasis is commonly profound. Bile flow may be stimulated with the choleretic ursodeoxycholic acid, but in many patients the pruritus continues unabated. Care should be taken to keep the skin hydrated with emollients, showers instead of long baths should be recommended, and fingernails should be trimmed. Therapy with antihistamines may provide some relief, but many patients require additional agents such as rifampin, cholestyramine, or naltrexone. Biliary diversion has been successful in a limited number of patients, but intractable pruritus continues to be an indication for transplantation in refractory patients.

Malnutrition and growth failure should be treated with aggressive nutritional therapy. There will be significant malabsorption of long-chain fat, and therefore formulas supplemented with medium-chain triglycerides have some nutritional advantage. Fat-soluble vitamin deficiency is present to a varying degree in most patients. Vitamin D, E, and A levels should be routinely monitored and prothrombin time/partial thromboplastin time (PT/PTT) should be monitored as an indicator of vitamin K deficiency (an inability to correct coagulopathy in some patients may of course indicate severe synthetic liver dysfunction). Multivitamin preparations may not provide the correct ratio of fat-soluble vitamins, and thus vitamins are best administered as individual supplements. Administration of vitamin A is not generally recommended because toxicity is largely hepatic. Individuals with splenomegaly should be fitted for a spleen guard, and this should be worn for physical activities. In general, extreme contact sports should be avoided by patients with significant splenomegaly.

Liver transplantation is indicated in those patients with synthetic liver dysfunction, intractable portal hypertension, bone fractures, severe pruritus, xanthomata, and growth failure. Transplantation becomes necessary in 21% to 50% of patients with hepatic manifestations in infancy, with post-transplantation survival rates ranging from 79% to 100%. These results indicate that individuals with AGS are good candidates for transplantation although morbidity and mortality post-transplantation are influenced by the degree of cardiopulmonary involvement.

The usefulness of baseline cranial magnetic resonance imaging with or without angiography has not been clinically evaluated in a large cohort of individuals with AGS. However, in light of the increasing number of reports of vascular anomalies and bleeds in this population, the presence of neurologic signs or symptoms or a traumatic head injury should prompt careful neurologic evaluation and appropriate imaging.

APPROACH TO THE CASE

In any infant presenting with conjugated hyperbilirubinemia and elevated GGT, the most important diagnosis to exclude in a timely fashion is extrahepatic biliary atresia. The outcome of the Kasai procedure (hepatic portoenterostomy) is significantly optimized by performing surgery before 60 days. A hepatobiliary scan

Table 26-2 Overview of Therapeutic Modalities in Alagille Syndrome		
Symptom	Pharmacologic Therapy	Dietary and Other Therapies
Fat malabsorption	Medium-chain triglycerides	Optimize carbohydrate and protein intake
Fat-soluble vitamin deficiency	Vitamin K (oral/intramuscular) Vitamin D (oral/intramuscular) (absorption of vitamin D may be enhanced by administration of d-α-tocopherol polyethylene glycol-1000 succinate [TPGS]) Vitamin E (oral) (TPGS-soluble preparation)	
Pruritus	Ursodeoxycholic acid Antihistamines Rifampin Cholestyramine Naltrexone	Hydrate skin with emollients Avoid baths Trim fingernails Biliary diversion
Decreased bone density/ osteoporosis	Calcium supplements	Annually monitor bone density with DEXA scans

DEXA, Dual-energy x-ray absorptiometry.

scan may assist in differentiating biliary atresia from other causes (see Table 26-1), although nonexcretion of tracer to the bowel may also occur in other conditions such as AGS. A liver biopsy will be most helpful in furthering the diagnosis.

In this case a liver biopsy was performed, which revealed bile duct paucity. The presence of the cardiac murmur warranted an echocardiogram, which detected peripheral pulmonary stenosis. The patient had an ophthalmologic evaluation and spinal x-rays that did not show any abnormalities.

SUMMARY

AGS is a multisystem developmental disorder caused by mutations in *JAG1*. AGS primarily affects the liver, heart, face, skeleton, and eyes, with renal and neurovascular manifestations as well. The AGS phenotype demonstrates variable expressivity with effects ranging from subclinical to life threatening. Although it had been hoped that genetic studies would reveal a correlation between the genetic mutation and phenotype to explain the clinical variability, this has generally not been the case. The lack of consistent phenotypes both within and between families with the same *JAG1* mutations suggests that there are modifiers of the AGS phenotype. The reported mortality of AGS is highly variable. Cardiac, hepatic, and central nervous system diseases account for the majority of deaths. The presence of complex intracardiac disease at diagnosis is the only predictor of excessive early mortality. Hepatic complications account for most of the later mortality, although recent series demonstrate significant mortality from intracranial bleeding.

MAJOR POINTS

AGS is typically manifested by:
- Cholestastic liver disease and bile duct paucity on liver biopsy
- Right-sided cardiac lesions, usually peripheral pulmonary stenosis
- Unique facies
- Butterfly vertebrae
- Posterior embryotoxon
- Renal anomalies, vascular abnormalities/events

AGS results from mutations in *JAG1*.
AGS is characterized by highly variable expressivity.

SUGGESTED READINGS

Alagille D, Estrada A, Hadchouel M, et al: Syndromic paucity of interlobular bile ducts (Alagille syndrome or arteriohepatic dysplasia): Review of 80 cases. J Pediatr 110:195-200, 1987.

Berard E, Sarles J, Triolo V, et al: Renovascular hypertension and vascular anomalies in Alagille syndrome. Pediatr Nephrol 12:121-124, 1998.

Cardona J, Houssin D, Gauthier F, et al: Liver transplantation in children with Alagille syndrome: A study of twelve cases. Transplantation 60:339-342, 1995.

Crosnier C, Driancourt C, Raynaud N, et al: Mutations in JAGGED1 gene are predominantly sporadic in Alagille syndrome. Gastroenterology 116:1141-1148, 1999.

Danks DM, Campbell PE, Jack I, et al: Studies of the aetiology of neonatal hepatitis and biliary atresia. Arch Dis Child 52:360-367, 1977.

Deprettere A, Portmann B, Mowat AP: Syndromic paucity of the intrahepatic bile ducts: Diagnostic difficulty; severe morbidity throughout early childhood. J Pediatr Gastroenterol Nutr 6:865-871, 1987.

Emerick KM, Rand EB, Goldmuntz E, et al: Features of Alagille syndrome in 92 patients: Frequency and relation to prognosis. Hepatology 29:822-829, 1999.

Emerick KM, Whitington PF: Partial external biliary diversion for intractable pruritus and xanthomas in Alagille syndrome. Hepatology 35:1501-1506, 2002.

Hoffenberg EJ, Narkewicz MR, Sondheimer JM, et al: Outcome of syndromic paucity of interlobular bile ducts (Alagille syndrome) with onset of cholestasis in infancy. J Pediatr 127:220-224, 1995.

Kamath BM, Bason L, Piccoli DA, et al: Consequences of JAG1 mutations. J Med Genet 40:891-895, 2003.

Kamath BM, Loomes KM, Oakey RJ, et al: Facial features in Alagille syndrome: Specific or cholestasis facies? Am J Med Genet 112:163-170, 2002.

Karrer FM, Price MR, Bensard DD, et al: Long-term results with the Kasai operation for biliary atresia. Arch Surg 131:493-496, 1996.

Krantz ID, Colliton RP, Genin A, et al: Spectrum and frequency of jagged1 (JAG1) mutations in Alagille syndrome patients and their families. Am J Hum Genet 62:1361-1369, 1998.

McDaniell R, Warthen DM, Sanchez-Lara PA, et al: NOTCH2 mutations cause Alagille syndrome, a heterogenous disorder of the notch signaling pathway. Am J Hum Genet 79:169-173, 2006.

Novotny NM, Zetterman RK, Antonson DL, et al: Variation in liver histology in Alagille's syndrome. Am J Gastroenterol 75:449-450, 1981.

Piccoli DA, Spinner NB: Alagille syndrome and the Jagged1 gene. Semin Liver Dis 21:525-534, 2001.

Quiros-Tejeira RE, Ament ME, Heyman MB, et al: Variable morbidity in Alagille syndrome: A review of 43 cases. J Pediatr Gastroenterol Nutr 29:431-437, 1999.

Rachmel A, Zeharia A, Neuman-Levin M, et al: Alagille syndrome associated with moyamoya disease. Am J Med Genet 33:89-91, 1989.

Rosenfield NS, Kelley MJ, Jensen PS, et al: Arteriohepatic dysplasia: Radiologic features of a new syndrome. AJR Am J Roentgenol 135:1217-1223, 1980.

Spinner NB, Colliton RP, Crosnier C, et al: Jagged1 mutations in Alagille syndrome. Hum Mutat 17:18-33, 2001.

Warthen DM, Moore EC, Kamath BM, et al: Jagged1 mutations in Alagille syndrome: Increasing the mutation detection rate. Hum Mutat 27:436-443, 2006.

Woolfenden AR, Albers GW, Steinberg GK, et al: Moyamoya syndrome in children with Alagille syndrome: Additional evidence of a vasculopathy. Pediatrics 103:505-508, 1999.

Alpha₁-Antitrypsin Deficiency

PHILLIP P. LE

JOSHUA R. FRIEDMAN

Disease Description
Case Presentation
Epidemiology
Pathophysiology
Differential Diagnosis
Diagnostic Testing
Treatment
Approach to the Case
Summary
Major Points

DISEASE DESCRIPTION

Alpha₁-antitrypsin (α_1-AT) deficiency is an autosomal recessive disorder that causes lung and liver disease. In the lungs the absence of functional α_1-AT leads to excessive neutrophil elastase activity, and the resulting tissue destruction culminates in emphysema. In the liver, injury is the result of intracellular accumulation of the mutant α_1-AT protein. α_1-AT deficiency is the most common genetic cause of neonatal liver disease and the most frequent genetic diagnosis necessitating pediatric liver transplantation. Patients with hepatic manifestations of α_1-AT deficiency often present in the neonatal period with persistent jaundice and altered liver enzymes. Although the jaundice generally resolves, the liver injury may progress toward cirrhosis at a variable rate. There is no standard medical therapy for α_1-AT deficiency. Liver transplantation is reserved for those with end-stage liver disease.

CASE PRESENTATION

T.L. is a full-term newborn white male product of an uncomplicated pregnancy and vaginal delivery who is noted to be mildly jaundiced at 8 days of life. He is otherwise feeding and acting well. The stools are yellow. On physical examination, the growth percentiles are 50% for both weight and height. The baby is jaundiced but is otherwise well developed and in no distress. There is no hepatosplenomegaly and the examination is otherwise unremarkable. Laboratory evaluation includes a total bilirubin of 11.0 mg/dL, with a conjugated bilirubin of 3.1 mg/dL. The alanine aminotransferase (ALT), aspartate aminotransferase (AST), albumin, and prothrombin time (PT) are normal. Laboratory evaluation results for galactosemia, tyrosinemia, and hypothyroidism are all negative, as are blood and urine cultures. A diisopropyl iminodiacetic acid (DISIDA) scan shows normal hepatic uptake of radiotracer, but there is no excretion into the gallbladder or small bowel within 24 hours. An abdominal ultrasound is normal. The child is admitted to the hospital for liver biopsy.

EPIDEMIOLOGY

α_1-AT deficiency is one of the most common inherited disorders worldwide, although most patients do not have severe disease. The two most common mutant alleles encode the protease inhibitor S (PIS) and Z (PIZ) types, whereas the normal protein is the M type (PIM). The classic form of α_1-AT deficiency occurs in patients homozygous for the PIZ allele (known as PIZZ individuals); a small number of other more rare alleles have also been associated with liver disease. The PIS allele itself is associated with lung but not liver disease, although liver disease does occur in PISZ compound heterozygotes. In the United States, the PIZ allele frequency is approximately 14.5 per 1000, with lower rates among Asians, African Americans, and Latinos and higher rates among whites. Overall, the PIZZ genotype is estimated to occur once in every 4775 births in the United States, with similar rates occurring in Europe, Australia, and New Zealand.

A large-scale prospective study conducted in Sweden indicates that only about 10% of PIZZ individuals will have evidence of liver disease by age 40.

PATHOPHYSIOLOGY

α_1-AT is a 52-kd protein composed of 394 amino acid residues and its gene is located on the long arm of chromosome 14. The protein is a member of the serpin family of *ser*ine *p*rotease *in*hibitors. It is synthesized by the liver and released into the circulation, where it is the main inhibitor of neutrophil proteases. In the lungs of PIZZ individuals, the loss of α_1-AT function and the resulting unopposed activity of destructive enzymes such as elastase, cathepsin G, and proteinase 3 result in progressive emphysema. Lung disease generally becomes symptomatic after the age of 30, and is accelerated by smoking.

In contrast with the mechanism of lung disease in α_1-AT deficiency, liver disease is the result of a gain of function in the PIZ protein. This is clearly shown by null mutant α_1-AT alleles in which no α_1-AT is synthesized; patients homozygous for these alleles develop lung but not liver disease. Furthermore, transgenic mice expressing the human PIZ protein develop liver disease despite having normal production of the wild-type mouse α_1-AT. The gain of function in the PIZ is the result of a mutation that substitutes lysine for glutamate at residue 342 of the protein. The mutant protein is retained in the endoplasmic reticulum (ER), and is much more likely to form polymers than the wild-type protein. This polymerized α_1-AT is the source of the periodic acid–Schiff (PAS)-positive, diastase-resistant globules seen in histologic examinations of liver biopsy sections from PIZZ individuals. It is unclear whether polymerization results in retention in the ER or vice versa. It is also unclear how retention of PIZZ leads to hepatocyte injury, although electron micrographic studies indicate that injury to mitochondria may play a role. It also has been suggested that the variability of clinical disease in PIZZ patients (see later) reflects differences in the protein degradation pathways that allow the cell to eliminate the PIZZ globules.

The natural history of α_1-AT deficiency–related liver disease has been described in a prospective screening study of 200,000 Swedish infants, in which 127 PIZZ individuals were identified. Twenty-two of these patients had evidence of liver disease during infancy, primarily prolonged neonatal jaundice. Two infants died during childhood; both had cirrhosis. In contrast, approximately 85% had no symptoms of liver disease and normal aminotransferases by their late teens; the remainder had only elevated aminotransferases without other symptoms. Beyond infancy, liver disease in α_1-AT deficiency can manifest at any age with elevated aminotransferases, portal hypertension, or progressive hepatic failure and cirrhosis. Thus, it is clear that other genetic and environmental factors modify the extent of liver damage. Finally, patients with α_1-AT deficiency are at increased risk of developing hepatocellular carcinoma, although this is likely secondary to the development of cirrhosis.

DIFFERENTIAL DIAGNOSIS

The differential diagnosis depends on age at presentation (Tables 27-1 and 27-2). In the classic neonatal presentation with jaundice, the other diagnoses to consider most urgently include biliary atresia, other sources of extrahepatic obstruction, galactosemia, tyrosinemia, and congenital infections, because these may require prompt therapeutic intervention. At other ages, a broad differential including infectious, autoimmune, and metabolic causes should be considered.

DIAGNOSTIC TESTING

The diagnosis of α_1-AT deficiency is established by protease inhibitor typing, in which electrophoresis is used to separate the α_1-AT forms present in the serum.

Table 27-1 Differential Diagnosis of Neonatal Conjugated Hyperbilirubinemia and Neonatal Hepatitis

Category	Causes
Anatomic	Biliary atresia
	Choledochal cyst
	Neonatal sclerosing cholangitis
Infectious	Cytomegalovirus
	Herpesvirus
	Rubella virus
	Enterovirus
	Hepatitis viruses
	Adenovirus
	Bacterial sepsis
Metabolic	α_1-AT deficiency
	Tyrosinemia
	Galactosemia
	Bile acid synthetic disorders
	Lipidoses
	Peroxisomal disorders
Endocrine	Hypothyroidism
	Panhypopituitarism
Other inherited causes	Alagille syndrome
	Familial intrahepatic cholestasis
	Cystic fibrosis
	Neonatal iron storage disease

Table 27-2	Differential Diagnosis of Elevated Aminotransferases, Portal Hypertension, and Liver Failure in Children and Young Adults
Category	Causes
Anatomic	Cholelithiasis
	Choledochal cyst
Infectious	Cytomegalovirus
	Epstein-Barr virus
	Hepatitis A
	Chronic hepatitis B
	Chronic hepatitis C
Metabolic	α_1-AT deficiency
	Hereditary fructose intolerance
	Glycogen storage disease
	Fatty acid oxidation defect
	Wilson's disease
	Lipidoses
Toxic	Ethanol
	Acetaminophen
	Other medications
Autoimmune	Autoimmune hepatitis
	Primary sclerosing cholangitis
Other inherited	Alagille syndrome
	Cystic fibrosis
	Congenital hepatic fibrosis
	Familial intrahepatic cholestasis
	Benign recurrent intrahepatic cholestasis

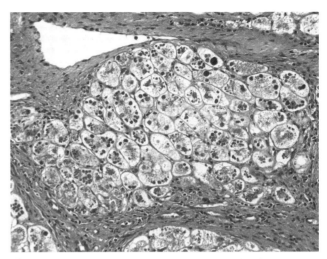

Figure 27-1 *(See also Color Plate 27-1.)* Explant liver section from a patient with α_1-AT deficiency and cirrhosis stained with periodic acid–Schiff (PAS). The hepatocytes within the cirrhotic nodule are slightly swollen and contain numerous PAS-positive globules. (Magnification ×200) (Courtesy Eduardo Ruchelli, MD, Children's Hospital of Philadelphia.)

Measurement of the total serum α_1-AT level also may be useful because it is low (10% to 15% of normal) in the majority of PIZZ patients. However, α_1-AT is an acute phase reactant, so levels can be artificially elevated by inflammation. Deoxyribonucleic acid (DNA)–based diagnosis of the most common α_1-AT mutations has been developed and is commercially available.

Histologic analysis of liver biopsy specimens usually reveals PAS-positive, diastase-resistant globules in the endoplasmic reticulum of hepatocytes (Fig. 27-1), although this is not specific for α_1-AT deficiency and is not sufficient to establish the diagnosis. Other findings may include varying degrees of bile duct injury, bile duct paucity, inflammatory infiltrates, portal fibrosis, or cirrhosis.

TREATMENT

There is currently no medical therapy that has been shown to be effective in the treatment of α_1-AT deficiency-related liver disease. Avoidance of smoking is crucial in reducing lung damage. Intravenous infusion of α_1-AT purified from human plasma is used in patients with severe lung disease, but this would not be expected to ameliorate liver injury due to the accumulation of the mutant α_1-AT. Investigational approaches to the treatment of α_1-AT deficiency include the use of cyclosporine A to prevent mitochondrial damage, chemical chaperones to prevent misfolding of the mutant protein, and modifiers of glycosylation to improve α_1-AT secretion. As with exogenous α_1-AT treatment, gene therapy may eventually be used to prevent lung disease in α_1-AT deficiency; however, this therapy would not be expected to affect the liver disease unless the host mutation is itself corrected.

Orthotopic liver transplantation is curative of liver disease and prevents further progression of emphysema in α_1-AT deficiency, but it is reserved for patients with severe complications of cirrhosis or portal hypertension. In fact, the disease may progress very slowly, and patients with cirrhosis and portal hypertension may not require transplantation for many years.

APPROACH TO THE CASE

The liver biopsy reveals bile ductular proliferation, with some bile plugging. PAS-positive, diastase-resistant globules are present within hepatocytes. There is mild bridging fibrosis, with no inflammation. α_1-AT protease inhibitor (PI) typing reveals the PIZZ phenotype, establishing the diagnosis of α_1-AT deficiency.

Over the next month the conjugated bilirubin rose to 5.5 mg/L, and the ALT and AST rose to 152 and 216 IU/L, respectively. The gamma-glutamyl-transferase was elevated at 1480 IU/L. An intraoperative cholangiogram was performed to rule out extrahepatic biliary obstruction. This revealed a normal gallbladder and extrahepatic biliary tree, with free flow of contrast into the duodenum.

The child continued to feed and grow well, and over the next few months the jaundice completely resolved. The bilirubin, albumin, and PT have remained normal, and the ALT and AST have remained elevated through 3 years of follow-up. The patient has continued to grow and develop normally.

This case illustrates the need to evaluate patients who present with neonatal cholestasis for biliary atresia and other causes of early liver disease that require urgent intervention. The initial evaluation should include an abdominal ultrasound and laboratory testing for infectious and metabolic causes. The DISIDA scan is also useful in ruling out biliary atresia, although an abnormal result is not specific for this disease. Indeed, as illustrated in this case, there may be no excretion of tracer material in patients with α_1-AT deficiency. If the results of protease inhibitor (PI) typing are not available, an intraoperative cholangiogram may be performed to visualize the extrahepatic biliary system; this will be normal in PIZZ individuals.

SUMMARY

α_1-AT deficiency is a common genetic disorder that results in varying degrees of hepatic and pulmonary dysfunction. It occurs in approximately 1 in 4775 live births in the United States and, affected individuals often present with persistent neonatal jaundice. Presentation during childhood and later is characterized by elevated aminotransferases with or without cirrhosis or portal hypertension. The liver disease is caused by accumulation of the PIZ form of the protein within hepatocytes, whereas the resulting decreased serum levels of the protein are the primary cause of the lung disease. The diagnosis is made by protease inhibitor typing or by DNA-based testing. Although the majority of affected individuals appear to have no to mild liver disease, the full spectrum of disease extends to cirrhosis, liver failure, and portal hypertension. There is no evidence to support medical therapy for the liver disease; orthotopic liver transplantation is reserved for the most severe cases.

SUGGESTED READINGS

Braun A, Meyer P, Cleve H, et al: Rapid and simple diagnosis of the two common alpha 1-proteinase inhibitor deficiency alleles Pi*Z and Pi*S by DNA analysis. Eur J Clin Chem Clin Biochem 34:761-764, 1996.

Burrows JA, Willis LK, Perlmutter DH: Chemical chaperones mediate increased secretion of mutant alpha 1-antitrypsin

MAJOR POINTS

α_1-AT deficiency is a relatively common autosomal recessive genetic disorder, occurring in approximately 1:4775 live births in the United States.
Presentation is variable and depends on age.
In the neonate, it often manifests with prolonged neonatal jaundice.
Only about 10% of affected individuals experience clinically significant liver disease.
Liver disease is caused by the inability to secrete α_1-AT, resulting in hepatocellular damage through an unknown mechanism.
Lung disease is caused by low levels of serum α_1-AT, resulting in excessive destructive protease activity.
The diagnosis can be made by protease inhibitor typing using protein electrophoresis or DNA analysis.
In PIZZ individuals, serum levels of α_1-AT are low (10% to 15% of normal), whereas PIS and PISZ individuals have intermediate levels.
Histologically, PAS-positive, diastase-resistant globules are seen in hepatocytes.
Treatment is mostly supportive and should include smoking cessation. Liver transplantation is reserved for the most severe cases. Some investigational therapies appear to be promising.

(alpha 1-AT) Z: A potential pharmacological strategy for prevention of liver injury and emphysema in alpha 1-AT deficiency. Proc Natl Acad Sci U S A 97:796, 2000.

Carlson JA, Rogers BB, Sifers RN, et al: Accumulation of PiZ alpha 1-antitrypsin causes liver damage in transgenic mice. J Clin Invest 83:1183, 1989.

Carrell RW, Lomas DA: Alpha1-antitrypsin deficiency: A model for conformational diseases. N Engl J Med 346:45, 2002.

de Serres FJ: Worldwide racial and ethnic distribution of alpha1-antitrypsin deficiency: Summary of an analysis of published genetic epidemiologic surveys. Chest 122:1818, 2002.

de Serres F, Blanco I, Fernandez-Bustillo E: Genetic epidemiology of alpha-1 antitrypsin deficiency in North America and Australia/New Zealand: Australia, Canada, New Zealand and the United States of America. Clin Genet 64:382, 2003.

Dycaico MJ, Grant SG, Felts K, et al: Neonatal hepatitis induced by alpha 1-antitrypsin: A transgenic mouse model. Science 242:1409, 1988.

Lomas DA, Evans DL, Finch JT, et al: The mechanism of Z alpha 1-antitrypsin accumulation in the liver. Nature 357:605, 1992.

Perlmutter DH: Alpha-1-antitrypsin deficiency: Diagnosis and treatment. Clin Liver Dis 8:839, 2004.

Sveger T: Liver disease in alpha1-antitrypsin deficiency detected by screening of 200,000 infants. N Engl J Med 294:1316, 1976.

Sveger T, Eriksson S: The liver in adolescents with alpha 1-antitrypsin deficiency. Hepatology 22:514, 1995.

CHAPTER 28

Autoimmune Hepatitis

UDEME EKONG

KARAN M. EMERICK

Disease Description
Case Presentation
Epidemiology
Pathophysiology
Differential Diagnosis
Diagnostic Testing
Treatment
Approach to the Case
Summary
Major Points

DISEASE DESCRIPTION

Autoimmune hepatitis (AIH) is an unresolving inflammation of the liver characterized histologically by dense mononuclear cell infiltrates within the portal tracts, interface hepatitis, and serologically by the presence of nonorgan and liver-specific autoantibodies in the absence of a known etiology. Two types of AIH are recognized according to the presence of smooth muscle and/or antinuclear antibody (SMA/ANA, type 1 AIH) or liver kidney microsomal antibody type 1 and/or liver cytosol antibody type 1 (LKM1/LC1, type 2 AIH).

CASE PRESENTATION

A 10-year-old girl presents with a 2-week history of jaundice. She developed nausea with vomiting while on vacation in Florida, 2 months before presentation. Similar gastrointestinal symptoms have occurred, without jaundice, in two older siblings, which resolved spontaneously. There is no history of fever. A 2-pound weight loss has been noted over the past 1 to 2 months. Her family denies herbal preparation intake, prior transfusion of blood/ blood products, travel abroad, and use of any medications. The patient is usually in a good state of health with no past history of jaundice. There is a family history of type 1 diabetes mellitus. Physical examination reveals a well-grown girl with scleral icterus and spider angiomas over her face. She has hepatomegaly with liver edge 6 cm below the subcostal margin, palpable spleen, and no ascites.

EPIDEMIOLOGY

The mean annual incidence of AIH among white Northern Europeans is 1.9 per 100,000, with a point prevalence of 16.9 per 100,000; it accounts for approximately 2% to 5% of chronic liver disease in children, with a relative incidence in childhood of 1.2%.

PATHOPHYSIOLOGY

The underlying mechanism of this condition is believed to be autoimmune, such that the presence of autoantibodies is one of the main diagnostic criteria. In AIH type 1, the putative target antigens of ANA include single- and double-stranded deoxyribonucleic acid (DNA), histones, small nuclear ribonucleoproteins, and centromere. SMA is directed against F-actin. In AIH type 2, the target antigen of LKM1 is human cytochrome P450 of the 2D subfamily CYP2D6, and the molecular target of LC1 has been identified as formiminotransferase cyclodeaminase (FTCD).

In addition to the diagnostic autoantibodies (ANA, SMA, LKM1), which are routinely determined by most clinical immunology laboratories, patients with AIH have a wide range of autoantibodies, such as liver-specific lipoprotein (LSP), soluble liver antigen (SLA), and liver pancreas antigen (LP). Studies on a large series of patients have shown that not only are anti-SLA antibodies highly specific markers of AIH, and particularly useful in the diagnosis of patients without conventional antibodies, they are also related to relapse of the inflammatory process after corticosteroid withdrawal.

A complex of environmental and genetic factors likely determines susceptibility to AIH. Studies suggesting a higher risk of AIH in women and monozygotic twins have contributed to the focus on genetic vulnerability. Genetic polymorphisms constituting the susceptible host involve variations in the major histocompatibility complex (MHC) genes. In a population of Northern European origin, (HLA)-DRB1 03 is the primary susceptibility allele associated with the development of AIH. Other subtypes linked to AIH in different populations include DRB1* 0405 in Argentina and Japan and DRB1 0404 in Mexico. In children, risk factors in type 1 AIH are DRB1* 03 and 13, with DRB1* 07 and 03 alleles being associated with type 2 AIH. Because HLA-DQB1* 0201 is in strong linkage imbalance with DRB1* 03 and 07, it has been recently proposed that the HLA-DRB1 gene is the major determinant in the HLA class II region for children with type 1 AIH, and HLA-DQB1 in children with type 2 AIH. An individual genotype does not by itself predict the development of clinical disease; however, the expression of the clinical phenotype is manifested after the vulnerable host encounters some additional environmental factors or combination of factors.

AIH is also associated with autoimmune endocrinopathies such as type 1 diabetes or autoimmune thyroid diseases, as well as nonendocrine disorders (vitiligo) more frequently than the general population. The incidence of AIH among children with autoimmune polyendocrinopathy-candidiasis-ectodermal dystrophy (APECED) is about 20%. This is a rare autosomal recessive condition involving mutations within the autoimmune regulator gene, located on chromosome 21q22.3, and is characterized by hypoparathyroidism, Addison's disease, and mucocutaneous candidiasis with a peak age of onset at 12 years. Distinct molecular targets distinguish AIH from the liver disease associated with APECED. Antibody to CYP1A2 is a specific (100%) but insensitive (50%) marker for APECED-associated liver disease, yet it is not detected in patients with AIH.

DIFFERENTIAL DIAGNOSIS

The diagnosis of AIH is guided by the presence of hypergammaglobulinemia, circulating autoantibodies, periportal and interface hepatitis on histology, and the exclusion of other causes of chronic hepatitis. However because AIH can occur in all age-groups, conditions that should be specifically excluded depend on the age of the child (Table 28-1). Significant biliary changes do not typically occur in AIH, and their presence would suggest an alternative diagnosis, such as primary sclerosing cholangitis (PSC), autoimmune cholangiopathy, primary biliary cirrhosis (PBC), or an "overlap" syndrome. Overlap syndromes are conditions in which clinical, histologic, or serologic features of AIH overlap with features of PBC or PSC. The overlap syndrome between AIH and PSC has been reported in children. It is not clear whether these conditions are two separate autoimmune diseases that occur in the same patient or if they are part of a broader spectrum of autoimmune liver disease.

Three clinical patterns of disease have been observed in children (Table 28-2). In the preceding review, six children (11.5%) developed acute hepatic failure, with five of these children having the LKM1 antibody. From gathering information on AIH over the years, the International Autoimmune Hepatitis Group (IAHG) has proposed a scoring system for the diagnosis of AIH based on clinical, laboratory, and histologic features (Table 28-3).

Table 28-1	Differential Diagnosis by Age Group
Older children	Hepatitis A, B, and C, Epstein-Barr virus infection, α_1-antitrypsin deficiency, Wilson's disease, choledochal cyst, Caroli's disease, sclerosing cholangitis, drug-induced liver disease
Younger children	Hepatocellular injury secondary to metabolic, genetic, and infectious causes

Table 28-2	Clinical Patterns of Disease in Autoimmune Hepatitis	
Pattern 1	Malaise, nausea, vomiting, anorexia, abdominal pain followed by jaundice, dark urine, pale stools, indistinguishable from acute viral hepatitis	Seen in 50% of patients with ANA/SMA and 65% of patients with LKM1
Pattern 2	Insidious onset with progressive fatigue, relapsing jaundice, headache, anorexia, weight loss lasting 6 months to 2 years before diagnosis	Seen in 38% of patients with ANA/SMA and 25% of patients with LKM1
Pattern 3	Present with complications of chronic liver disease, including hematemesis from esophageal varices, bleeding diathesis, chronic diarrhea, weight loss, and vomiting	Seen in 6 of 52 children (11.5%), with 2 children having LKM1

ANA, antinuclear antibody; SMA, smooth muscle antibody; LKM1, anti-liver, kidney, microsomal 1 antibody.
(From Gregorio GV, Mieli-Vergani G: Autoimmune liver disease in childhood. Indian J Gastroenterol 16:60-63, 1997.)

Table 28-3 Scoring System for Autoimmune Hepatitis	
Parameter/Features	Score
Female sex	+2
Alkaline Phosphatase: AST (or ALT) Ratio	
<1.5	+2
1.5-3.0	0
>3	−2
Serum Globulin or IgG Above Normal	
>2	+3
1.5-2.0	+2
1.0-1.5	+1
<1	0
ANA, SMA, or LKM1	
>1:80	+3
1:80	+2
1:40	+1
<1:40	0
AMA positive	−4
Hepatitis Viral Markers	
Positive	−4
Negative	+3
Drug History	
Positive	−4
Negative	+1
Average Alcohol Intake	
<25g daily	+2
>60g daily	−2
Liver Histology	
Interface hepatitis	+3
Predominantly lymphoplasmacytic	+1
Resetting of liver cells	+1
None of the above	−5
Biliary changes	−3
Other changes	−3
Other autoimmune diseases	+2
Optional Additional Parameters	
Seropositive for other defined autoantibodies	+2
HLA DR3 or DR4	+1
Response to Therapy	
Complete	+2
Relapse	+3
Interpretation of Aggregate Score	
Pretreatment	
Definite autoimmune hepatitis (AIH)	>5
Probable AIH	10-15
Post-treatment	>7
Definite AIH	12-17
Probable AIH	

ALT, alanine transaminase; AMA, antimitochondrial antibody; ANA, antinuclear antibody; AST, aspartate transaminase; IgG, immunoglobulin G; LKM1, anti-liver, kidney, microsomal 1 antibody; SMA, smooth muscle antibody.

DIAGNOSTIC TESTING

Although the diagnostic criteria outlined in Table 28-3 by the IAHG apply, some practical guidelines are as follows:

- The patient should be seronegative for markers of a current infection with hepatitis A, B, and C.
- Total serum globulin should be greater than 1.5 times the upper limit of normal.
- Alcohol consumption should be less than 25 g/day, and there should be no history of recent use of hepatotoxic drugs.
- Seropositivity for ANA, SMA, or anti-LKM1 should be present at titers greater than 1:80. Lower titers may be significant for children.
- Evidence of liver cell injury must be present and other causes of liver disease excluded. Interface hepatitis of moderate or severe activity should be present on liver biopsy without biliary lesions, well-defined granuloma, or other findings that would be consistent with another diagnosis.

A minority of children are negative for ANA, SMA, and LKM1 at presentation; however, if other biochemical or histologic features strongly support AIH, the presence of anti-SLA/LP may support the diagnosis of AIH (Table 28-4). As with adults, type 1 AIH occurs in the majority of children, with girls being more commonly affected, accounting for up to 75% of patients. Patients with LKM1 present at a younger age (median age, 7.4 vs. 10.5 years) and are more likely to present with acute liver failure. Patients with ANA/SMA are more commonly cirrhotic at presentation (69% vs. 38%), with severe impairment of hepatic synthetic function (53% vs. 30%) compared with LKM1 patients. Pediatric series report a similarly severe disease in patients who are positive for ANA/SMA or LKM1.

TREATMENT

Table 28-5 illustrates the most common treatment protocol taken from several experiences.

Corticosteroids: This is considered standard treatment for AIH. The mechanism of action is not fully understood, but it is known to inhibit lymphocyte activation and cytokine secretion. Prednisone is the most frequently administered form in the treatment of AIH. Initial treatment consists of 2 mg/kg/day, maximum 60 mg/day. The dose is then gradually decreased over 4 to 8 weeks, by 5 mg every 2 weeks when serum aminotransferase activity is less than twice the normal values. The patient is then maintained on the minimal dose of prednisone necessary to keep the serum aminotransferase level normal (2.5 to 5 mg/day, depending on age).

Table 28-4	Frequency of Autoantibodies in Autoimmune Hepatitis	
AIH Type	Auto Antigens	Frequency (%)
1	SMA	90-100
	ANA	0-10
	SMA/ANA	40-60
2	LKM1	40-45
	LC1	20-25
	LKM1/LC1	35-40

(From Alvarez F: Autoimmune hepatitis. In Suchy FJ, Sokol RJ, Balistreri WF (eds): Liver Disease in Children, 2nd ed. Philadelphia, Lippincott Williams and Wilkins, 2001, pp 429-442.)

Azathioprine: The exact mechanism of action is not known, but maturation of lymphocyte precursors is blocked and synthesis of DNA, RNA, and proteins is inhibited. Dosage is 1.5 to 2 mg/kg/day.

Cyclosporine has been used successfully in patients with AIH who failed prednisone/azathioprine therapy, and had severe side effects. There is report of short-term use of cyclosporine in 32 children to control the inflammatory process, subsequently followed by low-dose corticosteroids and azathioprine, with the achievement of more than 90% complete response. Although side effects associated with short-term cyclosporine treatment were mild, longer follow-up clearly needed to establish the safety of the cyclosporine regimen.

Mycophenolate mofetil has been successfully used in adult as well as pediatric patients who did not tolerate or were unresponsive to azathioprine. The main difficulty is the cost and the lack of accessible laboratories able to test for its blood levels.

During the first 6 to 8 weeks of therapy, liver indices should be checked weekly to allow a constant fine-tuning of the treatment and avoidance of severe corticosteroid-related side effects. In most children, an 80% decrease in initial serum transaminases is achieved within 6 weeks, although complete resolution of liver test abnormality may take several months. Pediatric series report normalization of serum aminotransferase levels occurring at a median of 0.5 years (0.2 to 7 years) in children with ANA/SMA and 0.8 years (0.02 to 3.2 years) in children with LKM1. Relapse on treatment necessitating a temporary increase in the dose of prednisone affects 40% of children.

Discontinuation of treatment should be considered after 1 year of normal liver function tests and minimal or absence of inflammatory changes in liver biopsy tissue. A pediatric series reports successful withdrawal of treatment in 6 of 13 children after a median treatment duration of 3.2 years (range 1 to 11 years) with remission being sustained for 9 to 13 years. All six children had ANA/SMA. The remaining seven children relapsed between 1 and 15 months following drug withdrawal (median interval, 2 months), three of these patients had ANA/SMA, and four had LKM1. This indicates that most children with AIH, particularly those with LKM1, will require lifelong immunosuppressive therapy.

Despite the efficacy of current treatment, severe hepatic decompensation may develop after many years of good biochemical control. Bahar and colleagues from the University of California, Los Angeles and the University of California, San Francisco, report that 55% of their patients followed over a median time of 8 years required liver transplantation; however, this represents data from large pediatric referral centers rather than those representing the general population. In their series, though a larger percentage of African Americans required liver transplantation than did Hispanic or white patients, this difference did not approach statistical significance. They also saw no significant differences between type 1 and type 2 AIH with regard to the need for liver transplantation. A high rate of disease recurrence among children and adults following liver transplantation for AIH has been reported, but there does not appear to be a significant relationship between disease type and recurrence after liver transplantation.

APPROACH TO THE CASE

In this case, liver function should be evaluated by measuring serum aminotransferases and protein and albumin levels. Liver synthetic function should be further evaluated through measurement of prothrombin time and International Normalized Ratio.

As alluded to in the section on differential diagnosis, infectious etiologies should be excluded by checking serologies for hepatitis A, B, C, and Epstein-Barr virus. Wilson's disease and α_1-antitrypsin deficiency also

Table 28-5	Treatment Regimen for Autoimmune Hepatitis		
Initial Regimen	Maintenance Regimen	End Point	
Prednisone 2 mg/kg daily (up to 60 mg/day), either alone or in combination with azathioprine 1-2 mg/kg daily	Prednisone, taper over 6-8 weeks to 0.1-0.2 mg/kg daily or 5 mg daily. Azathioprine at constant dose if added initially	Normal liver tests for 1-2 years during treatment. No flare during entire interval Liver biopsy examination discloses no inflammation	

(From Czaja AJ, Freese DK: Diagnosis and treatment of autoimmune hepatitis. Hepatology 36:479-497, 2002.)

should be excluded by measuring serum ceruloplasmin levels and an ophthalmologic examination looking for the presence of Kayser-Fleischer rings, and α_1-antitrypsin level and phenotype. The conventional repertoire of antibodies implicated in autoimmune hepatitis, and easily available in most commercial laboratories (ANA, SMA, LKM1) also should be measured. It is prudent to perform a liver biopsy, the safest route for this being determined by the patient's coagulation profile and the presence of ascites.

SUMMARY

Autoimmune hepatitis is a chronic, necroinflammatory liver disease affecting children of all ages. It should be considered in the differential diagnosis of all children presenting with clinical or biochemical evidence of hepatocellular injury. The presence of autoimmune markers in blood with compatible histologic findings is necessary for diagnosis. A short duration of symptoms should not delay the diagnosis of AIH in children. Prednisone and azathioprine can control symptoms and normalize serum transaminases in most children.

MAJOR POINTS

AIH is a chronic inflammatory disease of the liver, characterized by loss of tolerance against liver tissue with resultant destruction of hepatic parenchyma.

It is most prevalent among females and displays an immunogenetic association with HLA-DR3 or DR4 haplotype and extrahepatic syndromes.

Diagnosis is guided by the presence of hypergammaglobulinemia, circulating autoantibodies, periportal and interface hepatitis on histology, and the exclusion of other causes of chronic hepatitis.

Although autoantibody profiles are used to subclassify AIH, they do not define distinct therapeutic subgroups.

AIH is generally responsive to immunosuppressive therapy, with corticosteroids and azathioprine remaining the standard therapy.

Liver transplantation is the ultimate therapeutic option when irreversible and life-threatening complications ensue.

Recurrence following liver transplantation may occur in nearly 50% of patients.

Overlap syndromes are conditions in which clinical, histologic, or serologic features of AIH overlap with features of PBC or PSC.

SUGGESTED READINGS

Aaltonen J, Bjorses P, Sandkuijl L, et al: An autosomal locus causing autoimmune disease: Autoimmune polyglandular disease type I assigned to chromosome 21. Nat Genet 8:83-87, 1994.

Alvarez F: Treatment of autoimmune hepatitis: Current and future therapies. Curr Treat Options Gastroenterol 7:413-420, 2004.

Alvarez F, Berg PA, Bianchi FB, et al: International Autoimmune Hepatitis Group Report: review of criteria for diagnosis of autoimmune hepatitis. J Hepatol 31:929-938, 1999.

Alvarez F, Ciocca M, Canero-Velasco C, et al: Short-term cyclosporine induces a remission of autoimmune hepatitis in children. J Hepatol 30:222-227, 1999.

Baeres M, Herkel J, Czaja AJ, et al: Establishment of standardised SLA/LP immunoassays: Specificity for autoimmune hepatitis, worldwide occurrence, and clinical characteristics. Gut 51:259-264, 2002.

Bahar RJ, Yanni GS, Martin MG, et al: Orthotopic liver transplantation for autoimmune hepatitis and cryptogenic chronic hepatitis in children. Transplantation 72:829-833, 2001.

Boberg KM, Aadland E, Jahnsen J, et al: Incidence and prevalence of primary biliary cirrhosis, primary sclerosing cholangitis, and autoimmune hepatitis in a Norwegian population. Scand J Gastroenterol 33:99-103, 1998.

Czaja AJ: Natural history, clinical features, and treatment of autoimmune hepatitis. Semin Liver Dis 4:1-12, 1984.

Czaja AJ, Cassani F, Cataleta M, et al: Antinuclear antibodies and patterns of nuclear immunofluorescence in type 1 autoimmune hepatitis. Dig Dis Sci 42:1688-1696, 1997.

Czaja AJ, Donaldson PT, Lohse AW: Antibodies to soluble liver antigen/liver pancreas and HLA risk factors for type 1 autoimmune hepatitis. Am J Gastroenterol 97:413-419, 2002.

Czaja AJ, Kruger M, Santrach PJ, et al: Genetic distinctions between types 1 and 2 autoimmune hepatitis. Am J Gastroenterol 92:2197-2200, 1997.

Davidson A, Diamond B: Autoimmune diseases. N Engl J Med 345:340-350, 2001.

Debray D, Maggiore G, Girardet JP, et al: Efficacy of cyclosporin A in children with type 2 autoimmune hepatitis. J Pediatr 135:111-114, 1999.

Devlin J, Donaldson P, Portmann B, et al: Recurrence of autoimmune hepatitis following liver transplantation. Liver Transpl Surg 1:162-165, 1995.

Djilali-Saiah I, Renous R, Caillat-Zucman S, et al: Linkage disequilibrium between HLA class II region and autoimmune hepatitis in pediatric patients. J Hepatol 40:904-909, 2004.

Goldstein NS, Rosenthal P, Sinatra F, Dehner LP: Liver disease in polyglandular autoimmune disease type one: Clinicopathologic study of three patients and review of the literature. Pediatr Pathol Lab Med 16:625-636, 1996.

Gotz G, Neuhaus R, Bechstein WO, et al: Recurrence of autoimmune hepatitis after liver transplantation. Transplant Proc 31:430-431, 1999.

Gregorio GV, Mieli-Vergani G: Autoimmune liver disease in childhood. Indian J Gastroenterol 16:60-63, 1997.

Gregorio GV, Portmann B, Karani J, et al: Autoimmune hepatitis/sclerosing cholangitis overlap syndrome in childhood: A 16-year prospective study. Hepatology 33:544-553, 2001.

Gregorio GV, Portmann B, Reid F, et al: Autoimmune hepatitis in childhood: A 20-year experience. Hepatology 25:541-547, 1997.

Gueguen M, Yamamoto AM, Bernard O, Alvarez F: Anti-liver-kidney microsome antibody type 1 recognizes human cytochrome P450 db1. Biochem Biophys Res Commun 159: 542-547, 1989.

Hyams JS, Ballow M, Leichtner AM: Cyclosporine treatment of autoimmune chronic active hepatitis. Gastroenterology 93:890-893, 1987.

Jackson LD, Song E: Cyclosporin in the treatment of corticosteroid resistant autoimmune chronic active hepatitis. Gut 36:459-461, 1995.

Johnson PJ, McFarlane IG: Meeting report: International Autoimmune Hepatitis Group. Hepatology 18:998-1005, 1993.

Kanzler S, Weidemann C, Gerken G, et al: Clinical significance of autoantibodies to soluble liver antigen in autoimmune hepatitis. J Hepatol 31:635-640, 1999.

Lapierre P, De Guise S, Muir DC, et al: Immune functions in the Fisher rat fed beluga whale *(Delphinapterus leucas)* blubber from the contaminated St. Lawrence estuary. Environ Res 80:S104-S112, 1999.

Ma Y, Peakman M, Lobo-Yeo A, et al: Differences in immune recognition of cytochrome P4502D6 by liver kidney microsomal (LKM) antibody in autoimmune hepatitis and chronic hepatitis C virus infection. Clin Exp Immunol 97:94-99, 1994.

Maggiore G, Veber F, Bernard O, et al: Autoimmune hepatitis associated with anti-actin antibodies in children and adolescents. J Pediatr Gastroenterol Nutr 17:376-381, 1993.

Manns MP, Gerken G, Kyriatsoulis A, et al: Characterisation of a new subgroup of autoimmune chronic active hepatitis by autoantibodies against a soluble liver antigen. Lancet 1:292-294, 1987.

Manns MP, Johnson EF, Griffin KJ, et al: Major antigen of liver kidney microsomal autoantibodies in idiopathic autoimmune hepatitis is cytochrome P450db1. J Clin Invest 83:1066-1072, 1989.

Manns MP, Kruger M: Immunogenetics of chronic liver diseases. Gastroenterology 106:1676-1679, 1994.

Marcos Y, Fainboim HA, Capucchio M, et al: Two-locus involvement in the association of human leukocyte antigen with the extrahepatic manifestations of autoimmune chronic active hepatitis. Hepatology 19:1371-1374, 1994.

McFarlane IG, Eddleston AL, Williams R: Lymphocyte subpopulations in chronic liver disease. Clin Exp Immunol 30:1-3, 1977.

Meyer zum B, Miescher PA. Liver specific antigens: Purification and characterization. Clin Exp Immunol 10:89-102, 1972.

Mieli-Vergani G, Vergani D: Autoimmune hepatitis in children. Clin Liver Dis 6:335-344, 2002.

Obermayer-Straub P, Perheentupa J, Braun S, et al: Hepatic autoantigens in patients with autoimmune polyendocrinopathy-candidiasis-ectodermal dystrophy. Gastroenterology 121: 668-677, 2001.

Prados E, Cuervas-Mons V, de la Mata M, et al: Outcome of autoimmune hepatitis after liver transplantation. Transplantation 66:1645-1650, 1998.

Richardson PD, James PD, Ryder SD: Mycophenolate mofetil for maintenance of remission in autoimmune hepatitis in patients resistant to or intolerant of azathioprine. J Hepatol 33:371-375, 2000.

Seki T, Ota M, Furuta S, et al: HLA class II molecules and autoimmune hepatitis susceptibility in Japanese patients. Gastroenterology 103:1041-1047, 1992.

Squires RH Jr: Autoimmune hepatitis in children. Curr Gastroenterol Rep 6:225-230, 2004.

Stechemesser E, Klein R, Berg PA: Characterization and clinical relevance of liver-pancreas antibodies in autoimmune hepatitis. Hepatology 18:1-9, 1993.

Stechemesser E, Strienz J, Berg PA: Serological definition of new subgroup of patients with autoimmune chronic active hepatitis. Lancet 1:683, 1987.

Vazquez-Garcia MN, Alaez C, Olivo A, et al: MHC class II sequences of susceptibility and protection in Mexicans with autoimmune hepatitis. J Hepatol 28:985-990, 1998.

Vogel A, Strassburg CP, Obermayer-Straub P, et al: The genetic background of autoimmune polyendocrinopathy-candidiasis-ectodermal dystrophy and its autoimmune disease components. J Mol Med 80:201-211, 2002.

Wies I, Brunner S, Henninger J, et al: Identification of target antigen for SLA/LP autoantibodies in autoimmune hepatitis. Lancet 355:1510-1515, 2000.

Cholelithiasis

DANA BOCTOR

Disease Description
Case Presentation
Epidemiology
Pathophysiology
Differential Diagnosis
Diagnostic Testing
    Laboratory Testing
    Imaging
Treatment
    Symptomatic Cholelithiasis
    Asymptomatic Patients
Approach to the Case
Summary
Major Points

DISEASE DESCRIPTION

Although cholelithiasis, or gallstones, is an uncommon finding in healthy children, there are several associated predisposing diseases (Table 29-1). Typically, gallstones are asymptomatic and picked up incidentally by abdominal ultrasound. Children with symptomatic gallstone disease may present with biliary colic or other symptoms related to complications of cholelithiasis. Biliary colic typically manifests as sudden onset, recurrent epigastric or right upper quadrant (RUQ) pain that can radiate to the back or right shoulder. Often there is a steady epigastric—"colicky" or crampy—pain that lasts 1 to 3 hours. The severity and interval between episodes can be variable. Episodes are commonly accompanied by nausea and vomiting and may be accompanied by fever in younger children. Often the pain develops without precipitating factors, and fat intolerance is not a consistent feature.

CASE PRESENTATION

Maria, a 13-year-old Mexican American, presents with a 6-month history of chronic recurrent abdominal pain. The pain is usually crampy and occurs in the periumbilical, right and left lower quadrants. The pain occurs several times a week for several minutes to an hour and there are no obvious aggravating or alleviating factors. She did have one episode of intense epigastric pain lasting for a couple of hours. By the time she reached the local emergency department, she was feeling better and the bloodwork and abdominal radiograph done were reportedly normal. She was told to start on ranitidine but has not noticed any relief with this. She tends to have a low-fiber, high-fat diet with an emphasis on refined carbohydrates. A high-fat meal does not seem to cause her any discomfort. She has one bowel movement every 2 days, which at times requires straining. She has some occasional knee pain and is known to have obstructive sleep apnea. Otherwise, she is healthy, and the family history is unremarkable for gallstones but positive for peptic ulcer disease in her mother. Physical examination reveals a morbidly obese adolescent with a body mass index (BMI) of 36 kg/m^2 and a normal abdominal examination. Stool is palpated in the left lower quadrant and on digital rectal examination she has hard stool in a dilated rectal vault that is negative for occult blood. Abdominal ultrasound done in the emergency department reveals a solitary 3-cm stone in the gallbladder and no dilation of the biliary tree.

EPIDEMIOLOGY

Epidemiologic studies in the United States and in Italy report 10% to 20% of adults have cholelithiasis, and only 20% to 30% go on to develop symptoms. It has been estimated that the risk of developing symptoms or complications is approximately 2% to 4% per year. Gallstones

Table 29-1 Conditions Predisposing to Gallstones and Biliary Sludge

Black stones
- Chronic hemolytic disease
  - Sickle cell anemia
  - Congenital spherocytosis
  - Thalessemia: major and minor
  - Pyruvate kinase deficiency
  - Glucose-6-phosphate dehydrogenase deficiency
  - Autoimmune hemolytic disease
- Total parenteral nutrition
- Cirrhosis and chronic cholestasis

Cholesterol stones
- Obesity
- Precipitous weight loss
- Pregnancy
- Female gender

Brown stones
- Infections: parasites and flukes
  - *Ascaris lumbricoides*
  - *Clonorchis sinesis*
  - *Fasciola hepatica*

Cholesterol or pigment stones*
- Ileal resection
- Jejunoileal bypass
- Ileal Crohn's disease
- Cystic fibrosis

Gallbladder sludge
- Infants born to morphine abusers
- Ceftriaxone
- Total parenteral nutrition (TPN)

* Both types of stones have been reported with these conditions.

are more common with increasing age and BMI. Women are twice as likely as men to develop gallstones. The lowest frequency of gallstones is seen among sub-Saharan Africans and Canadian Inuit. Native American Indians, Swedes, Chileans, Czechs, and Hispanic Americans have the highest frequency of gallstones. In particular, among Pima Indians in whom obesity is endemic, there is a prevalence of 50% among the population older than 15 years of age. Cholesterol gallstones are more common in Western cultures. In the United States, cholesterol stones account for 70% to 90% of adult stones, whereas pigment stones are more typical among Asian populations, in whom a common cause is fluke or parasite infestation.

In contrast to adults, less is known about the epidemiology of cholelithiasis in children because it is less common and studies have limited numbers of patients. It is difficult to determine the exact prevalence of gallstones because the majority of patients are asymptomatic. In children and adolescents, the prevalence rates are reported to be 0.1% to 0.6%. The female predisposition seen in adulthood emerges during adolescence. Among Western children, there has been an increase in the prevalence of gallstones and the incidence of cholecystectomy over the past three decades. It is not clear if this reflects improved ultrasonographic detection or true increases in predisposing factors such as obesity, prematurity, parenteral nutrition, and teenage pregnancy. In Pima Indians ages 15 to 24 years, the prevalence of gallstones is 5.9% in females and 0% in males. In children, the majority of stones are pigment type (70%), with cholesterol stones making up a smaller proportion (15% to 20%) until adolescence, when cholesterol stones become the dominant type in Western societies.

Although the increasing prevalence of obesity and obesity-related diseases in children is well recognized, the implications for development of cholelithiasis and related morbidity are not yet known. A recent study of 493 obese children and adolescents previously treated for obesity, had a 2% prevalence of cholelithiasis by ultrasound, and none of the 95 prepubertal children had cholelithiasis. The patients with cholelithiasis had more severe obesity. Medical conditions with an increased prevalence of gallstone disease include chronic hemolytic disease, chronic cholestasis, cirrhosis, ileal resection, jejunoileal bypass, ileal Crohn's disease, cystic fibrosis, pregnancy, and parasitic infestation. Children with Down syndrome and survivors of cancer are at increased risk for cholelithiasis but the mechanisms are unknown.

PATHOPHYSIOLOGY

There are two major types of gallstones: cholesterol and pigment stones (black and brown pigment types) (Table 29-2). The disease process relates to the type of stone produced. Gallstone formation occurs with an alteration in the composition of bile. This can occur as an increase in the composition of a biliary component that exceeds its solubility or a decrease in a solubilizing component. There are three main factors contributing to gallstone formation: first, cholesterol supersaturation, when the amount of cholesterol exceeds the carrying capacity of bile acids and phospholipids in bile; second, accelerated nucleation, whereby the precipitation of cholesterol crystals from the supersaturated bile may be accelerated by certain proteins; and third, stasis related to gallbladder hypomotility, which alters the bile composition and allows crystal precipitation. Certain bacterial species may promote the initial precipitation of bilirubin salts and serve as a nidus for stone formation. In addition, gallstones may become colonized with bacteria, leading to bilirubinate salts or the remodeling of preexisting stones. Biliary sludge is believed to represent the early stages of gallstone formation. Sludge is made up of microscopic precipitates of cholesterol or calcium bilirubinate. It may evolve into gallstones or may disappear spontaneously. Cholesterol stones contain more than 50% cholesterol and varying amounts of protein and calcium salts. Pigmented stones contain less cholesterol, as well as insoluble calcium salts such as

Table 29-2	Types of Gallstones		
Features	Cholesterol	Black	Brown
Composition	>50% Cholesterol Protein Calcium salts	<10% Cholesterol Pigment polymer Calcium salts	10%-30% Cholesterol Calcium bilirubinate Calcium soaps
Consistency	Crystalline	Hard	Greasy, soft
Location	Gallbladder ± Common duct	Gallbladder Bile ducts	Common bile duct
Radiodensity	85% stones radiolucent	50% stones radiopaque	100% stones radiolucent
Clinical associations	Metabolic	Hemolysis Cirrhosis	Infection Inflammation Infestation

calcium bilirubinate, calcium phosphate, and calcium carbonate. Cholesterol and black pigment stones are typically found in the gallbladder, whereas brown pigment gallstones are commonly found in the extrahepatic ducts and possibly in the intrahepatic ducts.

Cholesterol is excreted from the body through secretion into the bile directly as cholesterol or as bile salts. The formation of cholesterol gallstones involves hypersecretion of cholesterol into bile, decreased gallbladder motility, increased production of mucin by the gallbladder, increased conversion of primary bile salts to the more hydrophobic secondary bile salts, and increased formation of cholesterol crystals. Cholesterol stones can be solitary or multiple and may vary in size from a few millimeters to a few centimeters. Cholesterol stones are associated with female gender, obesity, pregnancy, and a positive family history of cholelithiasis. In obese individuals, there is marked cholesterol supersaturation of bile and gallbladder hypomotility. In addition, obese individuals who have had rapid weight loss are prone to the development of gallstones because of the increased mobilization of cholesterol from the adipose tissue being secreted into the bile.

The main pathophysiologic feature of black pigment stone formation relates to bilirubin supersaturation in the bile. Bacterial enzymes deconjugate bilirubin from glucuronic acid and hydrolyzed phospholipids, providing excess bilirubin and free fatty acids to precipitate with calcium (calcium bilirubinate). There is an excessive secretion of unconjugated bilirubin into the bile with hemolytic diseases, disorders of erythropoiesis and diseases in which there is excess unconjugated bilirubin undergoing enterohepatic circulation. Approximately one third of all pediatric gallstones are hemolysis-derived black pigment stones. The prevalence of pigment stones increases with age in patients with hemolytic disorders. In sickle cell anemia, the frequency of stones is 14% in children younger than 10 years of age, 36% in 10- to 20-year-olds, 50% by age 22, and 60% to 85% by age 33. Total parenteral nutrition (TPN) and fasting also predispose to sludge and black pigment stone formation. There is some suggestion that neonates and adult patients with sludge associated with prolonged TPN may go on to develop gallstones. The use of even minimal enteral nutrition, allowing for increased gallbladder contraction reduces the rate of sludge appearance. Patients with cirrhosis and chronic cholestasis also are at increased risk for black pigment stones for unclear reasons. Hypersplenism-related hemolysis, or a limited solubilizing capability of bile due to decreased concentrations of biliary bile acids may play a role. Most brown stone formation occurs in obstructed bile ducts and is associated with infection and parasitic infestation. Uncommon in the Western Hemisphere, brown stones are rare in infants and children, but in the Pacific Rim these stones are seen with *Ascaris lumbricoides* infestation.

Diseases such as cystic fibrosis, Crohn's disease, and distal small bowel resections are prone to have bile salt malabsorption in the terminal ileum and subsequent interruption of the enterohepatic cycling of bile salts. The exact mechanism of how this leads to cholelithiasis is unclear. In adults, it is believed that bile acid pool contraction and biliary cholesterol supersaturation lead to the noted cholesterol stones. In children, pigmented stones tend to be reported with these diseases. Although cholesterol supersaturation in children with ileal resection has not been noted, biliary supersaturation develops after puberty. Of note, in general, only one type of stone forms at a given time.

A number of medications are associated with cholelithiasis and biliary sludge. Progestins, oral contraceptives, and octreotide impair gallbladder emptying, thus promoting sludge and stone formation. Biliary sludge is also seen in infants born to morphine abusers. Ceftriaxone, which is excreted into bile, may precipitate with calcium to form sludge or pseudolithiasis. Nearly 25% of children treated with high-dose ceftriaxone have been reported to develop ultrasound abnormalities. However, this is not believed to cause clinical complications, and these stones tend to resolve over weeks to months. Calcium carbonate, normally found in bones and teeth, forms stones in a rare condition called milk of calcium cholelithiasis. The appearance of these can be quite impressive on radiographs. The etiology and pathophysiology of these stones are unknown.

There are limited data on stone characterization of pediatric gallstones. A review of 693 cases of pediatric gallstones found that 72% of the stones were pigmented, whereas 17% were cholesterol stones. It appears that black stones predominate until adolescence when cholesterol stones begin to account for the majority of stones. A recent 5-year study assessed the stone composition in 20 consecutive children who underwent cholecystectomy for cholelithiasis. Seven children were found to have stones containing at least 90% calcium carbonate, which are very rarely found in adults. Five of the 7 children had a history of neonatal surgery and TPN use. Surgical neonates may have multiple factors predisposing them to gallstone formation such as prematurity, lack of enteral feeds, TPN, surgery, blood transfusion, sepsis, and diuretic administration.

DIFFERENTIAL DIAGNOSIS

When a patient is suspected to have biliary colic, several other causes for epigastric or RUQ pain should be considered (Table 29-3), including complications of cholelithiasis. Stones lodged in the neck of the gallbladder or cystic duct result in distention and inflammation of the gallbladder wall (cholecystitis), which can be further complicated by a secondary bacterial infection, empyema, gangrene, or perforation. When stones are impacted in the common bile duct (choledocholithiasis), patients present with obstructive jaundice and may develop pancreatitis or an ascending inflammation of the bile ducts (cholangitis). Symptoms identical to those caused by cholelithiasis can be caused by the passage of sludge out of the gallbladder into the cystic duct and common bile duct. Sludge can be associated with biliary colic, pancreatitis, cholangitis, and cholecystitis. Inflammation of the gallbladder in the absence of gallstones is referred to as acalculous cholecystitis or gallbladder hydrops. Acute acalculous cholecystitis is associated with streptococci, and gram-negative (salmonella, *Leptospira interrogans*) and parasitic (*Ascaris lumbricoides, Giardia lamblia*) infections and post-trauma or burn injury.

DIAGNOSTIC TESTING

Laboratory Testing

Laboratory tests are often normal in patients with cholelithiasis and episodes of biliary colic. In a small number of patients, there may be a transient elevation in serum

Table 29-3 Differential Diagnosis for Biliary Colic

Disease	Distinguishing Features
Cholecystitis	• RUQ pain usually lasting more than 3 hours, fever, RUQ mass, positive Murphy's sign; leukocytosis, thickened gallbladder wall with pericholecystic fluid
Choledocholithiasis	• Jaundice, elevated bilirubin, AP and GGT, CBD dilatation on ultrasound, and absent gallbladder on scintigraphy
Acalculous cholecystitis	• Associated with bacterial and parasitic infections, post-trauma/burn injury • RUQ/generalized tenderness, absence of gallbladder on scintigraphy
Pancreatitis	• Epigastric pain of varying duration, elevated amylase and lipase, pancreatic inflammation on sonography
Peptic ulcer disease	• Positive family history, anemia, epigastric dull ache/burning pain (minutes-hours), nocturnal pain, relief with antacids
Gastritis	• Anemia, epigastric burning, relief with antacids
Acute hepatitis	• Associated viral symptoms, markedly elevated transaminases
Appendicitis	• Fever, leukocytosis, migration of pain to RLQ
Irritable bowel syndrome	• Associated diarrhea ± constipation, exacerbated by stress, other functional symptoms
Pneumonia	• Fever, tachypnea, hypoxia, positive pulmonary examination, and chest x-ray

AP, alkaline phosphatase; CBD, common bile duct; GGT, gamma-glutamyl-transferase; RLQ, right lower quadrant; RUQ, right upper quadrant.

bilirubin, aminotransferase, and alkaline phosphatase. In complications of cholelithiasis such as acute cholecystitis, cholangitis, or pancreatitis-associated cholelithiasis, there may be leukocytosis or mild elevations in transaminases. Elevations in gamma-glutamyl-transferase (GGT), alkaline phosphatase, and bilirubin are seen with biliary obstruction.

Imaging

Plain abdominal x-rays should not be considered a first-line investigation in assessing for cholelithiasis. However, calcified gallstones (cholesterol stones with a calcified shell or pigment stones composed of calcium bilirubinate or calcium carbonate) are radiopaque and may be picked up incidentally. In children, 20% to 47% of gallstones are radiopaque. Transabdominal ultrasonography is the initial imaging modality that should be used to diagnose cholelithiasis (Fig. 29-1) and sludge (Fig. 29-2). Abdominal ultrasonography has a sensitivity and specificity of more than 95%. It is also useful for measurement of the thickness of the gallbladder wall, indicating chronic

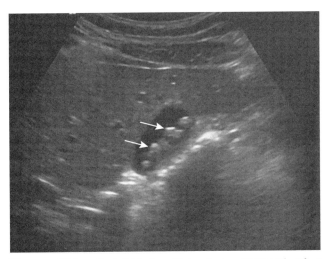

Figure 29-1 Cholelithiasis. Abdominal ultrasound of a 10-year-old Native American female presenting with pancreatitis and mild hepatitis found to have numerous small hyperechoic foci with shadowing (*arrows*) in the gallbladder representing multiple gallstones.

infection or acalculous cholecystitis. The sensitivity of ultrasound drops to about 30% to 40% for detection of common bile duct stones, but these should be suspected if dilated intrahepatic and common ducts are noted.

Occasionally, other imaging modalities may be indicated (Tables 29-4 and Fig. 29-3). Abdominal computed tomography (CT) is less sensitive than ultrasonograpy in diagnosing sludge and stones but may be useful in confirming the extent and nature of complications of acute cholecystitis. Magnetic resonance cholangiopancreatography (MRCP) should be considered when bile duct obstruction is suspected but not visualized on sonography or when more detailed diagnostic information is required for treatment planning. The high sensitivity (>90%) and specificity (>97%) of MRCP make it useful as a noninvasive diagnostic modality, particularly when the pretest probability of stones is low or in an obese patient in whom sonography may be more of a challenge. Endoscopic retrograde cholangiopancreatography (ERCP) also provides excellent imaging of the extrahepatic and

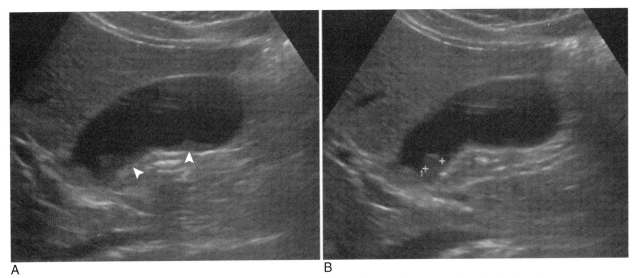

Figure 29-2 Biliary sludge. A 9-year-old girl with hereditary spherocytosis. Longitudinal supine sonographies demonstrate low-level echoes layering in the dependent portion of the gallbladder (*arrowheads* in **A** and *cursors* in **B**). (Courtesy Xingchang Wei, MD, Alberta Children's Hospital).

Table 29-4 Imaging Methods

Disease Process	Ultrasound	Scintigraphy	CT	MRCP
Cholelithiasis	+++			
Acute cholecystitis	+++	++		
Acute acalculous cholecystitis	++	+		
Chronic acalculous cholecystitis	+	+++		
Bile duct obstruction	+++	++	++	+++

Adapted from Broderick A, Sweeney BT: Gallbladder disease. In Walker WA, Goulet O, Kleinman RE, et al (eds): Pediatric Gastrointestinal Disease. Hamilton, Ontario, BC Decker, 2004.

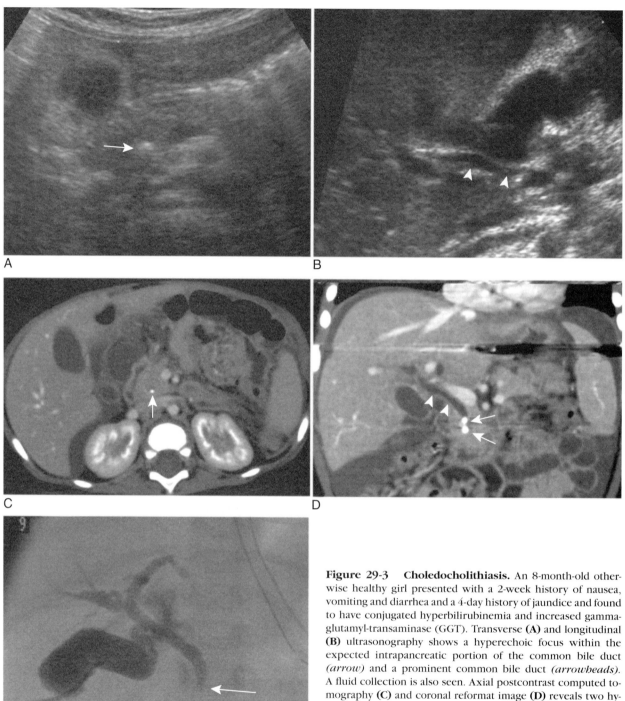

Figure 29-3 Choledocholithiasis. An 8-month-old otherwise healthy girl presented with a 2-week history of nausea, vomiting and diarrhea and a 4-day history of jaundice and found to have conjugated hyperbilirubinemia and increased gamma-glutamyl-transaminase (GGT). Transverse **(A)** and longitudinal **(B)** ultrasonography shows a hyperechoic focus within the expected intrapancreatic portion of the common bile duct *(arrow)* and a prominent common bile duct *(arrowheads)*. A fluid collection is also seen. Axial postcontrast computed tomography **(C)** and coronal reformat image **(D)** reveals two hyperdense calculi *(arrows)* within the distal common bile duct *(arrowheads)*. Fluid is seen in Morison's pouch, the porta hepatis, and the subdiaphragmatic space. Intraoperative cholangiography **(E)** confirms distal biliary obstruction *(arrow)*. (Courtesy Xingchang Wei, MD, Alberta Children's Hospital).

pancreatic duct systems as well as providing opportunity for therapeutic intervention such as impacted stone retrieval and sphincterotomy (see Fig. 29-3).

The main role for radionuclide imaging or scintigraphy is when ultrasonographic findings are equivocal for acute cholecystitis or if the diagnosis of alcalculous cholecystitis is suspected. After a period of fasting, the patient is given an intravenous injection of technetium-99m–labeled iminodiacetic acid derivative, which is excreted into the bile ducts and then sequentially imaged by a gamma camera. An abnormal study is failure to visualize the gallbladder within 90 minutes.

In adults, endoscopic ultrasound (EUS) can detect more than 90% of common bile duct stones. In a recent adult study, EUS was able to detect cholelithiasis or choledocholithiasis in 77% of patients with recurrent idiopathic pancreatitis and negative previous results with CT, ultrasound, or ERCP. This tool is not yet routinely used in pediatrics.

TREATMENT (Table 29-5)

Symptomatic Cholelithiasis

Once an episode of biliary colic has occurred, there is a high chance of repeat episodes. Early adult studies indicated a 38% to 50% incidence rate of recurrent biliary pain per year and a risk of developing biliary complications to be 1% to 2% per year. Although it may be difficult to predict the likelihood of an attack in an individual patient, the patient and the family may want to proceed with definitive treatment—cholecystectomy. Ultimately, the management plan will depend on the patient's surgical candidacy. Laparoscopic cholecystectomy is the procedure of choice for children requiring cholecystectomy. For hemodynamically stable patients with acute cholecystitis, an early laparoscopic cholecystectomy (within 24 to 48 hours) is preferable. The management of common bile duct (CBD) stones is more controversial.

If the patient is identified to also have choledocholithiasis, there is a higher risk of complications, and stone extraction should be considered by cholecystectomy or ERCP should there be local expertise. In adults, if a patient is suspected to have choledocholithiasis and is presenting with jaundice, obstructive cholangitis, or an obstructed CBD by sonography, an immediate preoperative ERCP and possible sphincterotomy and stone extraction can be done, followed by a routine laparoscopic cholecystectomy within a few days. If the index of suspicion for choledocholithiasis is low, many surgeons will proceed directly to laparoscopic surgery with an intraoperative cholangiography to rule out choledocholithiasis. If a CBD stone is found, it can be removed intraoperatively or postoperatively by ERCP. A recent Cochrane Database review of 13 trials assessed surgical versus endoscopic treatment of choledocholithiasis and concluded that ERCP was less successful than open surgery in CBD stone clearance. However, laparoscopic CBD stone clearance was as efficient as pre- or postoperative ERCP for bile duct clearance in patients undergoing laparoscopic cholecystectomy. The use of ERCP did not have an apparent advantage over surgical exploration, but the use of ERCP may incur an increased number of procedures per patient.

Such volume of data with ERCP is not available in pediatrics, and the indications for ERCP are not clearly defined. One small study of 21 children reported high ERCP complication rates (21%: 6 with pancreatitis and 1 with bleeding). A more recent larger, but still small, study of 116 children compared with adults found similar, low complication rates (3.4% vs. 2.5%, respectively) and similar success rates (97% vs. 98%, respectively). Likely this reported variability relates to the experience of the endoscopist. The long-term results of endoscopic sphincterotomy are not available and for this reason some favor a more conservative approach. It has been suggested that in children with choledocholithiasis, a laparoscopic exploration be done first, and if there is residual obstruction following flushing of the CBD, a postoperative ERCP and sphincterotomy can be performed. As well, a retrospective study of 100 children undergoing cholecystectomy noted that spontaneous passage of stones was common pre- and postoperatively with only 2 out the 13 patients with choledocholithiasis requiring postoperative ERCP. Currently, there is a lack of consensus on whether a suspected CBD stone warrants a preoperative ERCP, whether an intraoperative cholangiogram should be performed routinely, and on the management of CBD stones seen on intraoperative cholangiogram. Thus, these decisions are made on an individual basis with a collaborative approach.

Table 29-5 Approach to Treatment

Clinical Scenario	Therapeutic Options
Asymptomatic Cholelithiasis	
1. <1 cm and suspected to be cholesterol stones	• Consider ursodeoxycholic acid* • Expectant management
2. <2 cm	• Expectant management
3. >2 cm	• Consider elective cholecystectomy
4. Any size in a patient with hemolytic disease	• Elective cholecystectomy
Symptomatic Cholelithiasis	
1. Biliary colic	• Elective laparoscopic cholecystectomy
2. Cholecystitis	• Laparoscopic cholecystectomy within 24-48 hours
3. Biliary colic and CBD stone	• Laparoscopic cholecystectomy ± ERCP
4. Biliary colic and suspected CBD stone	• Laparoscopic cholecystectomy ± ERCP

*Efficacy not yet proved in children.
CBD, common bile duct; ERCP, endoscopic retrograde cholangiopancreatography.

Asymptomatic Patients

In adults, although elective cholecystectomy has a low morbidity and mortality, there is no great advantage to prophylactic cholecystectomy given the low risk of developing gallstone-related symptoms. However, in certain high-risk patients, emergency operations may be technically challenging and possibly lead to significant complications, and thus it has been suggested that elective cholecystectomy be considered in these patients. The high-risk criteria proposed for elective cholecystectomy in adults include life expectancy of more than 20 years, calculi more than 2 cm in diameter, calculi less than 3 cm and a patent cystic duct, radiopaque calculi, polyps in the gallbladder, a nonfunctioning or calcified ("porcelain") gallbladder, concomitant diabetes, women younger than 60 years, and individuals in geographic regions with a high prevalence of gallbladder cancer.

There have been no pediatric studies following the natural history of silent stones or guidelines published for the management of cholelithiasis in children. Generally, the practice is expectant management for healthy children with stones less than 2 cm. Larger gallstones (greater than 2 cm) may carry a greater risk for carcinoma of the gallbladder, and under these circumstances a cholecystectomy may be warranted. In infants and children with hemolytic disease, gallstones are expected to worsen with increasing age. In patients with sickle cell anemia; gallstone formation, cholecystitis, and adhesions increase with increasing age, and thus it is recommended that a cholecystectomy be performed once gallstones are identified.

Dissolution therapy by use of oral bile acid such as ursodeoxycholic acid can be used in patients with patent cystic ducts and small noncalcified stones (<1 cm) composed of cholesterol. The intake of these bile salts leads to a decrease in cholesterol secretion into the bile and thus the bile becomes less saturated with cholesterol. The therapy tends to be slow and has a dissolution rate of 40% at 2 years. The success is limited by a recurrence rate of 10% per year with cessation of therapy. There have not been any pediatric studies on the efficacy of dissolution therapy. A recent study of adult patients with highly symptomatic gallstones awaiting cholecystectomy failed to find any improvement in biliary symptoms compared with placebo.

Lithotripsy is not approved for used in children.

APPROACH TO THE CASE

The patient is constipated, which likely accounts for her lower abdominal symptoms. It is explained to the family that Maria is predisposed to gallstones by virtue of her ethnicity and because she is obese. It is likely that the cholelithiasis is responsible for the episode of more severe upper abdominal pain and she is at risk for a subsequent attack. Given that the stone is 3 cm in size, dissolution therapy is unlikely to be successful and the stone may not pass spontaneously. However, it is possible that the stone is an incidental finding and that the pain instead represented gastritis, peptic ulcer disease, or functional abdominal pain, with pancreatitis being less likely with the short duration of the episode of pain. The family elected to wait and see if she has another severe attack before referral to a surgeon. Maria was asked to follow a high-fiber, low-fat diet and to increase physical activity. Fast weight loss was discouraged. She was also instructed to take polyethylene glycol 3350 (MiraLax) once daily.

Six months later, Maria was seen in follow-up. Dietary changes were minimal but she managed to take the MiraLax 4 or 5 days a week. Her BMI of 36 kg/m^2 was maintained and she reports being pain free for the preceding 4 months with a normalization of her bowel movements. With this success, the family decided to hold off on pursuing treatment for the cholelithiasis.

Two years later, over the period of 1 month, Maria presented with two episodes of severe RUQ abdominal pain radiating to the back, accompanied by nausea and nonbilious, nonbloody vomiting. She did not seek medical attention with the first episode because she was afraid of the possibility of surgery. During the second episode, she was seen in the emergency department. On examination she was mildly anicteric and afebrile but tachycardic. Her BMI was now 38 kg/m^2. Her abdomen was soft and nontender with a negative Murphy's sign. Bloodwork revealed a normal complete blood count, amylase, and lipase. She had an elevated conjugated bilirubin of 3.0 mg/dL, aspartate transaminase (AST) of 80, alanine transaminase (ALT) of 90, GGT of 250, and AP of 300. Abdominal ultrasound revealed a 3-cm stone in the gallbladder and a dilated common bile duct. An MRCP demonstrated a 4-mm stone in the common bile duct. Maria finally agreed to undergo a laparoscopic cholecystectomy, during which a small stone was dislodged from the CBD; a postoperative ERCP was not required. She was seen in follow-up 3 months later. There was no recurrence of the epigastric abdominal pain, but she did have occasional lower abdominal and periumbilical pain and irregular bowel movements. Subsequently, attention was turned to lifestyle issues related to her morbid obesity and the regularization of her bowels.

SUMMARY

Gallbladder stones are infrequent in children and are usually asymptomatic. Ethnicity, age, and female gender are predisposing factors for cholelithiasis as well as several medical conditions. Gallstones occur with cholesterol

MAJOR POINTS

Gallbladder stones are infrequent in children and usually asymptomatic.

Populations with high prevalence rates of cholelithiasis include Swedes, Chileans, Czechs, Hispanic Americans, and Native Americans, especially Pima Indians.

Conditions predisposing to cholelithiasis include hemolytic diseases, obesity, prolonged TPN use, chronic cholestasis, cirrhosis, cystic fibrosis, pregnancy, parasitic infections, Crohn's disease, and other diseases interrupting the enterohepatic circulation.

Gallstones occur with cholesterol supersaturation of the bile, precipitation of cholesterol, and gallbladder hypomotility.

Cholesterol stones, which are associated with obesity, are most common in Western cultures, black pigment stones are seen with hemolytic diseases, and brown pigment stones are associated with infection and inflammation.

In children, black stones predominate in childhood until adolescence, when cholesterol stones emerge as the main type.

Symptomatic gallstones or biliary sludge can manifest as biliary colic, obstructive jaundice or complications such as cholecystitis, cholangitis, and pancreatitis.

Biliary colic is characterized by recurrent severe, steady abdominal pain in the right upper quadrant or epigastrium, and in children is not typically provoked by a fatty meal.

Laboratory tests in biliary colic are usually normal unless the colic is accompanied by obstructive jaundice or pancreatitis.

Abdominal ultrasound is the investigation of choice in diagnosing gallbladder disease and only occasionally are other imaging modalities required.

MRCP should be considered when bile duct obstruction is suspected but stones are not visualized by sonography or when more detailed diagnostic information is required for planning of management.

Asymptomatic stones or sludge can be managed expectantly.

An elective cholecystectomy can be considered in stones larger than 2 cm.

An elective cholecystectomy should be done in patients with hemolytic disease once stones of any size are identified.

Ursodeoxycholic acid has been used for slow dissolution of cholesterol stones less than 1 cm in adults. However, in younger children the majority of stones are pigmented stones and there are no longitudinal pediatric studies on efficacy.

Symptomatic stones should be managed by laparoscopic cholecystectomy.

Laparoscopic cholecystectomy should be done within 24 to 48 hours in patients with cholecystitis

ERCP is useful in the management of CBD stones, but caution should be exercised until larger and more long-term studies are available.

---

supersaturation of the bile, precipitation of cholesterol, and gallbladder hypomotility. Cholesterol stones, which are associated with obesity, are most common in Western cultures, black pigment stones are seen with hemolytic diseases, and brown pigment stones are seen with infection and inflammation. In children, black stones predominate from childhood until adolescence, when cholesterol stones emerge as the main type of stone. Symptomatic gallstones or biliary sludge can manifest as biliary colic, obstructive jaundice, or as complications such as cholecystitis, cholangitis, or pancreatitis. Abdominal pain is a frequent complaint in pediatrics. A detailed characterization of abdominal pain in children who have also been identified as having cholelithiasis is important in distinguishing biliary colic from other possible sources of abdominal pain. Laboratory tests are usually normal in patients with biliary colic unless there is accompanying obstructive jaundice or pancreatitis. Abdominal ultrasound is the investigation of choice in diagnosing gallbladder disease and only occasionally are other imaging modalities required. MRCP can be considered if bile duct obstruction is suspected but stones are not visualized on sonography or when more detailed diagnostic information is required for planning of management. Asymptomatic stones or sludge can be managed expectantly. An elective cholecystectomy should be done in patients with hemolytic disease once stones of any size are identified and can be considered in healthy children with stones larger than 2 cm. Ursodeoxycholic acid can be considered for small stones with the knowledge that dissolution of cholesterol stones is slow, that there is a high recurrence rate, and that longitudinal pediatric studies have not yet been published. Symptomatic stones should be managed by laparoscopic cholecystectomy. ERCP can be useful in the management of CBD stones, but caution should be exercised until larger and more long-term studies are available.

SUGGESTED READINGS

Ahmed A, Cheung RC, Keeffe EB: Management of gallstones and their complications. Am Family Phys 61:1673, 2000.

Baker S, Barlow S, Cochran W, et al: Overweight children and adolescents: A clinical report of the North American Society for Pediatric Gastroenterology, Hepatology and Nutrition. J Pediatr Gastroenterol Nutr 40:533-543, 2005.

Broderick A, Sweeney BT: Gallbladder disease. In Walker WA, Goulet O, Kleinman RE, et al (eds): Pediatric Gastrointestinal Disease. Hamilton, Ontario, BC Decker, 2004.

Colombo C, Apostolo MG, Ferrari M, et al: Analysis of risk factors for the development of liver disease associated with cystic fibrosis. J Pediatr 124:393-399, 1994.

Davidoff AM, Ranum GD, Murray EA, et al: The technique of laparoscopic cholecystectomy in children. Ann Surg 215:186-191, 1992.

Friesen CC, Roberts CC: Cholelithiasis: Clinical characteristics in children. Case analysis and literature review. Clin Pediatr 28:294-298, 1989.

Heubi JE, O'Connell NC, Setchell KDR: Ileal resection/dysfunction in childhood predisposed to lithogenic bile after puberty. Gastroenterology 103:636-640, 1992.

Heubi JE, Lewis LG, Pohl JF: Diseases of the gallbladder in infancy, childhood and adolescence. In Suchy FJ, Sokol RJ, Balistreri WF (eds): Liver Disease in Children, 2nd ed. Philadelphia, Lippincott Williams & Wilkins, 2001.

Kaechele V, Wabitsch M, Thiere D, et al: Prevalence of gallbladder stone disease in obese children and adolescents: Influence of the degree of obesity, sex and pubertal development. J Pediatr Gastroenterol Nutr 42:66-70, 2006.

Lemberg D, Day AS, Wyeth B: Biliary colic: Is it gallstones? J Pediatr Child Health 41:291-293, 2005.

Lui C, Lo C, Chan JKF, et al: EUS for detection of occult cholelithiasis in patients with idiopathic pancreatitis. Gastrointest Endosc 51:28-32, 2000.

Martin DJ, Vernon DR, Toouli J: Surgical versus endoscopic treatment of bile duct stones (review). Cochrane Database Syst Rev, 3, 2006.

Matos C, Avni ER, Van Gansbeke D, et al: Total parenteral nutrition and gallbladder disease in neonates. J Ultrasound Med 6:243-248, 1987.

Messing B, Bories C, Kunstlinger F, et al: Does total parenteral nutrition induce gallbladder sludge formation and lithiasis? Gastroenterology 84:1012-1019, 1983.

Patino JF, Quintero GA: Asymptomatic cholelithiasis revisited. World J Surg 22:1119-1124, 1998.

Prasil P, Laberge LJ, Barkum A, et al: Endoscopic retrograde cholangiopancreatography in children: A surgeon's perspective. J Pediatr Surg 36:733-735, 2001.

Salen G, Tint GS, Shafer S: Treatment of cholesterol gallstone with litholytic bile acids. Gastroenterol Clin North Am 20:171-182, 1991.

Sampliner RE, Bennett PH, Comess LJ, et al: Gallbladder disease in Pima Indians: Demonstration of high prevalence and early onset by cholecystography. N Engl J Med 283:1358, 1970.

Shea JA, Berlin JA, Escare JJ, et al: Revised estimates of diagnostic test sensitivity and specificity in suspected biliary tract disease. Arch Intern Med 154:2573-2581, 1994.

Stringer MD, Taylor DR, Soloway RD: Gallstone composition: Are children different? J Pediatr 142:435-440, 2003.

Toscano E, Trivellini V, Amdria G: Cholelithiasis in Down's syndrome. Arch Dis Child 85:242-243, 2001.

Vanneman NG, Besselink MGH, Keulemans YCA, et al: Ursodeoxycholic acid exerts no beneficial effect in patients with symptomatic gallstones awaiting cholecystectomy. Hepatology 43:1276-1283, 2006.

Varadarajulu S, Wilcox CM, Hawes RH, et al: Technical outcomes and complications of ERCP in children. Gastrointest Endosc 60:367-367, 2004.

Waldhausen JH, Benjamin DR: Cholecystectomy is becoming an increasingly common operation in children. Am J Surg 177:364, 1999.

Wesdorp I, Bosman D, de Graaff D, et al: Clinical presentations and predisposing factors of cholelithiasis and sludge in children. J Pediatr Gastroenterol Nutr 31:411-441, 2000.

Wu SS, Casas AT, Abraham SK, et al: Milk of calcium cholelithiasis in childhood. J Pediatr Surg 36:644-647, 2001.

CHAPTER 30

Congenital Hepatic Fibrosis

KATHLEEN M. LOOMES
MATTHEW J. RYAN

Disease Description
Case Presentation
Pathophysiology
    Embryology of the Intrahepatic Bile Ducts
    Ductal Plate Malformation
    Congenital Hepatic Fibrosis
    Autosomal Recessive Polycystic Kidney Disease
        Genetics
    Caroli's Disease and Caroli Syndrome
    Autosomal Dominant Polycystic Kidney Disease
        Genetics
    Congenital Hepatic Fibrosis Nephronophthisis
    Isolated Polycystic Liver Disease
    Other Inherited Disorders Associated with Ductal
        Plate Malformation
    Cilia
Differential Diagnosis
Diagnostic Testing
Management
Approach to the Case
Summary
Major Points

DISEASE DESCRIPTION

Congenital hepatic fibrosis (CHF) is characterized by ductal plate malformation and hepatic fibrosis, resulting in portal hypertension and an increased risk of ascending cholangitis. Ductal plate malformation is a developmental abnormality of the hepatic architecture defined by failure of remodeling of embryonic duct structures. Congenital hepatic fibrosis is best considered a single disorder with a wide spectrum of manifestations most commonly associated with autosomal recessive polycystic kidney disease (ARPKD).

CASE PRESENTATION

The patient is a 4-year-old previously healthy white male who has presented to the emergency department with two episodes of hematemesis. The history is negative for upper respiratory tract symptoms, fever, pruritus, jaundice, bleeding, bruising, weight loss, or fatigue. He has not taken any medications or herbal remedies, and the history is negative for any accidental caustic or foreign body ingestion. Birth history reveals an unremarkable pregnancy with no complications of pregnancy, labor, or delivery. Past medical history is unremarkable, and family history is negative for any individuals with gastrointestinal bleeding or liver or kidney disease. In the emergency department, nasogastric lavage reveals 250 mL of bright red blood and clots before finally clearing. (Refer to Table 30-1 or Chapter 10 for the differential diagnosis of upper gastrointestinal [GI] bleeding.)

On physical examination, the patient is pale and tachycardic with a heart rate of 130 beats per minute. Abdominal examination is remarkable for a firm, nontender spleen tip palpated 4 cm below the left costal margin. The liver span is 8 cm at the right costal margin. The liver is also palpated in the midline at 4 cm below the sternum. Extremities are warm, but capillary refill is slightly delayed at 2 to 3 seconds. The remainder of the physical examination is unremarkable. Laboratory workup is significant for a white blood cell (WBC) count of 4,000/µL, hemoglobin of 4.3 g/dL, platelet count of 90,000/µL, and an elevated International Normalized Ratio (INR) of 1.4. Liver enzymes are within the normal limits.

The patient is admitted to the pediatric intensive care unit for further volume resuscitation and stabilization. Abdominal ultrasound with Doppler reveals mildly abnormal hepatic echotexture, splenomegaly, normal portal venous flow, and modestly enlarged kidneys with

Table 30-1 Causes of Hematemesis
Esophagitis/gastritis
Mallory-Weiss tears
Peptic or duodenal ulcers
Esophageal or gastric varices
Vascular anomalies
Vasculitis
Gastrointestinal duplication cysts
Caustic ingestion
Foreign bodies
Crohn's disease
Nongastrointestinal sources (e.g., epistaxis or hemoptysis)

increased echogenicity. There is no evidence for cavernous transformation of the portal vein.

PATHOPHYSIOLOGY

Embryology of the Intrahepatic Bile Ducts

To fully understand the ductal plate malformations, one must review the formation of the intrahepatic biliary tree. The ductal plate starts to develop at the fifth week of gestation. It is formed from bipotential hepatoblasts adjacent to the portal tract. These hepatoblasts develop into a continuous layer of cuboidal, biliary cells. Over the next several weeks this continuous layer of cells divides into a double layer that surrounds the portal tract. At week 12 of gestation, distinct tubular spaces are created through a process of remodeling and apoptosis. These tubules then migrate centrally into the portal tracts (Fig. 30-1). This complicated process begins at the liver hilum and extends out toward the periphery of the liver. The development of the intrahepatic bile ducts therefore starts at the fifth week of gestation and continues into the first month of life.

Ductal Plate Malformation

First coined by Jorgensen in 1977, the term *ductal plate malformation* (DPM) refers to a characteristic structural abnormality of the intrahepatic bile ducts, associated with many inherited pediatric liver disorders. Ductal plate malformation results from incomplete or arrested remodeling of the ductal plate during development. Because of the abnormal development, the bile ducts form dilated channels in an interrupted ring around the perimeter of the portal tracts. These abnormal biliary channels dilate and become cystic with time. The lumens of the cystic biliary channels communicate with the entire biliary tree. The close association of ductal plate malformation with many renal cystic disorders leads us to believe that the etiopathogenesis of ductal plate malformation is probably closely linked to the same genes that cause cystic lesions in the kidneys.

Congenital Hepatic Fibrosis

CHF refers to a developmental liver disorder with the characteristic hepatopathology of the ductal plate malformation. Clinically, these patients are at risk for portal hypertension and ascending cholangitis. CHF may occur in isolation, or in association with a number of disorders, most commonly in the setting of autosomal recessive polycystic kidney disease. A point of controversy exists regarding whether CHF and ARPKD are two separate disease entities or whether they represent a wide spectrum of clinical severity in the same disease. Typically, CHF patients present with hepatic manifestations of the disease, and may have minor renal abnormalities. In contrast, patients with ARPKD are more likely to present early in life with severe renal disease, and hepatic manifestations, although present, may not be clinically relevant. The recent identification of *PKHD1* as the disease gene for ARPKD will enable more exact classification of these disorders.

The most common clinical presentation in CHF is portal hypertension within the first two decades of life. Many patients may present with the sudden onset of gastrointestinal (GI) bleeding, manifesting as either hematemesis or melena. Others may have hepatomegaly and/or splenomegaly detected on routine physical examination. Hypersplenism also may be present, causing leukopenia and thrombocytopenia. Cholangitis also may be a presenting symptom of CHF. As a result of dilated intrahepatic bile ducts and biliary stasis, these patients may develop acute or chronic cholangitis or biliary calculi. Severe episodes of cholangitis may lead to sepsis and liver failure, contributing greatly to morbidity and mortality in this disease.

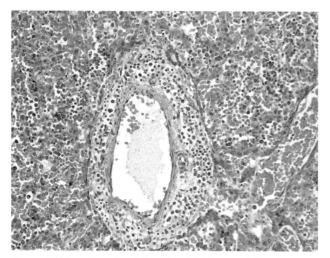

Figure 30-1 *(See also Color Plate 30-1.)* Normal ductal plate in a human fetal liver at 22 weeks' gestation. (H&E staining, 400×)

Autosomal Recessive Polycystic Kidney Disease

ARPKD is estimated to occur in 1 in 20,000 live births. Pathologically, ARPKD is characterized by fusiform dilatation of renal collecting ducts and DPM. In keeping with the wide clinical spectrum of these disorders, the severity of renal disease in ARPKD patients is highly variable. The most severely affected infants pre-sent in the neonatal period with massively enlarged cystic kidneys, renal failure, and pulmonary compromise. Up to 30% of patients die as neonates as a result of respiratory complications secondary to varying degrees of pulmonary hypoplasia. Patients who survive the neonatal period may go on to develop hypertension and chronic renal insufficiency. Up to 45% of patients develop end-stage renal disease within 15 years. Later in the first decade, these patients also may develop complications of liver disease, including signs of portal hypertension.

Genetics

In 2002, two research groups independently identified the ARPKD disease gene as *PKHD1*, located on chromosome 6p21.1-p12 (Table 30-2 is a summary of the genetics of polycystic liver diseases). Ward and colleagues demonstrated mutations in ARPKD patients in the human ortholog of the gene mutated in a rat model of polycystic kidney disease. Using a different approach, Onuchic and associates narrowed the critical region on chromosome 6 by positional cloning, and then screened for mutations in candidate genes highly expressed in the kidney. *PKHD1* is a relatively large gene of about 470 kb, encoding the protein fibrocystin (also termed polyductin). Fibrocystin is believed to represent a novel integral membrane protein with a highly glycosylated extracellular portion, a single transmembrane-spanning domain, and a short intracytoplasmic tail. The function of fibrocystin is unknown, but several of the extracellular domains are similar to those found in the hepatocyte growth factor receptor (HGFR). To date, many different mutations have been identified in *PKHD1*. Mutations are more likely to be identified in severe ARPKD patients, whereas patients presenting with a more mild phenotype or with liver disease alone are less likely to have a mutation detected. There is some genotype-phenotype correlation in that of patients carrying two truncating mutations in *PKHD1*, all had a very severe clinical presentation leading to death in the perinatal period. Overall, it seems that missense mutations are less severe, but several missense mutations also lead to severe disease and early death. Ongoing studies will help to elucidate further genotype-phenotype correlations.

Caroli's Disease and Caroli Syndrome

Caroli's disease is defined as a congenital dilatation of the large intrahepatic bile ducts in the absence of any other features. These dilated ducts may be visible on prenatal or postnatal ultrasound. The relation between Caroli's disease and type V choledochal cyst is controversial because there is clinical overlap between the two disorders. Caroli syndrome refers to the combination of congenital hepatic fibrosis and macroscopic dilatation of the large intrahepatic bile ducts. Patients with either variant are predisposed to bile stasis and repeated attacks of cholangitis. Figure 30-2 shows a magnetic resonance cholangiogram image from a patient with Caroli syndrome, demonstrating the diffuse dilatation of the intrahepatic bile ducts.

Autosomal Dominant Polycystic Kidney Disease

Autosomal dominant polycystic kidney disease (ADPKD) is the most common inherited renal disorder, occurring in as many as 1 in 400 to 1 in 1000 individuals. This disorder is characterized by cysts in the liver and kidneys that increase in size and number with age. Although patients usually present clinically as adults, cysts may be apparent in the pediatric age range as well. Hepatic cysts are lined with biliary epithelium, but unlike the lesions in ARPKD, they are noncommunicating with the biliary tree and do not contain bile. In a subset of patients,

Table 30-2 Inherited Polycystic Diseases

Disease	Inheritance	Gene Locus	Gene Name	Gene Product
ARPKD	AR	6p21.1-p12	*PKHD1*	Fibrocystin/polyductin
ADPKD	AD	16p13.3-p13.12	*PKD1*	Polycystin 1
		4q21-q23	*PKD2*	Polycystin 2
PCLD	AD	19p13.2-p13.1	*PRKCSH*	Hepatocystin
			SEC63	

AD, autosomal dominant; *ADPKD*, autosomal dominant polycystic kidney disease; *AR*, autosomal recessive; *ARPKD*, autosomal recessive polycystic kidney disease; *PCLD*, polycystic liver disease.

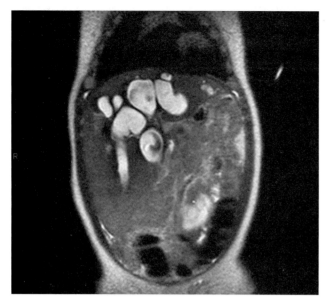

Figure 30-2 Magnetic resonance cholangiogram in a patient with Caroli syndrome shows massively dilated intrahepatic bile ducts.

DPM-like lesions may be present in the portal tracts. In older patients, hepatic complications may arise from progressively enlarging cysts; the most common complications include infection, cholangiocarcinoma, portal hypertension, and compression of other organs due to massive hepatomegaly. Renal tubular cysts enlarge over time, and eventually result in chronic renal insufficiency in many patients. As many as 30% of patients also may have arterial aneurysms in the cerebral circulation or elsewhere.

Genetics

To date, two disease genes have been identified for ADPKD: *PKD1* and *PKD2*, encoding polycystin-1 and polycystin-2. *PKD1* has been implicated in 86% of cases of ADPKD, whereas mutations in *PKD2* are found in 5% of patients, leaving speculation that a third locus exists. The focal nature of the cysts and the increasing numbers of cysts over time in this autosomal dominant disorder are consistent with the two-hit hypothesis. Somatic mutations in the normal copy of the disease gene lead to cyst formation arising from individual cells in the liver and kidney. Both polycystin-1 and polycystin-2 are expressed in the primary cilia of the renal epithelium and are believed to function in a common biologic pathway regulating mechanosensation of fluid flow in the renal tubule.

Congenital Hepatic Fibrosis Nephronophthisis

Nephronophthisis, a genetically heterogeneous group of autosomal recessive cystic kidney disorders, is the most common genetic cause of chronic renal failure in children. The renal lesion in nephronophthisis is distinct from that seen in ARPKD, and is characterized by inflammation, fibrosis, tubular atrophy, cyst formation, and glomerulosclerosis. About 10% of these patients have coincident retinitis pigmentosa (Senior-Loken syndrome). A subset of patients also demonstrate hepatic lesions similar, but not identical to, the ductal plate malformation. To date, five genes have been identified for nephronophthisis *(NPHP1-5)*, all of which are expressed in the primary cilia of the renal epithelium. Further studies of these genes will shed light on the role of cilia in renal and hepatic development and will help to categorize this complex group of disorders.

Isolated Polycystic Liver Disease

Polycystic liver disease (PCLD) is an autosomal dominant disorder characterized by the formation of fluid-filled biliary cysts in the liver in the absence of renal involvement. The disease typically remains asymptomatic until the fifth or sixth decade of life, when patients may present with abdominal pain or other symptoms of liver enlargement and compression of neighboring organs. Rarely, severe hepatic enlargement may lead to compression of the inferior vena cava and portal hypertension. Women are affected more severely than men, with larger and more numerous cysts. Recent studies have shown that many PCLD patients remain entirely asymptomatic throughout their lives. Positional cloning has identified two disease genes for polycystic liver disease: *PRKCSH* and *SEC63*. Both of these genes encode proteins that are involved in the translocation, folding, and processing of newly synthesized glycoproteins in the endoplasmic reticulum. Interestingly, in contrast to most of the other disease genes identified for hepatorenal cystic disorders, neither *PRKCSH* nor *SEC63* is expressed in cilia.

Other Inherited Disorders Associated with Ductal Plate Malformation

Phosphomannose isomerase deficiency, classified as congenital disorder of glycosylation type 1b, is an autosomal recessive disorder characterized clinically by chronic diarrhea, protein-losing enteropathy, coagulopathy, and hepatomegaly. Liver biopsy, if performed, demonstrates the features of DPM. This finding is fascinating in light of the fact that interactions with glycoproteins are believed to be important for the remodeling of the ductal plate during embryonic development. Table 30-3 describes other congenital malformation syndromes also associated with DPM, the most important of which are Meckel-Gruber syndrome, Jeune syndrome, Joubert syndrome, and Bardet-Biedl syndrome.

Cilia

A common thread through many of these renal cystic diseases is the involvement of the cilia. Either cilia or flagella are present on the majority of cells in the human

Table 30-3 Disorders Associated with Ductal Plate Malformation

Disorders Associated with Ductal Plate Malformation (DPM)
Congenital hepatic fibrosis
Autosomal recessive polycystic kidney disease (ARPKD)
Autosomal dominant polycystic kidney disease (ADPKD)
Caroli syndrome
Congenital hepatic fibrosis (CHF) nephronophthisis
Congenital disorder of glycosylation type 1b (phosphomannose isomerase deficiency)
Extrahepatic biliary atresia (occasional association)
Congenital malformation syndromes

Congenital Malformation Syndromes Associated with DPM
Syndromes frequently associated with DPM
  Meckel-Gruber syndrome
    Cystic renal disease
    Postaxial polydactyly
    Occipital encephalocele
  Jeune syndrome (asphyxiating thoracic dystrophy)
    Malformation of the thoracic rib cage
    Secondary pulmonary insufficiency
    Cystic renal and pancreatic disease
  Bardet-Biedl syndrome
    Retinal dystrophy
    Obesity
    Mental retardation
    Cystic renal disease
  Joubert syndrome
    Hypoplasia of the cerebellar vermis
    Retinal dystrophy
    Subset with medullary cystic disease of the kidney and CHF
    Genetically heterogeneous, can be caused by homozygous deletion of the *NPHP1* gene, also the disease gene for nephronophthisis type 1
  Ivemark syndrome
    Cystic dysplasia of the kidneys, liver, and pancreas
    With or without asplenia or laterality defects
Syndromes rarely reported to be associated with DPM
  Tuberous sclerosis
  COACH syndrome (cerebellar hypoplasia, oligophrenia, ataxia, coloboma, hepatic fibrosis)
  Ellis-van Creveld syndrome
  Trisomy 9
  Trisomy 13

body. These cilia function in motility and transport, as well as mechanoreception. The structure of a cilium consists of nine sets of doublet microtubules arranged circumferentially with two single microtubules in the center. Nonmotile cilia in the renal tubules and biliary epithelium lack the central two microtubules. The microtubules and their associated proteins make up the axoneme, which is the internal framework of the cilia. The basal body of the cilium, containing the centriole, forms the template for the assembly of the axoneme.

Centrioles are also the key elements in centrosomes. The centrosome, of course, plays an integral role as the center for the cytoplasmic microtubules during the interphase stage of mitosis. Each centrosome must contain a pair of centrioles in order to function. The connection between cilia, centriole, and centrosome is best observed in the fact that cells with a single cilium and two centrioles need to disassemble the cilium so both centrioles are available for mitosis. All the genes associated with nephronophthisis, ARPKD, and ADPKD are localized in cilia, basal bodies, or centrosomes, highlighting the importance of either the cilia themselves or the interplay between cilia, centriole, and centrosome in the formation of renal and hepatic cysts.

DIFFERENTIAL DIAGNOSIS

Table 30-3 lists the differential diagnosis of the genetic disorders associated with the finding of ductal plate malformation.

DIAGNOSTIC TESTING

An approach to diagnostic testing of CHF is detailed in Table 30-4. Serologic testing may include a complete blood count (CBC) to assess for signs of anemia or hypersplenism and prothrombin time/partial thromboplastin time (PT/PTT) to assess liver synthetic function. Liver enzymes are frequently within normal limits, but changes from baseline may be helpful in assessing for possible cholangitis. Imaging studies may include an abdominal ultrasound with Doppler to evaluate for hepatosplenomegaly, liver echotexture, and portal blood flow. The kidneys should also be examined for any cystic changes. Computed tomography (CT) or magnetic resonance imaging/magnetic resonance (MRI/MR) cholangiogram of the abdomen and biliary tree may be useful in the evaluation of enlarging hepatic cystic structures or bilomas. Magnetic resonance angiography may also have a role in the assessment of portal hypertension and collateral circulation. Finally, a liver biopsy demonstrates the characteristic features of the DPM, and may establish a definitive diagnosis. The gross appearance of the liver in CHF shows wide bands of white-gray fibrous tissue dissecting the parenchyma. Microscopically, wide bands of bridging fibrosis are seen encircling nodules of normal liver parenchyma. Around the periphery of the enlarged fibrotic portal tracts, dilated, abnormally shaped duct profiles are present, and the normal intrahepatic bile ducts are often absent (Fig. 30-3).

MANAGEMENT

The clinical management of congenital hepatic fibrosis is mainly supportive. Periodic monitoring of liver function and coagulation factors is warranted. Much of

Table 30-4 Diagnostic Studies Useful in the Evaluation of Congenital Hepatic Fibrosis

Radiologic

Ultrasound with Doppler	Can evaluate liver echotexture and signs of portal hypertension; also to visualize the kidneys for cysts
Magnetic resonance cholangiogram	Noninvasive imaging of the biliary tree to evaluate for strictures or bilomas

Serologic

Complete blood count (CBC)	Look for signs of hypersplenism, such as thrombocytopenia. Evaluate for anemia, especially if varices or chronic disease
Liver function tests (LFTs)	Look for cholestasis, liver inflammation, and overall synthetic function of the liver
PT/PTT/INR	Evaluate the synthetic function of the liver
Basic metabolic panel (BMP)	Assess renal function
Fat-soluble vitamin levels	If cholestasis is present

Invasive

Liver biopsy	Assess the degree of hepatic fibrosis
Esophagogastroduodenoscopy	To look for and treat varices either through band ligation or sclerotherapy

INR, International Normalized Ratio; PT, prothrombin time; PTT, partial thromboplastin time.

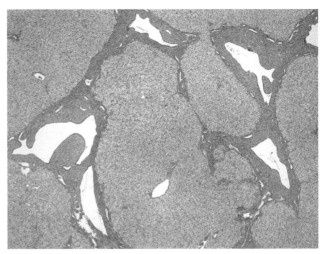

Figure 30-3 *(See also Color Plate 30-3.)* Typical features of ductal plate malformation include persistence of embryonic ductal structures surrounding the periphery of the portal tracts, dilated cystic ducts and increased fibroconnective tissue. (H&E staining, 100×)

the management deals with addressing the complications associated with DPM, including extensive fibrosis and dilated ductal structures. The two most common complications are portal hypertension with esophageal varices and cholangitis caused by the abnormal bile duct structure and stagnant bile flow.

Portal hypertension can lead to esophageal varices in a substantial number of patients. Studies have shown that in children with cirrhosis, up to two thirds can develop varices. The overall mortality from variceal bleeding in children is much lower than in adults (15% to 30% in adults vs. 0% to 8% in children). Once the varices form, they can be managed medically, endoscopically, or surgically. Prophylactic medical therapies include propranolol, which constricts splanchnic vessels and decreases portal blood flow. There is no recommended dose of propranolol for varices in children, but the goal is a 20% to 25% reduction in heart rate. Patients who have developed variceal bleeding are managed with endoscopic banding or sclerotherapy, with repeat sessions scheduled depending on the size, number, and severity of the varices.

If the bleeding cannot be controlled through these therapies, the patient can be evaluated for portosystemic shunting. There are several different options for shunts and the correct shunt depends on the anatomy of the patient and the experience of the surgeon. The goal of a shunt is to direct the portal blood flow into the systemic circulation and thereby lower the pressure in the portal system. Examples of portosytemic shunts include the splenorenal, portocaval, and mesocaval shunts. The recently developed mesentericoportal bypass or Rex shunt is effective only for patients with extrahepatic portal hypertension, such as portal vein thrombosis. Finally, a transjugular intrahepatic portosystemic shunt (TIPS) can be performed endovascularly, but has a high rate of thrombosis and is often not a long-term solution. The type of shunt and the actual procedure should be performed by, or in consultation with, a transplant surgeon in case the patient does progress to liver transplantation. Post-shunt encephalopathy has been reported, but the incidence is extremely low.

Cholangitis is another major complication associated with CHF and can lead to liver failure. Fevers or new elevations in transaminases or inflammatory markers should warrant a workup for infection and prophylactic antibiotic coverage. Patients are often treated with ursodeoxycholic acid to improve bile flow. Ursodeoxycholic acid, along with prophylactic antibiotic administration, may prevent ascending cholangitis by improving bile flow, reducing inflammation, and protecting against invading organisms, but neither has been sufficiently studied in CHF and cholangitis.

In patients who progress to chronic liver failure, have multiple episodes of bleeding from varices and poor coagulation, or suffer from multiple episodes of cholangitis, liver transplantation becomes an option. The patient may be evaluated for a combined liver/renal transplant depending on the extent of the renal disease.

APPROACH TO THE CASE

Our case involves a previously healthy patient presenting with an acute upper GI bleed. His physical examination is remarkable for hepatosplenomegaly, and his laboratory results demonstrate severe anemia, along with leukopenia, thrombocytopenia, and mild coagulopathy. These data, in combination with the ultrasound finding of abnormal hepatic echotexture, are concerning for underlying portal hypertension and possible esophageal varices as a cause of the GI bleeding. Once the patient was stabilized, an upper endoscopy was performed to confirm the source of the bleeding and provide treatment if possible. Multiple large varices were visualized with no active bleeding at the time of endoscopy (see Fig. 30-4). Three of the largest varices were sclerosed with 1-mm injections of sodium morrhuate. No further bleeding was noted. (Refer to Table 30-5 for the differential diagnosis of portal hypertension in children.)

Over the next several days, a workup was initiated to investigate the etiology of the portal hypertension. Multiple serologic studies were sent to evaluate for infection, autoimmune disease, and other potential causes of underlying liver disease. When the patient was clinically stable, a liver biopsy was performed to complete the diagnostic workup.

The patient's liver biopsy is shown in Figure 30-5. The important features are expanded portal tracts and proliferating, cystic bile ducts. There are also areas of bridging fibrosis. The liver biopsy shows the typical findings of ductal plate malformation, consistent with the diagnosis of congenital hepatic fibrosis.

The patient was discharged home without complications. Repeat endoscopy in 2 months showed one large varix, which was injected. He continued to have prophylactic sclerotherapy over the next 6 months with no further bleeds. During the hospitalization, a sample was obtained for genetic testing. The patient was found to be a compound heterozygote for two unique missense mutations in *PKHD1*, confirming the diagnosis of CHF/ARPKD. Both parents were tested and each parent was found to be heterozygous for one of the mutations.

Table 30-5 Differential Diagnosis of Portal Hypertension

Prehepatic
  Cavernous transformation of the portal vein
  Splenic vein thrombosis
Intrahepatic
  Congenital hepatic fibrosis (CHF)
  Sclerosing cholangitis
  Autoimmune hepatitis
  Infection
  Inherited disorders
  Cystic fibrosis
  α_1-Antitrypsin deficiency
  Cholestasis syndromes
  Wilson's disease (rare to present at age 4)
  Metabolic liver disease (e.g., tyrosinemia, glycogen storage disease)
  Cryptogenic cirrhosis
Posthepatic
  Budd-Chiari syndrome
  Congestive heart failure
  Veno-occlusive disease

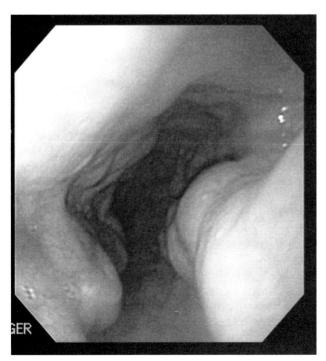

Figure 30-4 *(See also Color Plate 30-4.)* Esophageal varices.

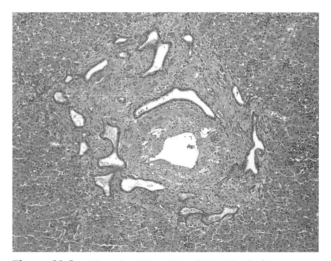

Figure 30-5 *(See also Color Plate 30-5.)* Needle biopsy, congenital hepatic fibrosis (CHF) (cytokeratin stain). Wide bands of bridging fibrosis are seen encircling nodules of normal liver parenchyma. Portal tracts are expanded with proliferation of abnormal dilated bile ducts. (H&E staining, 100×)

SUMMARY

CHF is a global term describing a developmental abnormality of the bile ducts characterized by the histologic finding of DPM. CHF is genetically heterogeneous, and may be associated with a number of different inherited disorders, most commonly ARPKD. Of the known genetic defects in disorders associated with ductal plate malformation, all of the genes are expressed in the primary cilia of the renal tubular and biliary epithelia, indicating a role for the cilia in cyst formation and biliary development.

The histologic lesion of CHF is associated with increased connective tissue in the portal tracts, leading to portal hypertension, and dilated bile ducts, which may predispose to bile stasis and recurrent cholangitis. The most common clinical presentations of CHF include hepatosplenomegaly or upper GI bleeding as a result of portal hypertension. Diagnostic testing may include abdominal ultrasound with Doppler, MR cholangiogram, and liver biopsy showing the typical findings of DPM. Management of patients with CHF is mainly supportive, directed toward preventing and treating potential complications of the disease.

MAJOR POINTS

- CHF is a global term describing a developmental abnormality of the bile ducts characterized by the histologic finding of DPM.
- CHF is associated with a number of different inherited disorders, most commonly ARPKD.
- Of the known genetic defects in disorders associated with DPM, all of the genes are expressed in the primary cilia of the renal tubular and biliary epithelia. This indicates a role for the cilia in cyst formation and biliary development.
- Clinical presentations of CHF would commonly include hepatosplenomegaly or upper GI bleeding as a result of portal hypertension.
- Diagnostic testing may include abdominal ultrasound with Doppler, MR cholangiogram, and liver biopsy showing the typical findings of DPM.
- Common complications of CHF include portal hypertension and cholangitis.
- Management of patients with CHF is mainly supportive, directed toward preventing and treating potential complications of the disease.

SUGGESTED READINGS

Al-Bhalal L, Akhtar M: Molecular basis of autosomal dominant polycystic kidney disease. Adv Anat Pathol 12:126-133, 2005.

Bergmann C, Senderek J, Sedlacek B, et al: Spectrum of mutations in the gene for autosomal recessive polycystic kidney disease (ARPKD/PKHD1). J Am Soc Nephrol 13:76-89, 2003.

Botha JF, Campos BD, Grant WJ, et al: Portosystemic shunts in children: A 15-year experience. J Am Coll Surg 199:179-185, 2004.

Davila S, Furu L, Gharavi AG, et al: Mutations in *SEC63* cause autosomal dominant polycystic liver disease. Nat Genet 36:575-577, 2004.

Desmet, VJ: Pathogenesis of ductal plate abnormalities (Ludwig Symposium on Biliary Disorders-Part I). Mayo Clin Proc 73:80-89, 1998.

Drenth JPH, Martina JA, van de Kerkhof R, et al: Polycystic liver disease is a disorder of co-translational protein processing. Trends Mol Med 11:37-42, 2005.

Drenth JP, Tahvanainen E, te Morsche RH, et al: Abnormal hepatocystin caused by truncating PRKCSH mutations leads to autosomal dominant polycystic liver disease. Hepatology 39:924-931, 2004.

Everson GT, Taylor MR, Doctor RB: Polycystic disease of the liver. Hepatology 40:774-782, 2004.

Freeze HH: Congenital disorders of glycosylation. Semin Liv Dis 21:501-515, 2001.

Harris PC, Rossetti S: Molecular genetics of autosomal recessive polycystic kidney disease. Mol Genet Metab 81:75-85, 2004.

Hildebrandt F, Otto E: Cilia and centrosomes: A unifying pathogenic concept for cystic kidney disease? Nat Rev Genet 6:928-940, 2005.

Johnson CA, Gissen P, Sergi C: Molecular pathology and genetics of congenital hepatorenal fibrocystic syndromes. J Med Genet 40:311-319, 2003.

Molleston JP: Variceal bleeding in children. J Pediatr Gastroenterol Nutr 37:538-545, 2003.

Nauli SM, Alenghat FJ, Luo Y, et al: Polycystins 1 and 2 mediate mechanosensation in the primary cilium of kidney cells. Nat Genet 33:129-137, 2003.

Onuchic LF, Furu L, Nagasawa Y, et al: PKHD1, the polycystic kidney and hepatic disease 1 gene, encodes a novel large protein containing multiple immunoglobulin-like plexin-transcription-factor domains and parallel beta-helix 1 repeats. Am J Hum Genet 70:1305-1317, 2002.

Pan J, Wang Q, Snell WJ: Cilium-generated signaling and cilia-related disorder. Lab Invest 85:452-463, 2005.

Piccoli DA, Russo P: Disorders of the intrahepatic bile ducts. In Walker WA, Goulet O, Kleinman RE, et al (eds): Pediatric Gastrointestinal Disease: Pathophysiology, Diagnosis, Management, Lewiston, NY, BC Decker, 2004.

Ruchelli, ED: Developmental anatomy and congenital anomalies of the liver, gallbladder, and extrahepatic biliary tree. In Russo P, Ruchelli E, Piccoli DA (eds): Pathology of Pediatric Gastroenterology and Liver Disease, New York, Springer, 2004.

Ward CJ, Hogan MC, Rossetti S, et al: The gene mutated in autosomal recessive polycystic kidney disease encodes a large, receptor-like protein. Nat Genet 30:259-269, 2002.

Hemochromatosis

PATRICIA A. DERUSSO

Disease Description
Case Presentation
Etiology
Pathophysiology
Differential Diagnosis
Diagnosis
   Neonatal Hemochromatosis and Hereditary Hemochromatosis
Treatment
   Medical Therapies
      Antioxidant Therapy
      High-Dose Immunoglobulin Therapy in Pregnancy
Surgical Therapy
   Liver Transplantation
Approach to the Case
Summary
Major Points

DISEASE DESCRIPTION

Neonatal hemochromatosis (NH) is a rare disorder characterized by severe liver disease of intrauterine onset and marked iron deposition in multiple organs including the liver.

CASE PRESENTATION

The patient is a 1-day-old infant born in the 29th week of pregnancy by cesarean section to a 27-year-old G3P1 mother with a history of two stillborn pregnancies associated with hydrops fetalis. The pregnancy was complicated by polyhydramnios and premature rupture of membranes. Apgar scores were 3 and 7, at 1 and 5 minutes, respectively. The infant developed respiratory distress and required mechanical ventilation. There was no urine output despite fluid resuscitation and furosemide. He was hypotensive, requiring dopamine infusion. Laboratory findings were remarkable for hemoglobin of 8 g/dL, platelets of 28,000 mm^3, reticulocyte count of 5.6%, and direct Coombs' test was negative. The alanine transaminase (ALT) was 10 IU/L, aspartate transaminase (AST) 56 IU/L, albumin 1.0 g/dL, total bilirubin 3.7 g/dL, direct bilirubin 0.4 g/dL, prothrombin time International Normalized Ratio (INR) 1.5, and partial thromboplastin time was 79.3 seconds.

ETIOLOGY

The disease usually manifests within hours of birth, although there are reports in which the disorder manifested later in infancy. The neonates are critically ill and the disorder is often fatal due to hepatic or renal failure unless liver transplantation is performed. The etiology has not yet been identified. No gene has been implicated and there is no clear pattern of inheritance. NH has been recognized by a phenotype with the diagnosis based on clinical and pathologic findings. Iron is deposited primarily in parenchymal cells with reticuloendothelial sparing. Iron accumulation is seen primarily in the liver, endocrine glands, and heart. Whether the disorder is a primary defect in iron metabolism or whether fetal liver injury results in abnormal accumulations of iron within hepatocytes has been debated. Recently, it has been hypothesized that the disorder may be an alloimmune disease. Other causes of neonatal liver failure must be excluded because hepatic iron overload is associated with several neonatal liver diseases. NH is similar to hereditary hemochromatosis and other iron-loading disorders in that the distribution of iron is within the parenchymal cells of the liver and other organs.

PATHOPHYSIOLOGY

The pathophysiology of NH remains obscure. Several theories have been proposed to explain the phenotype of iron overload. There are a number of case reports in which iron overload was present in neonates with an infectious or metabolic disorder. This would suggest that injury to the fetal liver results in dysregulation of iron metabolism. Alternatively, a primary defect in iron metabolism involving fetoplacental iron handling may lead to iron overload. It should be noted that biosynthesis of transferrin receptor and ferritin is appropriately regulated by iron in fibroblasts from neonates with the disorder. In addition, mothers of neonates with NH have normal iron studies. The occurrence of NH in multiple siblings without a clear pattern of genetic inheritance has led to a theory of possible alloimmune disease. The immune-mediated theory proposes that the mother is exposed during pregnancy to a fetal liver antigen that results in sensitization and production of a specific immune response. Immunoglobulins of the IgG class recognize and bind antigens as well as cross the placenta to the fetus. In the fetal circulation IgG would bind the liver antigen and possibly interfere with a vital function of a protein related to iron metabolism or result in immune injury of the fetal liver. Results of treatment of pregnant women with immune globulin are promising.

DIFFERENTIAL DIAGNOSIS

There are historic clues that may suggest a diagnosis of NH. A history from the mother of prior fetal loss should raise the suspicion of NH, because there is a high rate of recurrence in offspring of women who have had affected infants. It has been reported that there is approximately an 80% probability that each subsequent baby born to the same mother will be affected. A history of hydrops fetalis on fetal ultrasound also suggests the diagnosis of NH. The fetal insult from this disorder results in newborns that are born prematurely, have intrauterine growth restriction, and edema associated with hypoalbuminemia. Hepatic iron overload has been reported in other causes of liver failure that may present at birth and need to be excluded (Table 31-1). In addition, NH has been associated with other disorders.

Physical examination of an infant with NH reveals severe liver failure. Infants are edematous because of impaired synthetic function and hypoalbuminemia. Some will have respiratory and renal insufficiency secondary to decreased perfusion and poor oncotic pressure. The liver size is either normal or small as a result of hepatic necrosis. Splenomegaly may be present from portal hypertension.

DIAGNOSIS

There is no laboratory test available to establish the diagnosis of NH. Elevated serum ferritin concentrations have been found in neonates with this disorder with ranges usually increased to 2000 to 3000 µg/L. Higher ferritin concentrations have been reported in eight patients with NH (median ferritin levels were 4180 µg/L with a range of 1650 to 40,000 µg/L; normal range 110 to 503 µg/L) although infections were also present in two patients. Elevated ferritin levels can be present in other causes of severe hepatocellular injury in neonates and therefore cannot be diagnostic of the disorder. The transferrin saturation is usually elevated until 2 months of age and is therefore less helpful.

There is a classic pattern of chronic end-stage liver disease at birth. Rather than markedly elevated aminotransferases often seen in acute infections, serum transaminases are characteristically normal or low, reflecting long-standing liver injury. Severe coagulopathy, conjugated hyperbilirubinemia, hypoalbuminemia, thrombocytopenia, and hypoglycemia are common, reflecting marked hepatocellular injury.

The diagnosis of NH is based on clinical and pathologic findings and requires the exclusion of all other causes of neonatal liver failure. In an infant suspected of having NH on the basis of clinical findings or family history, the demonstration of iron deposition in multiple organs is necessary for definitive diagnosis. In individuals with NH, excessive parenchymal iron has been seen in the liver, pancreas, heart, and other organs with sparing of the spleen, bone marrow, and other sites of the reticuloendothelial system. Markedly elevated serum ferritin concentrations would be supportive but not definitive of NH. Infants with NH are severely ill and coagulopathic, which usually precludes a percutaneous liver biopsy because of bleeding risk. When liver biopsy is not feasible, lip or gingival biopsy of minor salivary glands to assess for iron deposition has been suggested. Six of seven infants with NH had positive biopsy findings of iron deposition in salivary glands, whereas there were four infants without NH who did not have iron present. Abdominal magnetic resonance imaging (MRI) has been performed to look for evidence of iron overload in hepatic and extrahepatic tissues.

Neonatal Hemochromatosis and Hereditary Hemochromatosis

There are four types of primary iron overload disorders in adults with parenchymal iron accumulation classified by the Online Mendelian Inheritance in Man. These include *HFE*-related hereditary hemochromatosis, juvenile hereditary hemochromatosis subtypes A and B,

Table 31-1	Disorders of Neonatal Liver Failure with High Iron Deposition in the Liver and Other Organs with Reticuloendothelial Sparing		
Disease Category	Disease	Hepatic Iron Content	Diagnostic Tests
Metabolic	Neonatal Hemochromatosis	+++	Salivary gland or liver biopsy Hepatic and extrahepatic iron overload on magnetic resonance imaging (MRI) Serum ferritin
	Delta^4-3-oxosteroid 5β-reductase deficiency	+++	Urinary bile acid analysis by fast atom-bombardment mass spectroscopy
	Tyrosinemia	++	Urine succinylacetone Plasma quantitative amino acids Alpha-fetoprotein
Storage disease	Zellweger syndrome	+	Quantitative very long-chain fatty acids
Infections	Echovirus 9	+++	Culture from pharynx or blood Polymerase chain reaction
	Cytomegalovirus	+++	Buffy coat antigen Polymerase chain reaction
	Herpes simplex virus	++	Cultures from nasopharynx, rectal swab and lesions
	Parvovirus B19	+	IgM Polymerase chain reaction
	Rubella	+	IgM Culture from urine or nasopharynx
Other	Mitochondrial cytopathy	++	Muscle or liver biopsy for analysis of respiratory chain enzyme defect Lactic acidosis

+, ++, and +++ indicate minimal, moderate, and high relative quantities of iron in liver tissue, respectively.
From Murray KF, Kowdley KV: Neonatal hemochromatosis. Pediatrics 108:960-964, 2001.

and TfR2-related hereditary hemochromatosis. Our understanding of the pathophysiology of these iron-loading disorders is much greater than our understanding of NH. The gene and gene product for each of these disorders have been identified. (See article by Pietrangelo in "Suggested Readings" for complete review.) Unlike NH, the pattern of inheritance has been established as autosomal recessive. NH is the only disorder in which symptomatic disease occurs in the neonate. The main similarities among these disorders are that iron deposition is found in the parenchymal cells rather than reticuloendothelial cells and the predominant organs of iron accumulation include the liver, endocrine glands, and heart.

The most common form of hereditary hemochromatosis is associated with mutation of the *HFE* gene, which is located on chromosome 6. In the majority of cases, the mutation is a single-base change that results in the substitution of tyrosine for cysteine at position 282 of the HFE protein (C282Y). Homozygosity for the C282Y mutation is found in approximately 1 of every 200 people of Northern European descent. Approximately 1% to 2% of individuals who are compound heterozygote for C282Y and H63D (aspartic acid replaces histidine at position 63) seem predisposed to disease expression.

Although the metabolic defect is present at birth, HFE-hereditary hemochromatosis rarely manifests before adulthood, because it usually takes many years of excessive iron absorption in the intestinal mucosa before toxic accumulation occurs in the liver and other organs. Furthermore, not all individuals will develop disease. Expression of the disease is variable and is in part influenced by dietary iron intake and by physiologic and pathologic blood loss. Women are affected less frequently than men, probably because menstruation and childbearing decrease the iron burden. The natural history of the disease is unknown, although gradual progression of iron accumulation seems to occur with symptoms of unexplained fatigue or joint pain generally seen in midlife.

Children of individuals diagnosed with hemochromatosis may be taken to a physician because parents are concerned that their child will inherit the disease. Genetic testing for mutations in HFE is readily available, and children who have inherited the mutations can be identified.

Further testing with laboratory markers of iron overload, transferrin saturation, and ferritin should be done to assess and monitor for iron overload. Treatment for individuals with iron overload due to HFE-hereditary hemochromatosis is phlebotomy. Studies in adults have established that early diagnosis and treatment are essential to prevent complications of liver cirrhosis, organ failure, and primary hepatocellular carcinoma.

Because the function of HFE involves interacting with transferrin receptor, and HFE was shown to interact with the transferrin receptor in human placenta, it raises the possibility that HFE may play a role in NH. In several families with neonatal hemochromatosis, however, molecular analysis of the HFE gene found no evidence of pathogenic mutations segregating with the disease phenotype. Furthermore, we are not aware of any reports of women with HFE-hereditary hemochromatosis giving birth to infants with NH.

TREATMENT

Medical Therapies

Antioxidant Therapy

A regimen of iron chelation and antioxidant therapy (Table 31-2) has been given to infants with NH. This therapy has not been tested in a randomized controlled trial because the disease is rare, treatment at a single institution with few patients is impossible, and placebo control would be difficult. Iron chelation therapy in the form of subcutaneous deferoxamine in one individual revealed no changes in clinical, biochemical, or histologic findings, and the infant subsequently died at 3 months of age. More favorable results were reported in three individuals treated with a combination of iron chelation and antioxidant therapy. N-acetylcysteine, alpha-tocopherol polyethylene glycol succinate (TPGS) and selenium in addition to prostaglandin E_1 and deferoxamine were given between 1 and 14 days of age in infants, with improvement noted within 3 days of therapy and subsequent recovery. A subsequent study revealed that in eight patients treated with an antioxidant-chelation cocktail, seven died before liver transplantation and one stabilized on therapy but never recovered and ultimately required liver transplantation. The authors also noted that prostaglandin infusion and deferoxamine administration were not entirely benign in their small group of patients. Several infants apparently had pulmonary fluid overload associated with patency of the ductus arteriosus with prostaglandin infusion. In addition, there was a concern that a fatal infection in one infant was related to use of deferoxamine.

High-Dose Immunoglobulin Therapy in Pregnancy

A promising therapy to prevent subsequent pregnancies resulting in an infant with NH is to give pregnant females high-dose immunoglobulins. In 15 women whose most recent pregnancy ended in documented NH, 1 g/kg weekly intravenous immunoglobulin was given during 16 pregnancies starting at 18 weeks until the end of gestation. Twelve of these infants reportedly had some liver dysfunction; 11 infants had elevated ferritin and alpha-fetoprotein concentrations. Seven infants with liver dysfunction or biopsy-proved liver injury with iron overload were treated with a chelation and antioxidant cocktail. Four neonates had no evidence of liver injury, and it is unclear whether NH would have developed. All 16 infants survived and were healthy at 6 months' follow-up.

SURGICAL THERAPY

Liver Transplantation

Orthotopic liver transplantation has been successful in NH. In 14 patients diagnosed with NH between 1985 and 1995, 60% of transplanted patients survived more than 1 year. It is generally recognized that children with fulminant hepatic failure would be considered for liver transplantation and management focused on supporting the patient, including the consideration of the antioxidant and chelation regimen, until either clear recovery occurs or transplantation is performed.

APPROACH TO THE CASE

Assessment was that the infant had neonatal liver failure. Initial considerations were (1) metabolic disorders such as hemochromatosis, delta^4-3 oxosteroid 5B-reductase deficiency, tyrosinemia and mitochondrial cytopathy; (2) infections, including cytomegalovirus,

Table 31-2 Deferoxamine Chelation Therapy and Antioxidant Cocktail

d-alpha tocopherol polyethylene glycol succinate (TPGS) 25 IU/kg/day orally for 6 weeks
N-acetylcysteine 140 mg/kg oral loading dose, then 70 mg/kg every 4 hours for 19 doses
Prostaglandin-E_1 0.4 μg/kg/hour intravenously (IV) for maximum of 2 weeks
Selenium 3 μg/kg/day IV with deferoxamine 30 mg/kg/day IV until serum ferritin <500 ng/mL

echovirus, herpes simplex virus, parvovirus B19, adenovirus; and (3) bacterial infection.

Studies considered were serum ferritin level, urinary bile acid atom-bombardment, urine succinylacetone and alpha-fetoprotein, lactate, cytomegalovirus polymerase chain reaction (CMV PCR), culture from pharynx, echovirus 9 PCR, rectal swab for herpes culture, parvovirus B19 PCR, and blood and urine cultures. Acyclovir was suggested because of the possibility of herpesvirus infection.

Serum ferritin concentration was greater than 2000 μg/L. Liver biopsy was not attempted because of worsening coagulopathy. A lower lip biopsy was performed, and stainable iron was found in the minor salivary glands, consistent with the diagnosis of NH. The patient was supported by medical management and listed for orthotopic liver transplantation. Antioxidant therapy was initiated but the infant subsequently developed sepsis and died.

Autopsy revealed pronounced iron overload in parenchymal cells of the liver, pancreas, and heart with sparing of the spleen and other sites of the reticuloendothelial system. The mother was referred to a center for evaluation of high-dose immunoglobulin therapy for subsequent pregnancies.

SUMMARY

NH is a rare condition in which iron accumulates in the liver and extrahepatic sites in the fetus and is associated with neonatal liver failure. Other etiologies of liver failure need to be considered. A complete history including previous fetal deaths should be obtained because therapy for subsequent pregnancies may prove helpful.

MAJOR POINTS

NH usually manifests within hours of birth.
Neonates are critically ill and the disorder is often fatal as a result of hepatic or renal failure unless liver transplantation is performed.
Physical examination of an infant with NH reveals severe liver failure.
There is approximately an 80% probability that each subsequent baby born to the same mother will be affected.
There is no laboratory test available to establish the diagnosis of NH.
NH demonstrates a classic pattern of chronic end-stage liver disease at birth.
The diagnosis of NH is based on clinical and pathologic findings and requires the exclusion of all other causes of neonatal liver failure.

A buccal biopsy should be considered to identify iron overload in extrahepatic tissues when severe coagulopathy precludes liver biopsy. Medical treatment, including iron chelation has been used as well as liver transplantation in cases of no improvement. High-dose immunoglobulin during pregnancy for recurrent neonatal hemochromatosis has been given with promising results.

SUGGESTED READINGS

Cheung PC, Ng WF, Chan AK: Neonatal haemochromatosis associated with Down syndrome. J Paediatr Child Health 31:249-52, 1995.

Flynn DM, Mohan N, McKiernan P, et al: Progress in treatment and outcome for children with neonatal haemochromatosis. Arch Dis Child Fetal Neonatal Ed 88:124-127, 2003.

Jaaskelainen J, Martikainen A, Vornanen M, Heinonen K: Neonatal haemochromatosis combined with duodenal atresia. Eur J Pediatr 154:247-248, 1995.

Johal JS, Thorp JW, Oyer CE: Neonatal hemochromatosis, renal tubular dysgenesis, and hypocalvaria in a neonate. Pediatr Dev Pathol 1:433-437, 1998.

Jonas MM, Kaweblum YA, Fajaco R: Neonatal hemochromatosis: Failure of deferoxamine therapy. J Pediatr Gastroenterol Nutr 6:984-988, 1987.

Kelly AL, Lunt PW, Rodrigues F, et al: Classification and genetic features of neonatal haemochromatosis: A study of 27 affected pedigrees and molecular analysis of genes implicated in iron metabolism. J Med Genet 38:599-610, 2001.

Kershisnik MM, Knisely AS, Sun C-C J, et al: Cytomegalovirus infection, fetal liver disease, and neonatal hemochromatosis. Hum Pathol 23:1075-1080, 1992.

Knisely AS, Harford JB, Klausner RD, Taylor SR: Neonatal hemochromatosis: The regulation of transferrin-receptor and ferritin synthesis by iron in cultured fibroblastic-line cells. Am J Pathol 134:439-445, 1989.

Knisely AS, O'Shea PA, Stocks JF, Dimmick JE: Oropharyngeal and upper respiratory tract mucosal gland siderosis in neonatal hemochromatosis: An approach to biopsy diagnosis. J Pediatr 113:871-874, 1988.

Lee WS, Mckiernan PJ, Kelly DA: Serum ferritin level in neonatal fulminant liver failure. Arch Dis Child Fetal Neonatal Ed 85:F226, 2001.

Lund DP, Lillehei CW, Kevy S, et al: Liver transplantation in newborn liver failure: Treatment for neonatal hemochromatosis. Transplant Proc 25:1068-1071, 1993.

Metzman R, Anand A, DeGiulio PA, Knisely AS: Hepatic disease associated with intrauterine parvovirus B19 infection in a newborn premature infant. J Pediatr Gastroenterol Nutr 9:112-114, 1989.

Morris S, Akima S, Dahlstrom JE, et al: Renal tubular dysgenesis and neonatal hemochromatosis without pulmonary hypoplasia. Pediatr Nephrol 19:341-334, 2004.

Murray KF, Kowdley KV: Neonatal hemochromatosis. Pediatrics 108:960-964, 2001.

Niederau C, Fischer R, Purschel A, et al: Long-term survival in patients with hereditary hemochromatosis. Gastroenterology 110:1107-1119, 1996.

Oddone M, Bellini C, Bonacci W, et al: Diagnosis of neonatal hemochromatosis with MR imaging in duplex Doppler sonography. Eur Radiol 9:1882-1885, 1999.

Parizhskaya M, Reyes J, Jaffe R: Hemophagocytic syndrome presenting as acute hepatic failure in two infants: Clinical overlap with neonatal hemochromatosis. Pediatr Dev Pathol 2:360-366, 1999.

Parkhila S, Waheed A, Britton RS, et al: Association of the transferrin receptor in human placenta with HFE, the protein defective in hereditary hemochromatosis. Proc Natl Acad Sci U S A 94:13198-202, 1997.

Pietrangelo A: Hereditary hemochromatosis: A new look at an old disease. N Engl J Med 350:2383-2397, 2004.

Rand EB, McClenathan DT, Whitington PF: Neonatal hemochromatosis: Report of successful orthotopic liver transplantation. J Pediatr Gastroenterol Nutr 15:325-329, 1992.

Roberts EA: Neonatal hepatitis syndrome. Semin Neonatol 8:357-374, 2003.

Rochette J, Pointon JJ, Fisher CA, et al: Multicentric origin of hemochromatosis gene (HFE) mutations. Am J Hum Genet 64:1056-1062, 1999.

Schoenlege J, Buyon JP, Zitelli BJ, et al: Neonatal hemochromatosis associated with maternal autoantibodies against Ro/SS-A and La/SS-B ribonucleoproteins. Am J Dis Child 147:1072, 1993.

Shamieh I, Kibart PK, Suchy FJ, Freese D: Antioxidant therapy for neonatal iron storage disease (NISD). Pediatr Res 33:109A, 1993.

Shneider BL, Setchell KDR, Whitington PF, et al: Delta 4-3-oxosteroid 5 beta-reductase deficiency causing neonatal liver failure and hemochromatosis. J Pediatr 124:234-238, 1994.

Sigurdsson L, Reyes J, Kocoshis SA, et al: Neonatal hemochromasosis: Outcomes of pharmacologic and surgical therapies. J Pediatr Gastroenterol Nutr 26:85-89, 1998.

Smith SR, Shneider BL, Magid M, et al: Minor salivary gland biopsy in neonatal hemochromatosis. Arch Otoloaryngol Head Neck Surg 130:760-763, 2004.

Taucher SC, Bentjerodt R, Hubner ME, Nazer J: Multiple malformations in neonatal hemochromatosis. Am J Med Genet 50:213-214, 1994.

Verloes A, Lombet J, Lambert Y, et al: Tricho-hepato-enteric syndrome: Further delineation of a distinct syndrome with neonatal hemochromatosis phenotype, intractable diarrhea, and hair anomalies. Amer J Med Genet 68:391-395, 1997.

Whitington PF, Hibbard JU: High-dose immunoglobulin during pregnancy for recurrent neonatal haemochromatosis. Lancet 364:1690-1698, 2005.

Whitington PF, Malladi P: Neonatal hemochromatosis: Is it an alloimmune disease? J Pediatr Gastroenterol Nutr 40:544-549, 2005.

CHAPTER 32

Metabolic Liver Disease: Tyrosinemia, Galactosemia, and Hereditary Fructose Intolerance

RANDOLPH P. MATTHEWS

Disease Description
Case Presentation
Epidemiology
   Tyrosinemia
   Galactosemia
   Hereditary Fructose Intolerance
Pathophysiology
   Tyrosinemia
   Galactosemia
   Hereditary Fructose Intolerance
Differential Diagnosis
Diagnostic Testing
Treatment
   Tyrosinemia
   Galactosemia
   Hereditary Fructose Intolerance
Approach to the Case
Summary
Major Points

DISEASE DESCRIPTION

Inborn errors of metabolism are important causes of liver disease in children, particularly infants. Tyrosinemia, galactosemia, and hereditary fructose intolerance are metabolic disorders caused by defects in the breakdown of tyrosine, galactose, and fructose, respectively. The genetic lack of specific enzymes in these breakdown pathways results in the accumulation of toxic byproducts and/or a disruption of normal metabolism that causes the manifestations of the specific diseases. These conditions are amenable to treatment with diet, and in the case of tyrosinemia, with medication as well.

CASE PRESENTATION

Our patient presented at the age of 4 months with hepatosplenomegaly. She was the product of a normal full-term pregnancy notable only for the presence of an elevated alpha-fetoprotein in her mother. The patient was doing well until the age of 2 months, when she was admitted to a local hospital for dehydration following a viral illness. She was noted at that time to have thrombocytopenia. Her pediatrician monitored this after discharge, and the patient was subsequently noted to have abdominal distention and hypoalbuminemia. She was never noted to be jaundiced or fussy, and she was gaining weight on breast milk and soy formula. Her mother is of mixed European ancestry, and her father is Jewish.

On presentation, her weight and length are at the 75th percentile. She is well appearing and her examination is notable for the abdominal distention, with the liver 4 to 5 cm below the right costal margin and the spleen palpable 5 cm below the left costal margin. Laboratory studies are notable for normal transaminases, moderately elevated gamma-glutamyl-transpeptidase, and markedly elevated alkaline phosphatase, prothrombin time, and partial thromboplastin time. She also has mild unconjugated hyperbilirubinemia and the hypoalbuminemia previously noted. She continues to have thrombocytopenia but is not anemic and has a normal white blood cell count. Her urine is abnormal, with trace amounts of glucose and protein. An abdominal ultrasound shows a "coarse" liver and some abdominal fluid but is otherwise unremarkable. The decision is made to admit her to the hospital for further evaluation and correction of her coagulopathy.

EPIDEMIOLOGY

Tyrosinemia

Tyrosinemia is an autosomal recessive disorder, with an estimated birth rate of 1 in 100,000 to 1 in 120,000 worldwide. The disease is significantly more common in Quebec and Scandinavia, with a rate of 1 in approximately 17,000 in Quebec and 1 in approximately 1900 in the Saguenay–Lac–St.-Jean area of Quebec. Tyrosinemia type I is caused by a lack of the enzyme fumarylacetoacetate hydrolase (FAH), whereas the less common type II is caused by a lack of the enzyme tyrosine aminotransferase. Tyrosinemia type III is even less common, and is caused by a defect in 4-hydroxyphenylpyruvate dioxygenase; liver disease in both type II and type III is exceedingly rare. Several mutations in the *FAH* gene have been identified in patients with tyrosinemia type I, one of which is common in patients from northern Quebec.

Galactosemia

The most common defect causing galactosemia, another autosomal recessive disorder, is a defect in galactose-1-phosphate uridyl transferase. There have been more than 150 distinct mutations described in this gene. Of these mutations, several lead to the severe "classic" form of galactosemia, whereas others lead to milder forms, the most common of which is the "Duarte" variant. The rate of classic galactosemia is 1 in 50,000 live births, whereas the rate for all forms of galactosemia is around 1 in 10,000 live births. Galactokinase deficiency, which also results in galactosemia, is significantly less common than the transferase deficiency form of the disease, and it does not lead to liver disease. Uridine diphosphate galactose-4-epimerase deficiency also results in galactosemia and is similarly rare, but it does occasionally lead to liver disease similar to the transferase deficiency.

Hereditary Fructose Intolerance

Hereditary fructose intolerance is caused by a lack of the enzyme fructose-1-phosphate aldolase. This condition is also an autosomal recessive disorder, affecting the aldolase B gene, with a frequency of 1 in 20,000.

PATHOPHYSIOLOGY

Tyrosinemia

The cardinal features of tyrosinemia include chronic liver disease and cirrhosis, acute liver failure (liver "crisis"), renal Fanconi syndrome, neurologic crises involving paresthesias and paralysis, and a risk of hepatocellular carcinoma. Tyrosine, a nonessential amino acid, is important in protein synthesis and is the precursor of several neurotransmitters. Tyrosine may be obtained directly from the diet or may be synthesized from phenylalanine by phenylalanine hydroxylase, the enzyme that is deficient in phenylketonuria. Fumarylacetoacetate hydrolase (FAH) is the final step in the breakdown of tyrosine, catalyzing the breakdown of fumarylacetoacetate into fumarate and acetoacetate (Fig. 32-1). Blockage of FAH leads to the accumulation of fumarylacetoacetate as well as its upstream precursor maleylacetoacetate, and the alternative breakdown products of fumarylacetoacetate, succinylacetone, and succinylace-

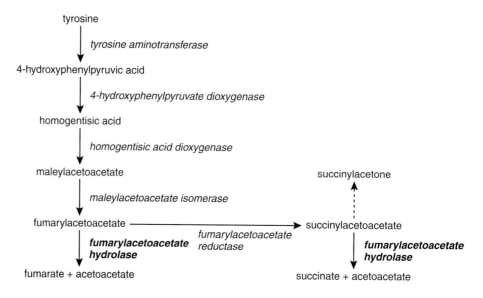

Figure 32-1 Metabolism of tyrosine. The breakdown of tyrosine is depicted. Enzymes are indicated in italics. Cofactors in certain steps are omitted to simplify the diagram. The defective enzyme in type I tyrosinemia is depicted in bold italics. N-TBC inhibits 4-hydroxyphenylpyruvate dioxygenase.

toacetate. It is likely that at least some of these compounds are responsible for the pathologic features of tyrosinemia. Tyrosinemia type II and type III affect more upstream enzymes, and thus are not associated with elevations of succinylacetone and the consequent liver and kidney damage.

A trigger such as a viral illness generally precipitates liver crises. Typical symptoms of a crisis are hepatomegaly, ascites, and coagulopathy, occasionally with overt bleeding. The degree of prolongation of the prothrombin time and partial thromboplastin time is almost always out of proportion to the increase of the aminotransferases. The compounds upstream of FAH, in particular fumarylacetoacetate itself, are most likely causative; rarely, serum tyrosine and phenylalanine levels will rise, but these compounds are not toxic even in excess. Cirrhosis is likely the result of chronic exposure to fumarylacetoacetate and succinylacetone. Interestingly, fumarylacetoacetate and maleylacetoacetate resemble maleic acid, which has been shown to cause renal Fanconi syndrome; these compounds also are associated with a decrease in glutathione and thus greater susceptibility to liver damage by other compounds.

Neurologic crises, involving pain and/or paralysis, are caused by succinylacetone and its effect on the porphoryin pathway. Succinylacetone inhibits the enzyme delta-aminolevulinic acid dehydratase, and elevated delta-aminolevulinic acid is toxic and leads to neurologic crises. Finally, the nodules and potential hepatocellular carcinoma likely result from fumarylacetoacetate, which is a mutagen. The nodules are areas of normal liver that have reverted to wild-type secondary to a mutation and thus have a growth advantage. Over time, the mutagenic activity can lead to hepatocellular carcinoma, which can occur in patients as young as 15 months and may have an incidence as high as 37%.

Galactosemia

The normal metabolism of galactose is depicted in Figure 32-2. Deficiency of the galactose-1-phosphate uridyl transferase enzyme results in the buildup of galactose-1-phosphate, as well as the alcohol and amine forms of galactose, galactitol, and galactosamine. Accumulation of these compounds in specific tissues leads to the pathologic changes associated with galactosemia. The clinical manifestation of liver disease is typically the early development of jaundice and hepatomegaly. Galactosemic patients may present with vomiting and diarrhea, failure to thrive, and/or a hemolytic anemia. In addition to the liver, patients with galactosemia may have problems in the brain, kidney, lens, and ovary. These manifest as more long-term sequelae of galactosemia, as mental retardation, renal tubular dysfunction leading to renal Fanconi syndrome, cataracts, and infertility. Additionally, these patients are at greater risk for infection by *Escherichia coli*, especially in the neonatal period.

Because a large amount of galactose metabolism occurs in the liver, defects in the transferase enzyme lead to ready accumulation of toxic metabolites after exposure to galactose. Although it is not clear precisely which metabolite results in liver damage, buildup of these metabolites is associated with liver damage. Galactitol accumulates in the brain, which probably accounts for the longer-term changes in the brain such as developmental delay and mental retardation. Although there may be defects in the transferase enzyme in the intestine, vomiting and diarrhea are more likely secondary to effects of metabolite accumulation in the brain and nervous system. In the kidney, accumulation of galactose-1-phosphate appears to be responsible for causing the renal tubular dysfunction, whereas galactitol and the resulting water accumulation appear to be the cause of the cataracts. The mechanism by which ovarian failure occurs is unclear,

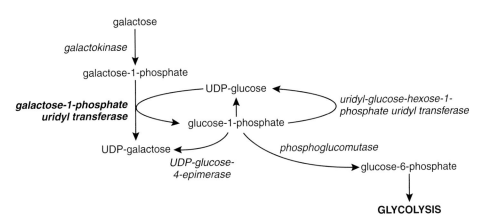

Figure 32-2 Metabolism of galactose. The breakdown of galactose is depicted. Enzymes are indicated in italics. Cofactors in certain steps are omitted to simplify the diagram, but uridine diphosphate (UDP) glucose is included as it is an intermediate as well. The enzymatic defect in galactosemia is noted in bold italics.

although the cause appears to be hypogonadotropic hypogonadism. The increased susceptibility to *E. coli* infection is likely a result of impaired bactericidal activity of leukocytes deficient in transferase activity in the presence of galactose.

Hereditary Fructose Intolerance

The pathogenesis of hereditary fructose intolerance is related to the age of the patient and the degree of exposure to fructose. Although galactose is a component of lactose and is thus present in milk, the primary exposure to fructose in infancy is from fruit or from sucrose (glucose plus fructose) found in baby foods. The normal metabolism of fructose is depicted in Figure 32-3. As suggested by the figure, a defect in aldolase results in accumulation of fructose-1-phosphate, which appears to be the toxic metabolite in hereditary fructose intolerance. Accumulation of fructose-1-phosphate in the liver, kidneys, and small intestine—tissues in which aldolase B is present—results in the pathologic features found in hereditary fructose intolerance. In addition to hepatic failure, hereditary fructose intolerance is associated with abdominal pain, vomiting, and diarrhea. As with the preceding conditions, these patients also may have a renal Fanconi syndrome; they also develop hypoglycemia, hypophosphatemia, hyperuricemia, and elevated lactic acid.

The pathology of hereditary fructose intolerance results from accumulation of the metabolites upstream of the enzymatic block, in this case accumulation of fructose-1-phosphate. Because fructose-1-phosphate cannot be metabolized, phosphate metabolism is impaired and adenosine triphosphate (ATP) is depleted. Depletion of ATP results in purine degradation and hyperuricemia, and probably results in the liver toxicity because of impaired energy metabolism. Hypoglycemia likely results from an inhibition of glycogenolysis and gluconeogenesis by fructose-1-phosphate itself. The renal dysfunction is likely secondary to the loss of ATP in the kidney tubules.

DIFFERENTIAL DIAGNOSIS

Our patient presented with hepatosplenomegaly and signs of liver failure, specifically hypoalbuminemia and coagulopathy. Although that presentation is certainly not specific for metabolic liver disease, there are clues in the presentation that suggest metabolic disease. Metabolic liver disease, defined as liver disease associated with an underlying disease that affects biochemical pathways of energy metabolism, can present as congenital ascites, neonatal cholestasis, fulminant liver failure, or a more indolent course. Clues suggestive of metabolic liver disease associated with any of these presentations are listed in Table 32-1.

Metabolic causes of indolent hepatic failure, as seen in the presentation of our patient, are listed in Table 32-2. More severe neonatal hepatic failure may be caused by overwhelming infection, neonatal iron storage disease, lysosomal storage disease, or a mitochondropathy. Of the causes of a more indolent hepatic failure listed in Table 32-2 and not discussed elsewhere, α_1-antitrypsin deficiency results in the accumulation of α_1-antitrypsin within the hepatocytes and may have any type of presentation of liver disease, including failure, and may manifest at any age. There are several types of bile acid synthetic disorders, some of which may cause indolent hepatic failure. Congenital disorders of glycosylation are a heterogeneous group of rare disorders that also manifest in a variety of presentations at any age, though failure is more common in infants than in older children.

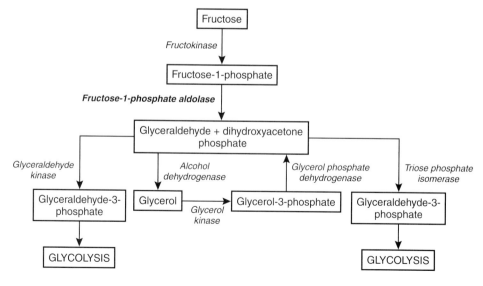

Figure 32-3 Metabolism of fructose. The breakdown of fructose is depicted. Enzymes are indicated in italics. Cofactors in certain steps are omitted to simplify the diagram. The enzymatic defect in hereditary fructose intolerance is noted in bold italics.

Table 32-1 Clues to a Metabolic Etiology of Liver Disease
Historical Clues
Paroxysmal nature of disease
Irritability or increased fussiness
Coma, lethargy, or increased sleepiness
Seizures
Vomiting
Poor feeding
Failure to thrive
Family history
Physical Examination Clues
Abnormal odor
Coma
Hypotonia
Hepatomegaly without splenomegaly
Hepatosplenomegaly without jaundice
Ascites
Dysmorphic features
Screening Laboratory/Diagnostic Study Clues
Hypoglycemia
Low serum bicarbonate/lactic acidosis
Coagulopathy or hypoalbuminemia with only mild hepatitis or hyperbilirubinemia
Anemia
Concurrent *Escherichia coli* infection
Abnormal urinalysis (especially glucosuria or proteinuria)
Abnormal echotexture of liver on ultrasound

Table 32-2 Metabolic Causes of Indolent Hepatic Failure in Children

	Infant	Child	Adolescent
α_1-Antitrypsin deficiency	x	x	x
Bile acid synthetic disorder	x	x	x
Cystic fibrosis	x	x	x
Congenital disorders of glycosylation	x	x	
Fatty acid oxidation disorder		x	
Galactosemia	x		
Glycogen storage disease	x	x	
Hereditary fructose intolerance	x		
Neonatal iron storage disease	x		
Tyrosinemia	x	x	
Wilson's disease		x	x
Wolman's disease	x		

Fatty acid oxidation disorders, the most common of which is medium-chain acyl-coenzyme A dehydrogenase (MCAD) deficiency, may present with hepatic failure in the older infant or young child, typically with encephalopathy as a cardinal feature. Cystic fibrosis may lead to hepatic failure at any age, although this presentation is more common if there is another cause of liver disease as well, which is also the case for α_1-antitrypsin deficiency. There are many types of glycogen storage disease, but it is principally type IV, or a defect in the debranching enzyme, that results in neonatal or infantile hepatic failure; other types, particularly types I and II, are more associated with hepatomegaly and hypoglycemia. Neonatal iron storage disease is an idiopathic form of neonatal liver failure that is usually fulminant, in which there is a large amount of iron deposited in the liver and other tissues; there is no relation between this condition and hemochromatosis. Wilson's disease is a disorder of copper metabolism in which copper builds up in the liver, eyes, and brain, and does not present until school age at the earliest. Wolman's disease is a disorder of cholesterol metabolism caused by a deficiency of lysosomal acid lipase A, which results in severe neonatal liver failure and adrenal calcification.

Many of these diseases have associated features that may distinguish them. Although some features, such as the neurologic disease of tyrosinemia or *E. coli* infection in galactosemia, are more specific, other associated findings, such as renal Fanconi syndrome, are somewhat less specific. Renal Fanconi syndrome is a form of renal tubular dysfunction in which the tubules leak glucose, phosphate, uric acid, and amino acids. Causes of renal Fanconi syndrome in which liver disease is also present are listed in Table 32-3. From these tables, the differential diagnosis of the case presented includes tyrosinemia, galactosemia, hereditary fructose intolerance, and perhaps glycogen storage disease type IV.

The typical presentation of a child with tyrosinemia, galactosemia, or hereditary fructose intolerance is of a

Table 32-3 Causes of Renal Fanconi Syndrome and Liver Disease
Galactosemia
Glycogen storage disease
Hereditary fructose intolerance
Mitochondrial disorders
Tyrosinemia
Wilson's disease

child in hepatic failure, as is the case for the presentation here. As stated, associated findings, such as vomiting, diarrhea, and failure to thrive, also are occasionally present. Tyrosinemia and galactosemia generally present in the neonatal or infant period, and neonates in particular can be severely affected. The presentation of hereditary fructose intolerance in particular is more variable and is age dependent, with generally milder symptoms more common in older children. In such milder presentations, the differential diagnosis includes various storage diseases and other causes of liver disease in older children.

DIAGNOSTIC TESTING

The threshold for suspicion for metabolic liver disease should be low, especially when features noted in Table 32-1 are present in a child with hepatic failure. General screening laboratory tests can provide clues to metabolic diseases, and more specialized screening studies should be performed in any patient in whom metabolic disease is even remotely suspected. Routine and specialized screening tests, along with the findings suggesting specific metabolic disorders, are listed in Table 32-4. Many of these studies will screen for metabolic disorders that only rarely if ever affect the liver; these disorders are not discussed here. More importantly, some of these tests are only abnormal during an acute exacerbation of the metabolic disorder. Other tests performed routinely on patients with liver disease, such as an ultrasound, may be helpful occasionally, because tyrosinemia, in particular, occasionally demonstrates a nodular or coarse appearance on ultrasound, even in the early stages.

In addition to the screening laboratory studies mentioned, more specific blood and urine tests may be performed to evaluate for tyrosinemia, galactosemia, or hereditary fructose intolerance. Blood and urine may be screened for succinylacetone, the toxic metabolite in tyrosinemia, as well as for galactitol, a toxic metabolite found in galactosemia. There is no blood or urine test for fructose-1-phosphate, but the diagnosis may be established by a fructose tolerance test. In this test, patients are given intravenous fructose in a con-

Table 32-4 Screening Tests for Metabolic Diseases

Test	Abnormal Result	Disorder
Screening Labs		
Basic chemistry panel	Metabolic acidosis	Organic acidurias, primary lactic acidemias
Glucose	Hypoglycemia	Fatty acid oxidation disorders, some primary lactic acidemias, some organic acidurias, glycogen storage diseases, hereditary fructose intolerance
Magnesium	Below normal	Hereditary fructose intolerance
Phosphate	Below normal	Hereditary fructose intolerance
Ammonia	Elevated	Hepatic encephalopathy, urea cycle disorders
Urinalysis	Ketonuria	Organic acidurias, primary lactic acidemias
	Renal tubular acidosis, proteinuria, glucosuria	Renal Fanconi syndrome
	Positive reducing substances (and no glucosuria)	Galactosemia, hereditary fructose intolerance
Metabolic Labs		
Lactate/pyruvate	Elevated	Primary lactic acidemia
Serum amino acids	Elevation of specific amino acids	Tyrosinemia, others
Acylcarnitine profile	Elevation of specific components	Fatty acid oxidation disorders
Urine amino acids	Elevation of specific amino acids	Renal Fanconi syndrome
Urine organic acids	Elevation of specific organic acids	Disorders of amino acid metabolism, others
Specific Tests		
Urine and/or blood succinylacetone	Elevated	Tyrosinemia
Liver or skin fumarylacetoacetate hydrolase activity	Decreased or absent	Tyrosinemia
Urine and/or blood galactitol	Elevated	Galactosemia
Blood galactose-1-phosphate uridyl transferase activity	Decreased or absent	Galactosemia
Liver or intestinal aldolase B activity	Decreased or absent	Hereditary fructose intolerance
Fructose tolerance test	Abnormal	Hereditary fructose intolerance
Blood genetic testing	Specific mutation	Tyrosinemia, galactosemia, or hereditary fructose intolerance

trolled setting, and blood levels of glucose and phosphate are drawn serially; if the levels fall, the patient is diagnosed with hereditary fructose intolerance.

Tests of enzymatic activity for tyrosinemia, galactosemia, and hereditary fructose intolerance have been the standard diagnostic tests for definitive establishment of the diagnosis. Fumarylacetoacetate hydrolase activity can be tested on liver tissue or on cultured skin fibroblasts, whereas galactose-1-phosphate uridyl transferase activity can be measured in red blood cells. Aldolase B activity is most frequently measured on liver tissue from a percutaneous biopsy, although an intestinal biopsy could also be used. In general, a liver biopsy is not often required for diagnosis of metabolic liver disease, but it can be helpful to exclude other causes of liver disease and to look for storage diseases, and to perform testing for specific enzyme activities. Furthermore, it may be helpful to gauge the degree of liver damage, and biopsies can be performed serially to monitor the response to treatment.

Genetic testing for tyrosinemia, galactosemia, and hereditary fructose intolerance is becoming used more frequently. Specific mutations can be tested for, and this technique is most useful in the diagnosis of hereditary fructose intolerance, because of the lack of a screenable metabolite. In general, however, the diagnoses of these conditions can be made using the tests mentioned earlier. The standard diagnostic test for tyrosinemia is the presence of succinylacetone in the urine or blood, whereas the clinching test for galactosemia is considered to be decreased activity of the galactose-1-phosphate uridyl transferase enzyme in blood. The definitive diagnosis of hereditary fructose intolerance is the fructose tolerance test, although decreased aldolase B activity in liver or intestinal tissue or the mutation analysis may establish the diagnosis as well.

Because of rapidly improving technology allowing sophisticated testing on a small sample of blood, many states in the United States are able to offer and thus require extensive newborn screens. All states require screening for galactosemia and most require testing for tyrosinemia. No state requires testing for hereditary fructose intolerance, most likely because of technical difficulties in screening for a condition in which there is no neonatal exposure to the offending agent. Table 32-5 lists the diseases screened by each state, but many hospitals offer more testing than is required.

Table 32-5 Newborn Screens in the United States by State

Alabama—B, C, F, G, Hy, P, S, TMS
Alaska—B, C, F, G, Hy, M, Ma, O, P, S, T, TMS
Arizona—B, C, F, G, Ho, Hy, M, O, P, S, T, TMS
Arkansas—G, Hy, P, S
California*—C, F, G, Hy, O, P, S, T, TMS
Colorado—B, C, Cf, F, G, Hy, O, P, S, T, TMS
Connecticut—B, C, F, G, Ho, Hy, M, O, P, S, T, TMS
Delaware—B, C, F, G, Ho, Hy, M, O, P, S, T, TMS
District of Columbia—B, F, G, G6, Hy, Ho, M, O, P, S, T, TMS
Florida—C, F, G, Hy, O, P, S, T, TMS
Georgia—B, C, Cf, F, G, Ho, Hy, M, O, P, S, T, TMS
Hawaii—B, C, F, G, Hy, M, Ma, O, P, S, T, TMS
Idaho—B, C, Cf, F, G, Hy, M, Ma, O, P, S, T, TMS
Illinois—B, C, F, G, Hy, M, Ma, O, P, S, T, TMS
Indiana—B, C, F, G, Ho, Hy, M, O, P, S, T, TMS
Iowa*—B, C, Cf, F, G, Hy, M, Me, O, P, S, T, TMS
Kansas—G, Hy, P, S
Kentucky—B, C, Cf, F, G, Hy, O, P, S, T, TMS
Louisiana—B, C, F, G, Hy, O, P, S, T, TMS
Maine—B, C, G, Ho, Hy, M, O, Me, P, S, T, TMS
Maryland—B, C, Cf, F, G, Hy, M, O, P, S, T, TMS
Massachusetts*—B, C, G, Ho, Hy, M, P, S, TMS
Michigan—B, C, F, G, Hy, M, Me, O, P, S, T, TMS
Minnesota—B, C, Cf, F, G, Hy, M, O, P, S, T, TMS
Mississippi—B, C, Cf, F, G, Hy, M, Ma, O, P, S, T, TMS
Missouri—C, Cf, F, G, Hy, O, P, S, T, TMS
Montana—G, Hy, P
Nebraska—B, C, Cf, G, Hy, Me, P, S
Nevada—B, C, F, G, Hy, M, Ma, O, P, S, T, TMS
New Hampshire—B, C, G, Ho, Hy, M, P
New Jersey—A, B, C, Ci, Cf, F, G, Hy, M, O, P, S
New Mexico—B, C, Cf, F, G, Hy, O, P, S, T, TMS
New York—B, C, Cf, F, G, Ho, Hy, M, O, P, S, T, TMS
North Carolina—B, C, F, G, Hy, M, O, P, S, TMS
North Dakota—B, C, Cf, F, G, Hy, Me, O, P, S, T, TMS
Ohio—B, C, Cf, F, G, Hy, M, O, P, S, T, TMS
Oklahoma—G, Hy, Me, P, S
Oregon—B, C, Cf, F, G, Hy, M, Ma, O, P, S, T, TMS
Pennsylvania*—C, G, Hy, M, P, S
Rhode Island—B, C, Cf, F, G, Ho, Hy, M, O, P, S, T, TMS
South Carolina—B, C, Cf, F, G, Ho, Hy, M, O, P, S, T, TMS
South Dakota—B, C, Cf, F, G, Ho, Hy, M, O, P, S, T, TMS
Tennessee—B, C, F, G, Hy, M, O, P, S, TMS
Texas—B, C, F, G, Ho, Hy, M, O, P, S, T, TMS
Utah—B, C, F, G, Ho, Hy, M, O, P, S, T, TMS
Vermont—B, C, F, G, Hy, M, O, P, S, T, TMS
Virginia—B, C, Cf, F, G, Ho, Hy, M, Me, O, P, S, T, TMS
Washington—B, C, G, Ho, Hy, M, Me, P, S
West Virginia—G, Hy, P, S
Wisconsin—A, B, C, Cf, Ci, F, G, Ho, Hy, M, O, P, S, T, TMS
Wyoming—B, C, Cf, F, G, Ho, Hy, O, P, S, T, TMS

*Offers additional testing for numerous conditions in select hospitals.
A, arginosuccinic aciduria; B, biotinidase deficiency; C, congenital adrenal hyperplasia; Cf, cystic fibrosis; Ci, citrullinemia; F, fatty acid oxidation disorders (including Me, medium-chain acyl-CoA dehydrogenase deficiency); G, galactosemia; G6, G6PD; Ho, homocystinuria; Hy, hypothyroidism; M, maple syrup urine disease; Ma, malonic aciduria; O, organic acid disorders; P, phenylketonuria; S, sickle cell disease and hemoglobinopathies; T, tyrosinemia; TMS, tandem mass spectrometry, which tests for numerous other disorders as well.
For more current information, see the National Newborn Screening Status Report, which is updated regularly. State screening protocols change periodically due to changes in technology and state laws.

TREATMENT

Tyrosinemia

Historically, the mainstay of therapy for tyrosinemia has been diet modification, with a low-phenylalanine/low-tyrosine diet. Another part of this therapy is an attempt to minimize protein catabolism by maximizing caloric intake. These measures are somewhat effective in limiting kidney and liver damage, but will not prevent the development of cirrhosis or hepatocellular carcinoma.

The medication N-TBC [2-(2-nitro-4-trifluoromethylbenzoyl)-1, 3-cyclohexanedione] has greatly facilitated the medical treatment of tyrosinemia. This compound inhibits 4-hydroxyphenylpyruvate dioxygenase, and thus blocks tyrosine metabolism upstream of the defect in tyrosinemia, preventing the accumulation of succinylacetone. N-TBC is administered along with dietary therapy, and the N-TBC dose is titrated to keep blood and urine succinylacetone levels undetectable. N-TBC treatment prevents acute liver and neurologic crises, and may delay the progression of cirrhosis and the development of hepatocellular carcinoma. The most common side effect is the development of corneal opacities, a common feature in 4-hydroxyphenylpyruvate dioxygenase deficiency (tyrosinemia type III).

Long-term monitoring of patients with tyrosinemia involves screening for cirrhosis and for the development of dysplasia or frank hepatocellular carcinoma. The latter involves periodic ultrasounds and monitoring of serum alpha-fetoprotein, a marker of hepatocellular carcinoma, as well as liver biopsies. The treatment for cirrhosis that is not responding to medical therapy is liver transplantation, which has the added benefit of serving as partial gene therapy because the transplanted liver will contain wild-type fumarylacetoacetate hydrolase. The treatment of hepatocellular carcinoma is transplantation as well. Liver transplantation in children has a relatively high success rate, with a current 5-year graft survival of approximately 65% and patient survival of 75% to 80%, although there is variability between diseases and between transplantation centers.

Galactosemia

The primary treatment of galactosemia is dietary therapy. This involves the use of lactose-free formulas and complete elimination of dairy products. This is not sufficient, however, because many fruits and vegetables contain galactose as well, and many foods that may not seem to contain dairy products in fact do. It also appears that there is a fair amount of endogenous production of galactose, which clearly complicates efforts to eliminate galactose from the diet.

Despite complications in restricting the diet, the acute manifestations of galactosemia, such as hepatic failure and cataracts, clearly respond to the dietary elimination of galactose. Mental retardation, however, does not respond quite as well, and many well-controlled galactosemic patients have remaining deficits, although they are often mild. Ovarian failure also appears to persist despite good dietary control.

Hereditary Fructose Intolerance

The mainstay of therapy in hereditary fructose intolerance is dietary elimination of fructose. Total elimination of fructose is exceedingly difficult, especially in Western diets, given the large amount of consumption of sucrose and high-fructose corn syrup. Sorbitol must be avoided as well, because it is converted to fructose. The dietary therapy, though, can be liberalized in early childhood, because fructose tolerance appears to improve by age 3.

Recovery from the effects of hereditary fructose intolerance appears to be age related as well. Younger infants recover slowly after removal of fructose, and the liver damage may be extensive enough that liver transplantation must be performed. A liver transplant may also be required for chronic liver damage that has not responded to dietary therapy or in patients in which adequate dietary therapy has not been achieved. The long-term outlook of patients with hereditary fructose intolerance is excellent after early childhood, although these patients are always at risk of serious illness following exposure to large amounts of fructose or sorbitol.

APPROACH TO THE CASE

During her hospital stay, our patient was provided with supportive care for her coagulopathy and ascites. Based on her presentation and the coarse appearance of the liver on ultrasound, metabolic disease was suspected. A liver biopsy was performed, but the pathology was nondiagnostic. Screening metabolic laboratory studies demonstrated elevation of serum tyrosine and phenylalanine, and succinylacetone was present in the urine. The diagnosis of type I tyrosinemia was confirmed by low activity of fumarylacetoacetate hydrolase from the liver biopsy.

She was placed on a low-phenylalanine/low-tyrosine diet, and was started on N-TBC. Unfortunately, her liver disease had progressed enough that it could not be reversed, and she required a liver transplant. She is now well, 5 years after transplantation.

SUMMARY

Metabolic disease is an important, though rare, etiology of liver disease in children. Inborn errors of metabolism should always be considered in the differential diagnosis of acute or chronic liver failure and neonatal cholestasis, but are more likely if there are characteristic features. The evaluation of metabolic liver disease includes suggestive findings on general screening laboratory studies, more specialized metabolic screening laboratory studies, and tests for specific metabolic diseases. Tyrosinemia, galactosemia, and hereditary fructose intolerance are three of the most common causes of metabolic liver disease, and are relatively amenable to treatment. The pathogenesis of all three of these conditions arises from the buildup of harmful metabolites upstream of the characteristic enzymatic defect.

MAJOR POINTS

- Always include metabolic disease in the differential diagnosis of acute liver failure, chronic liver failure, and neonatal cholestasis.
- Consider metabolic disease more likely if the patient has a change in mental status, seizures, vomiting, or failure to thrive, or if hypotonia or ascites are noted on examination.
- Consider metabolic disease more likely if the patient has hypoglycemia, low serum bicarbonate, or an abnormal urinalysis (especially a renal Fanconi syndrome).
- Consider metabolic disease more likely if physical examination or laboratory studies seem more abnormal than expected from the clinical history.
- Many inborn errors of metabolism are routine assays in state newborn screens in the United States.
- Tyrosinemia, a defect in amino acid metabolism that leads to the accumulation of succinylacetone, is an important cause of metabolic liver disease, and affects the kidneys as well.
- Tyrosinemia can be controlled by the medication N-TBC, but may require liver transplantation.
- Patients with tyrosinemia are at higher risk for hepatocellular carcinoma.
- Galactosemia, a defect in the breakdown of galactose that leads to accumulation of galactitol and other metabolites, is an important cause of metabolic liver disease that also affects the kidneys, brain, and lenses of the eyes.
- Galactosemia is associated with *E. coli* sepsis in neonates.
- Hereditary fructose intolerance, a defect in metabolism of fructose that only appears after exposure to fructose, is an important cause of metabolic liver disease, especially of acute liver failure in infants.
- Both galactosemia and hereditary fructose intolerance are treated by diet therapy, although the long-term outlook of hereditary fructose intolerance is generally better than that of galactosemia.

SUGGESTED READINGS

Ali M, Rellos P, Cox TM: Hereditary fructose intolerance. J Med Genet 35:353, 1998.

Burton BK: Inborn errors of metabolism in infancy: A guide to diagnosis. Pediatrics 102:E69, 1998.

Clayton PT: Diagnosis of inherited disorders of liver metabolism. J Inherit Metab Dis 26:135, 2003.

Galactosemia (230400). Online Mendelian Inheritance in Man. www.ncbi.nlm.nih.gov.

Ghishan FK, Ballew MP: Inborn errors of carbohydrate metabolism. In Suchy FJ, Sokol RJ, Balistreri WF (eds): Liver Disease in Children, 2nd ed. Philadelphia, Lippincott Williams & Wilkins, 2001.

Grompe, M: The pathophysiology and treatment of hereditary tyrosinemia type I. Semin Liver Dis 21:563, 2001.

Hereditary fructose intolerance (229600). Online Mendelian Inheritance in Man. www.ncbi.nlm.nih.gov.

Kvittingen EA, Rootwelt H, Berger R, et al: Self-induced correction of the genetic defect in tyrosinemia type I. J Clin Invest 94:1657, 1994.

Leslie ND: Insights into the pathogenesis of galactosemia. Ann Rev Nutr 23:59, 2003.

Levy HL, Sepe SJ, Shih VE, et al: Sepsis due to *Escherichia coli* in neonates with galactosemia. N Engl J Med 297:823, 1977.

Mitchell GA, Larochelle J, Lambert M, et al: Neurologic crises in hereditary tyrosinemia. N Engl J Med 322:432, 1990.

Mitchell GA, Russo P, Dubois J, Alvarez F: Tyrosinemia. In Suchy FJ, Sokol RJ, Balistreri WF (eds): Liver Disease in Children, 2nd ed. Philadelphia, Lippincott Williams & Wilkins, 2001.

State-specific newborn screening. www.savebabies.org.

Tyrosinemia, Type 1 (276700). Online Mendelian Inheritance in Man. www.ncbi.nlm.nih.gov.

Waggoner DD, Buist NR, Donnell GN: Long-term prognosis in galactosemia: Results of a survey of 350 cases. J Inherit Metab Dis 13:802, 1990.

ACKNOWLEDGMENT

The author thanks Ralph Deberardinis, MD, PhD, for his critical review of the manuscript.

CHAPTER 33

Jaundice

MURALIDHAR JATLA
BARBARA A. HABER

Disease Description
Case Presentation
Epidemiology
    Indirect Hyperbilirubinemia
    Direct Hyperbilirubinemia
Diagnostic Testing
    Laboratory Investigations
        Body Fluids
        Radiologic Studies
        Liver Biopsy
Treatment
    Difficulties of Growth and Nutrition
    Ursodeoxycholic Acid, Steroids, and Antibiotics
Approach to the Case
Summary
Major Points

DISEASE DESCRIPTION

Neonatal jaundice is one of the most common problems encountered by pediatricians. Up to 60% of term infants may have clinical jaundice in the first days of life, but few have significant underlying disease. The challenge for the clinician is to determine when clinical jaundice needs further evaluation. Jaundice in the newborn period can be associated with serious illnesses such as hematologic disorders, metabolic diseases, endocrine diseases, infections, and diseases of the liver or the biliary tree. It is critical to know when to pursue an evaluation and to know what tests to order.

Almost all jaundice in the first days of life is due to indirect bilirubin and is a physiologic self-resolving problem. Physiologic hyperbilirubinemia develops as a combination of increased bilirubin production, decreased ability to eliminate bilirubin, and a significant enterohepatic circulation of bilirubin. On a per-kilogram basis, the average newborn produces almost 2.5 times as much bilirubin as an adult.

At times, the pediatrician is presented with a neonate who warrants further analysis, thus the need to approach the problem expeditiously.

CASE PRESENTATION

The patient is a 6-week-old boy who has a new onset of jaundice. He is the 7-pound, 12-ounce product of a normal, uncomplicated pregnancy and delivery. He is exclusively breastfed. The parents have noted a yellow tinge to the whites of his eyes. He has normal growth and development. The review of systems is unremarkable. His stools are soft and pale yellow. He has not been on any medication. Physical examination reveals scleral icterus. The breath sounds are clear, and there is no heart murmur. The abdomen is soft. The liver span is 6 cm, and the edge is soft. The spleen tip is palpable at the right anterior axillary line. Rectal examination is heme negative. Skin examination is without petechiae, bruising, or abnormal vascular pattern.

Laboratory evaluation revealed an elevated total bilirubin of 9.2 mg/dL with 6.3 mg/dL of direct bilirubin. Alanine aminotransferase (ALT) is 80 U/L, aspartate transaminase (AST) is 110 U/L, gamma-glutamyl-transferase (GGT) is 850 U/L, alkaline phosphatase is 342 U/L, and albumin is 4.1 g/dL. Prothrombin time is 15 seconds. Ultrasound reveals no gallbladder, otherwise normal. The patient was admitted for further evaluation and correction of his coagulopathy.

EPIDEMIOLOGY

The conditions causing hyperbilirubinemia are divided into those that result in an increased indirect bilirubin and those with increased direct bilirubin. A total and direct bilirubin should be obtained whenever clinical jaundice is identified.

Indirect Hyperbilirubinemia

Jaundice at 2 weeks of age is a relatively common finding, observed in 2.4% to 15% of newborns. Breastfeeding increases the likelihood of jaundice. Recently, jaundice was found in 9% of breastfed infants at 4 weeks of age, but in fewer than 1 in 1000 formula-fed infants. Clinical jaundice is observed when bilirubin pigment deposits in the skin and mucous membranes. Depending on the underlying etiology, jaundice may present at different stages of infancy. Unconjugated hyperbilirubinemia is most commonly encountered by general pediatricians and primary care providers. Most cases are self limited. The conditions that need to be evaluated when indirect bilirubin levels continue to rise to abnormal levels on the American Academy of Pediatrics (AAP) nomogram for designation of risk include hemolytic disease, red cell membrane defects, red cell enzyme deficiencies, extravasated blood, inborn errors of metabolism, and increased enterohepatic circulation such as pyloric stenosis or intestinal obstruction. When these etiologies are excluded, the cause is often elusive. Recent studies have suggested that some of these problems are due to genetic defects of hepatobiliary transporters. A study of Scottish newborns showed that 31% of breastfed infants with total bilirubin exceeding 5.8 mg/dL on day 28 of life were homozygous for Gilbert's mutation.

The purpose of early evaluation and treatment is to prevent kernicterus. Bilirubin levels typically increase during the first week of life, often not peaking until 96 hours and beyond. A list of causes of unconjugated hyperbilirubinemia is provided in Table 33-1. The remainder of this chapter focuses on the definition, causes, features, and therapies for conjugated hyperbilirubinemia in the neonate.

Direct Hyperbilirubinemia

Direct hyperbilirubinemia affects 1 in 2500 infants. Direct hyperbilirubinemia should be suspected when jaundice persists beyond 2 weeks of life. At that point clinical jaundice is evaluated by total and direct bilirubin. When the direct bilirubin exceeds 1 mg/dL or more than 20% of the total bilirubin, underlying pathology is suspected and a larger evaluation is undertaken.

Much of the evaluation of direct hyperbilirubinemia is driven by a single disease: biliary atresia. In biliary atresia the outcome is believed to be related to the timeliness of diagnosis. Thus, many tests are undertaken simultaneously rather than in the typical stepwise fashion often found in medicine.

Table 33-1 Causes of Indirect Hyperbilirubinemia

Hemolytic Causes
Fetal hydrops
ABO or minor blood group incompatibility
Spherocytosis
Glucose-6-phosphate dehydrogenase (G6PD) deficiency
Hemoglobinopathy
Infections

Nonhemolytic Causes
Birth trauma
Intraventricular hemorrhage
Polycythemia
Physiologic jaundice
Breastfeeding jaundice
Pyloric stenosis
Ileus

Decreased Conjugation
Breast milk jaundice
Prematurity
Hypothyroidism
Gilbert's disease
Crigler-Najjar syndrome (types 1 and 2)

Biliary atresia is a progressive fibro-obliterative disease of unclear etiology that starts in the extrahepatic biliary tree and progresses to the intrahepatic tree. A birth prevalence rate of 1 in 12,000 to 20,000 live births is found and it is the single most common pediatric liver disease leading to liver transplantation. Other diagnostic considerations are numerous (Table 33-2). As our understanding of the hepatobiliary system has evolved over the past decades, numerous genetic and metabolic diseases have been identified. Neonatal hepatitis, once believed to be the second most common cause of neonatal direct hyperbilirubinemia, is now an orphan disease of those cases with no identifiable underlying etiology. The pathology of neonatal hepatitis has a characteristic histology of giant cell transformation, cholestasis, extramedullary hematopoiesis, and inflammation.

Biliary atresia occurs most commonly without any other associated anomalies in a healthy neonate who develops jaundice after a jaundice-free period for the first week or two of life. The disease progresses and is considered uniformly fatal by 2 years of life if no intervention is taken. With surgical intervention (the Kasai hepatoportoenterstomy) the chance of transplantation is 50% at 2 years of age and 75% by young adulthood. Despite intervention, inflammation continues in the biliary tree for unknown reasons. The consequence of this disease progression is biliary cirrhosis, portal hypertension, malabsorption, and ultimately liver failure. In approximately 20% of cases with biliary atresia

Table 33-2 Causes of Direct Hyperbilirubinemia

Extrahepatic Biliary Disease
Biliary atresia
Choledochal cyst
Bile duct stenosis
Spontaneous perforation of the bile duct
Choledocholithiasis
Neonatal sclerosing cholangitis
Neoplasm

Intrahepatic Biliary Disease
Bile duct paucity
Syndromic form—Alagille syndrome
Nonsyndromic forms
Congenital hepatic fibrosis
Caroli's disease
Hepatic cysts
Langerhans' cell histiocytosis
Inspissated bile

Hepatocellular Disease
Metabolic and genetic diseases
Disorders of amino acid metabolism
Tyrosinemia
Disorders of lipid metabolism
Fatty acid oxidation defect
Respiratory chain disorder/mitochondrial
Niemann-Pick cell disease
Gaucher's disease
Wolman's disease
Disorders of carbohydrate metabolism
Galactosemia
Glycogen storage disease type IV
Hereditary fructose intolerance
Peroxisomal disorders
Zellweger syndrome
Endocrine disorders
Hypothyroidism
Panhypopituitarism
Familial/uncategorized
Neonatal hemochromatosis
Neonatal hepatitis
Dubin-Johnson syndrome

Hepatocellular Disease—cont'd
Rotor syndrome
Aagenaes syndrome (hereditary cholestasis with lymphedema)
Defective canalicular secretion and transport
PFIC1 familial intrahepatic cholestasis-1 (FIC1)
PFIC2 bile salt export pump deficiency (BSEP)
PFIC3 multidrug resistance protein 3 deficiency (MDR3)
Defective bile acid synthesis
3-Oxosteroid-5 β-reductase deficiency
3 β-hydroxy-C27-steroid oxidoreductase deficiency [3-HSD]
Oxysterol 7 α-hydroxylase deficiency
Bile acid transporter deficiency
Defective protein synthesis
α_1-Antitrypsin deficiency
Altered ion transport
Cystic fibrosis
Chromosomal disorders
Turner's syndrome
Trisomy 18
Trisomy 21
Infectious
Viral
Hepatitis B
Hepatitis C
Cytomegalovirus
Rubella
Herpes
Adenovirus
Enterovirus
Parvovirus B19
Other
Toxoplasmosis
Tuberculosis
Syphilis
Iatrogenic
Total parenteral nutrition
Miscellaneous
Shock or hypoperfusion

---

there are associated anomalies. The most common group of anomalies are situ anomalies. A variety of terms have been used to describe this group including embryonic biliary atresia, heterotaxy, and biliary atresia splenic malformation syndrome. In this specific group, there can be a midline liver, malrotation, interrupted inferior vena cava (IVC), asplenia or polysplenia, and cardiac anomalies. The remaining infants with congenital anomalies have a wide array of findings, but none has yet provided clues to the ultimate etiology for this devastating disease. The diagnosis of biliary atresia is suspected when percutaneous liver biopsy shows biliary inflammation and bile duct proliferation. In the operating room, visualization of the biliary tree often shows a shriveled fibrotic biliary system, and a cholangiogram, the definitive test, shows a lack of patency of the biliary system. Helpful tests include hepatobiliary scintigraphy and ultrasound. In the former, lack of excretion suggests biliary obstruction and the latter is used to eliminate other structural defects such as a stone or a choledochal cyst.

α_1-Antitrypsin deficiency comprises roughly 10% of cases. Defective storage and intracellular processing of the mutant PiZZ protein in the endoplasmic reticulum is associated with significant liver disease in a proportion of affected individuals. A paucity of protease inhibitor in the systemic circulation leads to pulmonary damage from cigarette smoke and environmental pollution. Many variants of protease inhibitors (Pi) exist including normal (M), and mutant (Z or S). Inherited in an autosomal recessive manner, carriers (MZ or MS) are rarely symptomatic. Five percent of affected (ZZ or SZ) infants will suffer serious liver disease within the first year of life. Cirrhosis, jaundice, and poor weight gain are common manifestations. Affected adults have up to a 30% to 40% chance of cirrhosis and liver malignancy.

Alagille syndrome, progressive familial intrahepatic cholestasis (PFIC) 1, 2, and 3, and bile acid synthetic disorders comprise 25% of cases. Alagille syndrome, or arteriohepatic dysplasia, is characterized by bile duct hypoplasia (<0.5 bile duct-portal triad), chronic cholestasis, and characteristic facies. The genetic defect in Alagille syndrome is a mutation in the *Jagged1* gene that encodes for Notch, a protein involved in cell fate determination. Dominantly inherited, more than 60% of *Jagged1* mutations are spontaneous. Histologically, bile-duct proliferation is absent, periportal fibrosis is nonprogressive, and cirrhosis is uncommon in the absence of recurrent cholangitis.

PFIC 1 through 3 represents disorders of canalicular secretion and transport with three distinct gene mutations. PFIC1, also known as familial intrahepatic cholestasis-1 (FIC1) gene deficiency was previously referred to as Byler's disease. FIC1 is characterized by jaundice, pruritus, chronic watery diarrhea, and failure to thrive in the first few months of life. GGT levels are normal or low in this disorder. Liver biopsy reveals bland intracanalicular cholestasis, portal tract fibrosis, and bile ductular proliferation. The only distinguishing feature is the presence of coarse granular bile in the canaliculus when tissue is examined by electron microscopy.

PFIC 2, also known as bile salt export pump deficiency (BSEP), represents a spectrum, with benign recurrent intrahepatic cholestasis (BRIC type 2) being a mild manifestation. Pruritus, jaundice, failure to thrive, splenomegaly, and hepatomegaly are common. Histology is that of giant cell hepatitis with canalicular and hepatocellular cholestasis. Liver transplantation is required in many cases.

PFIC 3, also known as multidrug resistance protein 3 deficiency (MDR3), affects canalicular membrane transport and secretion. As a result, toxic phosphatidylcholine-poor bile is formed. Significant phenotypic variation is seen in humans, including hepatic gallstone formation, biliary fibrosis, and intrahepatic cholestasis of pregnancy. Similar to other forms of PFIC, MDR3 deficiency manifests with cholestatic liver disease early in life. The characteristic difference between manifest who have MDR3 deficiency and those who have PFIC1 and PFIC2 is that MDR3 deficiency manifests with an elevated level of GGT in serum. Ursodeoxycholic acid (UDCA) is less toxic and more hydrophilic than bile acid and is found to be helpful in patients who have a missense MDR3 mutation. Patients who do not respond to UDCA should be considered for liver transplantation.

A variety of other disorders account for the remainder of cases, including extra-hepatic obstruction from common duct gallstone or choledochal cyst (prevalence of 1:150,000 live births), infection, and other rare disorders. Metabolic disorders such as tyrosinemia, galactosemia, hypothyroidism, and inborn errors of bile acid metabolism comprise another 20% of cases.

DIAGNOSTIC TESTING

The threshold for suspicion of hyperbilirubinemia should be low, and particularly for direct hyperbilirubinemia if certain features in the history or physical examination (Table 33-3) are present. Any infant noted to be jaundiced at 2 weeks of age should be evaluated with measurement of total and direct serum bilirubin. The American Academy of Pediatrics recommends testing if jaundice is accompanied by dark urine or light stool or if it persists beyond 3 weeks. Evaluation must be driven by the need to reach a diagnosis in a timely manner. There is great overlap between these conditions and a physician's diagnostic acumen cannot be reliably applied. Workup should proceed from identifying those conditions that are most amenable to treatment to those that are currently untreatable, and not in the order of incidence.

The clinical landmarks of neonatal direct hyperbilirubinemia are independent of etiology and include icterus, acholic stools, and a characteristic dark urine occurring in the first 3 months of life. Other associated problems may include pruritus, xanthomas, ascites, portal hypertension, lethargy, growth failure, and hepatosplenomegaly. Regrettably, the individual signs and

Table 33-3 Physical Examination Clues for Causes of Direct Hyperbilirubinemia

Hepatomegaly	Storage disease, cirrhosis, or vascular obstruction
Splenomegaly	Portal obstruction, cirrhosis, hemolysis, storage diseases
Acholic stools	Biliary obstruction
Unusual odor	Metabolic disease
Systolic heart murmur	Pulmonic stenosis or left-sided heart defects
Heme-positive stool	Coagulopathy
Broad forehead, pointed chin Elongated nose with bulbous tip	Facies seen in Alagille syndrome

symptoms of direct hyperbilirubinemia will not differentiate with certainty intrahepatic from extrahepatic disease. The infant may appear ill or healthy. Only by combining several historical and physical findings can the clinician begin to establish the etiology of the direct hyperbilirubinemia. The presence of nonhepatic findings may provide helpful clues to a specific diagnosis. For example, peripheral pulmonic stenosis, vertebral anomalies, posterior embryotoxon, and abnormal facies are associated with Alagille syndrome. Poor muscular tone is anticipated with Zellweger syndrome. Cataracts and brain calcifications are suggestive of some perinatal infections. Multiple organ involvement, hypotonia, nystagmus, and seizures might suggest mitochondrial disease.

Laboratory Investigations

The diagnostic evaluation of an infant with direct hyperbilirubinemia (Table 33-4) is aimed at making an expedient and accurate diagnosis. Because of this urgency, the workup is rarely tailored. Once the clinical diagnosis of direct hyperbilirubinemia has been made by physical examination and the finding has been confirmed by measurement of the serum direct bilirubin, a more detailed workup is undertaken that can be divided into three areas: (1) evaluation of body fluids, (2) radiologic examination, and (3) liver biopsy.

Body Fluids

The routine blood tests, complete blood count, liver enzyme analysis, and clotting studies are not diagnostic. They are useful for identifying cholestasis, differentiating biliary from hepatocellular disease, and following the course of hepatic function. The complete blood count may have an elevated white cell count or platelet count suggestive of an infection. An anemia or increased red cell distribution width may be from primary hemolytic disease or may be secondary to red cell alterations resulting from an increased cholesterol-to-phospholipid ratio. Hepatic enzyme determinations are obtained for evidence of hepatocellular disease and identification of biliary inflammation. Synthetic function assays (prothrombin time, albumin) are particularly useful for establishing the sufficiency of hepatic function. A decrease in the production of these proteins suggests a loss of functional hepatocytes.

More specific tests are needed to exclude metabolic diseases, infections, and anatomic origins of neonatal cholestasis. (See Table 33-4 for the tests that should be obtained in this initial phase of evaluation.)

Certain pitfalls of these tests must be noted. α_1-Antitrypsin deficiency should be evaluated by a serum α_1-antitrypsin level as well as protease inhibitor typing. The α_1-antitrypsin protein accounts for most of

Table 33-4 The Diagnostic Evaluation of an Infant with Direct Hyperbilirubinemia

History and physical examination
Screening assessment of patient's general status and liver sufficiency
Complete blood count, smear, reticulocyte count
Liver enzymes—aspartate and alanine aminotransferases, alkaline phosphatase, and gamma-glutamyl-transferase
Total protein and albumin
Prothrombin and partial thromboplastin times
Stool pigment
Body fluid examination for etiologic identification
Blood
Serology or polymerase chain reaction (PCR) cytomegalovirus, herpes, rubella, toxoplasmosis, rapid plasma reagin test, hepatitis B, hepatitis C
α_1-Antitrypsin level with protease inhibitor typing
Thyroxine and thyroid-stimulating hormone
Plasma amino acids
Blood culture
Maternal antibodies for toxoplasmosis, other infections, rubella, cytomegalovirus infection, and herpes simplex (TORCH) infections
Urine
    Urine analysis
    Urine culture
    Urine reducing substances
    Urine organic acids
    Urine succinylacetone
    Urine bile acids
Sweat chloride test
Intestine
Stool culture
Radiologic examination
Ultrasound with Doppler
Radionuclide examination
Operative cholangiogram if operated on for extrahepatic obstruction
Liver biopsy
Percutaneous or operative
Electron microscopy for familial intrahepatic cholestasis-1 (FIC1), mitochondrial
Immunostaining for bile salt export pump deficiency (BSEP), multidrug resistance protein 3 deficiency (MDR3)

the alpha-globulin fraction by serum protein electrophoresis. Levels less than 40% of normal will identify most patients with α_1-antitrypsin deficiency and the ZZ phenotype, but will miss approximately two thirds of the SZ phenotype. In addition, α_1-antitrypsin is an acute phase reactant.

The urine examination for reducing substance should always be obtained while the infant is receiving the offending dietary agent. Thus, lactose, a glucose-galactose disaccharide, needs to be part of the diet when urine is checked for reducing substances to rule out galactosemia. Quantification of urine bile acids can help rule out a bile acid synthetic disorder, as long as the sample was not obtained while the patient was taking a choleretic agent such as ursodiol. Plasma amino acid levels have maximal value in the detection of tyrosinemia early in the disease. As liver disease progresses, the amino acid pattern alters, such that elevations of straight chain amino acids (particularly methionine, phenylalanine, tyrosine, free tryptophan, aspartate, and glutamate) in the two- to fourfold range are found. This makes interpretation difficult once significant liver pathology is present. Finally, gene tests for various conditions are likely to become available as they become standardized.

Radiologic Studies

Ultrasound is helpful in the identification of processes such as tumors, biliary stones, cysts, obstruction, and inhomogeneity of liver tissue and can help facilitate prompt medical intervention. The absence of a gallbladder may suggest biliary atresia. Because this test is noninvasive and because of the reported coexistence of certain cholestatic diseases (for example, α_1-antitrypsin and biliary atresia), we advocate that all cholestatic infants undergo this diagnostic test.

Radionuclide scans allow evaluation of hepatocellular function as well as biliary anatomy. Injected radioactive material is normally excreted through the biliary tree into the intestine. On injection, the radionuclide is rapidly taken up by hepatocytes and secreted into bile. Nonvisualization of radioactivity within the intestine (in the scanning field comprising the intestines) 24 to 48 hours after injection is considered to be an abnormal result, indicating biliary obstruction or hepatocellular dysfunction. Hepatitis is characterized by slow uptake but normal excretion kinetics, whereas biliary atresia is characterized by normal uptake and absent excretion into the gut lumen. Unfortunately, the infant with biliary atresia at 4 to 6 weeks of age may have documented excretion of the tracer that is subsequently absent at 10 weeks. Conversely, nonexcretion of hepatic radioactivity does not necessarily indicate extrahepatic obstruction, because severe intrahepatic cholestasis can prevent excretion of the tracer.

Liver Biopsy

Percutaneous liver biopsy can be helpful in the diagnosis of biliary atresia. The interpretation of a single liver biopsy in a child with neonatal cholestasis can be limited because many cholestatic conditions evolve over time. If obstruction is suggested on biopsy, an operative exploration and cholangiogram are indicated. If no obstruction is suggested, etiologies such as cytomegalovirus (CMV), Alagille syndrome, or α_1-antitrypsin deficiency may be seen, thereby avoiding a visit to the operating room. Liver biopsy specimens obtained early in the course of biliary atresia may be indistinguishable from hepatitis. In addition to being able to visualize the hepatocanalicular cholestasis and injury, the liver biopsy also can provide disease-specific findings. Examples include periodic acid–Schiff (PAS)–positive, diastase-resistant granules in α_1-antitrypsin deficiency, ductal paucity in Alagille syndrome, necroinflammatory duct lesions in sclerosing cholangitis, and other findings that are relatively specific for metabolic and storage diseases. Liver biopsy can be performed safely and expeditiously in young infants and is useful in establishing specific diagnoses. A liver biopsy should be performed in almost all infants with undiagnosed cholestasis, to be interpreted by a pathologist with expertise in pediatric liver disease. A percutaneous liver biopsy is recommended before performing a surgical procedure to diagnose biliary atresia. If done early in the course of the disease (before 6 weeks of age), the biopsy may have to be repeated if the results are equivocal. Electron microscopy can be performed on liver biopsy to evaluate for glycogen or lipid storage material, as well as coarse bile, as seen in FIC1 and mitochondrial diseases. Immunostains for many viruses and specialized immunostains for BSEP and MDR3 proteins can be performed to assess for PFIC2 and PFIC3.

TREATMENT

Consultation with a pediatric gastroenterologist is essential for infants with conjugated hyperbilirubinemia of unknown cause. Therapy for cholestasis is diverse and is based on the underlying mechanism. If an obvious extrinsic obstruction (such as choledochal cyst) is present, referral for surgery is warranted. If the biopsy shows findings consistent with obstruction, then surgical exploration is warranted as in this case. For biliary atresia, the first-line treatment is relief of the obstructive process with a Kasai portoenterostomy. Long-term care focuses on growth and nutrition. After correction of the underlying condition, if direct hyperbilirubinemia persists, the focus of treatment is geared toward nutrition.

Difficulties of Growth and Nutrition

The backbone of treatment is aggressive nutritional supplementation and vitamin replacement. Malnutrition and growth restriction result from a combination of factors including fat malabsorption from decreased intestinal bile salts, organomegaly, or ascites. The child might not be able to meet the increased metabolic demands of a liver with chronic inflammation. Typically, a formula high in medium-chain triglycerides (MCT) is chosen to overcome some of the fat malabsorption. Previously used formulas with more than 80% MCT were deficient in long-chain fatty acids, especially linoleic acid. The more recently developed formulas contain approximately 60% MCT and provide essential fatty acids. This choice will allow dietary fat to be absorbed without a substantial need for micelle formation, which may be impaired. When the child does not sustain adequate growth, supplementation is achieved by increasing the caloric density of the formula and if necessary, nasogastric feedings are implemented to guarantee intake. Infants may have caloric requirements in excess of 150 kcal/kg/day. Growth is monitored by following length, weight, and head circumference. However, there is good evidence that this may under recognize nutritional issues because of the issues of organomegaly and fluid retention. Midarm circumference and tricep skinfold measurements by a technician trained in anthropometry may be a better way to detect true lean body and fat mass.

Protein is typically not restricted from the diet of children unless there is encephalopathy. Protein intake aids in achieving positive nitrogen balance, and the type of casein protein typical of most infant formulas is well tolerated. Monitoring of proteins such as albumin, retinol binding protein, and prothrombin time (PT) provides an index of protein balance and hepatic synthetic function. Fat-soluble vitamins are closely monitored and supplemented as needed. Some institutions routinely provide supplements for vitamins A, D, E, and K until the total bilirubin is less than 2 mg/dL. However, no unified standard has been adopted. Vitamin A deficiency is rare, and its toxicity when given inappropriately has made this vitamin the one most commonly monitored and is supplemented only when deficient. The goal of therapy is low normal serum levels of 400 to 500 μg/mL. Vitamin D is normally ingested in the diet, but is highly dependent on bile salt solubilization for absorption. Dietary vitamin D is hydroxylated at the 25 position in the liver, followed by hydroxylation at the 1 position by the kidney to form the active hormone. Usual supplementation is with 25-OHD, which is the most common form found in the circulation. Because there is no impairment of the hydroxylation in the kidneys, this is the preferred and safer form. However, when there is rickets, the active hormone, 1,25-(OH)2D is given with close monitoring of calcium and phosphorus levels. Vitamin E deficiency is found in biliary atresia. Supplementation is successfully achieved with d-alpha-tocopherol polyethylene glycol (TPGS). Lastly, vitamin K is critical for activation of clotting factors II, VII, IX, and X. Two naturally occurring forms of vitamin K exist. K1 is of dietary origin and K2 is synthesized by intestinal bacteria. Monitoring PT is standard and an easy method of assessing vitamin K status. Other nutrients that may need to be monitored include iron, zinc, and cholesterol. Iron may become deficient due to inadequate dietary content, chronic inflammation with poor iron utilization, and gastrointestinal (GI) blood loss.

Zinc is sometimes depleted in malabsorptive states and has been associated with poor linear growth. Cholesterol is often elevated in chronic cholestasis, with some patients developing cutaneous deposits in the form of xanthomas, especially in Alagille syndrome.

Ursodeoxycholic Acid, Steroids, and Antibiotics

Ursodeoxycholic acid is routinely given to promote choleresis and prevent scarring. There is no documented efficacy in biliary atresia; however, it is considered a well-tolerated medicine with potential benefit. Its use stems from the literature regarding primary biliary cirrhosis, autoimmune hepatitis, and rat models of fibrosis. Ursodeoxycholic acid is a naturally occurring dihydroxy bile acid with known choleretic properties. It undergoes extensive enterohepatic recycling. Following conjugation and biliary secretion, the drug is hydrolyzed to active ursodiol. Several large well-designed studies in adults with primary biliary cirrhosis have demonstrated its usefulness and tolerability. UDCA significantly lowers serum levels of alkaline phosphatase, ALT, and AST at a dose of 13 to 15 mg/kg/day in adults with primary biliary cirrhosis (PBC). With this chemical improvement there has also been documented reduction in disease progression based on histology and mortality. Few subjects in these studies have had to discontinue the drug because of adverse events. The literature regarding its efficacy in preventing fibrosis is fledgling, but there has been demonstrated benefit in a bile duct–ligated rat model of fibrosis.

For biliary atresia there are some specific differences in management compared with other cases of cholestasis. In the initial postoperative period the major objective is to prevent postoperative cholangitis. A combination of antibiotics and possibly steroids is given. The use of steroids has been adopted from Japan, where steroids are routine. Prednisolone is given IV for 4 days followed by oral administration until the total bilirubin is less than 2 mg/dL. In the United States, there is a multicenter trial to determine an accurate risk benefit profile for this therapy. Progression of liver disease is also believed to be related to repeated bouts of cholangitis. Therefore, one clinical approach is to aggressively treat cholangitis. Cholangitis typically occurs in the first year of life. Reports from the 1980s suggest that the incidence of cholangitis ranges from 50% to more than 90%. Our more recent (not published) experience is significantly less. Some hospitals routinely use antibiotic prophylaxis for the first year of life. However, some argue that the risk of developing resistant intestinal flora outweighs any proved benefit. The diagnosis is made by percutaneous liver biopsy and confirmed by blood culture. The suspicion should be raised in any child with fever, irritability, leukocytosis, or an unexplained change in liver enzymes. Unfortunately the diagnosis is complicated by the frequency of childhood febrile diseases such as otitis media and viral illnesses. When no specific source is identified and there is clinical suspicion, broad-spectrum antibiotics should be used to cover enteric organisms.

APPROACH TO THE CASE

During the hospital stay, our patient was given IV vitamin K to normalize his prothrombin time. An ultrasound was performed that revealed no gallbladder, mild hepatomegaly, and no splenomegaly. A DISIDA scan revealed hepatocellular uptake but no visualization of tracer in the small bowel even on delayed images at 6 and 24 hours. Next, a liver biopsy was performed that revealed bile plugging, expansion of bile ducts, and mild fibrosis. Soon after, the patient had an intraoperative cholangiogram that was consistent with biliary atresia, and a Kasai hepatoportoenterostomy was performed. Seven days later the patient was discharged home on a protein hydrolysate formula, and was started on ursodiol; vitamins A, D, E, and K; and trimethoprim-sulfamethoxazole (Bactrim). He is now doing well, 13 months post-Kasai procedure.

SUMMARY

Hyperbilirubinemia is a common finding in the newborn period. Accurate and timely diagnosis of the etiology of neonatal direct hyperbilirubinemia is challenging and critically important. Many jaundiced infants will have to be tested to find the few infants with direct hyperbilirubinemia because of the gravity of the consequences of a missed diagnosis. High clinical suspicion is crucial in detecting these patients, and selecting appropriate and timely diagnostic testing based on the resources available, and referral to a pediatric gastroenterologist can optimize outcome. Unlike indirect hyperbilirubinemia, in which neurotoxicity is the greatest concern, morbidity and mortality associated with direct hyperbilirubinemia are due to the underlying disease process and resultant sequelae of malnutrition, hepatic failure, and portal hypertension. The differential diagnosis of direct hyperbilirubinemia is extensive and can be the result of disorders in different regions of the hepatobiliary and portovenous systems. It is essential that physicians obtain a thorough history, perform a complete physical examination, and understand the proper use of diagnostic tests and management options in order to provide timely, optimum care for patients who present with direct hyperbilirubinemia.

Percutaneous liver biopsy can be very helpful in evaluating direct hyperbilirubinemia. Because of the dynamic and progressive nature of extrahepatic biliary atresia, even this test can be misleading. Scintigraphy is useful in excluding extrahepatic obstruction. Sonographic evaluation is currently useful for excluding anatomic abnormalities.

Any infant noted to be jaundiced at 2 weeks of age should be evaluated for direct hyperbilirubinemia with measurements of total and direct serum bilirubin. Breast-fed infants who can be reliably monitored and who have an otherwise normal and physical examination may be seen at 3 weeks of age and, if jaundice persists, have measurements of total and direct serum bilirubin at that time. The primary cause of the acute problem should be sought and treated in ill infants. In well-appearing infants, direct hyperbilirubinemia should still be evaluated quickly, because the most common etiologies can be serious and treatable.

MAJOR POINTS

The timing of diagnosis and therapy in many causes of direct hyperbilirubinemia has a profound effect on long-term prognosis

Always fractionate the total bilirubin level when evaluating neonatal hyperbilirubinemia.

Consider metabolic disease in the differential diagnosis of direct hyperbilirubinemia.

Fat-soluble vitamin deficiencies are common sequelae of direct hyperbilirubinemia and often need to be repleted.

Nutritional needs are increased in direct hyperbilirubinemia as a result of malabsorption, and supplemental feedings with nasogastric or gastrostomy tubes may be necessary to maintain growth.

Infants with biliary atresia often appear well at initial presentation, and there is evidence that early diagnosis and Kasai portoenterostomy are associated with longer survival of the native liver.

The chance of transplantation is 50% at 2 years and 75% at young adulthood if Kasai portoenterostomy is performed before 60 days of age.

The evaluation of direct hyperbilirubinemia should be directed toward etiologies that are treatable.

SUGGESTED READINGS

American Academy of Pediatrics Subcommittee on Hyperbilirubinemia: Management of hyperbilirubinemia in the newborn infant 35 or more weeks of gestation. Pediatrics 114: 297-231, 2004.

Balistreri W, Bezerra J: Whatever happened to "neonatal hepatitis"? Clin Liver Dis 10:27-53, 2006.

Bhutani VK, Johnson L, Sivieri EM: Predictive ability of a predischarge hour-specific serum bilirubin for subsequent significant hyperbilirubinemia in healthy term and near-term newborns. Pediatrics 103:6-14, 1999.

Burton EM, Babcock DS, Heubi JE, et al: Neonatal jaundice: Clinical and ultrasonographic findings. South Med J 83:294-302, 1990.

Choo-Kang LR, Sun CC, Counts DR: Cholestasis and hypoglycemia: Manifestations of congenital anterior hypopituitarism. J Clin Endocrinol Metab 81:2786-2789, 1996.

Doumas BT, Wu TW: The measurement of bilirubin fractions in serum. Crit Rev Clin Lab Sci 28:415-450, 1991.

Fox VF, Cohen MB, Whitington PF, et al: Outpatient liver biopsy in children. J Pediatr Gastroenterol Nutr 23:213-216, 1996.

Garcia FJ, Nager AL: Jaundice as an early diagnostic sign of urinary tract infection in infancy. Pediatrics 109:846-851, 2002.

Haber B, Russo P: Biliary atresia. Gastroenterol Clin North Am 32:891-891, 2003.

Hussein M, Howard ER, Mieli-Vergani G, et al: Jaundice at 14 days of age: Exclude biliary atresia. Arch Dis Child 66:1177-1179, 1991.

Ikeda S, Sera Y, Yamamoto H, Ogawa M: Effect of phenobarbital on serial ultrasonic examination in the evaluation of neonatal jaundice. Clin Imag 18:146-148, 1994.

Kotb MA, Kotb A, Sheba MF, et al: Evaluation of the triangular cord sign in the diagnosis of biliary atresia. Pediatrics 108:416-420, 2001.

Lai MW, Chang MH, Hsu SC, et al: Differential diagnosis of extrahepatic biliary atresia from neonatal hepatitis: A prospective study. J Pediatr Gastroenterol Nutr 18:121-127, 1994.

Lin WY, Lin CC, Changlai SP, Shen YY: Comparison of Tc-99m disofenin cholescintigraphy with ultrasonography in the differentiation of biliary atresia from other forms of neonatal jaundice. Pediatr Surg Int 12:30-33, 1997.

Maggiore O, Hadchouel BM, Lemonnier A, Alagille D: Diagnostic value of serum γ-glutamyl transpeptidase activity in liver diseases in children. J Pediatr Gastroenterol Nutr 12:21-26, 1993.

Mowat AP, Davidson LL, Dick MC: Earlier identification of biliary atresia and hepatobiliary disease: Selective screening in the third week of life. Arch Dis Child 72:90-92, 1995.

Moyer V, Freese D, Whitington P, et al: Guideline for the evaluation of cholestatic jaundice in infants: Recommendations of the North American Society for Pediatric Gastroenterology, Hepatology and Nutrition [NASPGHAN Clinical Guidelines]. J Pediatr Gastroenterol Nutr 39:115-128, 2004.

Psacharopoulos HT, Mowat AP, Cook PJL, et al: Outcome of liver disease associated with a-1-antitrypsin deficiency (PiZ): Implications for genetic counseling and antenatal diagnosis. Arch Dis 58:882–887, 1983.

Shneider B, Brown M, Haber B, et al: A multicenter study of the outcome of biliary atresia in the United States, 1997 to 2000. J Pediatr 148:467-474, 2006.

Spivak W, Sarkar S, Winter D, et al: Diagnostic utility of hepatobiliary scintigraphy with 99mTc-DISIDA in neonatal cholestasis. J Pediatr 110:855-861, 1987.

CHAPTER 34

Primary Sclerosing Cholangitis

ELIZABETH RAND

MATTHEW J. RYAN

Disease Description
Case Presentation
Epidemiology
Pathophysiology
Differential Diagnosis
Diagnostic Testing
Treatment
Approach to the Case
Summary
Major Points

DISEASE DESCRIPTION

Primary sclerosing cholangitis (PSC) is a disorder of the hepatobiliary system characterized by inflammation of the intrahepatic and/or extrahepatic bile ducts that leads to periductular fibrosis with areas of alternating narrowing and dilatation. Often PSC is seen in association with inflammatory bowel disease (IBD), but can occur in the absence of IBD or in association with other disorders. Cholangitis related to stones, sludging, bacterial infection, surgery to biliary tract, ischemic injury, and neoplasm must be excluded for the designation of *primary* sclerosing cholangitis.

CASE PRESENTATION

J.M. is a 16-year-old male with 3-year history of ulcerative colitis. At routine gastrointestinal (GI) follow-up, he is being treated with mesalamine and a proton pump inhibitor. He reports two or three loose stools daily with no gross blood and denies abdominal pain but notices recent weight loss despite a good appetite. His only complaint is increased itching that he attributes to dry skin. His dentist also mentioned his sclera appeared yellow during his last dental visit 1 month ago.

On physical examination, his weight is 74.6 kg, height 180.4 cm, pulse 100, and blood pressure 108/58 mm Hg. Overall, he is well appearing but his sclera were mildly icteric. He has moist mucous membranes with no oral lesions. His abdomen is soft, nontender, and nondistended with no hepatosplenomegaly. There are areas of linear erythema from scratching, but no rashes or dry skin.

EPIDEMIOLOGY

PSC can occur at any age, although it primarily affects adults with a median age of 40. Males outnumber females 2:1 in the adult population. This male predominance is not seen in children. Initial symptoms in the pediatric age-group include fatigue, malaise, poor growth or weight loss, anorexia, and delayed puberty. Fifteen percent to 30% of patients are asymptomatic at the time liver enzyme abnormalities are first seen. Pruritus and intermittent jaundice are common in symptomatic patients as the disease progresses (additional clinical features are shown in Table 34-1). PSC is most often seen in conjunction with IBD, but can occur in the presence of any inflammatory condition, such as Langerhans' cell histiocytosis, immunodeficiencies, thyroid disorders, diabetes mellitus, or autoimmune disorders, or with no identifiable comorbidity.

The etiology behind the inflammation, fibrosis, and ultimate destruction of the bile ducts remains largely unknown. Primarily sclerosing cholangitis and autoimmune hepatitis may fall at opposite ends of a broad spectrum, with an overlap syndrome occurring that may have features of both. This overlap syndrome has been described as an autoantibody-positive sclerosing cholangitis or autoimmune sclerosing cholangitis. One study found that nearly one half of children who presented with

Table 34-1	Signs and Symptoms of Primary Sclerosing Cholangitis

Clinical Symptoms
Anorexia
Fatigue
Weight loss
Right upper quadrant pain
Jaundice
Pruritus
Delayed puberty
Gastrointestinal bleeding
Fever

Physical Signs
Hepatosplenomegaly
Ascites
Xanthomas

clinical, serologic, and histologic symptoms of autoimmune hepatitis (AIH) also had bile duct abnormalities on cholangiography. Overlap syndrome should be considered in AIH patients who do not respond to immunosuppressive therapy.

Several groups have attempted to further categorize PSC by age at onset and presence of comorbidity. Debray describes three major types: neonatal onset, postnatal with accompanying disease, and postnatal without accompanying disease. The onset is typically insidious; Debray found an average of 3 years from the onset of symptoms until a diagnosis. The neonatal form of PSC has been reported in as many as 10% of the total pediatric cases. The initial course is one of eventual resolution of the jaundice between 2 weeks and 1 year of age; however, in one series, all cases progressed to cirrhosis by 10 years of age.

PATHOPHYSIOLOGY

The pathogenesis of PSC is still not understood. Genetics as well as immune dysregulation likely play roles. Autoimmunity, infection and ischemia have also been implicated.

Arguments for an autoimmune etiology include the close association with other autoimmune or immune dysregulatory diseases such as ulcerative colitis, diabetes mellitus, and thyroid disorders. The close relation of PSC and ulcerative colitis (UC) may be due to shared antigens on the colonic epithelial cells and within the biliary tract. There are also a number of autoimmune serologic markers that may be positive in PSC. The most common of these serologic markers is perinuclear antineutrophil cytoplasmic antibody (pANCA), which occurs in up to 80% of cases of PSC. A large proportion of patients also may have antinuclear antibodies (ANA) or antismooth muscle antibodies, which makes distinguishing PSC from AIH difficult and raises the question of overlap syndrome in these particular patients. Children with both cellular and humoral immunodeficiencies can develop sclerosing cholangitis. Currently, there are no definitive laboratory studies for the diagnosis of PSC, although a disproportionately elevated gamma-glutamyl-transferase (GGT) in clinical context is suggestive. The diagnosis requires radiologic or histologic confirmation.

Genetic predisposition seems likely given that PSC has been observed in multiple family members. Prochazka and colleagues found an increased risk of severe, progressive disease in patients with HLA-Drw52a haplotype. It is likely that there is no single gene locus for PSC, but rather a predisposition to PSC through inheriting a certain combination of genetic polymorphisms. Cullen and colleagues found that susceptibility to PSC is associated with four HLA haplotypes.

DIFFERENTIAL DIAGNOSIS

The differential diagnosis of PSC is outlined in Table 34-2.

DIAGNOSTIC TESTING

Characteristic cholangiographic findings include focal narrowing and strictures of the common and hepatic bile ducts with intervening dilation producing the characteristic "beaded" appearance. Imaging of the intrahepatic ducts can reveal duct wall irregularities, peripheral duct destruction, filling defects, beading, and confluent strictures. The characteristic features of PSC cannot be diagnosed without direct imaging of the biliary tree. Unfortunately, damage and destruction of the bile ducts will only become apparent on imaging in the later stages or the large duct variant of the disease. Liver biopsy may be supportive in the diagnosis of PSC, but the diagnosis is made through imaging of the biliary tree, demonstrating multifocal structuring and intrahepatic/extrahepatic biliary dilation. In adults, cholangiocarcinoma should be ruled out, although this has not been reported in children.

The most useful diagnostic tests to be performed when considering PSC include (1) liver biopsy, (2) autoimmune markers, (3) magnetic resonance (MR) cholangiogram, (4) endoscopic retrograde cholangiopancreatography (ERCP), and (5) intraoperative cholangiogram. Table 34-3 outlines the advantages and disadvantages of these diagnostic modalities.

Table 34-2	Differential Diagnosis of an Adolescent with Cholestasis

Infectious
Cytomegalovirus
Epstein-Barr virus
Hepatitis A, B, and C
Human immunodeficiency virus
Influenza
Other viral causes
Infectious granulomatous hepatitides

Environmental/Toxic
Total parenteral nutrition
Acetaminophen
Antiepileptic agents
Heavy metals

Obstructive Lesions
Neoplasms
Gallstones
Choledochal cyst
Genetic/metabolic:
Cystic fibrosis
Wilson's disease
α_1-Antitrypsin deficiency
Disorders of lipid, carbohydrate, or amino acid metabolism
Progressive familial intrahepatic cholestasis
Mitochondrial disorders
Alagille syndrome
Benign recurrent intrahepatic cholestasis

Autoimmune
Autoimmune hepatitis
Primary sclerosing cholangitis
Secondary sclerosing cholangitis
Systemic lupus erythematosus (SLE)
Infiltrative:
Lymphoma/leukemia
Familial erythrophagocytic syndrome

Table 34-3 Diagnostic Options

	Pros	Cons
Liver biopsy	Examination of actual tissue	Invasive
Autoimmune markers	Noninvasive	Relatively nonspecific
Magnetic resonance cholangiogram	Images biliary tree	
Endoscopic retrograde cholangiopancreatography (ERCP)	Images biliary tree Allows for therapeutic intervention	Invasive
Intraoperative cholangiogram	Images biliary tree Allows for biopsy	Invasive

TREATMENT

Multiple studies have suggested improvement in biochemical markers or histologic grade of fibrosis with ursodeoxycholic acid (UDCA). Unconjugated UDCA is absorbed in the small intestine, undergoes hepatic conjugation with taurine or glycine, and is then excreted in the bile and enters the enterohepatic circulation. UDCA works through several mechanisms. First, it is a hydrophilic bile acid, which displaces the more toxic hydrophobic bile acids. Second, UDCA stimulates the secretion of bile acids and therefore has clinical applications in other cholestatic liver diseases, such as primary biliary cirrhosis, intrahepatic cholestasis of pregnancy, and parenteral nutrition–induced cholestasis. Finally, UDCA protects against apoptosis by stabilizing the mitochondrial membrane potential within hepatocytes.

A number of trials starting in the early 1990s evaluated the response of biochemical markers and histology following the use of UDCA. Dosages in these trials range from 15 to 30mg/kg/day. Even through multiple trials, a standard dose has yet to be determined and the actual role of UDCA in slowing the progression of PSC has yet to be established. Despite the questions, UDCA remains the only medical therapy effective in halting disease progression.

Given the theories of immune dysregulation being a causative factor for PSC, corticosteroids or newer immunomodulator agents would seem to be a logical choice in the treatment of PSC. No large clinical studies have evaluated the efficacy of corticosteroids, although a large number of patients are on steroids to control their ulcerative colitis and no improvement is observed. Corticosteroids continue to play a role in the treatment of overlap syndrome as immunosuppression has a proved benefit in autoimmune hepatitis. Studies have investigated the use of methotrexate, cyclosporine, and tacrolimus in the treatment of PSC. Aside from a single small study, none of the data has shown a benefit with the newer immunosuppressive agents. Current trials using antilymphocytic, anti–tumor necrosis factor-alpha (TNF-α) antifibrogenic agents are ongoing.

Focal strictures causing obstructive symptoms may be treated with balloon dilation during cholangiography (by ERCP or percutaneous cholangiography), but surgical repair of the biliary tree should be avoided. Endoscopic measures of either stenting or balloon dilation of dominant strictures allow for rapid improvement in the aspartate transaminase (AST), alkaline phosphatase, GGT, and bilirubin. ERCP also has a lower complication rate than percutaneous manipulation and should be the preferred approach if endoscopic access is possible. The development of bacterial infection related to stricture or manipulation can be difficult to manage, requiring drainage by ERCP or PTC as well as long-term antibiotics. Chronic infection and progression of biliary cirrhosis with end-stage liver disease are indications for liver transplantation. PSC recurrence after transplantation has been reported in children and adults, many centers will use Roux-en-Y rather than duct-to-duct biliary anastomoses in hopes of reducing the recurrence rate.

APPROACH TO THE CASE

Screening tests in this patient reveal mild elevations in conjugated bilirubin alanine aminotransferase, and AST. Alkaline phosphatase and GGT levels are markedly elevated, with a slight increase in his prothrombin time. Serum copper and ceruloplasmin levels also are elevated, common nonspecific findings in chronic cholestatic liver disease. Autoantibodies for autoimmune hepatitis are absent, and viral hepatitis markers are negative. Given his history of ulcerative colitis and now cholestasis, a percutaneous liver biopsy was performed. Characteristic focal concentric fibrosis around small and large bile ducts was observed, along with destruction of small bile ducts and a periportal inflammatory infiltrate. An MR cholangiogram done several days later confirmed the suspected diagnosis of PSC.

The classic histopathologic lesion associated with PSC is the concentric fibrosis and edema around the bile ducts termed "onion skinning." Other characteristic features include pericholangitis, fibro-obliterative lesions, and loss of bile ducts. Later stages occasionally show a proliferation of the remaining bile ducts. Over time, bile ducts are replaced by bands of connective tissue. Eventually, the inflammation and fibrosis progress to biliary cirrhosis.

SUMMARY

The pathogenesis of PSC is still poorly understood, making targeted therapies difficult to develop. Other causes of cholangitis must be ruled out before the diagnosis of PSC can be made. Overlap syndrome and autoimmune hepatitis should be considered. Although no definitive biochemical markers exist, classic histologic findings of concentric rings surrounding bile ducts and beading on MR cholangiogram are important factors in the diagnosis. Care is mainly supportive, with liver transplantation the only cure.

MAJOR POINTS

- PSC is an inflammatory fibrosing cholangiopathy in which inflammation leads to fibrosis, local duct narrowing, cholestasis, and ultimately biliary cirrhosis.
- Other causes of cholangitis (e.g., stones, infections, neoplasms) must be excluded before the diagnosis of PSC is made.
- Classic histologic findings include concentric fibrosis and edema around the bile ducts, and pericholangitis. Late findings may include fibro-obliterative lesions, leading to loss of bile ducts.
- Characteristic appearance on cholangiography includes biliary strictures alternating with areas of proximal dilation, filling defects and beading.
- Although laboratory findings may be suggestive of PSC, no specific single diagnostic test exists.
- UDCA may help slow the progression to cirrhosis, but currently no other medical therapy exists for PSC, and treatment is mainly supportive and aimed at management of obstruction and superinfection.

SUGGESTED READINGS

Cullen S, Chapman R: Primary sclerosing cholangitis. Autoimmunity Rev 2:305-312, 2003.

Cullen SN, Chapman RW: The medical management of primary sclerosing cholangitis. Semin Liver Dis 26:52-61, 2006.

Debray D, Pariente D, Urvoas E, et al: Sclerosing cholangitis in children. J Pediatr 124:49-56, 1994.

Gregorio GV, Portmann B, Karini J, et al: Autoimmune hepatitis/sclerosing cholangitis overlap syndrome in childhood: A 16-year prospective study. Hepatology 33:544-553, 2001.

Gilger MA, Gann ME, Opekun AR, et al: Efficacy of ursodeoxycholic acid in the treatment of primary sclerosing cholangitis in children. J Pediatr Gastroenterol Nutr 31:136-141, 2000.

McEvoy CF, Suchy FJ: Biliary tract disease in children. Pediatr Clin North Am 43:75-98, 1996.

Prochazka EJ, Terasaki PI, Park MS, et al: Association of primary sclerosing cholangitis with HLA-DRw52a. N Engl J Med 322:1842-1844, 1990.

Russo P, Ruchelli ED, Piccoli DA: Pathology of Pediatric Gastroenterology and Liver Disease. New York, Springer, 2004.

Suchy FJ, Sokol RJ, Balistreri WF: Liver Disease in Children, 2nd ed. Philadelphia, Lippincott Williams & Wilkins, 2001.

Van Milligen de Wit AW, van Deventer SJ, Tytgat GN: Immunogenetic aspects of primary sclerosing cholangitis: Implications for therapeutic strategies. Am J Gastroenterol 90:893-900, 1995.

CHAPTER 35

Viral Hepatitis

BARBARA HABER

Disease Description
Case Presentation—Hepatitis C
   Incidence
   Clinical Symptoms
   Acute Hepatitis C—Diagnosis and Treatment
   Chronic Hepatitis C—Diagnosis and Treatment
   Approach to the Case
Case Presentation—Hepatitis B
   Epidemiology and Natural History of Hepatitis B
   Pathophysiology
   Acute Hepatitis B
   Chronic Hepatitis B
   Treatment
   Approach to the Case
Summary
Major Points

DISEASE DESCRIPTION

Viral hepatitis is common. The viruses A through E are hepatotropic, and a number of other systemic viruses can cause hepatitis (Fig. 35-1). Hepatitis A and E are never chronic and are transmitted by the fecal–oral route. Hepatitis viruses B, C, and D are bloodborne and can often progress to chronic infection. Hepatitis A is the most common viral hepatitis, representing more than one half of all acute viral hepatitis presentations in the United States (National Health and Nutrition Examination Survey [NHANES] III data). The major treatment strategy is prevention by vaccination, handwashing, and careful hygiene in endemic areas. Hepatitis B and hepatitis C are the next most common causes of viral hepatitis. Hepatitis D can be found in up to 4% of all cases of acute hepatitis B, but almost always after travel to an endemic area. Hepatitis E is extremely rare in the United States. Because infections with hepatitis B and C can progress silently to chronic liver damage, it is important for the clinician to understand the natural history of each of these infections and to know how to screen and whom to treat. This chapter focuses on these two most common and significant forms of hepatitis.

CASE PRESENTATION—HEPATITIS C

A.W. is a 17-year-old boy who was notified of a positive hepatitis C antibody test result after donating blood. In 1987, he underwent cardiac repair for tetralogy of Fallot. He and his parents never suspected any other health issues. His growth and development were normal. He was an excellent student. He had neither signs nor symptoms of liver disease.

Incidence

Hepatitis C is common. Over the past decades this virus has insidiously entered our society through three major routes: (1) populations of people who have taken part in high-risk behaviors; (2) contaminated blood products used for medical purposes; and (3) émigrés who have brought the virus with them. Figure 35-2 shows who should be screened. Close to 4 million U.S. adults are chronically infected. Among children, there are an estimated one quarter of a million cases. The actual number may be much greater because many cases go undetected due to the lack of symptoms. Prevalence studies have found a seroprevalence of 0.2% for children under 12 years and 0.4% for those between 12 and 19 years (NHANES III data).

Clinical Symptoms

Hepatitis C causes both acute and chronic disease. Most commonly, the acute infection passes unnoticed. After inoculation, virus is found by polymerase chain

Differential Diagnosis of Viral Hepatitis
Hepatotropic Viruses
Hepatitis A virus (**HAV**)
Hepatitis B virus (**HBV**)
Hepatitis C virus (**HCV**)
Hepatitis D virus (**HDV**)
Hepatitis E virus (**HEV**)
Hepatitis G virus (**HGV**)
Systemic Viruses with Liver Involvement
Cytomegalovirus (**CMV**)
Epstein-Barr virus (**EBV**)
Herpes simplex virus (**HSV**)
Varicella-zoster virus (**VZV**)
Adenoviruses, enteroviruses, echoviruses, coxsackie-virus, rubella, human immunodeficiency virus (**HIV**)

Figure 35-1 Differential diagnosis of viral hepatitis.

reaction (PCR), typically within 1 to 2 weeks, with a range of 2 to 26 weeks. Symptoms, if present, occur approximately 2 months after exposure. Jaundice is mild and occurs in less than 20%. Other symptoms include malaise and nausea, symptoms that overlap with many viral illnesses, and thus many cases go undiagnosed. Silently, the patient enters a phase of chronic infection in upward of 80% of cases. The virus mutates rapidly, and, as a result, the body's immune surveillance is rarely effective.

The number of new cases of hepatitis C has fallen significantly since identification of the virus in the mid-1980s. The decline is primarily a result of effective screening of blood products. Contraction of hepatitis C from medical transfusions has been reduced to almost zero. Furthermore, programs aimed at education of high-risk populations such as IV drug abusers and incarcerated individuals and periodic screening of high-risk patients, have been pivotal in limiting the spread. Treatment is strongly encouraged for individuals with infection, to limit what has been targeted as a major health priority in our country. Unfortunately, therapies for hepatitis C are still relatively ineffective, with "cure" rates in the range of 50% for most patient populations (Fig. 35-3).

Acute Hepatitis C—Diagnosis and Treatment

Although it is quoted that acute hepatitis C accounts for 20% of all acute viral hepatitis, it is actually a rare presentation in the pediatric setting. Many cases go undiagnosed because of the mild symptoms. Without the prompt testing of abnormal liver enzymes, no evaluation is undertaken. However, on occasion a child is symptomatic, or an inadvertent exposure, such as a contaminated needlestick, prompts testing. In each case, it is important for the clinician to understand how to monitor and when to consider the possibility of treatment. Unlike many other infections, detection of antibody suggests ongoing infection rather than clearance of infection. There is no antibody pattern that allows one to determine past infection, present infection, or stage of infection. PCR is needed to determine the presence of ongoing infection, either acute or chronic (Fig. 35-4).

The distinction between acute hepatitis C virus infection and newly discovered chronic infection may not always be straightforward, because in both settings patients may have detectable hepatitis C virus ribonucleic acid (HCV RNA), detectable antibodies against hepatitis C, and elevated serum aminotransferases. Serologic markers, including HCV RNA and serum aminotransferases and antibodies with respect to a suspected exposure, are the most useful tools.

For the patient who presents with acute symptomatic disease, approximately 50% will have antibodies at the time of presentation and only 50% will go on to develop chronic infection. This group of patients will have elevated enzymes and a positive PCR. In the absence of any other causes of hepatitis and in the absence of a history of any behaviors associated with risk of exposure (see Fig. 35-2), the patient is presumed to have acute infection.

After an exposure through blood products, needlestick, razor, or sexual contact, testing is followed serially at 4-week intervals until 12 weeks after known exposure. Conversion from no antibody present to antibody present, along with positive viral titers, is diagnostic of an acute infection. For the patient who is not tested immediately after the exposure and antibody or viral titers, is found, circumstantial evidence is used to diagnose acute infection.

Because it is extremely likely that an acute infection will become chronic, early intervention has become a

Who Should Be Screened for Hepatitis C (adapted from CDC, AASLD, AND NIH guidelines)
Child born to infected mother
Child adopted from a country with a high incidence of infection
Patient with high-risk behaviors, e.g., IV drug use
Patient with exposure, e.g., needlestick or mucosal exposure
Patient with HIV
Patient with any evidence of liver disease
Patient whose sexual partner is infected
Patient with transfusion or organ transplant prior to 1992

Figure 35-2 Screening recommendations for hepatitis C. AASLD, American Association for the Study of Liver Diseases; CDC, Centers for Disease Control and Prevention; NIH, National Institutes of Health.

Treatment Efficacy, Pros, Cons	
Hepatitis C	**Hepatitis B**
Interferon alpha Efficacy: 17% (SVR) Pros: minimally effective Cons: side effect profile, shots 3 times weekly	Interferon alpha Efficacy: 30%-40% DNA loss Pros: durability of response 80%-90% Cons: side effect profile, shots 3 times weekly
Interferon alpha + ribavirin Efficacy: 30% in adults, approx. 60% in children <12 years Pros: relatively effective Cons: frequent injections, long course, side effects	Lamivudine Efficacy: 20%-40% DNA loss Pros: few side effects, convenient oral medicine Cons: frequently selects for mutant virus
Peginterferon + ribavirin (approved in adults/trials in children under way) Efficacy: 40%-60% in adults Pros: most effective current therapy Cons: long course of treatments, many side effects	Adefovir Efficacy: 23% eAg loss, 46% DNA decline Pros: few side effects, convenient oral medicine, less frequent mutants than lamivudine Cons: selects for mutant viruses, effective treatment may require 96-144 weeks of treatment

Figure 35-3 Pros and cons of current therapies for hepatitis B and C. DNA, Deoxyribonucleic acid; eAg, early antigen; SVR, sustained viral remission, defined as undetectable virus 6 months after completion of therapy.

focus of active research. A number of studies generated over the past 15 years have shown that high-dose interferon can be used early in the course of disease successfully. However, the toxicity of this intervention has led to cautious recommendations until further studies have been completed. Although it is not yet the standard of care, once timing and dosing are determined, clear guidelines will be generated for this population.

Chronic Hepatitis C—Diagnosis and Treatment

The risk of chronic infection after an acute episode of hepatitis C is extremely high. Reports suggest that upward of 80% and possibly as high as 100% will develop chronic infection among adults. As a general rule, most patients who are destined to spontaneously clear hepatitis C viremia do so within 12 weeks and usually no later than 20 weeks after the acute exposure. For most adults, spontaneous clearance after longer follow-up (as in the case of chronic hepatitis B) is believed to be unlikely.

Certain subpopulations are believed to have a relatively high rate of spontaneous clearance. This is most pertinent for the pediatrician. The most favorable group is neonates. These children, who typically acquire the infection at birth from their mother, may clear the virus in up to 75% by 2 years of age. The second most likely group is those who present with symptomatic acute hepatitis C. The reported chance of clearance is as high as 50%. A third group of young healthy teenagers and young adults is also likely to clear virus in almost one half of patients as shown by the Dionysos study from Italy.

The decision to treat is one that is reached after discussion among patients, parents, and the physician. The clinician must understand the natural history of the disease, toxicity of the therapy that will be used, and, effectiveness of the therapy (see Fig. 35-3). Prior to 1997, the American Association for the Study of Liver Diseases (AASLD) consensus was to offer treatment only to subjects with evidence of fibrosis. Now we consider therapy for all patients. The reasons behind this shift include the increased likelihood of responding to therapy in those with less significant liver damage and shorter duration of disease and because of the general concerns for spread of this virus within our society. Therapy can be offered to any patient older than 2 years (if younger than 2 years, interferon is contraindicated because of neurotoxicity). Interferon has U.S. Food and Drug Administration (FDA) approval for this indication in the population starting at 2 years of age and ribavirin is approved starting at age 3. Peginterferon, which has a more sustained half-life and convenience of once-weekly dosing will likely be approved after the completion of multicenter trials by several manufacturers.

Before initiating therapy, the clinician should thoroughly evaluate for viral genotype, viral quantitation, liver histology, and other causes of liver disease. With this information, the physician can appropriately present the pros and cons of treating (Fig. 35-5). Patients with low viral count, benign histology, and genotypes 2 or 3 are superb candidates for treatment and are more likely to respond. These positive factors need to be weighed against the hardships and complications associated with treatment. In the pediatric setting, the most important factors to consider are autoimmune disorders, because interferon may aggravate or induce such an illness in a predisposed individual. Other medical problems that influence the response to therapy or the course of disease and that should be screened for include: human immunodeficiency virus (HIV), blood dyscrasias, α_1-antitrypsin deficiency, Wilson's disease, and hemochromatosis. Other issues to consider when deciding to treat are depression, sexual activity, compliance and social concerns because this is an elective decision in most cases.

Overall, children are excellent candidates for therapy. A meta-analysis of reported pediatric trails suggests that children may have a two- to threefold higher response rate than adults. A number of factors probably contribute to this age effect, including shorter duration of disease, lower viral counts, benign liver histology, and age-related differences in immunity. Also, children tolerate therapy better than adults.

Approach to the Case

The first important information for the hepatologist is to determine if this child has chronic or acute hepatitis C. There is no laboratory test that will determine chronic versus acute infection; the medical history is the only clue. Most likely this child has chronic hepatitis C based on the lack of other risk factors and the knowledge that he had received a transfusion at a time in history when the blood supply was highly infected. Knowing that he is chronically infected is the most important factor to determine treatment. The patient's blood studies reveals that he has hepatitis C genotype 1a. His quantitative PCR viral load is 9×10^6 copies/mL of blood. His amino transferases and clotting studies are normal. He has no evidence of other medical problems that would complicate his treatment regimen; therefore, he was started on a 48-week course of once weekly

VIRAL HEPATITIS MARKERS AND THEIR SIGNIFICANCE

Marker		Significance
HbsAg	Hepatitis B surface antigen	Patient is infected with the virus
anti-HBs	Hepatitis B surface antibody	Patient is immune (from natural infection or vaccine)
HBeAg	Hepatitis B "e" antigen	Active viral replication; ongoing liver disease (usually); patient is highly infectious
anti-HBe (in presence of HBsAg)	Hepatitis B "e" antibody	Viral replication is reduced; inactive liver disease (usually); less infectious than if HBeAg were positive (rarely, anti-HBe may be associated with active viral replication)
HBV DNA	Hepatitis B virus-deoxyribonucliec acid	Active viral replication; ongoing liver disease (usually); patient is highly infectious
HBcAg	Hepatitis B core antigen	Never detectable in the serum
anti-HBc	Hepatitis B core antibody	Patient has been in contact with HBV and may or may not still be infected; may occasionally be a false positive in the absence of other markers
IgM anti-HBc	Immunoglobin M fraction of the hepatitis B core antibody	Signifies recent (within 6 months) infection with HBV; occasionally can persist in chronic carriers
anti-HCV	Hepatitis C virus antibody	Indicates past or present infection, but does not differentiate among acute, chronic, or past infections
HCV RNA (qualitative)	Hepatitis C virus ribonucleic acid	Detects presence or absence of virus and is more sensitive than quantitative PCR assays
HCV RNA (quantitative)	Hepatitis C virus ribonucleic acid	Determines concentration (viral load) of HCV

A

Figure 35-4 Significance of serum markers assayed for hepatitis B and hepatitis C. PCR, polymerase chain reaction. *(Figure continued on next page).*

Peginterferon and twice daily ribavirin. This case illustrates several points. Hepatitis C is an insidious virus. There were no overt signs of disease by physical examination, from symptoms or from a blood test. He was not screened even though he had received blood transfusions in 1987.

CASE PRESENTATION—HEPATITIS B

E.M. is an 8-year-old adopted boy from a Polish orphanage who was found to have hepatitis B during the screening adoption process. He is in the 25th percentile for height and weight. His physical examination is unremarkable and clinically he has no symptoms.

Epidemiology and Natural History of Hepatitis B

Despite the development and implementation of the hepatitis B vaccine, hepatitis B virus infection remains a global public health problem. There are more than 400 million hepatitis B carriers worldwide, of whom approximately 500,000 die annually from hepatitis B–related liver disease. In the United States, 1.25 million are chronically infected—surprisingly, the rate of HBV-related hospitalizations, cancers, and deaths have more than doubled during the past decade. There are three modes of transmission: perinatal, parenteral, and sexual. There are both acute and chronic forms of this disease.

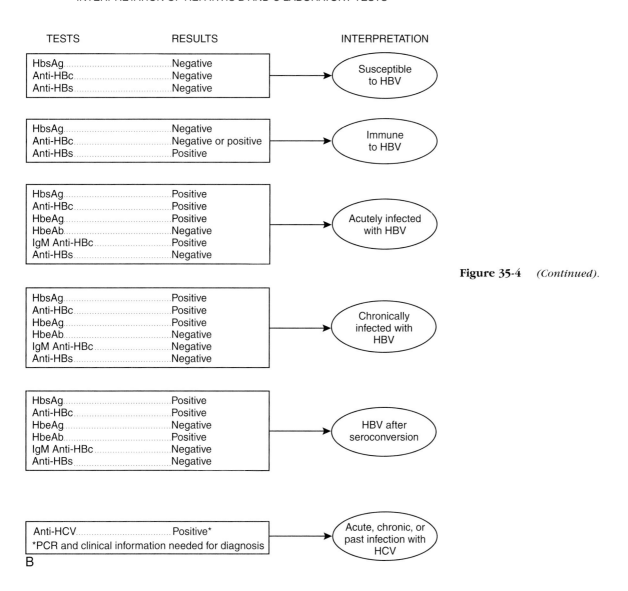

Figure 35-4 *(Continued).*

Factors Predictive of Treatment Response		
Factor	Hepatitis C	Hepatitis B
Pretreatment serum ALT	Does not predict response to therapy	Low/no response if ALT is normal
Pretreatment viral quantitation	Lower response PCR > 2×10^6	Lower response DNA > 200 pg/mL
Liver histology	Benign histology predicts better outcome	Active inflammation better response (but ALT a better predictor)
Age at treatment	Younger more likely to respond Younger tolerate IFN better	Younger more likely to be immune tolerant/no response
Genotype	Genotype 2,3 very likely response to treatment	Unclear relation to response to treatment

Figure 35-5 Interpretation of common laboratory test results for hepatitis B and hepatitis C. ALT, alanine transaminase; DNA, deoxyribonucleic acid; INF, interferon; PCR, polymerase chain reaction.

Pathophysiology

Hepatitis B can be either an acute or chronic infection. In the acute form the disease is self limited. After inoculation with the virus, there is a rapid development of the host immune response and clearance of the hepatitis B surface antigen and e antigen (HBeAg). For adults with robust immune systems, 95% will clear the virus. In children and in those with weaker immune systems, the chance of becoming a chronic carrier is much higher. In infants who acquire the infection in the perinatal period, 90% will develop a chronic infection. For those between the ages of 1 and 5 years, 20% to 50% will become chronically infected. The sequelae of chronic infection includes the possible development of cirrhosis and/or hepatocellular carcinoma. Infants who acquire this infection become cirrhotic much less frequently than those who acquire the infection at an older age. The risk of chronic damage increases with increased liver inflammation. For adults, about 30% of those with chronic infection develop cirrhosis.

Chronic hepatitis B has been classified into three different phases; the rate at which one moves through the phases is dependent on the age of initial infection and one's immune system. The first phase is an immune-tolerant phase. During this phase, liver enzymes are barely, if at all, elevated and viral titers are high. This phase is more prolonged in younger individuals and those who are immunosuppressed. The second phase is the immuno-elimination phase, characterized by the presence of e antigen with high levels of deoxyribonucleic acid (DNA) and elevated serum aminotransferases. There may or may not be symptoms. Most important, this phase is characterized by the body's recognition of the virus as foreign and the attempt of the immune response to eliminate the virus. The third phase is a nonreplicative phase, which is characterized by a negative e antigen, positive e antibody, low levels of hepatitis B DNA and normal alanine transaminase (ALT) levels. The goal of most therapies is to transition the patient to this third phase. The virus is not eliminated, but the child or adult is less contagious, and has a reduced risk of developing either cirrhosis or cancer. Understanding the interpretation of serum markers is important for identifying and interpreting the phase of liver infection.

Acute Hepatitis B

Acute hepatitis B infection remains a fairly common problem. Many cases occur in unvaccinated groups and in those exposed to a mutant virus. During the acute phase of the infection, signs and symptoms range from anicteric hepatitis (70%) to icteric hepatitis (30%) and, in rare cases, fulminant hepatitis (<0.5%). After exposure, symptoms develop 1 to 4 months later. Symptoms can include anorexia, nausea, jaundice, and right upper quadrant discomfort. Laboratory testing during the acute phase reveals elevations in the concentration of serum aminotransferases. The prothrombin time is the best indicator of prognosis. In patients who recover, serum aminotransferases return to normal within 1 to 4 months. Persistent elevation of serum alanine transferase for more than 6 months indicates progression to chronic hepatitis.

Among patients who recover from acute hepatitis B, it has been believed that the virus is completely cleared. However, traces of hepatitis B virus are often detectable in the blood by PCR for many years after clinical recovery from acute hepatitis, despite the presence of serum antibodies. One study found that hepatitis B DNA was detected in the liver tissues in 13 of 14 healthy liver transplant donors who were positive for anti-HB and antihepatitis B surface antibodies (anti-HBs). Persistent histologic abnormalities (including fibrosis and mild inflammation) were present as long as 10 years in another series focusing on 9 patients who demonstrated complete serologic recovery after acute infection.

These observations suggest that complete eradication of hepatitis B rarely occurs after recovery from acute HBV infection, even among those with positive antibodies. The major clinical issue to consider is that immunosuppression in such patients, as occurs after organ transplantation, can lead to reactivation of the virus.

Chronic Hepatitis B

The definition of chronic infection is detectable infection at two time points at least 6 months apart. Chronic infection occurs when the virus is not cleared by the immune system. Hence, people who are immunocompromised or very young are more likely to become chronically infected. Gender is also an influence, with more males becoming chronically infected.

Chronic infection is especially common in endemic areas. Alaska has a seroprevalence in excess of 8%. The lifetime risk of infection for children in this area is greater than 60%. The common mode of transmission is either vertical from mother to child or horizontal among household members. Similar patterns are seen in other endemic areas, including parts of Asia, Africa, and northern Canada. Outside these endemic areas infection occurs through high-risk behaviors and contact with infected individuals.

The importance of pediatric hepatitis B infection stems from the fact that the outcome of acute infection varies substantially depending on the age at which infection occurs. In children under 5 years of age, less than 5% of acute hepatitis B infections are symptomatic; however, chronic infection occurs in about 80% to 90% of infants infected during the first year of life and in about 20% to 50% of children infected between 1 and 5 years of age. In comparison, 30% to 50% of adults with acute hepatitis B infection are symptomatic, but only 2% to 10% develop chronic infection.

Treatment

Pediatric hepatologists wrestle with when, why, and which children with hepatitis B should be treated. The decision is complex and includes weighing many variables. The first and most effective treatment for hepatitis B is prevention. The vaccine provides 98% to 99% immunity with a series of three shots. Birth is the optimal time because the child is a captive audience, but for those who missed early vaccination, screening of the preteen population is mandated by many U.S. schools.

For those who are chronically infected, the medical goal of treatment is prevention of cirrhosis, prevention of liver failure, and prevention of hepatocellular carcinoma. In addition, the treatment is to alleviate the family and patient of many of the social concerns. Parents and patients struggle with whom to tell. Do they tell schools, children's parents, friends, babysitters, and sports coaches? For all of the aforementioned factors, families strongly consider treatment.

Effective treatment is measured by viral suppression and in some adult studies, by histologic improvement of the liver. Unfortunately, treatment rarely leads to viral eradication because of the viral structure. During treatment, the patient is monitored for conversion of e antigen to e antibody with concurrent fall in DNA by at least one log, but preferably below the level of detection. The patient in this condition is less contagious and less likely to have progression of liver disease. However, surface antigen is still made and there is no surface antibody. The virus is still in the host, but is only rarely able to produce a full viral particle. The patient still is at risk for hepatocellular carcinoma, just less so.

The decision to treat weighs two major factors: the chance of responding to intervention versus the risk of not treating. Over the past decade, it has become increasingly clear that many chronically infected children will clear their infection by young adulthood. We now believe 70% of those with perinatally acquired HBV will clear by young adulthood. This fact is weighed against the chance of responding to treatment. The factors that suggest a favorable response are the same as in adults. Treatment is effective only for those with serum alanine transferase elevations and is more favorable in those with low viral counts and inflammatory activity on liver histology (see Fig. 35-5).

There are three approved treatments for chronic HBV in the adult population (see Fig. 35-3). Comparisons of the three are limited by the fact that studies have not been done with head-to-head comparisons. Interferon-alfa (IFN-α) has both antiviral effects as well as immunomodulatory effects by activating macrophages, natural killer cells, and cytotoxic T cells. Six months of treatment results in clearance of virus in 30% to 40% of cases. The response in children is similar to that in adults. The major determinant is pretreatment ALT levels. Peginterferon might be more effective, but is currently in phase III trials. Interferon can precipitate or worsen liver failure and thus is contraindicated in the childs B or C cirrhosis. Duration is 6 months. Candidates for therapy are typically more than 2 years of age, have elevated transaminases, modest levels of hepatitis B DNA in serum, and histologic activity on liver biopsy. The problem is that this profile fits only a small portion of children with chronic hepatitis B. It is ineffective in children with normal liver enzymes.

Lamivudine is a nucleoside analog approved for the treatment of HIV and chronic hepatitis B that inhibits viral replication. It is given orally, unlike interferon, which is by subcutaneous injection, and has few side effects.In a previously published report in the *New England Journal of Medicine,* 358 Chinese patients with chronic hepatitis B were given lamivudine for 1 year. Approximately one half of patients responded with improved liver histology, and few side effects were noted. A problem with the drug, however, is that treatment appears to lead to the development of hepatitis B drug-resistant mutants. The most important mutation involves the YMDD locus of the reverse transcriptase domain of the polymerase gene. Drug mutations in a pediatric study documented 19% at the end of 1 year of therapy. In adults, 67% of subjects have mutations by the end of 5 years of therapy. Because of this limitation, a number of other antiviral agents are beginning to be marketed for adults with hepatitis B.

Adefovir has been approved in adults and is now in phase III investigations for children. It appears to have similar advantages as lamivudine, but without the same incidence of mutants. It has in vitro and in vivo activity against wild-type- and lamivudine-resistant hepatitis B. The major toxicities are renal tubular abnormalities and impaired renal function. Adefovir-resistant mutants occur in only 2% after 96 weeks of treatment, although that number seems to be increasing with more use. In all older patients, the diagnosis of hepatitis is divided into acute or chronic infection. The type of treatment and monitoring of the patient are dependent on understanding and interpreting the combination of laboratory tests, pattern of serologic studies, chronicity, and liver biopsy (see Fig. 35-4)

Approach to the Case

Blood tests showed elevated aminotransferases. Hepatits B surface antigen and e antigen were positive. His e antibody and surface antibody were negative. Liver biopsy was typical of pediatric hepatitis B and showed portal triads expanded by a lymphoplasmacytic infiltrate, associated with focal extension outside of the limiting plate (mild periportal inflammatory and piecemeal necrosis). No fibrosis was identified. He was started on a course of IFN-α treatment of three-time-weekly shots for 24 weeks.

SUMMARY

The two most significant therapeutic challenges in the pediatric population is the treatment of hepatitis B and C. These infections are common. Children in all settings—rich, poor, old, and young—have these infections. The affected individual is contagious; the therapies are only modestly effective. Treatment is of public importance. The physician needs to judiciously weigh and understand the pros and cons of treatment, timing of treatment, and the complex decisions.

MAJOR POINTS

- Patients with chronic hepatitis B and hepatitis C often:
  - Have no clinical symptoms
  - Have never been jaundiced
  - Have normal laboratory tests
- Screen all patients with risk factors regardless of symptoms or laboratory tests (see Fig. 35-2)
- Hepatitis C—all children with chronic infection should consider treatment
- Hepatitis B—only children with elevated liver enzymes should be considered for treatment

SUGGESTED READINGS

Alter MJ: Prevention of spread of hepatitis C. Hepatology 36: S93-S98, 2002.

Alter MJ, Mast EE: The epidemiology of viral hepatitis in the United States. Gastroenterol Clin North Am 23:437-455, 1994.

Barrera JM, Bruguera M, Ercilla MG, et al: Persistent hepatitis C viremia after acute self-limiting posttransfusion hepatitis C. Hepatology 21:639-644, 1995.

Beasley RP, Hwang LY, Lin CC, et al: Incidence of hepatitis B virus infections in preschool children in Taiwan. J Infect Dis 146:198-204, 1982.

Bellentani S, Tiribelli C: The spectrum of liver disease in the general population: Lesson from the Dionysos study. J Hepatol 35:531-537, 2001.

Ceci O, Margiotta M, Marello F, et al: High rate of spontaneous viral clearance in a cohort of vertically infected hepatitis C virus infants: What lies behind? J Hepatol 35:687-688, 2001.

Ceci O, Margiotta M, Marello F, et al: Vertical transmission of hepatitis C virus in a cohort of 2,447 HIV-seronegative pregnant women: A 24-month prospective study. J Pediatr Gastroenterol Nutr 33:570-575, 2001.

Cooksley WG, Piratvisuth T, Lee SD, et al: Peginterferon alpha-2a (40 kDa): An advance in the treatment of hepatitis B e antigen-positive chronic hepatitis B. J Viral Hepat 10:298-305, 2003.

Coursaget P, Yvonnet B, Chotard J, et al: Age- and sex-related study of hepatitis B virus chronic carrier state in infants from an endemic area (Senegal). J Med Virol 22:1-5, 1987.

Davis GL, Lau JY: Factors predictive of a beneficial response to therapy of hepatitis C. Hepatology 26:122S-127S, 1997.

Farci P, Alter HJ, Wong D, et al: A long-term study of hepatitis C virus replication in non-A, non-B hepatitis. N Engl J Med 325:98-104, 1991.

Farci P, Shimoda A, Coiana A, et al: The outcome of acute hepatitis C predicted by the evolution of the viral quasispecies. Science 288:339-344, 2000.

Farci P, Strazzera R, Alter HJ, et al: Early changes in hepatitis C viral quasispecies during interferon therapy predict the therapeutic outcome. Proc Natl Acad Sci U S A 99:3081-3086, 2002.

Fung SK, Lok AS: Treatment of chronic hepatitis B: Who to treat, what to use, and for how long? Clin Gastroenterol Hepatol 2:839-848, 2004.

Gonzalez-Peralta RP, Qian K, She JY, et al: Clinical implications of viral quasispecies heterogeneity in chronic hepatitis C. J Med Virol 49:242-247, 1996.

Haber BA: To treat or not to treat: That is the question. J Pediatr Gastroenterol Nutr 39:103-104, 2004.

Hoofnagle JH: Course and outcome of hepatitis C. Hepatology 36:S21-S29, 2002.

Hoofnagle JH: Therapy for acute hepatitis C. N Engl J Med 345:1495-1497, 2001.

Jacobson KR, Murray K, Zellos A, Schwarz KB: An analysis of published trials of interferon monotherapy in children with chronic hepatitis C. J Pediatr Gastroenterol Nutr 34:52-58, 2002.

Jonas MM, Mizerski J, Badia IB, et al: Clinical trial of lamivudine in children with chronic hepatitis B. N Engl J Med 346:1706-13, 2002.

Licata A, Di Bona D, Schepis F, et al: When and how to treat acute hepatitis C? J Hepatol 39:1056-1062, 2003.

Lok AS: New treatment of chronic hepatitis B. Semin Liver Dis 24(Suppl 1):77-82, 2004.

Maddrey WC: Hepatitis B: An important public health issue. J Med Virol 61:362-366, 2000.

Marusawa H, Uemoto S, Hijikata M, et al: Latent hepatitis B virus infection in healthy individuals with antibodies to hepatitis B core antigen. Hepatology 31:488-495, 2000.

Maynard JE: Hepatitis B: Global importance and need for control. Vaccine Suppl:S18-S20; discussion S21-S3, 1990.

McMahon BJ, Holck P, Bulkow L, Snowball M: Serologic and clinical outcomes of 1536 Alaska Natives chronically infected with hepatitis B virus. Ann Intern Med 135:759-768, 2001.

Nomura H, Sou S, Tanimoto H, et al: Short-term interferon-alfa therapy for acute hepatitis C: A randomized controlled trial. Hepatology 39:1213-1219, 2004.

Rehermann B, Ferrari C, Pasquinelli C, Chisari FV: The hepatitis B virus persists for decades after patients' recovery from acute viral hepatitis despite active maintenance of a cytotoxic T-lymphocyte response. Nat Med 2:1104-1108, 1996.

Sokal EM, Bortolotti F: Update on prevention and treatment of viral hepatitis in children. Curr Opin Pediatr 11:384-389, 1999.

Sokal EM, Conjeevaram HS, Roberts EA, et al: Interferon alfa therapy for chronic hepatitis B in children: A multinational randomized controlled trial. Gastroenterology 114:988-995, 1998.

Tabor E, Epstein JS: NAT screening of blood and plasma donations: evolution of technology and regulatory policy. Transfusion 42:1230-1237, 2002.

Tassopoulos NC, Papaevangelou GJ, Sjogren MH, et al: Natural history of acute hepatitis B surface antigen-positive hepatitis in Greek adults. Gastroenterology 92:1844-1850, 1987.

Thimme R, Oldach D, Chang KM, et al: Determinants of viral clearance and persistence during acute hepatitis C virus infection. J Exp Med 194:1395-1406, 2001.

Yotsuyanagi H, Yasuda K, Iino S, et al: Persistent viremia after recovery from self-limited acute hepatitis B. Hepatology 27:1377-1382, 1998.

Yuki N, Nagaoka T, Yamashiro M, et al: Long-term histologic and virologic outcomes of acute self-limited hepatitis B. Hepatology 37:1172-1179, 2003.

Wilson Disease

JAMES P. FRANCIOSI
KATHLEEN M. LOOMES

Disease Description
Case Presentation
Epidemiology
Pathophysiology
Differential Diagnosis
  Liver Disease
  Neuropsychiatric Disease
Diagnostic Testing
  Neuropsychiatric Disease
  Asymptomatic Relatives
  Genetic Testing
Treatment
Approach to the Case
Summary
Major Points

DISEASE DESCRIPTION

Wilson disease is a disorder of hepatic copper metabolism with protean manifestations and is an important cause of acute and chronic pediatric liver disease. It was first described in 1912 by neurologist Kinnear Wilson, who recognized the association of familial neurologic disease with liver disease. Wilson disease is fundamentally a defect in hepatic copper excretion due to mutations in the transmembrane protein ATP7B that results in systemic copper accumulation and toxicity.

Wilson disease, also termed hepatolenticular degeneration, can present with neurologic, psychiatric, or hepatic manifestations. Wilson disease should be considered in the differential diagnosis of any unexplained hepatic or neuropsychiatric disease. Timely diagnosis can prevent the need for liver transplantation, irreversible neurologic injury, and death. Hepatic Wilson disease can mimic autoimmune hepatitis and nonalcoholic steatohepatitis. Additional presenting signs of Wilson disease include, but are not limited to, Coombs'-negative hemolytic anemia, renal tubular dysfunction, pancreatitis, dysrhythmias, rickets, fractures, and amenorrhea.

On physical examination, Kayser-Fleischer rings are supportive of Wilson disease, but they are not pathognomonic or always present. Typical laboratory findings include a low alkaline phosphatase, an aspartate transaminase (AST) greater than alanine transaminase (ALT), and a low serum ceruloplasmin. However, a normal serum ceruloplasmin level does not exclude the diagnosis. In suspected cases, 24-hour urine copper collection and liver biopsy with copper quantification should be performed. No single diagnostic test is considered to be a perfect gold standard.

Untreated Wilson disease is fatal, and late diagnosis may result in irreversible sequelae or transplantation. In symptomatic patients, trientine has replaced D-penicillamine as the recommended chelation therapy. Zinc is recommended for asymptomatic patients. Lifelong compliance with therapy is essential for a favorable outcome. The most important step in establishing the diagnosis of Wilson disease is to consider it in the differential diagnosis.

CASE PRESENTATION

A 14-year-old previously healthy male presented to a local hospital with a 2-month history of vague intermittent abdominal pain, a 2-day history of black tarry stools, and one episode of hematemesis just prior to his evaluation in the emergency department. The patient was otherwise healthy, without recent infection, history of gastroesophageal reflux disease (GERD), bruising, bleeding, jaundice, weight loss, or pruritus. On presentation, the patient was pale and ill-appearing, but alert and oriented. His heart rate was 110 and blood pressure 115/70 mm Hg. His conjunctivae were pale and his sclerae were anicteric. Abdominal examination revealed normal active bowel sounds, no distention or tenderness, no hepatomegaly, and a spleen that was palpated 5 cm below the left costal margin. He was neurologically intact. Initial laboratories were notable for a white blood cell count of 2100/μL, a hemoglobin of 8.7 g/dL, and a platelet count of 97,000/μL. There was evidence of hemolysis on the peripheral blood smear, and a Coombs' antibody test was negative. His hepatic function panel demonstrated an AST of 87 U/L, an ALT of 57 U/L, a total bilirubin of 1.8 mg/dL, a conjugated bilirubin of 0 mg/dL, an albumin of 2.3 g/dL, and an alkaline phosphatase of 35 U/L. His coagulation profile was notable for a prothrombin time (PT) of 17.8 seconds and an International Normalized Ratio (INR) of 2.0.

EPIDEMIOLOGY

The prevalence of Wilson disease is estimated to be 1 in 30,000, and the carrier state occurs in approximately 1 in 90 people. Wilson disease is an autosomal recessive disorder that can present between 3 and 60 years of age, but the median age for children who present with liver disease is 12 years of age. Typically, the age at presentation correlates inversely with hepatic symptoms and directly with neuropsychiatric symptoms. Hepatic symptoms are present in 83% of patients between 3 and 9 years of age, 52% of patients between 10 and 18 years of age, and 26% of patients older than 18 years of age. Conversely, neuropsychiatric symptoms are present in 17% of patients between 3 and 9 years of age, 48% of patients between 10 and 18 years of age, and 74% of patients older than 18 years of age.

PATHOPHYSIOLOGY

A typical Western diet is replete with copper, and individuals typically consume an excess of copper relative to the standard metabolic needs. Foods that are particularly rich in copper include chocolate, nuts, shellfish, organ meats, and mushrooms. In normal copper metabolism, dietary copper is absorbed in the intestine and then removed from the body predominantly via the biliary system. The 20% of copper that is absorbed by the intestine travels from the portal vein into the hepatocyte and either is incorporated into ceruloplasmin or is transported into the biliary system and is excreted from the body in stool.

The defect in hepatic copper excretion in Wilson disease has been localized to the ATP7B copper transmembrane transport protein. This protein allows intracellular copper trafficking into the trans-Golgi network, where copper is incorporated into ceruloplasmin. In the presence of high intracellular copper concentrations, ATP7B translocates into vesicles and facilitates copper excretion into the bile canaliculus. In Wilson disease, the defect in ATP7B decreases copper excretion into the biliary system, and copper accumulates in the hepatocyte. Furthermore, copper incorporation into ceruloplasmin is impaired, and ceruloplasmin without copper, termed apoceruloplasmin, is rapidly degraded in the serum. This explains the low serum levels of ceruloplasmin often seen in patients with Wilson disease. Once toxic levels of hepatocyte copper are reached, hepatocyte death releases copper that is taken up by adjacent hepatocytes, resulting in a chain reaction of worsening parenchymal liver injury.

Once a certain level of copper-induced liver injury is reached, copper is then released into the systemic circulation and affects other organs such as the brain, eyes, heart, and kidneys (Table 36-1). Kayser-Fleischer rings are copper granules deposited in the corneal limbic region that are best appreciated with slit-lamp examination by an ophthalmologist. In approximately 15% of patients with Wilson disease, there is Coombs'-negative hemolytic anemia as a result of copper-induced oxidative stress. This also explains the finding of the AST being greater than ALT that is sometimes seen on the hepatic function panel.

DIFFERENTIAL DIAGNOSIS

Liver Disease

The differential diagnosis of pediatric liver disease is extensive, and is most accurately classified by type of hepatic disease, clinical presentation, and patient age. Hepatic involvement from Wilson disease can range from asymptomatic hepatomegaly to fulminant hepatic failure. Additional hepatic presentations of Wilson disease include acute self-limited hepatitis, fatty liver (steatohepatitis), ascites, cholestasis, chronic liver disease (cirrhosis), isolated splenomegaly, and pruritus.

There are broad differential categories for asymptomatic hepatosplenomegaly, cholestatic liver disease, acute hepatitis, acute liver failure, and chronic liver disease (cirrhosis) that are detailed in other chapters. In pediatric patients with Wilson disease, 70% present with jaundice, approximately 50% present in acute liver failure, 40% present with abdominal pain, 30% present with chronic active hepatitis, 30% present with hepato-

Table 36-1 Systemic Involvement in Wilson Disease

Hepatic	Neuropsychiatric	Ophthalmologic	Renal
Hepatitis Cirrhosis Hepatosplenomegaly Isolated splenomegaly Cholestasis Acute liver failure Chronic liver failure Fatty liver Ascites	Dystonia Movement disorders Depression Declining school performance Deteriorating handwriting Anxiety Schizophrenia Headaches Seizures Ataxia Tremors	Kayser-Fleischer ring Sunflower cataracts	Renal tubular dysfunction Proteinuria Hematuria Aminoaciduria Nephrolithiasis Glycosuria

Hematologic	Orthopedic	Cardiac	Other
Coombs'-negative hemolytic anemia Thrombocytopenia	Rickets Pathologic fractures Osteoporosis	Left ventricular hypertrophy Dysrhythmia	Amenorrhea

splenomegaly, and 25% present with acute hepatitis. Gastrointestinal bleeding can be a complication and presentation of cirrhosis and portal hypertension.

Acute self-resolving hepatitis is frequently attributed to a viral etiology, and can be missed as a presentation of Wilson disease. In Wilson disease–associated acute hepatitis, elevated serum copper can cause oxidative stress and renal tubular dysfunction that can manifest as Coombs'-negative hemolytic anemia, low uric acid, proteinuria, and microscopic hematuria. These findings are not typical for viral hepatitis.

Other liver diseases that resemble Wilson disease in presentation may include nonalcoholic steatohepatitis (NASH) and autoimmune hepatitis (AIH). NASH (commonly referred to as a "fatty liver") is liver steatosis that presents in obese children with elevated aminotransferases. Because NASH is a diagnosis of exclusion, any hepatitis in an obese child that is not responsive to diet and exercise should be considered to be Wilson disease until proved otherwise. In the setting of fulminant hepatic failure, Wilson disease can be very difficult to distinguish from autoimmune hepatitis. This distinction is critical because autoimmune hepatitis–associated liver failure may respond well to steroids, whereas Wilson disease–associated liver failure requires immediate evaluation for liver transplantation. In the setting of pediatric liver failure (elevated PT not responsive to vitamin K and low albumin), an urgent referral to a pediatric liver transplantation center is necessary.

Neuropsychiatric Disease

Although Wilson disease commonly manifests as liver disease in the pediatric age-group, patients can first come to medical attention with neuropsychiatric complaints. The neuropsychiatric manifestations of Wilson disease can be very subtle, and are often not appreciated in the differential diagnosis. Typical presentations such as movement disorders resembling Huntington's disease, dystonia resembling Parkinson's disease, severe depression, schizophrenia, declining school performance, and deteriorating handwriting should be investigated for Wilson disease.

DIAGNOSTIC TESTING

Diagnostic evaluation of any liver disease should begin with a hepatic function panel that includes AST, ALT, gamma-glutamyl-transferase (GGT), alkaline phosphatase, fractionated (total and conjugated) bilirubin, albumin, and total protein. Hepatic synthetic function is measured by the albumin and PT with INR. Aminotransferases in the 100 to 500 IU/L range (often with AST greater than ALT), a markedly elevated bilirubin, a low alkaline phosphatase, and a normal total serum protein level are laboratory findings suggestive of, but not diagnostic for, Wilson disease. An algorithm for investigating hepatic Wilson disease is adapted from the American Association for the

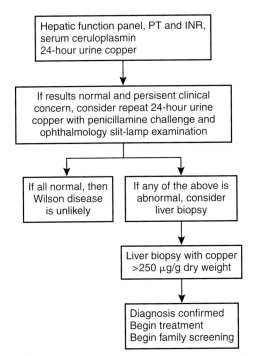

Figure 36-1 Algorithm for investigating hepatic Wilson disease. INR, International Normalized Ratio; PT, prothrombin time. (Adapted from Roberts EA, Schilsky ML: A practice guideline on Wilson disease. Hepatology 37: 1475, 2003).

Study of Liver Diseases (AASLD) 2003 guidelines and detailed in Figure 36-1.

Serum copper measurements are typically low, with values less than 20 μg/dL. However, copper levels may vary depending on disease activity, and serum copper is neither a sensitive nor specific marker for Wilson disease.

Serum ceruloplasmin testing alone has a sensitivity of approximately 80% and a specificity of 94% using the standard value of less than 200 mg/L (20 mg/dL). Although serum ceruloplasmin levels are typically low in Wilson disease, they may be normal. Any disorder that results in hepatic inflammation may elevate serum ceruloplasmin. Ceruloplasmin is also low in 20% of Wilson disease heterozygote carriers. Conversely, any disorder that reduces liver synthetic function may also reduce serum ceruloplasmin. Therefore, serum ceruloplasmin levels alone are inadequate to diagnose or rule out Wilson disease.

One of the most useful tests for Wilson disease is a 24-hour urine copper measurement. In these patients, typically, greater than 40 μg (0.6 μmol) of copper is excreted in a 24-hour collection. Levels between 40 μg and 100 μg constitute a gray zone for which further investigations are warranted. When the 24-hour urine copper is normal, penicillamine challenge may be helpful with a reported sensitivity of 88% and a specificity of 98%. In this test, 500 mg of D-penicillamine (not weight adjusted) is given orally at the beginning and at the 12-hour mark of the 24-hour urine copper collection. Values of greater than 1600 μg (25 μmol) of urine copper excreted in a 24-hour period are considered positive. Elevated urine copper may be seen in chronic liver disease and fulminant hepatic failure not attributed to Wilson disease. These findings warrant further investigation with liver biopsy.

In the appropriate setting, a liver biopsy can be very helpful in supporting the diagnosis of Wilson disease. On liver biopsy, light and electron microscopic findings of steatosis and mitochondrial changes may be clues to the diagnosis. Quantitative measurement of hepatic copper (>250 μg/g dry weight) on liver biopsy is the most important test. The specimen must be transported in a copper-free container. However, elevated hepatic copper is not unique to Wilson disease and may be seen in other chronic liver diseases such as biliary atresia and Alagille syndrome. In severe liver failure, the risk of liver biopsy may outweigh the benefit and cannot be safely performed.

Because of the relatively low sensitivity of the individual tests in Wilson disease, it is important to emphasize that no single diagnostic test is considered to be a perfect gold standard. Rather, it is the combination of select diagnostic testing with sound clinical judgment that leads to a correct diagnosis. A 24-hour urine copper collection and liver biopsy with copper quantification should be performed in suspected cases.

Neuropsychiatric Disease

Although classically described as a disorder involving the basal ganglia, Wilson disease can have a variety of neuropathologic findings. On computed tomography (CT) or magnetic resonance imaging (MRI), approximately 70% of patients can have ventricular dilation, and more than 60% can have cortical atrophy. Unlike patients presenting with isolated liver disease, approximately 95% of Wilson disease patients with neuropsychiatric symptoms have Kayser-Fleischer rings on slit-lamp examination. A hepatic function panel, a PT with INR, serum ceruloplasmin, a brain MRI, and a slit-lamp examination by a pediatric ophthalmologist would constitute an appropriate evaluation. Depending on the clinical situation, further investigations may be warranted (Fig. 36-2).

Asymptomatic Relatives

For asymptomatic relatives, screening should begin at 3 years of age. Investigation should include a complete history and physical examination, hepatic function panel with PT and INR, ceruloplasmin, slit-lamp

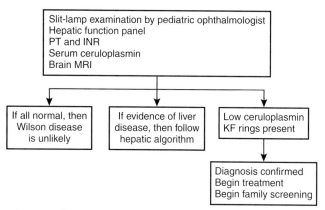

Figure 36-2 Algorithm for investigating neuropsychiatric Wilson disease. INR, International Normalized Ratio; KF, Kayser-Fleischer; MRI, magnetic resonance imaging; PT, prothrombin time. (Adapted from Roberts EA, Schilsky ML: A practice guideline on Wilson disease. Hepatology 37:1475, 2003).

examination by a pediatric ophthalmologist, 24-hour urine copper, and consideration for genetic testing.

Genetic Testing

In difficult diagnostic cases and for asymptomatic relatives, gene testing is available. The genetic defect in Wilson disease has been localized to the *ATP7B* gene on chromosome 13. Genetic mutations can be specific to different populations, and can help to target genetic screening. The large size of the gene and the presence of more than 200 unique mutations make direct screening difficult. More than 95% of individuals can have at least one mutation identified by complete sequencing of the *ATP7B* coding region. However, most patients are compound heterozygotes, which makes direct mutation analysis difficult. A number of patients with a clinical diagnosis of Wilson disease have had only one mutation identified. True heterozygotes, who do not require treatment, can be clinically challenging to distinguish from affected individuals because both can have low ceruloplasmin levels and elevated urinary copper levels. For prenatal diagnosis and family members, linkage analysis can be informative when proband mutations are unknown. Additionally, chromosome 13 haplotyping may be used to differentiate affected relatives from carriers if both mutations cannot be identified.

TREATMENT

Therapies are dependent on the clinical presentation and include diet modification, chelation, zinc, antioxidants, tetrathiomolybdate, and liver transplantation (Fig. 36-3). Without compliance to lifelong therapy, patients can expect a high likelihood of progression to liver failure or irreversible neurologic damage. Restriction of dietary copper (liver, shellfish, nuts, chocolate, mushrooms, and organ meats) is recommended for at least the first year of therapy. Other environmental sources of copper include well water and copper pipes. Water copper levels should be maintained at less than 0.1 part per million (ppm).

Copper chelation therapy was introduced in the 1950s with dimercaprol (BAL) followed by D-penicillamine and trientine. Dosing and laboratory testing for D-penicillamine and trientine are the same. Typical adult dosing for maintenance therapy is gradually increased weekly to 750 to 1000 mg divided two or three times per day with a maximum of 1500 mg/day. In children, dosing is approximately 20 mg/kg/day divided two or three times per day (rounded to the appropriate 250-mg tablet). Up to 30% of patients treated with D-penicillamine can

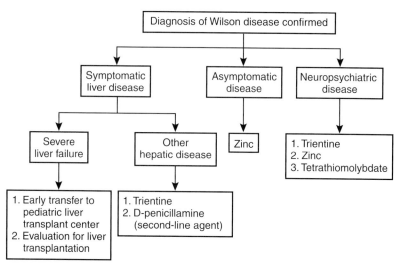

Figure 36-3 Therapy algorithm for Wilson disease. (Adapted from Roberts EA, Schilsky ML: A practice guideline on Wilson disease. Hepatology 37:1475, 2003).

develop severe adverse reactions that include hypersensitivity reactions, neutropenia, thrombocytopenia, proteinuria, and autoimmune disease. Similar reactions can occur with trientine, but occur in only 5% of patients. Therefore, many experts consider trientine as first-line therapy. Goals of therapy are determined by 24-hour urine copper between 200 and 500 μg (3 to 8 μmol) that is measured every 3 months for 2 years, then annually. Chronically elevated urine copper levels suggest noncompliance. Drug toxicity should be followed closely with complete blood count, hepatic function panel, creatinine, and urinalysis (every week for 1 month, every other week for 2 months, every month for 3 months, every 6 months for 2 years, and then annually). Pyridoxine (25 mg/day) also should be administered with both trientine and D-penicillamine therapies. Combination chelation and zinc therapy has been advocated by some experts, but this has not been studied in clinical trials and is not currently supported by the AASLD practice guidelines. Once again, lifelong compliance with medical therapy is essential for a favorable outcome.

In the asymptomatic patient, lifelong zinc therapy is recommended. Zinc inhibits copper uptake from the gastrointestinal tact, induces a metallothionein that competes for copper binding sites, and promotes copper excretion. Dosing of zinc therapy varies by age: 25 mg twice daily in patients younger than 6 years of age, 25 mg three times per day in patients 6 to 12 years of age (or <50 kg), and 50 mg three times per day in patients older than 12 years of age (>50 kg). The main side effect is gastritis, which occurs in approximately 10% of patients. Success of therapy is guided by 24-hour urine copper measurements every 3 months for 6 months, every 6 months for 2 years, and then yearly with a goal copper excretion of less than 75 μg (1.2 μmol) per 24 hours.

Antioxidants have been suggested as adjuvant therapy in many chronic liver diseases. In Wilson disease, there have been reports of low serum vitamin E levels and symptomatic improvement with vitamin E therapy. However, these data are limited, and vitamin E is no substitute for chelation or zinc therapies.

In severe hepatic failure, the most appropriate therapy is liver transplantation. In the setting of pediatric liver failure, Wilson disease should be managed in a referral center. As temporizing measures, plasmapheresis or renal dialysis may serve as useful bridges to liver transplantation, but should be used only under the direction of a pediatric hepatologist.

Patients that present with neuropsychiatric Wilson disease may be managed differently than those with hepatic manifestations. Many authors advocate for chelation therapy in patients with symptomatic neurologic disease. However, D-penicillamine and trientine have been reported to worsen neurologic disease in approximately 50% and 20% of patients, respectively. Controversy exists regarding initial choice of therapy; some authors suggest zinc therapy alone, whereas others believe that zinc acts too slowly and that trientine is the preferred medication. A newer therapy, tetrathiomolybdate, which functions by complexing with copper and blocking copper cellular uptake, may emerge as the first-line therapy for patients with neuropsychiatric disease. However, tetrathiomolybdate is not currently available in the United States. Severe, irreversible neurologic disease is a contraindication to liver transplantation. This further emphasizes the need for timely diagnosis and lifelong compliance with medical therapy.

APPROACH TO THE CASE

Once the patient was hemodynamically stabilized, he was transferred to a pediatric hepatology center. A nasogastric tube was placed and the stomach was lavaged with normal saline, yielding bright red blood and clots that cleared with room temperature saline irrigation. Packed red blood cells and fresh frozen plasma were administered in the intensive care unit. Medications included a proton pump inhibitor and intravenous vitamin K. Once volume resuscitated, the patient was taken to the operating room for upper endoscopy. The esophagus was remarkable for four large varices, and the stomach was notable for portal hypertensive gastropathy. Variceal ligation (banding) was performed on the esophageal varices. An ultrasound of the abdomen documented normal portal venous flow, a small nodular liver with ascites, and splenomegaly. The patient was screened for hepatitis A, B, and C, Epstein-Barr virus, cytomegalovirus, and autoimmune hepatitis. Serum and urine toxicology and metabolic screens were negative. Serum α_1-antitrypsin level was normal with an MM protease inhibitor-type. A serum ceruloplasmin level was 16 mg/dL, and a 24-hour urine copper collection was 174 μg. Additionally, Kayser-Fleischer rings were identified by a pediatric ophthalmologist. The diagnosis of Wilson disease was confirmed, and the patient was begun on trientine, pyridoxine, vitamin E, lansoprazole, and a low-copper diet.

SUMMARY

Wilson disease is a complex disorder of copper metabolism that requires excellent physician diagnostic and management skills. Appropriate testing may include serum ceruloplasmin, 24-hour urine copper, liver function tests, liver biopsy, and a slit-lamp examination by a pediatric ophthalmologist. Trientine and D-penicillamine are the current mainstays of liver disease therapy. Discontinuation of therapy can lead to irreversible hepatic failure. Zinc is recommended for asymptomatic patients. Any case of hepatic failure should be managed in a pediatric liver referral center. Early recognition, investigation, and treatment can mean the difference between a thriving child on minimal lifelong medications, to one requiring a liver transplantation, to death. Wilson disease should be part of the differential diagnosis in any patient with an unexplained hepatic or neuropsychiatric condition.

> **MAJOR POINTS**
>
> Wilson disease should be considered in the differential diagnosis of any unexplained hepatic or neuropsychiatric disease.
> Timely diagnosis can prevent the need for liver transplantation, irreversible neurologic injury, and death.
> No single diagnostic test is considered a gold standard.
> A 24-hour urine copper collection and liver biopsy with copper quantification should be performed in suspected cases.
> Liver enzyme measurements often show a low alkaline phosphatase and an AST greater than ALT.
> Kayser-Fleischer rings are supportive of Wilson disease, but they are not pathognomonic or always present.
> A normal serum ceruloplasmin level does not exclude the diagnosis.
> Hepatic Wilson disease can mimic autoimmune hepatitis and nonalcoholic steatohepatitis.
> Trientine has replaced D-penicillamine as the recommended chelation therapy for symptomatic patients with liver disease. Zinc is recommended for asymptomatic patients.
> Lifelong compliance with therapy is essential for a favorable outcome.

SUGGESTED READINGS

Ala A, Schilsky ML: Wilson disease: Pathophysiology, diagnosis, treatment, and screening. Clin Liver Dis 8:787, 2004.

Brewer GJ, Askari FK: Wilson disease: Clinical management and therapy. J Hepatol 42 Suppl(1): S13, 2005.

Cox DW, Roberts E: Wilson disease. www.genetests.org. Updated January, 2006.

Dhawan A, Taylor RM, Cheeseman P, et al: Wilson disease in children: 37-year experience and revised King's score for liver transplantation. Liver Transpl 11:441, 2005.

Feldstein AE, Chitkara DK, Plescow R, Grand RJ: Wilson disease. In Walker WA, Goulet O, Kleinman RE, et al (eds): Pediatric Gastrointestinal Disease: Pathophysiology, Diagnosis, Management, 2nd ed. Hamilton, Ontario, BC Decker, 2004.

Ferenci P, Caca K, Loudianos G, et al: Diagnosis and phenotypic classification of Wilson disease. Liver Int 23:139, 2003.

Integlia MJ, Pleskow RG, Grand RJ: Wilson's disease. In Altschuler SM, Liacouras CA (eds): Clinical Pediatric Gastroenterology. Philadelphia, Churchill Livingstone, 1998.

Jevon GP, Dimmick JE: Metabolic disorders in childhood. In Russo P, Ruchelli E, Piccoli DA (eds): Pathology of Pediatric Gastrointestinal and Liver Disease. New York, Springer, 2004.

Loudianos G, Gitlin JD: Wilson's disease. Semin Liver Dis 20:353, 2000.

Roberts EA, Schilsky ML: A practice guideline on Wilson disease. Hepatology 37:1475, 2003.

Sanchez-Albisua I, Garde T, Hierro L, et al: A high index of suspicion: The key to an early diagnosis of Wilson disease in childhood. J Pediatr Gastroenterol Nutr 28:186, 1999.

Schilsky ML: Diagnosis and treatment of Wilson disease. Pediatr Transplant 6:15, 2002.

Schilsky ML, Tavill AS: Wilson's disease. In Schiff ER, Sorrell MF, Maddrey WC (eds): Schiff's Diseases of the Liver. Philadelphia, Lippincott-Raven, 1999.

Sokol RJ, Narkewicz MR: Copper and iron storage disorders. In Suchy FJ, Sokol RJ, Balistreri WF (eds): Liver Disease in Children, 2nd ed. Philadelphia, Lippincott Williams & Wilkins, 2001.

Tanner S: Disorders of copper metabolism. In Kelly DA (ed): Diseases of the Liver and Biliary System in Children. Oxford, UK, Blackwell Science, 2004.

PANCREATIC DISORDERS

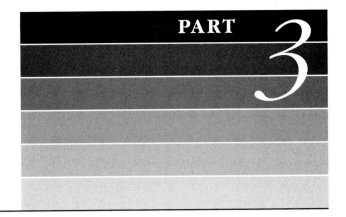

CHAPTER 37

Congenital Anomalies

RAMAN SREEDHARAN

PETAR MAMULA

Disease Description
Case Presentation
Development of the Pancreas
Pathophysiology and Epidemiology
    Pancreatic Agenesis, Hypoplasia, and Dysplasia
    Pancreas Divisum
    Common Channel Syndrome
    Annular Pancreas
    Heterotopic Pancreas
    Pancreatic Cysts
Differential Diagnosis
Diagnostic Testing
Treatment
Approach to the Case
Summary
Major Points

DISEASE DESCRIPTION

Congenital anomalies of the pancreas include pancreatic agenesis, pancreatic hypoplasia, pancreatic dysplasia, pancreas divisum, annular pancreas, and heterotopic pancreas (Table 37-1). Some of them are accompanied by clinical symptoms, but the majority are incidental findings during investigation for unrelated conditions, or at autopsy.

CASE PRESENTATION

A 15-year-old white girl was transferred to a pediatric gastroenterology service at a tertiary care hospital for management of recurrent episodes of pancreatitis. The problems started 10 months ago with abdominal pain, nausea, and vomiting. There was a history of collision and a fall during a basketball game at school a couple of days before the onset of the illness; otherwise she was a healthy child with no past major medical or surgical problems. She was referred to a local emergency department, where diagnosis of pancreatitis was made based on elevated serum amylase and lipase levels. She was admitted to the hospital and received intravenous (IV) fluids. Pain management required IV analgesics. With improvement in symptoms and a fall in the serum pancreatic enzyme levels, she was allowed clear fluids after 4 days. The diagnostic workup during the admission included an x-ray of the abdomen and chest, computed tomography (CT) scan of the abdomen, liver function tests, comprehensive metabolic panel, and urinalysis, all of which were normal. Before discharge from hospital, the pancreatic enzyme levels were near normal and an ultrasound of the abdomen looking for complications related to pancreatitis was reported to be normal. The patient was discharged from the hospital after a 2-week stay with a diagnosis of pancreatitis secondary to abdominal trauma, on oral analgesics as needed.

The symptoms of pain and nausea reappeared after 2 months, and blood testing revealed pancreatic enzyme elevation. The patient was readmitted to the hospital. A magnetic resonance cholangiopancreatography (MRCP) was performed but did not reveal any abnormality. A sweat test was also done during this admission and was reported as normal.

After the second hospital stay the patient's symptoms continued to recur, and outpatient pain management was becoming increasingly difficult. She had two further admissions at the local hospital, with similar symptoms and intermittent elevation of pancreatic enzymes. The repeat imaging studies with ultrasound and CT abdomen did not reveal any major abnormalities.

Subsequently, the patient was referred to a tertiary care pediatric hospital where nasojejunal tube feeding was initiated in an attempt to minimize the pancreatic

Table 37-1 Congenital Pancreatic Anomalies
Agenesis
Dysplasia
Hypoplasia
Pancreas divisum
Annular pancreas
Heterotopic pancreas
Common channel syndrome
Pancreatic cysts

stimulation. Extensive genetic testing for causes of pancreatitis was negative. The repeated imaging studies included ultrasound of the abdomen and MRCP, both of which were normal. Because of the persistence of the symptoms and elevated pancreatic enzyme levels, an endoscopic retrograde cholangiopancreatography (ERCP) was performed, which revealed the diagnosis of pancreas divisum.

DEVELOPMENT OF THE PANCREAS

Pancreatic development starts as early as the fourth week of gestation. The initial step in the development of pancreas is the appearance of a dorsal and a ventral outpouching from the endodermal lining of the primitive duodenum (Fig. 37-1). The dorsal anlage, which makes an early appearance compared with the ventral anlage, forms the superior part of the head, neck, body, and tail of the pancreas. The ventral anlage, which is situated more caudally and is anatomically closely related to the bile duct and hepatic diverticulum, develops into the inferior part of the head and uncinate process of the pancreas. An axial duct system develops during the same time in each of the anlages. The dorsal duct (duct of Santorini) arises directly from the duodenal wall and the ventral duct (duct of Wirsung) arises from the common bile duct.

By 7 weeks of gestation the dorsal and ventral anlages are brought into apposition by partial rotation of the duodenum and eventually fuse to form a single structure. At the time of fusion, the dorsal and ventral ducts fuse at the junction of the head and body of the pancreas to form the main pancreatic duct. In the majority of individuals the main excretory duct is the ventral duct or duct of Wirsung, which opens into the major papilla along with the common bile duct. The accessory duct, which is patent in 70% of individuals, is formed by the proximal part of the dorsal duct or duct of Santorini. The fusion of the ducts is complex and has many variations in the nature of the fusion and the openings of the ducts. The different cell types in the pancreas carry out its exocrine and endocrine functions. These cells originate from common pluripotent progenitor cells under the influence of different transcription factors. There are distinct developmental pathways such as Notch, Hedgehog, and tumor growth factor-beta (TGF-β) described; disruption of these pathways can lead to different congenital anomalies.

PATHOPHYSIOLOGY AND EPIDEMIOLOGY

Pancreatic Agenesis, Hypoplasia, and Dysplasia

Complete pancreatic agenesis is practically incompatible with life and is very rare. Partial pancreatic agenesis is usually due to an abnormal development of the dorsal anlage and leads to an altered size and shape of the

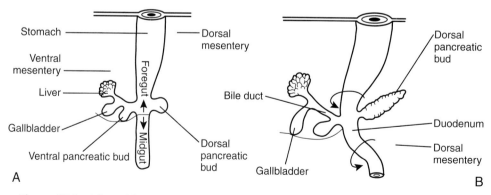

Figure 37-1 Adapted from Moore K, Persaud T: The Developing Human, 1982, with permission from Elsevier.)

pancreas. In pancreatic hypoplasia there is a reduction in ductal differentiation, and normal epithelial cells are replaced by fatty tissue. Pancreatic dysplasia is characterized by abundant fibromuscular tissue with disorganized ductal and parenchymal tissues. In these anomalies the exocrine and endocrine functions of the pancreas are affected in varying degrees. The clinical symptoms and manifestations depend on residual function of the pancreas. The different presentations include failure to thrive, fat malabsorption, and diabetes mellitus.

Pancreas Divisum

This is the most common congenital anomaly of the pancreas. The incidence of pancreas divisum reported in the literature, varies from 5% to 14% in autopsy specimens. Pancreas divisum occurs as a result of the incomplete fusion of the dorsal and ventral ducts during development, leading to persistence of two drainage systems in the pancreas. The duct of Wirsung or the ventral duct, which is normally the major duct system, drains only the head of the pancreas and opens via the major papilla. The duct of Santorini or the dorsal duct drains the rest of the pancreas and opens through a minor papilla that is positioned proximal to the major papilla. The minor papilla may be too small for the proper drainage of secretions from the major portions of the gland, which has been speculated as a mechanism for causing recurrent pancreatitis. Symptoms similar to a functional stenosis of the opening may manifest as recurrent abdominal pain.

Common Channel Syndrome

Common channel syndrome, like pancreas divisum, is a pancreatic duct anomaly. However, in this case it is the junction of the common bile duct and pancreatic duct that fails to develop appropriately. During development the junction progresses toward the duodenal wall, and is normally part of the wall. If this is interrupted the junction remains extraduodenal and not part of the usual sphincter system. The normal common channel is usually up to 5 mm in length, whereas the long channel exceeds 10 mm. The anomalous junction allows flow of pancreatic secretions into the common bile duct and vice versa. This may lead to development of choledochal cyst and recurrent pancreatitis.

Annular Pancreas

Annular pancreas is the second most common congenital anomaly of the pancreas and it occurs with a frequency of 1 in 20,000 births. A band of pancreatic tissue encircles the second part of the duodenum, producing varying degrees of obstruction in this region. Several theories have been put forward to explain this anomaly, which include failure of rotation due to fixation of the of the tip of the ventral anlage, persistence of the left segment of the ventral anlage that normally atrophy (Baldwin's theory), and hypertrophy of the two anlages, resulting in constriction of the duodenum.

The clinical manifestations depend on the degree of obstruction secondary to constriction. In complete constriction of the duodenum, pregnancy is complicated with polyhydramnios and the neonate presents with feeding difficulty, vomiting, and abdominal distention. The diagnosis is aided by the "double-bubble sign" on the abdominal x-ray. In less severe cases, the clinical manifestations could be subtle and diagnosis is usually delayed or incidental during investigation for unrelated conditions, or at autopsy. The feeling of postprandial fullness, nausea, and weight loss due to reduced intake are manifestations in some cases and could go on for years before diagnosis is made. Rarely, a manifesting symptom is gastrointestinal bleeding.

Heterotopic Pancreas

Heterotopic pancreas is ectopic pancreatic tissue without anatomic or vascular continuity to the main body of the pancreas. It is also known by different names like ectopic pancreas, pancreatic rest, accessory pancreas, and aberrant pancreas. The incidence of heterotopic pancreas has been reported to be 15% in autopsy specimens. The exact etiology is unknown, although one hypothesis involves ectopic migration of pancreas precursor. This is supported by expression of PDX1, marker of pancreatic progenitor cells in the stomach, duodenum, and small bowel, which is where heterotopic pancreas is most commonly seen (70% of cases), although it can be found anywhere in the intestinal tract. Extraintestinal locations include umbilicus and bronchopulmonary areas.

Heterotopic pancreas usually do not cause symptoms. However, nausea, vomiting, epigastric pain, dyspepsia, and abdominal distention can occur and may be related to obstruction. Gastrointestinal bleeding, intussusception, cholecystitis, and malignant changes are associated complications.

Pancreatic Cysts

Congenital pancreatic cysts are uncommon. Most do not cause symptoms, but depending on the size, may be associated with abdominal pain or pancreatitis. They may be isolated, associated with other organ cysts (kidney, liver), or as a part of a syndrome (i.e., von Hippel-Landau disease).

DIFFERENTIAL DIAGNOSIS

The differential diagnoses (Table 37-2) of congenital pancreatic anomalies can be divided into several subgroups depending on presenting signs and symptoms. The most common symptoms include abdominal pain, gastrointestinal bleeding, vomiting secondary to obstruction, and acute, chronic, or recurrent pancreatitis.

DIAGNOSTIC TESTING

Diagnostic testing for pancreatic congenital anomalies includes laboratory tests, radiologic, endoscopic studies, and histopathology (Table 37-3). Most commonly, the following blood tests are obtained: complete blood count, erythrocyte sedimentation rate or C-reactive protein, liver function tests, pancreatic enzymes, and comprehensive metabolic panel. Stool test for 72-hour fecal fat clearance can assess fat malabsorption, whereas serum glucose, urinalysis, and glucose tolerance tests investigate endocrine function. A sweat test is obtained if cystic fibrosis is suspected.

Table 37-2 Most Common Differential Diagnoses According to Symptoms

Abdominal Pain	Pancreatitis
Gastrointestinal infection	Idiopathic
Constipation	Traumatic
Gastroesophageal reflux	Structural (stone, stricture)
Functional abdominal pain	Metabolic (hyperlipidemia, cystic fibrosis)
Lactose intolerance	Medication
Inflammatory bowel disease	Hereditary
Celiac disease	Multisystem disease
Irritable bowel syndrome	
Hepatic pathology	**Obstruction/vomiting**
Urinary tract infection	Anatomic abnormalities (malrotation with atresia, stenosis)
Hemorrhage	
Peptic ulcer	Infectious
Duodenal ulcer	Appendicitis
Esophagitis	Neurologic
Mallory-Weiss tear	Renal
Gastritis	Metabolic
Esophageal varices	Incarcerated hernia
Vascular anomalies	Other

Table 37-3 Diagnostic Tests and Treatments for Pancreatic Congenital Anomalies

Anomaly	Diagnostic Tests	Treatment
Partial agenesis, hypoplasia, and dysplasia	Pancreatic exocrine function tests, fasting blood sugar, MRCP, angiography, and ERCP. Definitive diagnosis by laparotomy or at autopsy.	Supportive therapy, insulin, and pancreatic enzyme supplements.
Pancreas divisum	ERCP investigation of choice. MRCP with or without secretin stimulation is useful but not absolute.	ERCP procedures include sphincterotomy, balloon dilatation, and stent placement. Surgical procedures include sphincterotomy, sphincteroplasty, Puestow's procedure and Whipple's procedure.
Common channel syndrome	ERCP, MRCP, or transcutaneous cholangiogram.	When associated with choledochal cyst requires radical excision; otherwise, hepaticoenterostomy, pancreaticojejunostomy, or endoscopic sphincterotomy can be performed.
Annular pancreas	In severe cases with complete obstruction of duodenum "double bubble" sign on abdominal x-ray. Abdominal CT, MRCP, and ERCP can be helpful.	Bypass surgery.
Heterotopic pancreas	Usually seen at the time of endoscopy. Does not require further investigation unless diagnosis is in doubt or complications arise. Excision with biopsy diagnostic.	No treatment required unless complications arise, in which case surgical excision is performed.
Pancreatic cysts	Abdominal ultrasound or CT.	No treatment required unless complications arise, in which case surgical excision or endoscopic drainage can be performed.

CT, computed tomography; ERCP, endoscopic retrograde cholangiopancreatography; MRCP, magnetic resonance cholangiopancreatography.

Partial pancreatic agenesis, hypoplasia, and dysplasia are initially investigated by determining the functions of the endocrine and exocrine parts of the pancreas. The endocrine function is assessed by fasting blood sugar estimation. The exocrine functions can be assessed by cholecystokinin-secretin pancreatic stimulation test. Quantitative fecal fat estimation is an indirect method for the assessment of exocrine pancreatic function. Useful imaging studies of the pancreas include abdominal ultrasound, endoscopic ultrasound, CT scan of the abdomen, MRCP, angiography, and ERCP. Definitive diagnosis may be established at laparotomy or during autopsy, and through histologic analysis.

Pancreas divisum is diagnosed definitively by ERCP (Fig. 37-2). Other helpful imaging techniques include MRCP, endoscopic ultrasound, and CT scan of the abdomen, although they may be normal. MRCP with secretin stimulation is a dynamic study and has better yield than regular MRCP. Common channel syndrome can be detected on abdominal ultrasound, although ERCP, MRCP, and percutaneous cholangiogram are more sensitive diagnostic tools.

Annular pancreas causing complete obstruction at the duodenal level in a neonate will produce a "double bubble" sign on a plain abdominal x-ray. In minor degrees of obstruction, contrast study of the upper intestine shows an annular filling defect in the duodenum with prestenotic dilatation and reverse peristalsis. CT scan of the abdomen, MRCP, and ERCP are helpful tools but the definitive diagnosis is made at laparotomy.

Heterotopic pancreas is usually an incidental finding during endoscopy. It appears as yellowish nodules with

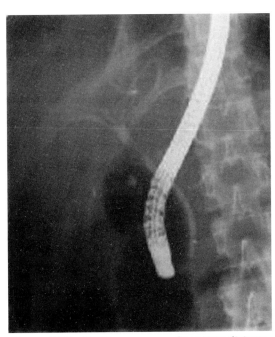

Figure 37-2 ERCP appearance of pancreas divisum.

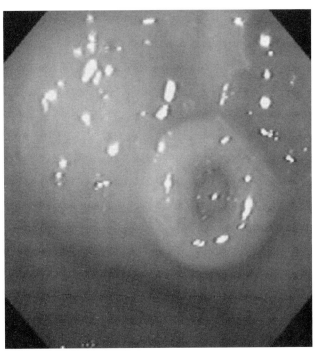

Figure 37-3 *(See also Color Plate 37-3.)* Endoscopic appearance of heterotopic pancreas (pancreatic rest) in the antrum of stomach.

a central umbilication of varying sizes (Fig. 37-3). Confirmation of the diagnosis is made by biopsy and histology. Pancreatic cysts can be detected by abdominal ultrasound or CT.

TREATMENT

Treatment of pancreatic anomalies depends on the type of anomaly, patient's symptoms, and complications (see Table 37-3). Management of hypoplasia and dysplasia depends on the exocrine and the endocrine involvement. Pancreatic enzyme supplements, insulin, and supportive care are the cornerstones of management.

Initial management of pancreas divisum with pancreatitis involves supportive care and pain management to stabilize the patient. Definitive management involves ERCP procedures or surgical procedures to improve the pancreatic drainage. The ERCP procedures include sphincterotomy of the minor papilla, balloon dilatation of the sphincter, and duct stent placement. Surgical interventions include sphincteroplasty, sphincterotomy, Puestow's procedure, and Whipple's procedure.

Treatment of common channel syndrome associated with choledochal cyst requires surgical therapy and surveillance for malignancy. Otherwise hepaticoenterostomy, pancreaticojejunostomy, or endoscopic sphincteroplasty may be curative.

Annular pancreas with complete obstruction of the duodenum is a surgical emergency in the neonatal period. The pancreatic band causing the obstruction cannot be released surgically because of major complications associated with surgical division of the pancreas, so bypass surgeries are the surgical treatment of choice. The bypass surgeries include duodenoduodenostomy and other extensive surgeries depending on the location and anatomy. A minor degree of obstruction that is difficult to manage medically, is surgically corrected as explained earlier.

Heterotopic pancreas does not require any intervention unless there are complications or if the diagnosis is in doubt. Surgical excision is the treatment of choice if required. Pancreatic cysts usually do not require therapy unless there are complications due to their size or location, in which case endoscopic drainage or surgery could be performed.

APPROACH TO THE CASE

Initially, patients with pancreatitis receive standard supportive therapy. This includes IV fluids, bowel rest, antacid therapy, pain management, and nutritional therapy including total parenteral nutrition (TPN), or possibly nasojejunal feedings. Early involvement of a pain team and a clinical psychologist is helpful in the management of pain.

Once stabilized, the patient is investigated thoroughly, looking for the etiology causing recurrent pancreatitis. Detailed workup to rule out different metabolic conditions causing pancreatitis should be undertaken. Genetic testing includes workup to rule out mutations of the cystic fibrosis transmembrane conductance regulator (CFTR) gene, cationic trypsinogen *(PRSS1)* gene, and pancreatic secretary trypsin inhibitor *(SPINK1)* gene. Relevant imaging studies include ultrasound of the abdomen, endoscopic ultrasound, CT scan of the abdomen, MRCP (if indicated with secretin stimulation), and ERCP. Endoscopic ultrasound is not frequently undertaken in children because of the size of the probe and the lack of expertise in children. MRCP is useful in many cases but is not as specific as ERCP to detect anomalies of the duct and may be difficult to interpret in small children, especially neonates and infants. MRCP with secretin stimulation is a dynamic study and identifies the duct structure better but is not commonly available for children. ERCP, even though invasive and associated with possible complications, is still the gold standard for identification of duct anomalies of the pancreas, including pancreas divisum. This procedure is frequently performed by an adult gastroenterologist who has expertise and experience with ERCP.

The management of pancreas divisum commonly involves ERCP. Sphincterotomy of the minor papilla at the time of ERCP is the procedure of choice. Also, balloon dilatation with stent placement can be attempted in order to improve the flow of pancreatic secretions. In some cases, surgery is required.

SUMMARY

Congenital pancreatic anomalies are fairly uncommon and comprise conditions ranging from completely asymptomatic and diagnosed incidentally, to those causing significant complications requiring extensive surgical therapy. The diagnostic process, as with any other condition, starts with a detailed history and physical examination. Based on the patient's symptoms, diagnostic workup is initiated and advanced from less invasive to more invasive procedures, like ERCP, which have a small but significant rate of complications. Depending on the type of anomaly, therapy is directed toward alleviating symptoms, first medical, then endoscopic, and finally surgical treatment.

MAJOR POINTS

Major aspects in the development of pancreas occur between the fourth and seventh weeks of gestation.

The congenital anomalies of the pancreas include agenesis of the pancreas, hypoplasia of the pancreas, dysplasia of the pancreas, pancreas divisum, annular pancreas, and heterotopic pancreas.

The majority of congenital pancreatic anomalies are clinically silent and are incidental findings during investigation for unrelated conditions or at autopsy.

In a case of recurrent or chronic pancreatitis, pancreas divisum as an etiology should be entertained.

SUGGESTED READINGS

Chen YC, Yeh CN, Tseng JH: Symptomatic adult annular pancreas. J Clin Gastroenterol 36:446-450, 2003.

Choi JY, Kim MJ, Kim JH, et al: Annular pancreas: Emphasis on magnetic resonance cholangiopancreatography findings. J Comput Assist Tomogr 28:528-532, 2004.

Cohen SA, Siegel JH: Pancreas divisum: Endoscopic therapy. Surg Clin North Am 81:467-477, 2001.

Duphare H, Nijhawan S, Rana S, Bhargava DK: Heterotopic gastric and pancreatic tissue in large bowel. Am J Gastroenterol 85:68-71, 1990.

Eisenberger CF, Gocht A, Knoefel WT, et al: Heterotopic pancreas: Clinical presentation and pathology with review of the literature. Hepatogastroenterology 51:854-858, 2004.

Hajivassiliou CA: Intestinal obstruction in neonatal/pediatric surgery. Semin Pediatr Surg 12:241-253, 2003.

Hamm M, Rottger P, Fiedler C: [Pancreas anulare as a rare differential diagnosis of duodenal stenosis in adulthood]. Langenbecks Arch Chir 382:307-310, 1997.

Jimenez JC, Emil S, Podnos Y, Nguyen N: Annular pancreas in children: A recent decade's experience. J Pediatr Surg 39:1654-1657, 2004.

Kamisawa T, Yuyang T, Egawa N, et al: A new embryologic hypothesis of annular pancreas. Hepatogastroenterology 48:277-278, 2001.

Khalid A, Slivka A: Pancreas divisum. Curr Treat Options Gastroenterol 4:389-399, 2001.

Klein SD, Affronti JP: Pancreas divisum, an evidence-based review: Part I, pathophysiology. Gastrointest Endosc 60:419-425, 2004.

Klein SD, Affronti JP: Pancreas divisum, an evidence-based review: Part II, patient selection and treatment. Gastrointest Endosc 60:585-589, 2004.

Lai R, Freeman ML, Cass OW, Mallery S: Accurate diagnosis of pancreas divisum by linear-array endoscopic ultrasonography. Endoscopy 36:705-709, 2004.

Laughlin EH, Keown ME, Jackson JE: Heterotopic pancreas obstructing the ampulla of Vater. Arch Surg 118:979-980, 1983.

Lin SZ: Annular pancreas: Etiology, classification and diagnostic imaging. Chin Med J (Engl) 102:368-372, 1989.

Lucandri G, Castaldo P, Meloni E, Ziparo V: [Ectopic pancreas with gastric localization: A clinical case and review of the literature]. G Chir 15:162-166, 1994.

Matos C, Metens T, Deviere J, et al: Pancreas divisum: Evaluation with secretin-enhanced magnetic resonance cholangiopancreatography. Gastrointest Endosc 53:728-733, 2001.

Mishra D, Singh R, Kohli A: Pancreas divisum: An uncommon cause of acute pancreatitis. Indian J Pediatr 70:593-595, 2003.

Nijs E, Callahan MJ, Taylor GA: Disorders of the pediatric pancreas: Imaging features. Pediatr Radiol 2004.

Pang LC: Pancreatic heterotopia: A reappraisal and clinicopathologic analysis of 32 cases. South Med J 81:1264-1275, 1988.

Paraskevas G, Papaziogas B, Lazaridis C, et al: Annular pancreas in adults: Embryological development, morphology and clinical significance. Surg Radiol Anat 23:437-444, 2001.

Ruangtrakool R, Mungnirandr A, Laohapensang M, Sathornkich C: Surgical treatment for congenital duodenal obstruction. J Med Assoc Thai 84:842-849, 2001.

Sencan A, Mir E, Gunsar C, Akcora B: Symptomatic annular pancreas in newborns. Med Sci Monit 8:CR434-CR437, 2002.

Shah KK, DeRidder PH, Schwab RE, Alexander TJ: CT diagnosis of dorsal pancreas agenesis. J Comput Assist Tomogr 11:170-171, 1987.

Slack JM: Developmental biology of the pancreas. Development 121:1569-1580, 1995.

Soehendra N, Kempeneers I, Nam VC, Grimm H: Endoscopic dilatation and papillotomy of the accessory papilla and internal drainage in pancreas divisum. Endoscopy 18:129-132, 1986.

Varshney S, Johnson CD: Surgery for pancreas divisum. Ann R Coll Surg Engl 84:166-169, 2002.

Wagner CW, Golladay ES: Pancreas divisum and pancreatitis in children. Am Surg 54:22-26, 1988.

Yagmurlu B, Erden A, Erden I: [Pancreas divisum: Diagnostic importance of MR cholangiopancreatography]. Tani Girisim Radyol 9:339-344, 2003.

CHAPTER 38

Cystic Fibrosis

VERA DE MATOS

MARIA MASCARENHAS

Disease Description
Case Presentation
Epidemiology
Pathophysiology
    Pancreatic Disease
    Liver Disease and the Biliary Tract
    Genotype-Phenotype Correlation
Gastrointestinal Complications in Patients with Cystic Fibrosis
    Meconium Ileus
    Distal Intestinal Obstruction Syndrome
    Intussusception
    Appendicitis
    Rectal Prolapse
    Small Bowel Bacterial Overgrowth
    Fibrosing Colonopathy
    Gastroesophageal Reflux Disease
    Delayed Gastric Emptying
    Constipation
Treatment
Approach to the Case
Summary
Major Points

DISEASE DESCRIPTION

Cystic fibrosis (CF) is the most common autosomal recessive genetic disease, with an incidence of 1 per 2500 to 1 per 4000 in the United States. The estimated carrier frequency in whites approaches 5%. There are more than 1000 different mutations of the cystic fibrosis transmembrane conductance regulator (CFTR) gene known. The CFTR gene is located in chromosome 7. CFTR is a cyclic adenosine monophosphate (cAMP)–dependent chloride channel located in the apical membrane of epithelial cells. It regulates electrolyte transport in secreting epithelia.

The most frequent mutation, a deletion of a pair base in exon 10, results in a deletion of phenylalanine at position 508 on the CFTR protein or ΔF508. In all known CFTR mutations, chloride reabsorption from sweat ducts is impaired and sweat chloride concentration is greater than 60 mmol/L. Changes in electrolyte transport impair fluid secretion and affect the respiratory epithelia, the pancreatic ducts, the intrahepatic and extrahepatic bile ducts, the intestinal epithelia, and the reproductive tract. Dehydrated and viscous secretions cause mucus obstruction in the bronchi and duct obstruction in the pancreas, explaining the classic presentation of the disease with pulmonary and pancreatic insufficiency. The disease is multisystemic, and although it affects more severely the pulmonary system and the pancreas, the liver, the gastrointestinal tract, and reproductive system also are affected. The diagnosis of CF is based on the clinical phenotype at presentation and the presence of an elevated sweat chloride concentration greater than 60 mmol/L. In some cases, genotyping is extremely helpful.

CASE PRESENTATION

A 12-year-old boy with cystic fibrosis (CF) presented with a 3-year history of recurrent episodes of severe midepigastric abdominal pain associated with bulky foul-smelling stools. Lactulose, enemas, and an oral "clean-out cocktail" (acetylcysteine [Mucomyst], mineral oil, and Coca-Cola) were tried, with only temporary improvement, in an effort to treat distal intestinal obstruction syndrome (DIOS). His gastrointestinal (GI) medications include ranitidine (Zantac) 150 mg twice a day and pancrelipase (Creon 20), 6145 lipase units/kg/meal. His past medical history was notable for a diagnosis of meconium ileus at birth and resection of 10 cm of his ileum. Because of persistent abdominal pain, an upper GI series with small bowel follow-through is performed to evaluate for a stricture, blind loop, adhesions, and partial small bowel obstruction. This study revealed an asymptomatic intussusception that was reduced. His abdominal pain did not resolve, and 1 month later he underwent an abdominal ultrasound that was normal (Table 38-1).

Because of a concern of possible ongoing malabsorption, he then underwent a fecal fat collection to document fat malabsorption, a lactulose breath test to look for bacterial overgrowth, and an abdominal x-ray to evaluate the amount and location of the stool. His pancreatic enzyme replacement therapy was optimized. The acetylcysteine dose was increased to 30 mL twice per day and he was started on a mixture of mineral oil and magnesium sulfate (Haley's M-O). Results of the above tests were significant for the following: A 3-day diet record showed a caloric intake of 2483 kcal/day, with 32% dietary fat, and excessive fat intake at lunch and dinner as well as the ingestion of very low-fat snacks. He had heme-negative stools and the coefficient of fat absorption was 84%. The lactulose breath test was not done for scheduling reasons and the abdominal x-ray showed a large amount of stool. Because of a concern that his initial upper GI series with small bowel follow-through was not adequate, he had a repeat study, which showed a persistently dilated loop of jejunum. His diet was changed. Fiber intake was increased and his fat intake was spread out throughout the day instead of being concentrated during his lunch and dinner meals.

Because of the results of the abdominal x-ray and upper GI series, he was treated with an oral clean-out cocktail and metronidazole for 2 weeks to treat DIOS and possible bacterial overgrowth, respectively. He did well for 1 month, but was subsequently admitted with severe abdominal pain due to DIOS. He received 2000 mL of a Gastrografin enema, with excellent results. The study was notable for the radiographic material refluxing into the terminal ileum.

After temporary improvement, he continued having persistent abdominal pain and was started on a daily treatment with lactulose and acetylcysteine and weekly with GoLYTELY. The GoLYTELY was discontinued 1 month later because of gagging and inability to tolerate the regimen. His abdominal pain persisted, so his dose of acetylcysteine was increased and he was prescribed another course of metronidazole for 4 weeks. Two months later the patient was doing better and all his medications were stopped except for daily lactulose. He was still following his prescribed diet, and his dose of pancreatic enzymes had slowly been decreased to Creon 20, 4248 lipase units (UL)/kg/meal.

EPIDEMIOLOGY

CF affects 1 in 2500 live births in white communities. It is less frequent in African Americans, with an incidence of 1 in 15,300 and is rare in Southeast Asians (1 in 100,000). The prevalence of CF in the United States was estimated to be 1 in 3000. The most common mutation, ΔF508, accounts for 66% of CF mutations worldwide. It is most frequent in northern Europeans (70% to 80%) and less frequent in southern Europeans (50% to 55%) and affects a minority of Ashkenazi Jews (30%).

PATHOPHYSIOLOGY

Pancreatic Disease

Pancreatic insufficiency (PI) is defined as insufficient lipase-colipase secretion resulting in fat malabsorption. The coefficient of fecal fat absorption obtained from a 3- to 5-day fat balance study is less than 93%. PI is present in patients with severe CFTR mutations (ΔF508 homozygotes or ΔF508 compound heterozygotes with another severe non-ΔF508 mutation) and it affects 80% to 90% of CF patients. The prevalence of PI increases with age; it affects 60% of neonates diagnosed with CF, 80% of children with CF ages 2 to 3 years, and 80% to 90% of children in late childhood. Several mutations confer milder disease, and these patients are usually pancreatic sufficient (PS). It is important to know the pancreatic phenotype because it determines the prognosis (Table 38-2). PS patients have a longer median survival age of 50 years compared with less than 30 years in the PI group. However, patients with PS can develop pancreatic insufficiency following episodes of recurrent acute pancreatitis. The complications of

Table 38-1 Causes of Abdominal Pain in Patients with Cystic Fibrosis

Location	Differential Diagnosis
Upper abdomen	Gastroesophageal reflux disease, peptic ulcer disease, *Helicobacter pylori* gastritis, constipation
Lower abdomen	Constipation, DIOS, colitis, malabsorption, renal disease, volvulus
Right side	Kidney disease, cholecystitis, gallstones, colitis, DIOS, appendicitis, *Yersinia* infection
Left side	Kidney disease, colitis, constipation
Generalized pain	DIOS, intussusception, volvulus, peptic ulcer disease, appendicitis, malabsorption, infections

DIOS, distal intestinal obstruction syndrome.

Table 38-2	Mutations of the CFTR Gene and Pancreatic Phenotype
Genotype	Percentage of Patients with PI or PS
ΔF508/ΔF508	99% PI, 1% PS
ΔF508/other	72% PI, 28% PS
Other/other	38% PS, 64% PS

PI, pancreatic insufficiency; PS, pancreatic sufficient.

pancreatic insufficiency are detailed in Table 38-3 and a list of PS mutations detailed in Table 38-4.

Recurrent episodes of pancreatitis, resulting in chronic pancreatitis, are a complication of CF and rarely can be the only manifestation of the disease. The frequency of common CFTR mutations in patients diagnosed with idiopathic chronic pancreatitis was four to six times higher than expected. It is important to screen for CFTR mutations in patients with recurrent episodes of acute pancreatitis or with established idiopathic chronic pancreatitis.

Liver Disease and the Biliary Tract

The CFTR gene is expressed in the epithelia of intrahepatic and extrahepatic bile ducts, and it is possibly involved in chloride and water secretion into the bile. Biliary obstruction from inspissation of biliary secretions in intrahepatic bile ducts leads to a decrease in bile flow and activates an inflammation response, gradually leading to portal fibrosis, focal biliary cirrhosis, multilobular biliary cirrhosis, and portal hypertension. There is no proven association between the CF genotype and the development of liver disease. However, it was shown that mutations of the mannose binder gene, the α_1-antitrypsin gene, and the hereditary hemochromatosis gene increased the risk of liver disease in CF patients. There is no effective therapy for liver fibrosis. Ursodiol has been used because it improves bile flow, decreases serum liver enzymes, and may be cytoprotective. Doses of 10 to 20 mg/kg/day were shown to be effective and are recommended.

Up to 17% of children with CF are estimated to have clinically significant liver disease. As the life expectancy of CF patients increases; clinically significant liver disease becomes more frequent. Neonatal cholestasis, hepatic steatosis, cholelithiasis, and rarely sclerosing cholangitis are other liver disorders associated with CF. Patients with gallstones should have a cholecystectomy if the gallstones are symptomatic or if liver function tests are abnormal.

Genotype-Phenotype Correlation

CFTR mutations are classified in four different types based on the characteristics of the CFTR protein (Table 38-5). Mutations of different classes produce different effects on the protein. The first two classes of mutations are associated with the more severe phenotypes because they are related to absence or abnormal localization of CFTR, whereas classes three and four are associated with varying degrees of residual CFTR activity.

Pancreatic involvement is closely related to the CFTR genotype. The pulmonary phenotype, however, seems to be modulated by other factors such as environment, compliance with therapy, and genetic factors inherited independently of the CFTR genotype. Liver expression also seems to be modulated by other genes inherited independently from the CFTR genotype. It is possible that the risk of meconium ileus and DIOS can also be influenced in a similar way. Genetic studies in mice and in human twins with CF determined a locus in chromosome 19 that modulates meconium ileus and DIOS expression.

GASTROINTESTINAL COMPLICATIONS IN PATIENTS WITH CYSTIC FIBROSIS

Meconium Ileus

Meconium ileus (MI) is the neonatal intestinal obstruction caused by thick inspissated intestinal secretions. The phenotype associated with MI and DIOS seems to be influenced by modifier genes and environ-

Table 38-3	Complications of Pancreatic Insufficiency
Protein maldigestion and malabsorption	Hypoproteinemia, edema
Fat maldigestion and malabsorption	Steatorrhea Wasting, poor growth Loss of bile acids and lithogenic bile cholelithiasis
Essential fatty acid deficiency	Thrombocytopenia Seborrheic dermatitis Poor wound healing
Fat-soluble vitamin malabsorption	**Vitamin A:** Benign intracranial hypertension Night blindness and xerophthalmia **Vitamin D:** Ricketts Osteomalacia **Vitamin E:** Hemolysis Peripheral neuropathy, ataxia, external ophthalmoplegia **Vitamin K:** Coagulopathy

Table 38-4 Mutations of the CFTR Gene and Phenotype

Sweat Test Disease Severity	Positive Sweat Test		Normal or Borderline Sweat Test
Severe Disease: Lung disease PI	R553X W1282X N1303K 395insT 1078delT 621+1G-to-T 1717+1G-to-A	ΔF508 G542X G551D Δ1507 R5603 S549N 3659delC G480C	
Mild Disease: Lung disease PS	R117H (5T) 3849+10kbC-to-T 2789+5G-to-A R334W G85EP G91R R347P R347H	R347L A455E Y563N P574H S945L L1065 D1152 F1286S	R117H(7T) 3849+10kb C-10 T G551S D1152H A455E

PI, pancreatic insufficiency; PS, pancreatic sufficient.

Table 38-5 Classification of CFTR Mutations in Relation to Properties of the CFTR Protein

Type	Defect	Mechanism	Gene Examples	Frequency
I	CFTR protein synthesis	Non-sense and frame shift mutations due to deletions or insertions that cause altered splicing	W1282X R553X G542X	Frequency >2% among all CF chromosomes
II	CFTR processing or maturation.	CFTR RNAm formed but the protein fails to traffic to the cell surface	ΔF508	Present in up to 80% of CF chromosomes from Northern Europe and America
III	Regulatory domains of the CFTR	The CFTR reaches the cell membrane but is not stimulated by cAMP	G551D	Frequent in Northern Europe
IV	Conductance of the Cl channel decreasing the time of channel opening	Missense mutations		

cAMP, cyclic adenosine monophosphate; CF, cystic fibrosis.

mental factors; MI affects 15% to 20% of neonates with CF. The diagnosis can be made in utero by ultrasound. It should be suspected in newborn infants who do not pass meconium within the first 2 days of life and who present with symptoms of small bowel obstruction. MI can be associated with malrotation, volvulus, intestinal atresia, and microcolon. The diagnosis is made with a Gastrografin enema, which can also be therapeutic in some instances. Surgical treatment in indicated for those infants with obstruction, perforation, and meconium cysts and includes resection of the affected intestine if indicated, lavage with saline and N-acetylcysteine, and placement of an ostomy (Table 38-6).

Distal Intestinal Obstruction Syndrome

Previously known as "meconium ileus equivalent," DIOS is a recurrent intestinal obstruction caused by an accumulation of stool, starting in the ileocecal region and extending throughout the colon. It is believed to be a

Table 38-6 Gastrointestinal and Liver Complications of Cystic Fibrosis

Gastrointestinal	Liver and Gallbladder	Pancreatic Disease
Meconium ileus Intussusception Constipation Rectal prolapse Bacterial overgrowth Fibrosing colonopathy GERD Dysmotility (delayed gastric emptying) Appendicitis	Liver congestion Steatosis Cholestasis Fibrosis and cirrhosis Portal hypertension Gallstones	Acute recurrent pancreatitis Pancreatic insufficiency

GERD, gastroesophageal reflux disease.

result of abnormal water and electrolyte transport, abnormal intestinal mucus, dysmotility, and inspissated secretions, among others. Precipitating factors include dehydration, diet changes, immobilization, respiratory infections, bacterial overgrowth, and perhaps inadequate pancreatic enzyme replacement. It is more frequent in adults than in children (16% versus 5%) and is associated with more severe genotypes. It can manifest as a palpable mass in the right lower quadrant, with or without pain, and can occur simultaneously with intussusception or with acute or chronic appendicitis (an ultrasound examination or a computed tomography (CT) scan of the abdomen helps differentiate DIOS from these two diagnoses). The treatment of DIOS depends on the degree of obstruction. Asymptomatic cases (palpable right lower quadrant abdominal mass and no pain) may be treated with oral lactulose. Patients with abdominal pain and right lower quadrant masses may need a clean-out with higher doses of lactulose, polyethylene glycol, or the oral clean-out cocktail. Patients with signs and symptoms of obstruction need to be given Gastrografin enemas. These patients should be well hydrated with intravenous fluids and the Gastrografin enema should be refluxed into the terminal ileum to prevent recurrent DIOS and hospitalizations. Some patients require a Gastrografin enema as well as GoLYTELY. Patients with recurrent DIOS and obstruction need to be evaluated for other causes of obstruction and for GI diseases such as: inflammatory bowel disease, celiac disease, bacterial overgrowth, and so on.

Intussusception

CF patients are at increased risk for intussusception. Intussusception can manifest with acute abdominal pain and symptoms of obstruction or it can be silent, chronic, and recurrent and seen incidentally on an upper gastrointestinal (UGI) series.

Appendicitis

Appendicitis occurs in 2% of CF patients, compared with an overall incidence of 7% in healthy subjects. The diagnosis of acute appendicitis in patients with CF is more difficult to make than in otherwise healthy subjects. It is often recognized late in the course of persistent or chronic abdominal pain, usually in a patient on antibiotic therapy for pulmonary disease. There is a high rate of complication with perforation and abscess formation. Furthermore, the radiologic criteria to diagnose appendicitis (appendiceal thickening and enlargement with a diameter greater than 6 mm), cannot be applied to CF patients. Actually, CF patients without abdominal complaints were found to have distended appendices on ultrasound measurements that were filled with mucoid material.

Rectal Prolapse

Rectal prolapse occurs in 5% to 10% of patients before the age of 5 years and is usually seen before treatment for CF is started. Rectal prolapse is associated with constipation and poor nutrition. All children presenting with rectal prolapse should have a sweat test determination. Treatment of rectal prolapse consists of manual reduction of the prolapse, stool softeners, and nutritional therapy. In rare cases, surgical therapy, such as sodium chloride sclerotherapy is indicated in recurrent episodes of prolapse unresponsive to medical therapy.

Small Bowel Bacterial Overgrowth

Small bowel bacterial overgrowth (SBBO) can be seen in CF patients. Predisposing factors include chronic antibiotic therapy or previous GI surgery with mechanical or functional stasis due to dysmotility. The diagnosis may be difficult to make because patients are frequently on antibiotic treatment, which prevents them from getting diagnostic breath tests.

Fibrosing Colonopathy

Fibrosing colonopathy was first described in the early 1990s. It consists of a noninflammatory fibrosing and stricturing process affecting the ascending colon, seen in CF patients on high-dose pancreatic enzyme replacement therapy (PERT). Clinical manifestations include abdominal pain, diarrhea, and hematochezia. The diagnosis is made when a stricture is identified on a contrast enema. Fibrosing colonopathy is associated with the use of potent pancreatic enzymes in high doses (>6000 UL/kg/meal for more than 6 months) and the presence of a modifier gene—the pancreatic trypsin inhibitor gene. Although the exact etiology is unknown, it is believed that high concentrations of pancreatic enzymes delivered to the colon accumulate in the cecum and cause mucosal damage. Predisposing factors include high doses of pancreatic enzymes and length of treatment, previous GI surgery, acid gastric blockade, and DNase therapies. Management includes decreasing the dose of pancreatic enzymes, evaluating for other GI diseases, nutritional support, and monitoring. Current recommendations for maximum daily PERT are 10,000 UL/kg/day or 2500 UL/kg/meal.

Gastroesophageal Reflux Disease

Gastroesophageal reflux disease (GERD) is estimated to occur in up to 25% of CF patients. The etiology of GERD in CF patients is multifactorial: severity of lung disease, chest physiotherapy, use of medications that relax the lower esophageal sphincter, delayed gastric emptying, and abnormal lower esophageal sphincter relaxation. The management of GERD is similar as that for non-CF patients. Dietary measures, including avoidance of foods that exacerbate symptoms and small frequent meals are recommended. Thickening formula and positioning may be helpful in infants. Medical treatment includes the use of acid blockers (H_2 receptor blockers and proton pump inhibitors), and prokinetic medications (cisapride, which is no longer available in the United States, erythromycin, and metoclopramide). Surgical therapy, Nissen fundoplication, is reserved for patients who have failed aggressive medical therapy and have severe GERD with failure to thrive, erosive esophagitis, esophageal strictures, or Barrett's esophagus.

Delayed Gastric Emptying

Gastric motility dysfunction and delayed gastric emptying are associated with CF. Poor gastric emptying contributes to GERD; promotes anorexia, fullness, and early satiety; and interferes with delivery of pancreatic enzymes in the duodenum. Clinically, gastric emptying can be evaluated with a scintigraphy study, and treatment includes prokinetics such as erythromycin and metoclopramide. Because SBBO can be associated with delayed gastric emptying, a search for bacterial overgrowth may be warranted.

Constipation

Chronic constipation is frequent in patients with CF and is probably multifactorial. Possible reasons include abnormal colonic mucus secretion, abnormal motility, poor fiber intake, and dehydration. Treatment consists of a high-fiber and high-fluid diet, stool softeners, lubricants, osmotic agents, and behavior modification such as toilet sitting, using a calendar, and setting up a reward system. In general, mineral oil is not used in patients with CF because it interferes with the absorption of fat-soluble vitamins. Patients with fecal impaction need more aggressive therapy with enemas, nasogastric polyethylene glycol solutions, or surgical disimpaction.

TREATMENT

The treatment of PI consists of:
1. A high-calorie diet with 30% to 40% calories from fat and an increase in salt intake (2 to 4 mEq/Kg/day).
2. PERT, 2000 to 4000 lipase units/120 mL of formula or per breastfeeding session in infancy, 1000 to 2500 lipase units/kg/meal for children 1 to 4 years of age, and 500 to 2500 lipase units/kg/meal for all patients older than 4 years. The total daily dose should be less than 10,000 lipase units/kg/day to avoid fibrosing colonopathy.
3. Use of medications that block gastric acid production. This results in a less acidic duodenal pH, improved function of PERT, and improved absorption of dietary nitrogen and fat.
4. Vitamin and mineral supplementation.

APPROACH TO THE CASE

The case study illustrates the causes of abdominal pain in a 12-year-old boy with PI and a history of intestinal surgery.

The differential diagnosis of chronic recurrent abdominal pain in a patient with CF and history of previous abdominal surgery includes DIOS, fat malabsorption, SBBO, constipation, intussusception, dysmotility (GERD, delayed gastric emptying), adhesions, chronic appendicitis, fibrosing colonopathy, peptic ulcer disease, renal stones, and gallbladder disease.

Investigations that would be helpful include a complete blood count with differential to look for changes associated with bacterial infections, liver function tests to assess for gallbladder disease, stool Hemoccult to look for mucosal damage from peptic ulcer disease, GERD, *Helicobacter pylori* gastritis, colitis, and fibrosing colonopathy. An abdominal x-ray is helpful to evaluate for signs of obstruction, presence of fecolith in the appendix, gallstones, and renal stones as well as severity of constipation or DIOS. An abdominal ultrasound can be used to look for gallbladder and renal stones, intussusception, and appendicitis. A CT scan of the abdomen is helpful in cases of chronic appendicitis, fibrosing colonopathy, and other causes of an acute abdomen. Gastrografin enemas used therapeutically for DIOS also provide some information about colonic anatomy. A UGI series with small bowel follow-through can determine small bowel anatomy and gross mucosal damage. Breath tests (lactulose and glucose) are useful to diagnose SBBO in patients not receiving chronic antibiotics. A 3-day fecal fat collection will determine the degree of fat malabsorption and effectiveness of PERT. The 3-day diet record determines not only caloric intake but also the distribution of fat content of meals and the doses of PERT used for meals and patterns of PERT use.

Our patient showed fat malabsorption despite a high dose of PERT. There was uneven distribution of dietary fat throughout the day, which probably contributed to his steatorrhea and escalation of PERT. Other contributors to the high dose of PERT and steatorrhea are the dilated jejunal loop with possible SBBO. Our patient improved after a 4-week course of metronidazole.

Our patient had heme-negative stools and the coefficient of fat absorption was 84%. The lactulose breath test was not done for scheduling reasons and the abdominal x-ray showed a large amount of stool. Due to a concern that his initial upper GI series with small bowel follow-through was not adequate, he had a repeat study which showed a persistently dilated loop of jejunum. His pancreatic enzyme replacement therapy was optimized. His diet was changed: fiber intake was increased and his fat intake was spread out throughout the day instead of being concentrated during his lunch and dinner meals. Because of the results of the abdominal x-ray and upper GI series, he was treated with an oral clean-out cocktail and metronidazole for 2 weeks to treat DIOS and possible bacterial overgrowth, respectively. He did well for 1 month, but was subsequently admitted with severe abdominal pain due to DIOS. He received 2000 mL of a Gastrografin enema with excellent results. The study was notable for the radiographic material refluxing into the terminal ileum.

After temporary improvement, he continued having persistent abdominal pain and was started on a daily treatment with lactulose and acetylcysteine and weekly treatments of GoLYTELY. The GoLYTELY was discontinued 1 month later because of gagging and inability to tolerate the regimen. His abdominal pain persisted, so his dose of acetylcysteine was increased and he was prescribed another course of metronidazole for 4 weeks. Two months later the patient was doing better and all his medications were stopped except for daily lactulose. He was still following his prescribed diet, and his dose of pancreatic enzymes had slowly been decreased to Creon 20, 4248 UL/kg/meal.

Our patient improved finally after successful treatment of SBBO and appropriate changes in his diet to treat the steatorrhea. These changes resulted in a decrease in his PERT dose. This case illustrates the importance of a careful history, a detailed dietary history, and a methodical approach to the evaluation and treatment of a patient with CF and intermittent abdominal pain.

SUMMARY

Cystic fibrosis affects approximately 1 out of every 2500 white Americans. Its complications involve not only the respiratory system but also the gastrointestinal system and other organs, including the small and large intestine, the liver, and the pancreas. It continues to be one of the most common autosomal recessive diseases that reduce the life spans of people in America. However, improved diagnostic and therapeutic techniques have led to reduced morbidity and mortality among people who have CF.

MAJOR POINTS

CF can affect the pancreas, the liver, and the gastrointestinal tract

Besides pancreatic insufficiency, the major clinical presentations include DIOS in children and adolescents and meconium ileus in neonates

Increased life expectancy results in increased prevalence of liver disease in CF patients

Other complicating features of CF include rectal prolapse, intussusception, appendicitis, fibrosing colonopathy, constipation, gastroesophageal reflux, and small bowel overgrowth

SUGGESTED READINGS

Aktay AN, Splaingard ML, Miller T, et al: Electrogastrography in children with cystic fibrosis. Dig Dis Sci 47:699-703, 2002.

Borowitz D, Baker RD, Stallings V: Consensus report on nutrition for pediatric patients with cystic fibrosis. J Pediatr Gastroenterol Nutr 35:246-259, 2002.

Borowitz DS, Grand RJ, Durie PR: Use of pancreatic enzyme supplements for patients with cystic fibrosis in the context of fibrosing colonopathy. Consensus Committee. J Pediatr 127:681-684, 1995.

Castaldo G, Fuccio A, Salvatore D, et al: Liver expression in cystic fibrosis could be modulated by genetic factors different from the cystic fibrosis transmembrane regulator genotype. Am J Med Genet 98:294-297, 2001.

Colombo C, Crosignani A, Assaisso M, et al: Ursodeoxycholic acid therapy in cystic fibrosis–associated liver disease: A dose-response study. Hepatology 16:924-930, 1992.

Corbett K, Kelleher S, Rowland M, et al: Cystic fibrosis-associated liver disease: A population-based study. J Pediatr 145:327-332, 2004.

Dray X, Bienvenu T, Desmazes-Dufeu N, et al: Distal intestinal obstruction syndrome in adults with cystic fibrosis. Clin Gastroenterol Hepatol 2:498-503, 2004.

Gaskin KJ: CFTR gene and cystic fibrosis. J Gastroenterol Hepatol 19:228, 2004.

Kerem E, Corey M, Kerem BS, et al: The relation between genotype and phenotype in cystic fibrosis: Analysis of the most common mutation (delta F508). N Engl J Med 323:1517-1522, 1990.

Lardenoye SW, Puylaert JB, Smit MJ, Holscher HC: Appendix in children with cystic fibrosis: US features. Radiology 232:187-189, 2004.

Macek M Jr, Mackova A, Hamosh A, et al: Identification of common cystic fibrosis mutations in African-Americans with cystic fibrosis increases the detection rate to 75%. Am J Hum Genet 60:1122-1127, 1997.

Mascarenhas MR: Treatment of gastrointestinal problems in cystic fibrosis. Curr Treat Options Gastroenterol 6:427-441, 2003.

McCarthy VP, Mischler EH, Hubbard VS, et al: Appendiceal abscess in cystic fibrosis: A diagnostic challenge. Gastroenterology 86:564-568, 1984.

Salvatore F, Scudiero O, Castaldo G: Genotype-phenotype correlation in cystic fibrosis: The role of modifier genes. Am J Med Genet 111:88-95, 2002.

Schappi MG, Roulet M, Rochat T, Belli DC: Electrogastrography reveals post-prandial gastric dysmotility in children with cystic fibrosis. J Pediatr Gastroenterol Nutr 39:253-256, 2004.

Scott RB, O'Loughlin EV, Gall DG: Gastroesophageal reflux in patients with cystic fibrosis. J Pediatr 106:223-227, 1985.

Sokol RJ, Durie PR: Recommendations for management of liver and biliary tract disease in cystic fibrosis. Cystic Fibrosis Foundation Hepatobiliary Disease Consensus Group. J Pediatr Gastroenterol Nutr 28(Suppl 1):S1-S13, 1999.

Waters DL, Dorney SF, Gaskin KJ, et al: Pancreatic function in infants identified as having cystic fibrosis in a neonatal screening program. N Engl J Med 322:303-308, 1990.

Wilcken B, Chalmers G: Reduced morbidity in cystic fibrosis. Lancet 1:439, 1986.

Witt H: Chronic pancreatitis and cystic fibrosis. Gut 52 (Suppl 2):ii31-ii41, 2003.

CHAPTER 39

Pancreatitis

RITU VERMA
TRACIE WONG

Disease Description
Case Presentation
Epidemiology
Pathophysiology
Acute Pancreatitis—Etiology
Chronic Pancreatitis—Etiology
Diagnostic Testing
   Acute Pancreatitis
   Chronic Pancreatitis
   Genetic Testing
Treatment of Acute Pancreatitis
   Severity and Grading Systems
   Complications
Treatment of Chronic Pancreatitis
Approach to the Case
Major Points

DISEASE DESCRIPTION

Pancreatitis in children differs significantly in prevalence and etiology from pancreatitis in adults. The disease is characterized by inflammation of the pancreas with abdominal pain and a rise in serum digestive enzymes. It can be categorized as acute or chronic. Chronic pancreatitis is a condition that is a sequela of progressive destructive and inflammatory changes in the organ from various causes. Complications of pancreatitis, such as pseudocyst formation and infected necrosis, are rare, but greatly influence the prognosis and treatment course of the disease.

CASE PRESENTATION

An 11-year-old girl presents with complaints of chronic abdominal pain and constipation for 3 months. Two months prior to presentation she was started on lactulose and omeprazole (Prilosec), with no improvement in her symptoms. Pain increased in the past week with development of nonbloody, nonbilious emesis that was not accompanied by fever or diarrhea.

On examination, she is afebrile, mildly tachycardic, and has normal blood pressure and respiratory rate. Examination is significant for a diffusely tender, nondistended abdomen with pain greatest in the epigastric area and level of the umbilicus, with no rebound or guarding.

Her laboratory evaluation reveals normal electrolytes, normal complete blood count, and elevated levels of amylase of 209 and lipase of 1607.

Ultrasound examination of the abdomen reveals increased echogenicity of the pancreas, an enlarged pancreatic duct, and enlarged common bile duct.

EPIDEMIOLOGY

Pancreatitis is probably more prevalent in childhood than was previously considered, with the number of reports in the pediatric literature increasing steadily over the years. However, it is still believed to occur less frequently than in adults. The male-to-female ratio can vary from 0.9 to 1.2, and the mean age of patients ranges from 6.9 to 9.4 years (Table 39-1).

Recurrent acute pancreatitis can be seen in about 10% of patients following an acute episode of pancreatitis. Possible etiologies include hereditary pancreatitis,

Table 39-1 Etiology of Pancreatitis			
	Study		
	DeBanto, et al Mild Cases	DeBanto, et al Severe Cases	Benifla and Weizman
Number	162	40	589
Age, mean	9.4	6.9	9.2
Male-to-female ratio	0.9	1	1.2
Etiology (%)			
Gallstone	7.4	2.5	0
Drug	11.1	7.5	12
Trauma	13	20	22
Familial	6.8	7.5	2
Systemic (e.g., HUS)	1.9	20	14
ERCP	3.1	0	0
Cystic fibrosis	3.1	0	0
Structural (divisum)	2.5	2.5	15
Hypercalcemia	3.1	0	1
Viral	2.5	2.5	10
Hypertriglyceridemia	0.6	2.5	1
DKA	1.2	0	0
Other	3.7	7.5	0
Unknown/Idiopathic	40.1	27.5	23

DKA, Diabetic ketoacidosis; *ERCP*, endoscopic retrograde cholangiopancreatography; *HUS*, hemolytic-uremic syndrome.

structural abnormalities, or idiopathic pancreatitis. Chronic pancreatitis has likewise been increasing in incidence. It is usually idiopathic or associated with atypical cystic fibrosis or hereditary pancreatitis, and the rising prevalence may be in part due to the increased incidence of acute pancreatitis.

PATHOPHYSIOLOGY

The basic functions of the pancreas include the production of digestive enzymes from its acinar cells, bicarbonate-rich fluid from its ductular cells, and insulin from its islet cells. The ductular cells also serve to connect the acinar cells to the duodenum and facilitate the clearance of secreted digestive enzymes out of the pancreas.

There are several protective mechanisms in the pancreas that have been elucidated and help explain the pathophysiology of pancreatitis. Many of these mechanisms are centered on trypsin, which is central in importance because it functions to activate many of the other digestive enzymes once they reach the duodenum. It is synthesized as the proenzyme trypsinogen, which requires activation to function. Under normal conditions, acinar cells are activated, and their intracellular concentration of calcium rises but remains within well controlled levels, prompting secretion of trypsinogen into the ductular lumen. The ductular cells secrete large amounts of bicarbonate-rich fluid and flush secreted enzymes out of the organ. Ductular cells depend on several transporters to carry out this function, especially the cystic fibrosis transmembrane regulator located on its apical membrane. Trypsinogen can be activated by enterokinase in the brush border of the duodenum, by trypsin, or by via its own slow ability to autoactivate. If trypsinogen is prematurely activated and not promptly cleared from the pancreas, the consequence can be autodigestion of the organ.

One protective mechanism is trypsin's ability to autoinactivate through autolysis, which is a process favored by a low-calcium environment within the acinar cell, but inhibited by the high-calcium environment of the ductular lumen and duodenum. Thus, if dysregulation occurs with hyperstimulation of calcium above critical levels within the acinar cell, it can result in sustained trypsin activation. Mutations in the *CFTR* gene that lead to decreased alkaline fluid secretion increase the risk of activated trypsin lingering in the pancreas.

Investigation of the autodestruct mechanism of trypsin has revealed that its first step depends on hydrolysis at a particular site on its side chain. This site is protected by calcium, which is consistent with the observation that an elevated calcium level supports continued trypsin activation. Some patients with hereditary pancreatitis have been found to possess a gene mutation in the trypsinogen *(PRSS1)* gene that results in an alteration at this site and thus have trypsin that cannot be autoinactivated. In addition, mutations in the trypsin gene itself can enhance trypsin activation and increase the likelihood of pancreatitis. Additional protection for the pancreas is afforded by the peptide serine protease inhibitor, Kazal type (SPINK 1). It serves to inhibit trypsin that has been activated within acinar cells. Mutations in this peptide are associated with some forms of familial and tropical pancreatitis.

ACUTE PANCREATITIS—ETIOLOGY

A high proportion of pancreatitis in adults is related to alcohol abuse and gallstones. Leading causes in the pediatric population are more expansive, including idiopathic pancreatitis, severe systemic illnesses, trauma, medications, structural abnormalities, and infections. Metabolic disorders such as inborn errors of metabolism, diabetic ketoacidosis (DKA), hypercalcemia, and hyperlipidemia are less common etiologies. Recent reviews have revealed a decrease in the number of idiopathic cases, perhaps due to better diagnostic testing of familial and gene mutation–associated pancreatitis.

Severe systemic diseases are an important cause of pancreatitis and include hemolytic-uremic syndrome (HUS) and postorgan transplantation pancreatitis. Trauma is also a leading basis for acute pancreatitis, and is usually blunt and accidental (e.g., bicycle handlebar injury or motor vehicle accident). However, child abuse also contributes to the number of traumatic cases.

Structural abnormalities such as pancreas divisum, choledochal cysts, and congenital sphincter of Oddi abnormality are risk factors for acute pancreatitis. In addition, choledocholithiasis is an important etiology that may require therapeutic endoscopic retrograde cholangiopancreatography (ERCP).

The most common infectious etiologies in North America are viral, with mumps, enterovirus, Epstein-Barr virus, hepatitis A, cytomegalovirus, rubella, coxsackie, varicella, rubeola, measles, and influenza cited as causes. Bacterial and parasitic infections, such as *Ascaris lumbricoides* also play a part, especially in less-developed parts of the world. Among human immunodeficiency virus (HIV)-positive patients, pancreatitis may develop from secondary infection by cytomegalovirus, *Mycobacterium avium intracellulare, Pneumocystis jiroveci,* or *Cryptosporidium parvum,* as well as from antiviral medications, such as didanosine.

Numerous medications in children have been linked to acute pancreatitis. The most commonly cited are valproate, prednisone, and L-asparaginase (Table 39-2).

Familial pancreatitis, which includes hereditary pancreatitis, is identified when the incidence of pancreatitis in a family is higher than the general population and cannot be explained by chance alone. Examples are patients with CFTR, SPINK 1 mutations, and those for whom no mutation has yet been identified.

Table 39-2 Medications Associated with Acute Pancreatitis

Acetaminophen
L-Asparaginase
Azathioprine/6-mercaptopurine
Cocaine
Fosphenytoin
Furosemide
Macrodantin
Metronidazole
Pentamidine
Phenytoin
Prednisone
Valproate

CHRONIC PANCREATITIS—ETIOLOGY

Most recent research suggests that chronic pancreatitis is a result of recurrent and chronic inflammation that started with acute pancreatitis and progressed to end-stage fibrosis with potentially irreversible loss of endocrine and exocrine function. In children, the most common etiologies are typical or atypical cystic fibrosis (CF), hereditary pancreatitis, and idiopathic causes.

Trypsinogen mutations are responsible for the majority of cases of hereditary pancreatitis, which usually manifests as recurrent acute pancreatitis between the ages of less than 1 and 60 years of age; one half of all cases become chronic pancreatitis. A notable clinical clue is a history of recurrent unexplained abdominal pain or pancreatitis in adults from the previous generation. This diagnosis can be confirmed by genetic testing of the *PRSS1* gene; however, 10% to 30% of smaller families with hereditary pancreatitis will not have identifiable mutations.

Cystic fibrosis is the most important cause of chronic pancreatitis in children. There are more than 1000 CFTR mutations, which can be categorized into mild-to-variable or severe classes, depending on their effect on the CFTR function. The heterozygous genotype composed of a severe allele with a mild-to-variable allele has been associated with idiopathic chronic pancreatitis. Also, a single CFTR mutation with other pancreatic susceptibility genes such as *SPINK,* or an environmental factor like alcohol may be a mechanism of disease. Idiopathic chronic pancreatitis can have early or late onset presentation. Early onset presentation is usually very painful and accompanied by slowly evolving calcification and endocrine insufficiency. In contrast, late presentation involves pain less frequently as a symptom (Table 39-3).

Table 39-3	Differential Diagnosis of Pancreatitis: Signs and Symptoms

Peptic ulcer disease
Acute cholecystitis
Biliary colic
Intestinal obstruction
Renal colic
Pneumonia (basilar)
Early acute appendicitis
Mesenteric vascular obstruction
Diabetic ketoacidosis

DIAGNOSTIC TESTING

Acute Pancreatitis

The diagnosis of acute pancreatitis can be difficult because there is no single definitive test. Currently, both clinical findings and laboratory values are used in combination. The findings of sudden-onset upper abdominal pain and elevation of amylase or lipase to at least three times the upper limit of normal are typical.

A clinical sign that should raise suspicion for pancreatitis is unexplained abdominal pain, usually epigastric or in the left or right upper quadrant that radiates to the back. It is also possible for back pain to occur alone. Nausea and vomiting are typical symptoms, and may be accompanied by fever, tachycardia, hypotension, or jaundice. In addition, examination of the abdomen may reveal rebound, guarding, and decreased bowel sounds. In the setting of systemically ill patients, intolerance of feeds is an important clue. Rarely, patients may present with an abdominal mass or ascites.

Laboratory values are not always reliable because enzyme levels can be normal in the setting of clear radiographic findings of pancreatitis, and enzymes may be elevated for reasons other than acute pancreatitis. In some patients, there is concurrent elevation of liver transaminases, which can also be a sign of biliary tract involvement. Evaluation of the patient should include calcium and triglyceride levels.

Imaging of the pancreas, by ultrasound or computed tomography (CT), is important for the diagnosis of inflammation, grading severity, and identifying complications such as pseudocysts. It can also help determine if chronic pancreatitis is present and elucidate if there are other concurrent pathologic processes.

On ultrasound, an enlarged pancreas with altered echogenicity may be seen. Other findings include a dilated pancreatic duct, gallstones, biliary sludge, dilated common or hepatic bile ducts, pancreatic calcifications,

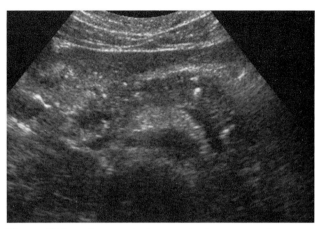

Figure 39-1 Ultrasound—increased echogenicity of pancreas with diffuse calcifications.

choledochal cysts, and peripancreatic or cystic fluid collections. A CT is usually not indicated until later in the course of the illness, when the patient has failed to improve. Instead of echogenicity, it will reveal decreased attenuation. Obtaining a magnetic resonance cholangiopancreatography (MRCP) may help to identify any ductal abnormalities. An ERCP is useful in cases of unexplained, recurrent pancreatitis, prolonged cases of pancreatitis with suspicion of duct disruption or structural defect, or in some cases of gallstone pancreatitis (Figs. 39-1, 39-2, and 39-3).

Chronic Pancreatitis

Chronic pancreatitis can be diagnosed by a combination of functional, morphologic, and histologic findings or by morphology and histology alone. Because pancreatic insufficiency can arise from other conditions without pancreatic inflammation, functional abnormalities

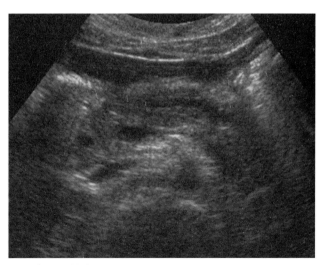

Figure 39-2 Ultrasound—pancreatic duct dilatation.

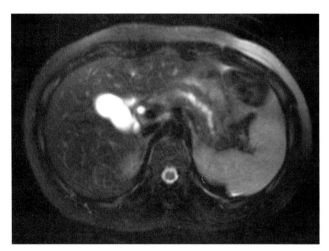

Figure 39-3. Magnetic resonance cholangiopancreatography—pancreatic duct dilatation.

in isolation are not adequate to diagnose chronic pancreatitis.

On abdominal radiography and transabdominal ultrasound, chronic pancreatitis with calcifications can make the diagnosis with 90% confidence. Other more sensitive modalities are CT, ERCP, MRCP, and endoscopic ultrasound (EUS); however, not all of these are widely available, and the roles of MRCP/MRI and EUS in evaluation of chronic pancreatitis are not yet clear. ERCP also has the unique advantage of offering a therapeutic as well as diagnostic option.

Both invasive and noninvasive tests of pancreatic exocrine function have limited usefulness. The functional reserve of the pancreas necessitates that there must be severe damage present before loss in function is evident clinically. The gold standard for testing exocrine pancreatic function is the invasive secretin-pancreozymin test, in which the response to injected secretin and pancreozymin is measured by collection of the duodenal aspirate, which is analyzed for pH, bicarbonate, and amylase content. It is, however, rarely performed, and results vary between institutions because the stimuli can vary.

A noninvasive test of pancreatic function is fecal elastase quantization. Unfortunately, this test lacks sensitivity and has a high false-positive rate. Fecal elastase quantification is the most sensitive for those patients with moderate to severe pancreatitis with concurrent steatorrhea. It is not as accurate with mild to moderate pancreatitis without steatorrhea.

Genetic Testing

Genetic testing is commercially available for the most common cationic trypsinogen (PRSS1) R122H and N291 mutations. Testing is indicated in patients who have recurrent idiopathic acute pancreatitis, idiopathic chronic pancreatitis, and for those who are symptomatic and come from a family with a known mutation. In addition, it may be useful in guiding patients in terms of lifestyle decisions (e.g., smoking, diet, and reproduction), given the risk of pancreatitis and potential for pancreatic cancer. Predictive testing (i.e., testing in patients without evidence for pancreatic disease) is generally not indicated in children, unless they have first-degree relatives who possess a PRSS1 mutation and can participate in the counseling and decision to test. At this time, most experts do not advocate genetic testing for SPINK1 mutations. Patients who present with idiopathic chronic pancreatitis should undergo full testing for CF; however, the CF gene panels test for the common CF-causing mutations and not the pancreatitis-causing mutations, which are often associated with lack of sinopulmonary disease and a negative sweat test. Further elucidation of the CFTR genotype–pancreatitis phenotype relationship is needed.

TREATMENT OF ACUTE PANCREATITIS

Medical management of acute pancreatitis centers on pancreatic rest, intravenous fluids, analgesia, and monitoring for complications. Because patients are usually kept nothing per mouth (NPO) and there can be intravascular fluid losses through third spacing and a capillary leak syndrome, it is important to pay attention to fluid balance. Use of a nasogastric (NG) tube to decompress the stomach in the setting of vomiting can also exacerbate losses. The early initiation of volume expansion can prevent pancreatic necrosis and contribute to cardiovascular stability. Pain control can be obtained by use of meperidine by intravenous or intramuscular administration.

Unless a prolonged or severe course of illness is anticipated, parenteral nutrition and enteral nutrition are not usually necessary. Antibiotics are likewise not used except in the most severe cases or if pancreatic necrosis is present.

Severity and Grading Systems

Although mortality from pancreatitis in children is not as high as in adults, pancreatitis can be life threatening. As a result of third spacing, vomiting, and the patient NPO, cardiovascular collapse can occur. Respiratory failure occurs when fluid leaks into alveolar spaces, accompanied by inflammation. Several scoring systems help determine the risk of a mild or severe clinical course; however, they are often not as useful as the physician's clinical assessment. The majority of cases can be categorized as mild pancreatitis, with minimal complications and a short clinical course.

Complications

Complications from acute pancreatitis can be both local and systemic. Examples of local complications include fluid collections, pancreatic abscesses, pancreatic duct rupture or strictures, bleeding, pseudocyst formation, and pancreatic necrosis. Necrosis occurs in less than 1% of cases, but is a serious concern. Its occurrence is a result of intravascular depletion, inflammation, and vascular leakage that lead to an increase in hematocrit and infarction of the pancreas. A contrast-enhanced CT demonstrating a segment of pancreas lacking perfusion establishes the diagnosis. The determination of infected necrosis versus sterile necrosis should be based on fine-needle aspiration and culture. Often necrosectomy is delayed for 2 weeks, allowing proper demarcation of pancreatic and peripancreatic necrosis. This decreases the risk of bleeding and minimizes loss of vital tissue.

Pancreatic pseudocysts, fibrous-walled cavities filled with enzymes, occur in about 13% of children and can resolve spontaneously by resorption, or may require drainage. Drainage may be done endoscopically or externally by interventional radiology or surgery. Abscesses can be treated with antibiotics and external drainage, and rarely require surgery. However, for traumatic rupture of the duct, surgery is usually necessary.

In cases in which the etiology of acute pancreatitis is gallstones or biliary sludge, cholecystectomy is indicated to prevent recurrence. In mild pancreatitis, surgery can be performed as soon as the patient has recovered. Severe cases may need to be delayed. In select cases, endoscopic sphincterotomy is an alternative to cholecystectomy.

TREATMENT OF CHRONIC PANCREATITIS

Preventing development of chronic pancreatitis should be addressed by determining etiology in patients with recurrent acute pancreatitis. Anatomic variants, for example, can often be corrected surgically or endoscopically.

In cases in which the etiology is an untreatable cause, such as hereditary pancreatitis, the associated development of type 1 diabetes mellitus is a concern. In some cases, islet cell transplantation may be an option; however, the long-term benefits are still in question. In the setting of chronic pancreatitis, chronic pain syndromes often become an issue. They are believed to arise from repeated exposure of nerve endings to growth factors associated with pancreatic inflammation.

Treatment of chronic pancreatitis centers on addressing the loss of pancreatic digestive enzymes, as well as providing adequate pain therapy and treating diabetes if it develops. Glucose intolerance occurs with some frequency in this population. Overt diabetes usually occurs late in the course of disease. Those patients with evidence of calcifying disease, and especially those with early calcification, develop diabetes more often than those with noncalcifying disease. Of note, diabetes in chronic pancreatitis differs from type 1 diabetes because the glucagon-secreting alpha cells are affected as well, conferring an increased risk of hypoglycemia.

Supplemental pancreatic enzymes should help normalize digestive function, and should accompany any fat- and protein-containing meals and snacks. Preparations that are enteric coated are preferred, because the enzymes are protected from acid degradation in the stomach and they are not associated with the oral and perianal excoriations that the uncoated formulations cause. The dosages may be adjusted based on the fat intake of the meal. Patients with CFTR mutations have a more acidic intestinal environment than those with other types of pancreatitis because of the lack of duodenal bicarbonate secretion. These patients may require more aggressive acid blockade with proton pump inhibitors. Conversely, patients without CF may retain significant pancreatic function, and may benefit from a more acidic duodenum with minimal gastric acid suppression to stimulate pancreatic fluid secretion.

Enzyme doses are calculated by the lipase content—a typical dose is 1000 to 2500 U lipase/kg/meal. Inadequate treatment should be suspected with occurrence of frequent, bulky, greasy stools, excessive bloating or flatus, and inadequate growth velocity.

Other complications besides diabetes and pain have been described. Bile duct obstruction, which may be accompanied by intestinal obstruction, can occur in 5% to 10% of patients with chronic pancreatitis. These problems may be recognized by increasing transaminases and hyperbilirubinemia or by postprandial pain and early satiety, respectively. They are caused by inflammation and fibrosis or a pseudocyst at the head of the pancreas, and occur most often in patients with dilated pancreatic ducts. In rare cases of disruption of the pancreatic duct, pancreatic ascites and pleural effusion may develop.

APPROACH TO THE CASE

The patient was hospitalized and treated with bowel rest until the pain improved and was kept on total parenteral nutrition until she started to tolerate clear liquids and a low-fat diet. During the course of the hospitalization, her enzymes decreased progressively. She was discharged after a 6-day stay.

At an outpatient follow-up visit, an ultrasound was repeated to evaluate the dilatation seen in the pancreatic and common bile duct on the patient's initial

MAJOR POINTS

Leading causes of acute pancreatitis in children include idiopathic pancreatitis, severe systemic illnesses, trauma, medications, structural abnormalities, and infection.

Recurrent acute pancreatitis occurs in 10% of patients following an acute episode of pancreatitis.

Cystic fibrosis is the most important cause of chronic pancreatitis in children.

The findings of sudden-onset upper epigastric abdominal pain radiating to the back and elevation of amylase or lipase to at least three times the upper limit of normal are typical criteria for acute pancreatitis

Medical management of pancreatitis includes bowel rest, intravenous fluids, analgesia, and monitoring for complications.

Complications of pancreatitis include fluid collections, pancreatic abscesses, pancreatic duct rupture or strictures, bleeding, pseudocyst formation, and pancreatic necrosis.

ultrasound. Both features were still present. She subsequently underwent an MRCP, which revealed a slightly full common bile duct but a normal pancreatic duct.

A month later the patient presented again with symptoms and signs of acute pancreatitis. Her evaluation included a sweat test and genetic testing for cystic fibrosis, which was negative. She was discharged without the development of any complications, but presented again 9 months later with another flare. Her pancreatic ultrasound at that time was remarkable for signs of chronic pancreatitis, including areas of parenchymal calcification and biliary sludge in her gallbladder and common bile duct. Genetic testing for hereditary pancreatitis was negative.

Following cholecystectomy and intraoperative cholangiogram, during which no filling defects in the ducts were appreciated, she was asymptomatic for several weeks. Her next presentation of pancreatitis necessitated an ERCP for removal of several pancreatic duct stones. She was started on pancreatic enzyme supplementation for her diagnosis of chronic pancreatitis of unknown etiology.

SUGGESTED READINGS

Aman ST, Bishop M, Curington C, Toskes PP: Fecal pancreatic elastase 1 is inaccurate in the diagnosis of chronic pancreatitis. Pancreas 13:226-230, 1996.

Applebaum-Shapiro SE, Finch R, Pfutzer RH, et al: Hereditary pancreatitis in North America: The Pittsburgh-Midwest Multi-Center Pancreatic Study Group Study. Pancreatology 1:439-443, 2001.

Benifla M, Weizman Z: Acute pancreatitis in childhood: Analysis of literature data. J Clin Gastroenterol 37:169-172, 2003.

Borowitz D, Baker RD, Stallings V: Consensus report on nutrition for pediatric patients with cystic fibrosis. J Pediatr Gastroenterol Nutr 35:246-259, 2002.

Cohn JS, Freidman KJ, Noone PG, et al: Relation between mutations of the cystic fibrosis gene and idiopathic pancreatitis. N Engl J Med 339:653-658, 1998.

DeBanto JR, Goday PS, Pedroso MR, et al: Acute pancreatitis in children. Am J Gastroenterol 97:1726-1731, 2002.

Dutta SK, Ting CD, Lai LL: Study of prevalence, severity and etiological factors associated with acute pancreatitis in patients infection with human immunodeficiency virus. Am J Gastroenterol 92:2044-2048, 1997.

Ellis I, Lerch MM, Whitcomb DC, Committee C: Genetic testing for hereditary pancreatitis: Guidelines for indications, counseling, consent and privacy issues. Pancreatology 1:401-411, 2001.

Howes N, Lerch MM, Greenhalf W, et al: Clinical and genetic characteristics of hereditary pancreatitis in Europe. Clin Gastroenterol Hepatol 2:252-261, 2004.

Layer P, Yamamoto H, Kaltoff L, et al: The different courses of early and late onset idiopathic and alcoholic chronic pancreatitis. Gastroenterology 107:1481-1487, 1994.

Lerner A, Branski, D, Lebenthal E: Pancreatic diseases in children. Pediatr Clin North Am 43:125-156, 1996.

Rowntree RK, Harris A: The phenotypic consequences of CFTR mutations. Ann Hum Genet 67: 471-485, 2003.

Simon P, Weiss FU, Sahin-Toth M, et al: Hereditary pancreatitis caused by a novel PRSS1 mutation (Arg122 → Cys) that alters autoactivation and autodegradation of cationic trypsinogen. J Biol Chem 21:21, 2001.

Steinberg W, Tenner S: Acute pancreatitis. N Engl J Med 330: 1198-1220, 1994.

Sutton R, Criddle D, Raraty MGT, et al: Signal transduction, calcium, and acute pancreatitis. Pancreatology 3:497-505, 2003.

Uhl W, Warshaw A, Imrie C, et al: IAP guidelines for the surgical management of acute pancreatitis. Pancreatology 2:565-573, 2002.

Werlin SL, Kugathasan S, Frautschy BC: Pancreatitis in children. J Pediatr Gastroenterol Nutr 37:591-595, 2003.

Whitcomb DC: Genetic Predispositions to acute and chronic pancreatitis. Med Clin North Am 84:531-547, 2000.

Whitcomb DC: How to think about SPINK and pancreatitis. Am J Gastroenterol 97:1085-1088, 2002.

CHAPTER 40

Shwachman-Diamond Syndrome

DAVID MACK

Disease Description
Case Presentation
Epidemiology
Pathophysiology
Differential Diagnosis
Diagnostic Testing
Treatment
Approach to the Case
Summary
Major Points

DISEASE DESCRIPTION

Shwachman-Diamond syndrome (SDS) is an autosomal recessive genetic disorder that most commonly manifests itself by dysfunction of the exocrine pancreas, dysfunction of the bone marrow, short stature, and skeletal abnormalities.

CASE PRESENTATION

A male patient is admitted to the hospital at 3 months of age with failure to thrive. He was born at 36 weeks gestation after an uneventful pregnancy and delivery. At birth, the length was 47.5 cm (20th percentile), the weight was 2988 g (20th percentile), and the head circumference was 43 cm (20th percentile). His intake has been good and there is no vomiting. Stools are described as loose, frequent, and bulky but without blood. He has developed a dry scaly rash with a mild erythematous base over his entire body. By 2 months of age his weight was at the 3rd percentile (4176 g) and by the third month of life there was a fall in weight from the previous month to 4119 g (Fig. 40-1), having being fed a cow's milk–based formula of 3 ounces every 3 hours (120 calories/kg/day). On admission to the hospital, general examination reveals the child is pale, he has a low-grade fever, and the thoracic chest is narrow (Fig. 40-2). There is a widespread fine scaly rash over the entire body. There is no organomegaly, and neurologic examination is normal.

The complete blood count was repeated a number of times and typically showed a normocytic, normochromic anemia with a hemoglobin ranging from 59 to 75 g/L, platelets were normal, and the total white count of 4.6 to 5.2×10^9 cells/L with a differential showing marked neutropenia (0.06 to 2.25×10^9 cells/L). The hemoglobin F was elevated at 25.6% (normal 5 to 20%) but other hematologic and routine biochemical blood tests were normal. Sweat chloride testing was normal. A chest x-ray was abnormal showing marked expansion of the anterior metaphyses of the ribs at the costochondral junctions (Fig. 40-3), but a skeletal survey was otherwise normal. The 72-hour fecal fat determination was elevated. The serum vitamin E was low at 11 μmol/L (normal 12 to 21), 25-OH vitamin D was normal, and the International Normalized Ratio (INR) was elevated at 1.4 with normal albumin and bilirubin levels (total and direct). The aminotransferases (aspartate transaminase [AST] = 66 U/L, alanine transaminase [ALT] = 61 U/L) were minimally elevated. During the hospital stay the child developed a respiratory syncytial virus infection and later a bacterial urinary tract infection. Based on the findings, the child was diagnosed with Shwachman-Diamond syndrome and started on pancreatic enzyme replacement therapy.

EPIDEMIOLOGY

SDS is a rare disorder with a wide heterogeneity of phenotypic expression on clinical presentation, and so the exact prevalence of the condition is unknown.

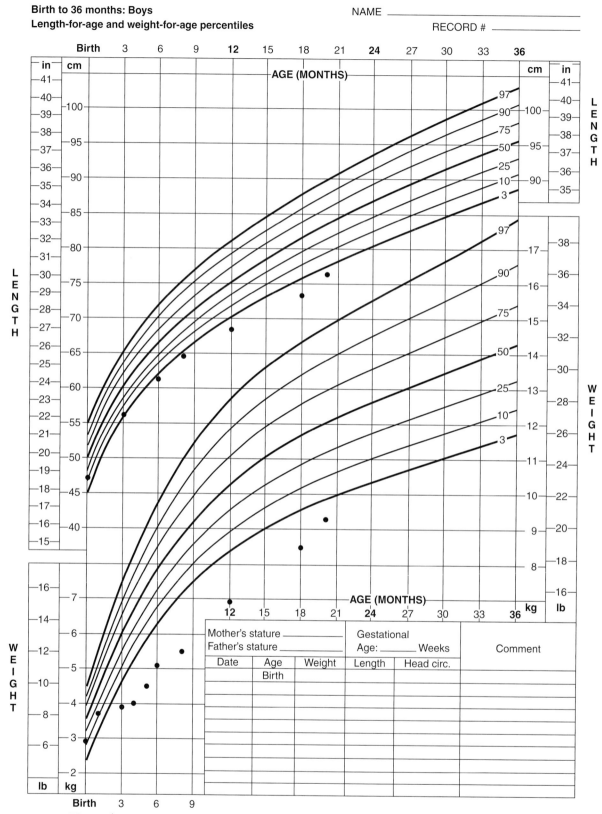

Figure 40-1 Height and weight chart for males between birth and 36 months of age (www.cdc.gov/growthcharts). The dots represent the patient's growth.

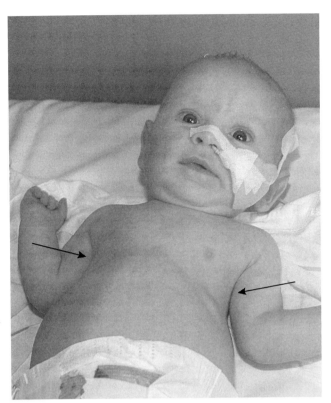

Figure 40-2 *(See also Color Plate 40-2.)* Thoracic dystrophy *(arrows)* can be noted. The patient also had a fine scaly rash over the entire body.

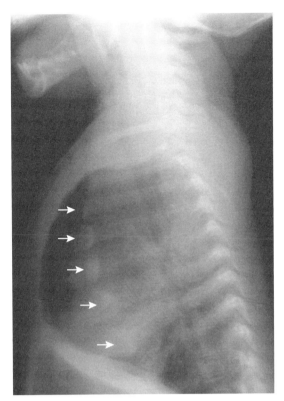

Figure 40-3 The *arrows* point to the marked expansion of the anterior metaphyses of the ribs at the costochondral junctions with the appearance of metaphyseal ends that are flared and irregular are seen in this lateral view of the chest. In addition, the ribs are abnormally short, consistent with the clinical observation of narrowing of the thorax. Note also the oval shape and globular appearance of vertebral bodies.

Estimates of the incidence of the condition are around 1 in 75,000 with a ratio of males to females of 1.7 to 1. It is the second most common cause of exocrine pancreatic insufficiency after cystic fibrosis and the third most common inherited cause of bone marrow failure after Fanconi's anemia and Diamond-Blackfan syndrome.

PATHOPHYSIOLOGY

This is a genetic disorder caused by mutations of the *SBDS* gene, and gene testing for the common mutations of the gene is now available. SBDS protein is widely expressed; however, its function is unknown. Indirect evidence has suggested orthologs may function in ribonucleic acid (RNA) metabolism with speculation that manifestation of disease occurs from loss of cellular function critical for development of the various organs involved in the phenotypic expression of this syndrome. The most common clinical manifestations are characterized by exocrine pancreatic dysfunction, bone marrow dysfunction, skeletal abnormalities, and short stature, with a number of other organ systems variably involved in reported cases (Table 40-1).

DIFFERENTIAL DIAGNOSIS

The differential diagnosis of SDS is listed in Table 40-2.

Exocrine pancreatic dysfunction is one of the common manifestations and present in all patients. However, enzyme secretion is not necessarily static because in a subset of patients, fecal fat balance testing and serum cationic trypsinogen testing have demonstrated age-related improvement. For some 30% to 50% of individuals with this condition, the 72-hour fecal fat balance studies will become normal, and serum cationic trypsinogen determinations can rise with approximately 20% having values in the normal range after the age of 3 years. Thus, these two tests alone may fail to provide confirmatory evidence of pancreatic dysfunction, complicating diagnosis. In contrast to serum trypsinogen, serum isoamylase values do not show age-related improvements in Shwachman-Diamond syndrome and thus can be used as a marker for pancreatic insufficiency in this syndrome. However, because pancreatic isoamylase normally has a slow rate of postnatal maturation, the sensitivity and

Table 40-1 Clinical Manifestations of Shwachman-Diamond Syndrome

Common Manifestations

Exocrine pancreatic dysfunction
  Pancreatic insufficiency, pancreatic sufficiency, pancreatic lipomatosis
Skeletal abnormalities
  Delayed appearance of secondary ossification centers, widening and irregularity of the metaphyses, thickening and irregularity of the growth plates, osteopenia, narrow rib cage, thoracic dystrophy, clinodactyly
Bone marrow dysfunction
  Leukopenia, persistent neutropenia, intermittent neutropenia, anemia, thrombocytopenia, aplastic anemia, myelodysplastic syndrome ± clonal cytogenetics, leukemia (AML, ALL)
Short stature
Other manifestations
  Infections (viral, bacterial, and fungal)
  Developmental delays and learning disorders
  Hepatomegaly and elevated aminotransferases in infants (usually improves by age 2 years)
  Delayed dentition of permanent teeth, dental dysplasia, increased risk of dental caries, periodontal disease
  Ichthyosis (usually associated with age-related improvement)
  Urologic (e.g., ureterocele, double ureter)
  Diabetes mellitus
  Myocardial fibrosis

All, acute lymphoblastic leukemia; AML, acute myelogenous leukemia.

specificity of this test for determination of exocrine pancreatic dysfunction should be limited to those patients older than 3 years. Quantitative pancreatic stimulation testing demonstrates that regardless of whether a patient is pancreatic insufficient (fecal fat losses exceed 15% of dietary fat intake for children younger than 6 months of age or exceed 7% of dietary fat intake for older children and require pancreatic enzyme replacement to correct maldigestion) or pancreatic sufficient (fecal fat losses are within the normal range for infants and children), the exocrine pancreas secretes significantly fewer enzymes than normal. Imaging studies of the pancreas can reveal pancreatic lipomatosis (Fig. 40-4) and histologic study of pancreas at autopsies has revealed fatty replacement of the acini with preserved ducts and ductules in keeping with the pathophysiology of the pancreatic defect being one of pancreatic acinar hypoplasia. In contrast, pancreatic nsufficiency in cystic fibrosis (see Chapter 38) occurs from damage arising from ductal plugging by macromolecules as a result of a deficit in ductular fluid secretion due to *CFTR* gene mutations.

Cross-sectional evaluation of the skeletal system can detect abnormalities in 50% of patients. Serial evaluations have shown skeletal changes are present in all patients but their localization varied without phenotype-genotype correlation. Chest abnormalities (see Fig. 40-1) are quite common in infants and children under the age of 2 years as is metaphyseal chondrodysplasia of the metacarpal, radial, and ulnar bones of the arms. In addition, there is age-related tendency toward normalization of epiphyseal maturation with worsening of the metaphyses and growth plates in the femur after 3 to 5 years of age and thus may lead to complications (Fig. 40-5).

Hematologically, SDS is characterized by varying degrees of cytopenia and a high risk of developing myelodysplastic syndrome plus or minus clonal cytogenetics and leukemia. Neutropenia is the most common abnormality, occurring in 88% to 100% of patients, is usually intermittent, and has been detected as early as the neonatal period. Immune dysfunction, along with a neutrophil chemotaxis defect makes SDS patients in early life particularly susceptible to viral, bacterial, and fungal

Table 40-2 Differential Diagnosis of Shwachman-Diamond Syndrome

Fanconi's anemia
Diamond-Blackfan anemia
Cystic fibrosis
Pearson's syndrome
Isolated pancreatic enzyme deficiency
Cartilage hair hypoplasia, rickets
Jansen-type metaphyseal chondrodysplasia
Schmid-type metaphyseal chondrodysplasia
Hepatomegaly (see Chapter 26)
Failure to thrive (see Chapter 7)

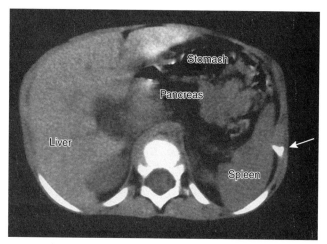

Figure 40-4 Computed tomography (CT) scan of the abdomen of another patient with Shwachman-Diamond syndrome revealing hypodensity in the region of the pancreas consistent with pancreatic lipomatosis. Note the abnormal anterior metaphysis of the rib *(arrow)*.

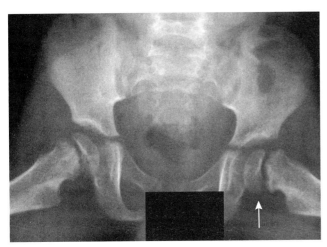

Figure 40-5 Hip radiograph of another patient with Shwachman-Diamond syndrome at 4 years of age. The patient is noted to have a slipped capital femoral epiphysis *(arrow)*. The femoral epiphysis is wide, irregular, and thickened. There is generalized osteopenia.

infections, with overwhelming sepsis a well-recognized fatal complication of this disorder, particularly in early life. Anemia with low reticulocytes and elevated fetal hemoglobin and thrombocytopenia are present in up to 80% of patients and similar to neutropenia; it is usually intermittent. The severity of the cytopenia does not always correlate with bone marrow cellularity; varying degrees of marrow hypoplasia and fat infiltration are the usual findings. The basis for the bone marrow disease is considered to be mulitfactorial in origin, with both stromal abnormalities and stem cell defects responsible. Pancytopenia when more severe in nature appears to carry a poor prognosis with a higher chance of developing severe aplasia, advanced myelodysplastic syndrome, or acute myelogenous leukemia. Cytogenetic abnormalities have been reported in SDS in various stages of malignant myeloid transformation, the most common being an isochrome 7q[I(7q)], but whether hematopoietic stem cell transplantation is indicated for patients with clonal marrow disease but without symptomatic cytopenia or increased blast counts is debatable. The risk of leukemia is around 15%, generally occurs in the second decade of life, and most often occurs in males; the type is predominantly acute myelogenous leukemia (AML), and SDS-related AML carries a poor prognosis.

Infants usually are born within the lower limits of normal birth length and weight but very quickly show subnormal growth velocity for both height and weight gain for the first 3 to 6 months of life, at a time when most patients are undiagnosed and are suffering from untreated steatorrhea. In contrast with other forms of maldigestion or pancreatic insufficiency that have acceleration of weight and height velocity following the addition of pancreatic enzyme replacement therapy, patients with SDS generally grow at a normal growth velocity after the age of 6 to 12 months and remain below the 5th percentile for height and weight. Similar to the age-related improvements in exocrine pancreatic function and growth velocity, liver aminotransferases, hepatomegaly, and skin rashes tend to resolve with age.

DIAGNOSTIC TESTING

Diagnostic testing for Shwachman-Diamond syndrome can be grouped into initial testing and periodic or maintenance testing. These tests are listed in Table 40-3.

TREATMENT

Pancreatic enzyme replacement therapy and supplemental fat-soluble vitamin administration is required for these pancreatic insufficient patients similar to patients with cystic fibrosis (see Chapter 38). For those patients with severe bacterial infections and neutropenia the addition of granulocyte-colony stimulating factor (G-CSF) may provide additional benefit to reduce the risk of overwhelming sepsis. Antibacterial mouthwashing during periods of profound neutropenia may help prevent periodontal disease. There are no specific therapies for the short stature or skeletal abnormalities, but orthopedic consultation may be required for those patients with impairment of function due to metaphyseal chondrodysplasia.

Table 40-3 Initial Evaluation of the Infant

Complete blood count (CBC) and differential, reticulocytes, and fetal hemoglobin
Liver aminotransferases, albumin, International Normalized Ratio, total and direct bilirubin
Fat-soluble vitamin serum determinations
Pancreatic function tests (serum cationic trypsinogen, serum pancreatic isoamylase [if patient is older than 3 years], fecal fat balance studies, imaging (ultrasound, computed tomography)
Radiographs of the chest and skeletal survey
Developmental assessment
Bone marrow biopsy and aspiration (assessment of cellularity, iron and cytogenetic abnormalities)
SBDS gene mutation analysis

Periodic Monitoring
CBC, differential and smear
Bone marrow biopsy and aspiration
Skeletal examinations and bone density evaluations
Dental checkup
Serum cationic trypsinogen (± fecal fat balance studies)

APPROACH TO THE CASE

The patient was initiated on regular infant formula with pancreatic enzyme replacement therapy. With fat-soluble vitamin supplementation, serum levels of vitamins A and E normalized along with the INR. A bone marrow biopsy and aspiration were performed that showed hypocellular marrow without cytogenetic abnormalities. Follow-up evaluation showed the child was growing with normal weight and height velocity for age but without catch-up growth (see Fig. 40-1) and with normal development. His skin rash disappeared by 8 months of age. Aminotransferases increased to about eight times normal levels before normalizing by three years of age. No other blood tests assessing liver dysfunction were present and there has been no evidence of hepatomegaly.

SUMMARY

Shwachman-Diamond syndrome is characterized by a widely variable phenotype affecting multiple organ systems occurring as a consequence to mutations of the *SBDS* gene. The hallmarks of the condition are exocrine pancreatic dysfunction, bone marrow dysfunction, and skeletal abnormities. Whereas some of the organ dysfunction such as that within the exocrine pancreas and liver tend to normalize with age, other organ systems that are involved, such as the skeletal and hematologic systems, may have progressive changes.

MAJOR POINTS

Shwachman-Diamond syndrome is a rare disorder.
It is the second most common cause of exocrine pancreatic insufficiency after cystic fibrosis.
It is the third most common inherited cause of bone marrow failure after Fanconi's anemia and Diamond-Blackfan syndrome.
This is a genetic disorder caused by mutations of the *SBDS* gene.
The most common clinical manifestations are characterized by exocrine pancreatic dysfunction, bone marrow dysfunction, skeletal abnormalities, and short stature.
Medical therapy includes pancreatic enzyme replacement therapy and supplemental fat-soluble vitamin administration.
There are no specific therapies for the short stature or skeletal abnormalities, but orthopedic consultation may be required for those patients with impairment of function due to metaphyseal chondrodysplasia.

SUGGESTED READINGS

Aggett PJ, Cavanagh NPC, Matthew DJ, et al: Shwachman's syndrome: A review of 21 cases. Arch Dis Child 55:331-347, 1980.

Boocock GRB, Morrison JA, Popovic M, et al: Mutations in *SBDS* are associated with Shwachman-Diamond syndrome. Nat Genet 33:97-101, 2002.

Dror Y, Freedman MH: Shwachman-Diamond syndrome. Br J Haematol 118:701-713, 2002.

Durie PR: Pancreatic aspects of cystic fibrosis and other inherited causes of pancreatic dysfunction. Med Clin North Am 84:609-620, 2000.

Ginzberg H, Shin J, Ellis L, et al: Shwachman syndrome: Phenotypic manifestations of sibling sets and isolated cases in a large patient cohort are similar. J Pediatr 135:81-88, 1999.

Ip W, Dupuis A, Ellis L, et al: Serum pancreatic enzymes define the pancreatic phenotype in patients with Shwachman-Diamond syndrome. J Pediatr 141:259-265, 2002.

Mack DR, Forstner GG, Wilschanski M, et al: Shwachman syndrome: Exocrine pancreatic dysfunction and variable phenotypic expression. Gastroenterology 111:1593-1602, 1996.

Makitie O, Ellis L, Durie PR, et al: Skeletal phenotype in patients with Shwachman-Diamond syndrome and mutations in SBDS. Clin Genet 65:101-112, 2004.

Index

Note: Page numbers followed by f indicate figures; those followed by t indicate tables.

A

Abdominal mass(es), 3-12
  case approach for, 11-12, 11f
  case presentation of, 3-4
  congenital and acquired
    choledochal cysts as, 7-8
    duplication cysts as, 8
    inguinal hernia as, incarcerated, 8
    pyloric stenosis as, 8
    umbilical hernia as, incarcerated, 8
  description of, 3
  diagnostic testing for, 4-5, 7f
  differential diagnosis of, 4, 4t-6t
  infectious and inflammatory, 4t, 7-8, 8-9
    abdominal wall abscesses as, 8
    appendicitis as, 8
    Crohn's phlegmon as, 8-9
    intussusception as, 9
    pancreatic pseudocysts as, 9
    tubo-ovarian abscess as, 9
    urachal remnant as, 9
  by location, 6t
  neoplastic, 4t, 9-11
    hepatic, 9
    lymphoma as, 9
    neuroblastoma as, 10
    ovarian, 10-11
    pancreatic, 10
    renal, 10
    sacrococcygeal teratoma as, 10
    sarcoma as, 10
Abdominal pain, differential diagnosis of, 134
Abdominal wall abscess(es), 8
Abscess(es)
  abdominal wall, 8
  hepatic, amebic, 173
  perirectal, 187, 189t
  pilonidal, 187, 189t
  tubo-ovarian, 9
Achalasia, 13-17
  case approach for, 17
  case presentation of, 13
  description of, 13
  diagnostic testing for, 15, 15f
  differential diagnosis of, 14-15, 14t, 15t
  etiology of, 13
  pathophysiology of, 13-14
  treatment of, 16-17
Acid ingestion(s). See Caustic ingestion(s).
Acid-lowering agents
  for gastroesophageal reflux disease, 82-84, 83t
  for gastrointestinal bleeding, 92

Aciphex (rabeprazole), for gastroesophageal reflux disease, 83t
Adefovir, for viral hepatitis, 291t, 296
Adenocarcinoma(s)
  esophageal, gastroesophageal reflux disease and, 75
  gastric, with Helicobacter pylori infection, 104
Adolescents. See also specific conditions.
  abdominal masses in, 5t
  celiac disease in, 25t
  gastroesophageal reflux disease in, 75
  growth of, 54
ADPKD. See Autosomal dominant polycystic kidney disease (ADPKD).
Aeroallergens, eosinophilic esophagitis and, 43-44
African American race, Helicobacter pylori infection and, 108
AGS. See Alagille syndrome (AGS).
AIH. See Autoimmune hepatitis (AIH).
Alacrima, 15
Alagille syndrome (AGS), 227-231
  case approach for, 230-231
  case presentation of, 227
  description of, 227
  diagnostic testing for, 229-230
  differential diagnosis of, 229, 229t
  epidemiology of, 227
  jaundice and, 279
  pathophysiology of, 227-229, 228f
  treatment of, 230, 231t
Alcohol abuse, pancreatitis and, 324
Alkali(s)
  in batteries, 67
  ingestion of. See Caustic ingestion(s).
Allergic disorders
  eosinophilic esophagitis and, 43-44
  Helicobacter pylori infection and, 106
Allgrove's syndrome, 15
Alosetron, for irritable bowel syndrome, 39
Alpha$_1$-antitrypsin (α_1-AT) deficiency, 233-236, 271
  case approach for, 235-236
  case presentation of, 233
  description of, 233
  diagnostic testing for, 234-235, 235f
  differential diagnosis of, 234, 234t, 235t
  epidemiology of, 233-234
  jaundice and, 278-279
  pathophysiology of, 234
  treatment of, 235
ALTEs. See Apparent life-threatening events (ALTEs).
Amebic infection(s), 172-176, 173f-175f
Amino acids, plasma levels of, in jaundice, 280-281

Aminosalicylates, for inflammatory bowel disease, 138
Amoxicillin
  for Helicobacter pylori infection, 107
  for infectious diarrhea, 129t
Anal atresia, 187
Anal fissures, 187, 189t
Ancylostoma duodenale infection(s), 184t
Anemia
  with Helicobacter pylori infection, 105-106
  in small bowel bacterial overgrowth, 219
Angiography
  in gastrointestinal bleeding, 91
  in Meckel's diverticulum, 159
Angiosarcomas, hepatic, 9
Anisakis infection(s), 184t
Annular pancreas
  pathophysiology and epidemiology of, 309, 310t, 311
  treatment of, 312
Anorectal manometry
  in chronic intestinal pseudo-obstruction, 204
  in constipation, 33t
Antacids, for gastroesophageal reflux disease, 82-83, 83t
Antibiotic(s)
  for chronic intestinal pseudo-obstruction, 207
  for Helicobacter pylori infection, 107
  for infectious diarrhea, 127, 129t
  for inflammatory bowel disease, 139
  for jaundice, 282-283
  for necrotizing enterocolitis, 166
  for small bowel bacterial overgrowth, 220-221
Antibiotic resistance, Helicobacter pylori treatment and, 107-108
Antibodies, in infectious diarrhea, 127t
Antiemetics, for chronic intestinal pseudo-obstruction, 207
Antigliadin antibody testing, for celiac disease, 25, 33t
Anti-IL-5 (mepolizumab), for eosinophilic esophagitis, 45-46
Antimotility agents, for infectious diarrhea, 127
Antioxidants
  for hemochromatosis, 264, 264t
  for Wilson disease, 303
Antireflux surgery, 84-85, 84t
Antroduodenal manometry, in chronic intestinal pseudo-obstruction, 202, 204, 205f
Anus, imperforate, 116, 187
APC gene, familial adenomatous polyposis and, 197
Apnea, gastroesophageal reflux disease and, 75

335

Apparent life-threatening events (ALTEs), gastroesophageal reflux disease and, 75
Appendicitis, 8
  cystic fibrosis and, 318
L-Arginine, for necrotizing enterocolitis, 166
ARPKD. *See* Autosomal recessive polycystic kidney disease (ARPKD).
Arteriohepatic dysplasia. *See* Alagille syndrome (AGS).
Arthritis, in inflammatory bowel disease, 133
Asacol (mesalamine)
  for inflammatory bowel disease, 139
  for ulcerative colitis, 138t
Ascaris lumbricoides infection(s), 176-178, 177f
α_1-AT deficiency. *See* Alpha$_1$-antitrypsin (α_1-AT) deficiency.
Atopy, eosinophilic esophagitis and, 43
Atrophy, *Helicobacter pylori* infection and, 101
Autoantibodies, in autoimmune hepatitis, 237-238
Autoimmune hepatitis (AIH), 237-241
  case approach for, 240-241
  case presentation of, 237
  description of, 237
  diagnostic testing for, 239, 240t
  differential diagnosis of, 238-239, 238t, 239t
  epidemiology of, 237
  overlap with primary sclerosing cholangitis, 248
  pathophysiology of, 237-238
  treatment of, 239-240, 240t
  Wilson disease *vs.*, 300
Autosomal dominant polycystic kidney disease (ADPKD), 255-256
  genetics of, 256
Autosomal recessive polycystic kidney disease (ARPKD), 254, 255
  genetics of, 255, 255t
Azathioprine (Imuran)
  for autoimmune hepatitis, 240, 240t
  for inflammatory bowel disease, 139-140
  for ulcerative colitis, 138t
Azithromycin, for infectious diarrhea, 129t

B

Balantidium infection(s), 181t
Bannayan-Riley-Ruvalcaba syndrome (BRRS), 193t, 195-196, 196t
Bardet-Beidl syndrome, 257t
Barium studies. *See also* Contrast studies.
  in achalasia, 15, 15f
  in chronic intestinal pseudo-obstruction, 202
  in constipation, 33t
  in gastroesophageal reflux disease, 77, 80t
  in Hirschsprung's disease, 116, 117f
Barrett's esophagus, gastroesophageal reflux disease and, 75
Basal metabolic panel (BMP)
  in congenital hepatic fibrosis, 258t
  in constipation, 33t
Battery ingestions
  case approach for, 71
  case presentation of, 64
  diagnostic testing and management for, 66-67, 67t
Beckwith-Wiedemann syndrome, 10
Bethanechol (Urecholine), for gastroesophageal reflux disease, 83t, 84
Bezoars, diagnostic testing and management for, 70-71, 71f
BICAP, for gastrointestinal bleeding, 93
Bile acids
  for cholelithiasis, 250
  jejunal, in small bowel bacterial overgrowth, 220t
Bile ducts
  intrahepatic
    embryology of, 254, 254f
    malformation of, 254, 256-257, 257t
    paucity of, in Alagille syndrome, 228, 228f
  obstruction of, 229t
    in pancreatitis, 327

Bile salt(s), malabsorption of, cholelithiasis and, 245
Bile salt export pump deficiency (BSEP), jaundice and, 279
Biliary anomalies, extrahepatic, malrotation with, 152
Biliary atresia, 277-279, 278t
Biliary disease, cystic fibrosis and, 316
Biliary sludge, 245, 246, 247f
Bipolar electrocoagulation, for gastrointestinal bleeding, 93
Birthweight, factors affecting, 54
Black pigment gallstones, 244, 244t, 245
Blastocystis hominis infection(s), 174-175, 175f
  diarrhea due to, treatment of, 129t
Bleeding
  gastrointestinal. *See* Gastrointestinal (GI) bleeding.
  intracranial, in Alagille syndrome, 229
Blind loop syndrome. *See* Small bowel bacterial overgrowth (SBBO).
Blood flukes, 179-181, 180f
Blood tests
  for detecting in gastrointestinal tract, 88
  in jaundice, 280
  for pancreatic anomalies, 310
BMP. *See* Basal metabolic panel (BMP).
Body packing, diagnostic testing and management for, 70
Bones, ingested, diagnostic testing and management for, 67
Botox injection, pyloric, for chronic intestinal pseudo-obstruction, 208
Botulinum toxin injections, for achalasia, 16
Breast milk, necrotizing enterocolitis and, 166
Breastfeeding, jaundice and, 277
β-Reductase deficiency, 263t
Brown pigment gallstones, 244, 244t, 245
BRRS. *See* Bannayan-Riley-Ruvalcaba syndrome (BRRS).
BSEP. *See* Bile salt export pump deficiency (BSEP).
Budesonide (Endocort; Entocort enema)
  for inflammatory bowel disease, 139
  for ulcerative colitis, 138t

C

Campylobacter jejuni infection(s), diarrhea due to, 124
  treatment of, 129t
Candida albicans infection(s), perianal, 187
Cardiac anomalies, Hirschsprung's disease and, 114
Cardiac disease, congenital, in Alagille syndrome, 228
Cardiac manifestations, in Wilson disease, 300t
Caroli syndrome, 255
Caroli's disease, 255
Cationic trypsinogen, serum, testing for, in Shwachman-Diamond syndrome, 331-332
Caustic ingestion(s), 19-23
  acid, 19, 20
  alkali, 19, 20
  case approach for, 22-23, 22f, 23f
  case presentation of, 19
  description of, 19
  diagnostic testing for, 21, 21t
  epidemiology of, 19-20
  evaluation of, 20-21
  pathophysiology of, 20
  signs and symptoms of, 20, 20t
  treatment of, 21, 21t
CBC. *See* Complete blood cell count (CBC).
^{14}C-bile acid test, in small bowel bacterial overgrowth, 220, 220t
Cefotaxime, for infectious diarrhea, 129t
Ceftriaxone, for infectious diarrhea, 129t
Celiac disease, 24-48
  case approach for, 27
  case presentation of, 24
  description of, 24
  diagnostic testing for, 25-26, 26f
  differential diagnosis of, 25, 25t

Celiac disease *(Continued)*
  epidemiology of, 24, 25t
  failure to thrive and, 60
  pathophysiology of, 24-25
  resources for, 27, 28t
  treatment of, 26-27, 26t-28t
Cellulase, for foreign body dissolution, 70
Centrioles, in centrosomes, in congenital hepatic fibrosis, 257
Centrosomes, centrioles in, in congenital hepatic fibrosis, 257
Ceruloplasmin, serum, measurement of, in Wilson disease, 301
Cestode infection(s), 183t-184t
CF. *See* Cystic fibrosis (CF).
CFTR gene, 314
  genotype-phenotype correlation in cystic fibrosis and, 316, 317t
Chagas' disease, 116
  achalasia *versus*, 14
Chelation therapy, for Wilson disease, 302-303
Children. *See also specific conditions.*
  abdominal masses in, 5t
  celiac disease in, 25t
  gastroesophageal reflux disease in, 75
  growth of, 54
Cholangiography, in primary sclerosing cholangitis, 286, 287t
Cholangitis, 246
  in congenital hepatic fibrosis, 258-259
  primary sclerosing. *See* Primary sclerosing cholangitis (PSC).
Cholecystectomy
  for cholelithiasis, 248
  for pancreatitis, 327
Cholecystitis, 246
  acalculous, 246
Choledochal cysts, 7-8
Choledocholithiasis, 246
Cholelithiasis, 243-251
  case approach for, 250
  case presentation of, 243
  cholesterol stones and, 244, 245t, 245
  description of, 243, 245t
  diagnostic testing for, 246-247
  differential diagnosis of, 246, 246t
  epidemiology of, 243-244
  pancreatitis and, 324
  pathophysiology of, 244-246, 245t
  pigment stones and, 244, 244t, 245
  in short bowel syndrome, treatment of, 214
  stone formation and, 244-245
  treatment of, 247-250
    for asymptomatic patients, 249-250
    for symptomatic patients, 247-249
Cholestasis, intrahepatic, familial, progressive, jaundice and, 279
Cholestasis syndrome, 229t
Cholesterol gallstones, 244, 245t, 245
Chronic intestinal pseudo-obstruction (CIPO), 200-209
  case approach for, 209
  case presentation of, 200
  description of, 200
  diagnosis of, 202, 204
  epidemiology of, 200-201, 201t
  outcome with, 209
  pathophysiology of, 201-202, 203t
  treatment of, 205-209, 208f
    nutritional, 205-206
    pharmacologic, 206-207, 208
    for small bowel bacterial overgrowth, 206
    surgical, 207, 208-209
Cilia, in congenital hepatic fibrosis, 256-257
Cimetidine (Tagamet)
  for gastroesophageal reflux disease, 83t
  in Meckel's diverticulum, 160
CIPO. *See* Chronic intestinal pseudo-obstruction (CIPO).
Ciprofloxacin
  for *Helicobacter pylori* infection, 107
  for infectious diarrhea, 129t

Cisapride (Propulsid), for gastroesophageal reflux disease, 83t, 84
Clarithromycin, for *Helicobacter pylori* infection, 107-108
Cloaca, persistent, malrotation with, 152
Cloacal anomalies, 189-190
Cloacal exstrophy, 187, 188
Clostridium difficile infection(s), diarrhea due to, 124
  treatment of, 129t
Clostridium difficile toxin assay, in infectious diarrhea, 127t
Coin ingestion(s), diagnostic testing and management for, 65-66, 66f, 66t
Colectomy, total, prophylactic, for familial adenomatous polyposis, 197-198
Colonic aganglionosis, total, treatment of, 119
Colonic manometry
  in chronic intestinal pseudo-obstruction, 204, 206f
  in constipation, 33t
Colonopathy, fibrosing, cystic fibrosis and, 319
Colonoscopy
  for gastrointestinal bleeding, 92, 93t
  in gastrointestinal bleeding, 92
  in inflammatory bowel disease, 135
  in Meckel's diverticulum, 159
  polyp removal at time of, 94-95, 94f, 95f
Colorectal carcinoma(s), familial adenomatous polyposis and, 197
Colostomy, for Hirschsprung's disease, 118-119
Common channel syndrome
  pathophysiology and epidemiology of, 309, 310t
  treatment of, 312
Complete blood cell count (CBC), in congenital hepatic fibrosis, 258t
Computed tomography (CT)
  for abdominal masses, 11, 11f
  of abdominal masses, 6-7
  in achalasia, 14
  in cholelithiasis, 247, 248t, 249f
  in Meckel's diverticulum, 159
  in pancreatitis, 325
Congenital hepatic fibrosis (CHF), 253-260
  case approach for, 259, 259f, 259t
  case presentation of, 253-254, 254t
  description of, 253
  diagnostic testing for, 257-258, 258f, 258t
  differential diagnosis of, 257, 257t
  management of, 258-259
  pathophysiology of, 254-257
    autosomal dominant polycystic kidney disease and, 255-256
    autosomal recessive polycystic kidney disease and, 254, 255
    Caroli's disease and Caroli syndrome and, 255, 256f
    cilia and, 257
    ductal plate malformation and, 254, 256-257, 257t
    embryology of intrahepatic bile ducts and, 254, 254f
    nephronolithiasis and, 256
    phosphomannose isomerase deficiency and, 256
    polycystic liver disease and, 256
Constipation, 30-35
  case approach for, 32-35
  case presentation for, 30
  cystic fibrosis and, 319
  description of, 30
  diagnostic testing for, 31, 32t, 33t, 34f-36f
  differential diagnosis of, 31, 31t, 32t
  epidemiology of, 31
  functional, 11
  pathophysiology of, 31
  retentive, functional, 34
  treatment of, 31-32, 37t
Contaminated small bowel syndrome. *See* Small bowel bacterial overgrowth (SBBO).
Contrast studies. *See also* Barium studies.
  of abdominal masses, 7
  in gastrointestinal bleeding, 90

Contrast studies *(Continued)*
  in intussusception, 143, 144f
  in malrotation, 154
  in Meckel's diverticulum, 159
Copper
  serum, measurement of, in Wilson disease, 301
  urine, 24-hour measurement of, 301
  Wilson disease and. *See* Wilson disease.
Cortenema (hydrocortisone), for ulcerative colitis, 138t
Corticosteroids
  for autoimmune hepatitis, 239, 240t
  for caustic ingestions, 21
  for eosinophilic esophagitis, 45
  for inflammatory bowel disease, 139
  for primary sclerosing cholangitis, 287
Cowden's syndrome (CS), 193t, 195-196, 196t
Crohn's disease. *See also* Inflammatory bowel disease (IBD).
  perianal manifestations of, 187, 189t, 190
  phlegmon in, 8-9
Cromolyn sodium, for eosinophilic esophagitis, 45
Cryptococcus DFA, in infectious diarrhea, 127t
Cryptosporidium infection(s), 175
  C. parvum, diarrhea due to, treatment of, 129t
CS. *See* Cowden's syndrome (CS).
CT. *See* Computed tomography (CT).
[14]C-xylose test, in small bowel bacterial overgrowth, 220, 220t
Cyclospora belli infection(s), diarrhea due to, treatment of, 129t
Cyclospora cayetanesis infection(s), 175-176
Cyclosporine
  for autoimmune hepatitis, 240
  for inflammatory bowel disease, 140
  for ulcerative colitis, 138t
Cyst(s). *See also* Pseudocyst(s).
  choledochal, 7-8
  duplication, 8
    intestinal, 116
    perianal, 187
    rectal, 116
  ovarian, 10
  pancreatic, pathophysiology and epidemiology of, 309, 310t
Cystadenocarcinomas, 10
Cystadenomas, 10
Cystic fibrosis (CF), 271, 314-320
  case approach for, 319-320
  case presentation of, 314-315, 315t
  description of, 314
  epidemiology of, 315
  gastrointestinal complications of, 316-319
    appendicitis as, 318
    constipation as, 319
    delayed gastric emptying as, 319
    distal intestinal obstruction syndrome as, 317-318
    fibrosing colonopathy as, 319
    gastroesophageal reflux disease as, 319
    intussusception as, 318
    meconium ileus as, 316-317, 318t
    rectal prolapse as, 318
    small bowel bacterial overgrowth as, 318-319
  pancreatitis and, 324
  pathophysiology of, 315-316
    genotype-phenotype correlation and, 316, 317t
    liver and biliary tract disease and, 316
    pancreatic disease and, 316-317, 316t, 317t
  treatment of, 319
Cytokines, proinflammatory, inflammatory bowel disease and, 132
Cytomegalovirus infection, neonatal liver failure and, 263t

D

Defecation, 31
Deferoxamine, for hemochromatosis, 264, 264t
Delayed gastric emptying, cystic fibrosis and, 319

Demystification, for constipation, 32
Denys-Drash syndrome, 10
Desipramine, for irritable bowel syndrome, 39
Desmoid tumors, ovarian, 10-11
Diabetes mellitus, in pancreatitis, 327
Diarrhea
  in *Giardia lamblia* infections, 171
  infectious. *See* Infectious diarrhea.
  in small bowel bacterial overgrowth, 218-219
Dicyclomine, for irritable bowel syndrome, 39
Dientamoeba fragilis infection(s), 174, 174f, 181t
Dietary fiber
  constipation and, 35
  for irritable bowel syndrome, 39, 40
Dietary therapy. *See* Nutritional therapy.
DIOS. *See* Distal intestinal obstruction syndrome (DIOS).
Diphyllobothrium latum infection(s), 183t
Direct injection therapy, for gastrointestinal bleeding, 92-93
Disaccharides, measurement of, in lactose intolerance, 149, 149f
Disofenin (DISIDA) scans, of abdominal masses, 7
Dissolution therapy, for cholelithiasis, 250
Distal intestinal obstruction syndrome (DIOS), cystic fibrosis and, 317-318
Diverticulitis, in Meckel's diverticulum, 159
Domperidone, for chronic intestinal pseudo-obstruction, 207
Doxycycline, for infectious diarrhea, 129t
DPM. *See* Ductal plate malformation (DPM).
Drug smuggling, body packing for, diagnostic testing and management for, 70
Drug therapy. *See also specific drugs and drug types.*
  for achalasia, 16
  for Alagille syndrome, 230, 231t
  for amebiasis, 173-174
  for *Ascaris lumbricoides* infections, 176, 178
  for autoimmune hepatitis, 239-240, 240t
  bezoar formation due to, 71
  for *Blastocystic hominis* infections, 175
  cholelithiasis associated with, 245
  for chronic intestinal pseudo-obstruction, 206-207, 208
  for Crohn's disease, 190
  for *Cryptosporidium* infections, 175
  for *Cyclospora cayetanesis* infections, 175-176
  for *Dientamoeba fragilis* infections, 174
  for *Enterobius vermicularis* infections, 179
  for gastroesophageal reflux disease, 82-84
    acid suppression and, 82-84, 83t
    prokinetic, 83t, 84
  for giardiasis, 172
  gluten in medications and, 27
  for hemochromatosis, 264, 264t
  for irritable bowel syndrome, 39, 39t
  for jaundice, 282-283
  for *Necator americanus* infections, 179
  for necrotizing enterocolitis, 166
  pancreatitis and, 324, 324t
  for primary sclerosing cholangitis, 287
  for *Schistosoma* infections, 181
  for small bowel bacterial overgrowth, 220-221
  for *Strongyloides stercoralis* infections, 176
  for *Trichuris trichuria* infections, 178
Drug-nutrient interactions, failure to thrive and, 56, 60t
Ductal plate malformation (DPM), 254
  inherited disorders assessment with, 256-257, 257t
Duhamel-Martin operation, for Hirschsprung's disease, 118, 118f
Dumping syndrome, following Nissen fundoplication, 84t
Duodenal aspirate and culture, in small bowel bacterial overgrowth, 219-220, 220t
Duplication cyst(s), 7
  intestinal, 116
  perianal, 187
  rectal, 116
Dysentery, 125-126

Dysphagia
　in achalasia, 14
　following Nissen fundoplication, 84t

E

Echovirus 9 infection, neonatal liver failure and, 263t
Ectopic tissue, in Meckel's diverticulum, 159
EES, for chronic intestinal pseudo-obstruction, 206–207
EGD. *See* Esophagogastroduodenoscopy (EGD).
EIA. *See* Enzyme immunoassay (EIA).
Elastase quantization, fecal, in pancreatitis, 326
Electrocoagulation
　bipolar, for gastrointestinal bleeding, 93
　thermal, for gastrointestinal bleeding, 93
Electrogastrography, in chronic intestinal pseudo-obstruction, 204
Elemental diet, for eosinophilic esophagitis, 43, 45
Embryotoxon, posterior, in Alagille syndrome, 230
Emesis
　of blood, 88–89
　contraindication to, in caustic ingestions, 21
　differential diagnosis of, 153, 154t
　in gastroesophageal reflux disease, 75
Endocort (budesonide)
　for inflammatory bowel disease, 139
　for ulcerative colitis, 138t
Endocrinopathies, autoimmune, autoimmune hepatitis and, 238
Endoscopic grading, of caustic ingestions, 21, 21t
Endoscopic retrograde cholangiopancreatography (ERCP), in cholelithiasis, 247, 248–249
Endoscopic therapy
　for caustic ingestions, 21, 22, 22f
　for foreign body removal, 66, 66f, 67, 70–71
　for gastrointestinal bleeding, 92, 93t
Endoscopic ultrasonography (EUS), in cholelithiasis, 247
Endoscopy, diagnostic
　in achalasia, 15
　in caustic ingestions, 21, 21t
　in celiac disease, 25, 26f
　in eosinophilic esophagitis, 44
　in gastrointestinal bleeding, 91–92, 92f
　in Meckel's diverticulum, 159
　video capsule, in gastrointestinal bleeding, 91
ENS. *See* Enteric nervous system (ENS).
Entamoeba histolytica infection(s), 172–174, 173f
　diarrhea due to, treatment of, 129t
Entamoeba histolytica test, in infectious diarrhea, 127t
Enteric nervous system (ENS), 201
Enterobius vermicularis infection(s), 178–179, 178f
Enteroclysis, in Meckel's diverticulum, 159
Enterocolitis
　Hirschsprung's, treatment of, 119
　in Hirschsprung's disease, 115
　necrotizing. *See* Necrotizing enterocolitis.
Entocort enema (budesonide)
　for inflammatory bowel disease, 139
　for ulcerative colitis, 138t
Enzyme immunoassay (EIA), for giardiasis, 171
EoE. *See* Eosinophilic esophagitis (EoE).
Eosinophilic esophagitis (EoE), 42–46
　case approach for, 46
　case presentation of, 42
　description of, 42
　diagnostic testing for, 44
　differential diagnosis of, 44
　epidemiology of, 42–43
　pathophysiology of, 43–44
　treatment of, 44–46
Epinephrine injections, for gastrointestinal bleeding, 92
ERCP. *See* Endoscopic retrograde cholangiopancreatography (ERCP).
Erythromycin, for gastroesophageal reflux disease, 83t, 84

Escherichia coli infection(s)
　enteroadherent, diarrhea due to, 124
　enteroinvasive, diarrhea due to, treatment of, 129t
　enterotoxigenic, diarrhea due to, 124
　　treatment of, 129t
　inflammatory bowel disease and, 132
Esomeprazole (Nexium), for gastroesophageal reflux disease, 83t
Esophageal adenocarcinoma(s), gastroesophageal reflux disease and, 75
Esophageal biopsy, in eosinophilic esophagitis, 44
Esophageal dilatation, for caustic ingestions, 22–23, 23f
Esophageal disorders
　familial clustering of, 76
　foreign body ingestions and. *See* Foreign body ingestion(s).
Esophageal manometry
　in achalasia, 15
　　intraoperative, 17
　in chronic intestinal pseudo-obstruction, 202
Esophageal varices
　bleeding, therapy for, 93–94, 93t, 94f
　in congenital hepatic fibrosis, 258
Esophagitis
　candidal, achalasia *versus*, 14–15
　eosinophilic. *See* Eosinophilic esophagitis (EoE).
　in gastroesophageal reflux disease, 75
Esophagogastroduodenoscopy (EGD)
　in congenital hepatic fibrosis, 258t
　in gastroesophageal reflux disease, 79, 80t, 81f
　for gastrointestinal bleeding, 92, 93t
　in inflammatory bowel disease, 135, 136f–138f
Esophagoscopy, in achalasia, 14
Ethanol injections, for gastrointestinal bleeding, 93
EUS. *See* Endoscopic ultrasonography (EUS).

F

Facies, in Alagille syndrome, 230
Failure to thrive, 48–63
　anthropometric measurements of nutritional and growth status and, 49, 52–54, 52t, 53t
　case approach for, 62
　case presentation of, 48–49, 50f–51f
　definition of, 49
　description of, 48
　diagnostic testing for, 60
　differential diagnosis of, 55
　intervention for, critical periods for, 54–55
　laboratory examination in, 60
　management of, 55, 56f–59f
　normal growth and, 54
　pathophysiology of, 54–55
　physical examination in, 60, 61f
　treatment of, 61–62
Familial adenomatous polyposis (FAP), 193t, 196t, 197–198, 197f, 198f
Famotidine (Pepcid), for gastroesophageal reflux disease, 83t
Fanconi syndrome, renal, 271, 271t
FAP. *See* Familial adenomatous polyposis (FAP).
Fatty acid(s), jejunal, in small bowel bacterial overgrowth, 220t
Fatty acid oxidation disorders, 271
Fecal fat balance studies, in Shwachman-Diamond syndrome, 331–332
Fecal impaction(s), 11
　removal of, 32
Fecal leukocyst test, in infectious diarrhea, 127t
Feeding
　family dynamic about, failure to thrive and, 60–61
　of premature infants, 164–165
Fiber
　constipation and, 35
　for irritable bowel syndrome, 39, 40
Fibrosing colonopathy, cystic fibrosis and, 319
Fish tapeworms, 183t

Flagyl (metronidazole)
　for Crohn's disease, 138t
　for *Helicobacter pylori* infection, 107–108
　for infectious diarrhea, 129t
　for inflammatory bowel disease, 139
Flora. *See also specific organisms.*
　intestinal. *See also* Small bowel bacterial overgrowth (SBBO).
　　normal, 218, 219t
Fluoroquinolones, for inflammatory bowel disease, 139
Fluoroscopic studies, of abdominal masses, 7
Food allergy(ies), eosinophilic esophagitis and, 43
Food impaction(s), diagnostic testing and management for, 69–70, 70f
Foreign body ingestion(s), 64–70
　case approach for, 71
　case presentation of, 64
　description of, 64
　diagnostic testing and management for, 65–70
　　for battery ingestions, 66–67, 67t
　　for body packing, 70
　　for coins, 65–66, 66f, 66t
　　for food impactions, 69–70, 70f
　　for lead objects, 69
　　for long or large objects, 68
　　for magnets, 69, 69f
　　for sharp bodies, 67–68, 68f
　epidemiology of, 64–65
　natural history of, 65
　symptoms of, 65
Fructose intolerance
　hereditary
　　epidemiology of, 268
　　pathophysiology of, 270, 270f
　　treatment of, 274

G

Galactosemia
　epidemiology of, 268
　pathophysiology of, 269–270, 269f
　treatment of, 274
Gall stones. *See* Cholelithiasis.
Gallium scans, of abdominal masses, 7
Ganglion cells, in Hirschsprung's disease, 115, 115f
Gas-bloat syndrome, following Nissen fundoplication, 84t
Gastric cancer, with *Helicobacter pylori* infection, 101, 104–105
Gastric emptying, delayed, cystic fibrosis and, 319
Gastric emptying studies, in gastroesophageal reflux disease, 78, 80t
Gastric hypersecretion, in short bowel syndrome, treatment of, 213–214, 214f
Gastric pacing, for chronic intestinal pseudo-obstruction, 208
Gastrinoma(s), 10
Gastritis, with *Helicobacter pylori* infection, 103, 104
Gastroccult test, 88
Gastroenterologic approach, to failure to thrive, 55, 56f
Gastroesophageal junction (GEJ), gastroesophageal reflux disease and, 75
Gastroesophageal reflux (GER), postmyotomy, 16
Gastroesophageal reflux disease (GERD), 74–85
　case approach for, 85
　case presentation of, 74–75
　clinical presentation of, 75
　cystic fibrosis and, 319
　description of, 74
　diagnostic testing for, 77–81, 80t
　　empiric testing as, 77
　　multichannel intraluminal impedance as, 81
　　nuclear scintigraphy as, 78
　　pH probe as, 79–80
　　upper endoscopy as, 79, 81f
　　upper gastrointestinal series as, 77
　　wireless pH monitoring as, 80–81
　differential diagnosis of, 76–77, 76t–79t

Gastroesophageal reflux disease *(Continued)*
  epidemiology of, 75
  Helicobacter pylori infection and, 106-107
  pathophysiology of, 75-76
  treatment of, 82-85
    dietary, 82
    lifestyle management for, 82
    pharmacologic, 82-84, 83t
    positioning therapy for, 82
    surgical, 84-85, 84t
Gastrointestinal (GI) bleeding, 87-95
  case approach for, 95
  case presentation of, 87
  description of, 87
  diagnostic testing for, 89-92, 90t, 91f, 91t, 92f
  differential diagnosis of, 88-89, 89t
  epidemiology of, 87
  lower, 89
  pathophysiology of, 87-88
  treatment of, 92-95, 93t, 94f, 95f
  upper, 88-89
Gastrostomy, for chronic intestinal pseudo-obstruction, 207
GEJ. *See* Gastroesophageal junction (GEJ).
Genetic screening, for polyposis syndromes, 198
Genetic testing
  in pancreatitis, 326
  for Wilson disease, 301
Gentamicin, for infectious diarrhea, 129t
Geographic location, failure to thrive and, 60
GER. *See* Gastroesophageal reflux (GER).
GERD. *See* Gastroesophageal reflux disease (GERD).
GI bleeding. *See* Gastrointestinal (GI) bleeding.
Giardia enzyme immunoassay, in infectious diarrhea, 127t
Giardia lamblia infection(s), 171-172, 172f, 173f
  diarrhea due to, 124
  treatment of, 129t
Gilbert's mutation, 277
Glioblastoma multiforme, in Turcot's syndrome, 197
Glucagon, in Meckel's diverticulum, 160
Glucose intolerance, in pancreatitis, 327
Gluten, in prescription medications, 27
Gluten intolerance. *See* Celiac disease.
Glycogen storage diseases, 271
Gold Probe, for gastrointestinal bleeding, 93
Granulosa-thecal cell tumors, 11
Group A-hemolytic streptococcal infection(s), perianal, 187
Growth
  anthropometric measurements of, 49, 52-54, 52t, 53t
  normal, 54
  phases of, 54
  retardation of
    in Alagille syndrome, 229
    with *Helicobacter pylori* infection, 105
Growth charts, 49, 50f-51f
  neonatal, 52
Guaiac, for detecting blood in gastrointestinal tract, 88

H

H$_2$ receptor antagonists
  for eosinophilic esophagitis, 45
  for gastroesophageal reflux disease, 77, 83, 83t
Hamartoma(s), embryonal, 9
Hamartomatous polyp(s), 193-197
  in Bannayan-Riley-Ruvalcaba syndrome, 193t, 195-196, 196t
  in Cowden's syndrome, 193t, 195-196, 196t
  juvenile, 193-194, 194f
  in juvenile polyposis syndrome, 193t, 194-195, 195f, 196t
  in Peutz-Jeghers syndrome, 193t, 196-197, 196f, 196t
H$_2$-blockers
  for eosinophilic esophagitis, 45
  for gastroesophageal reflux disease, 77, 83, 83t

Head circumference, measurement of, 49
Heart. *See* Cardiac *entries*.
Heartburn, in gastroesophageal reflux disease, 75
Height
  factors affecting, 54
  measurement of, 49
Helicobacter pylori infection(s), 98-108
  case approach for, 108
  case presentation of, 98-99
  clinical manifestations of, 103-107
    extragastric, 105-106
    gastroduodenal, 103-105
    gastroesophageal reflux and, 106-107
  description of, 98
  diagnosis of, 100-103
    gastrointestinal endoscopy and histology for, 100-101
  epidemiology of, 99
  pathophysiology of, 99-100
  serology for, 101-102
  stool antigen test for, 102-103
  treatment of, 107-108
  urea breath test for, 102
  urine antibody test for, 103
Heller myotomy, for achalasia, 16
Hemangioendothelioma(s), 9
Hematemesis, 88-89
Hematochezia, 89
Hematologic manifestations, in Wilson disease, 300t
HemeSelect test, 88
Hemoccult II test, 88
Hemoccult SENSA test, 88
Hemoccult test, 88
Hemochromatosis, 261-265
  case approach for, 264-265
  case presentation of, 261
  description of, 261
  diagnosis of, 262-264
  differential diagnosis of, 262, 263t
  etiology of, 261
  neonatal, 262-264, 263t, 271
  pathophysiology of, 262
  treatment of, 264, 264t
Hemorrhoids, 187
  external, 189t
Hepatic abscess(es), amebic, 173
Hepatic fibrosis, congenital. *See* Congenital hepatic fibrosis (CHF).
Hepatic neoplasms, 9
Hepatic portoenterostomy, 230
Hepatitis
  amebic, 173
  autoimmune. *See* Autoimmune hepatitis (AIH).
  neonatal, 229t
  viral, 289-296. *See also* Hepatitis B; Hepatitis C.
    description of, 289, 290f
    in Wilson disease, 300
Hepatitis A, 289
Hepatitis B, 293-296
  acute, 294-295
  case approach for, 296
  chronic, 295
  epidemiology and natural history of, 293
  pathophysiology of, 294
  treatment of, 291t, 295-296
Hepatitis C, 289-293
  acute, diagnosis and treatment of, 290-291, 291t, 292f-293f
  case approach for, 292-293
  case presentation of, 289
  chronic, diagnosis and treatment of, 291-292, 294f
  clinical symptoms of, 289-290, 291f
  incidence of, 289, 290f
Hepatitis D, 289
Hepatitis E, 289
Hepatobiliary disease, in inflammatory bowel disease, 133-134
Hepatobiliary inflammation, in small bowel bacterial overgrowth, 219
Hepatoblastoma(s), 9
  familial adenomatous polyposis and, 197

Hepatocellular carcinoma(s), 9
Hepatomegaly, in Alagille syndrome, 228
Hernia(s)
  incarcerated, 116
    inguinal, 8
    umbilical, 8
  paraesophageal, following Nissen fundoplication, 84t
Herpes simplex virus infection(s), neonatal liver failure and, 263t
Heterotopic pancreas
  pathophysiology and epidemiology of, 309, 310t, 311
  treatment of, 312
HFE gene, 263-264
Hirschsprung's disease, 114-121
  case approach for, 119-120, 120f
  case presentation of, 114
  constipation and, 34
  description of, 114
  diagnostic testing for, 116-118, 117f
  differential diagnosis of, 115-116, 115t
  epidemiology of, 114-115
  malrotation with, 152
  pathophysiology of, 115, 115f
  treatment of, 118-119, 118f
HLA-DQ2, celiac disease and, 25
HLA-DQ8, celiac disease and, 25
Hollow visceral myopathy, 116
Hookworms, 179
Hydrocortisone (Cortenema), for ulcerative colitis, 138t
Hydrogen breath test, in small bowel bacterial overgrowth, 220, 220t
Hyoscyamine, for irritable bowel syndrome, 39
Hyperbilirubinemia
  conjugated, in Alagille syndrome, 228
  direct, 277-279, 278t
  indirect, 277, 277t
Hypersensitivity
  eosinophilic esophagitis and, 43-44
  Helicobacter pylori infection and, 106
Hypolactasia, adult type, 147, 147t

I

IBD. *See* Inflammatory bowel disease (IBD).
ICCs. *See* Interstitial cells of Cajal (ICCs).
Idiopathic thrombocytopenic purpura (ITP), with *Helicobacter pylori* infection, 105
IFN-α. *See* Interferon-α (IFN-α).
IgA, for necrotizing enterocolitis, 166
IgA antiendomyseal antibody test, for celiac disease, 25, 33t
IgA antitissue transglutaminase antibody test, in celiac disease, 25
IgG, for necrotizing enterocolitis, 166
IL-5. *See* Interleukin-5 (IL-5).
Ileum, intussusception and. *See* Intussusception.
Imaging. *See specific imaging modalities*.
Immune function, inflammatory bowel disease and, 132
Immunoglobulin(s)
  for hemochromatosis, 264
  IgA, for necrotizing enterocolitis, 166
  IgG, for necrotizing enterocolitis, 166
Immunosuppressive agents, for primary sclerosing cholangitis, 287
Imperforate anus, 116, 187, 189
Imuran (azathioprine)
  for autoimmune hepatitis, 240, 240t
  for inflammatory bowel disease, 139-140
  for ulcerative colitis, 138t
Incarcerated hernias, 116
Index(ices), for growth status, 52-64, 52t, 63t
Infants. *See also specific conditions*.
  abdominal masses in, 5t
  celiac disease in, 25t
  gastroesophageal reflux disease in, 75
  growth of, 54
  newborn. *See* Newborns.

Infants (Continued)
    premature
        feeding, 164-165
        necrotizing enterocolitis in. See Necrotizing enterocolitis.
Infectious diarrhea, 123-130
    case approach for, 128, 130
    case presentation of, 123
    description of, 123
    diagnostic testing for, 125-126, 126t, 127t, 128f
    differential diagnosis of, 124-125, 125t, 126t
    epidemiology of, 123-124
    pathophysiology of, 124
    treatment of, 126-128
        antibiotic therapy for, 127
        oral rehydration therapy for, 126-127, 128t
        public health and, 127-128
        supplemental therapy for, 127
Infectious diseases. See also specific diseases and organisms.
    abdominal masses due to. See Abdominal mass(es).
    inflammatory bowel disease development and, 132
    inflammatory bowel disease versus, 134-135
    pancreatitis and, 324
    perirectal, 187
Inflammation
    abdominal masses due to. See Abdominal mass(es).
    hepatobiliary, in small bowel bacterial overgrowth, 219
    in Meckel's diverticulum, 159
    in necrotizing enterocolitis, 163, 165
Inflammatory bowel disease (IBD), 131-141
    case approach for, 140
    case presentation of, 131
    clinical features of, 132-134
    description of, 131
    diagnostic testing for, 135, 136f-138f
    differential diagnosis of, 134-135, 134t
    epidemiology of, 131-132
    pathophysiology of, 132
    treatment of, 135, 138-140, 138t
        nutritional therapy for, 135, 138
        pharmacologic, 139-140
        surgical, 140
Infliximab (Remicade)
    for inflammatory bowel disease, 140
    for ulcerative colitis, 138t
Inguinal hernia(s), incarcerated, 8
Insulinoma(s), 10
Interferon-α (IFN-α), for viral hepatitis, 291t, 295
Interleukin-5 (IL-5), eosinophilic esophagitis and, 43
Interstitial cells of Cajal (ICCs), 201
Intestinal atresia, 116
    malrotation with, 152
Intestinal biopsy, in chronic intestinal pseudo-obstruction, 204
Intestinal duplication cyst(s), 116
Intestinal failure, treatment of, 62
Intestinal malrotation, 152-157
    anomalies associated with, 152
    case approach for, 156
    case presentation of, 152
    description of, 152
    diagnostic testing for, 153-154, 155f
    differential diagnosis of, 153, 154t
    epidemiology of, 152
    pathophysiology of, 153, 153f
    treatment of, 154, 156
Intestinal manifestations, in Crohn's disease, 133
Intestinal metaplasia, Helicobacter pylori infection and, 101
Intestinal neuronal dysplasia, 116
Intestinal obstruction
    in Meckel's diverticulum, 159
    in pancreatitis, 327
Intestinal obstruction syndrome, distal, cystic fibrosis and, 317-318
Intestinal pseudo-obstruction. See Chronic intestinal pseudo-obstruction (CIPO); Hirschsprung's disease.
Intestinal stenosis, 116

Intestinal transplantation (IT), for chronic intestinal pseudo-obstruction, 208-209
Intestinal volvulus. See Volvulus.
Intracranial bleeding, in Alagille syndrome, 229
Intussusception, 9, 142-145
    case approach for, 144-145
    case presentation of, 142
    cystic fibrosis and, 318
    description of, 142
    diagnostic testing for, 143, 143f, 144f
    differential diagnosis of, 143, 143t
    epidemiology of, 142
    malrotation with, 152
    pathophysiology of, 142-143
    treatment of, 143-144
Iodoquinol, for infectious diarrhea, 129t
Iron chelation, for hemochromatosis, 264, 264t
Iron deposition. See Hemochromatosis.
Iron-deficiency anemia, with Helicobacter pylori infection, 105-106
Irritable bowel syndrome, 35-39
    case approach for, 39-40
    case presentation of, 35-36
    diagnostic testing for, 37, 38t
    differential diagnosis of, 37, 38t
    epidemiology of, 36-37
    pathophysiology of, 37
    treatment of, 38-39, 39t
Isosorbide dinitrate, for achalasia, 16
Isospora belli infection(s), 181t
    diarrhea due to, treatment of, 129t
IT. See Intestinal transplantation (IT).
ITP. See Idiopathic thrombocytopenic purpura (ITP).
Ivemark's syndrome, 257t

J

Jaundice, 276-283
    case approach for, 283
    case presentation of, 276
    description of, 276
    diagnostic testing for, 279-281, 279t, 280t
    epidemiology of, 276-279
        direct hyperbilirubinemia and, 277-279, 278t
        indirect hyperbilirubinemia and, 277, 277t
    treatment of, 281-283
        nutritional, 281-282
        pharmacologic, 282-283
Jejunal bile acids, in small bowel bacterial overgrowth, 220t
Jejunal fatty acids, in small bowel bacterial overgrowth, 220t
Jejunostomy, for chronic intestinal pseudo-obstruction, 207
Jeune's syndrome, 257t
Joubert's syndrome, 257t
JPS. See Juvenile polyposis syndrome (JPS).
Juvenile polyp(s), 193-194, 194f
Juvenile polyposis syndrome (JPS), 193t, 194-195, 195f, 196t

K

Kasai procedure, 230
Kernicterus, prevention of, 277
Kidney, ureter, and bladder (KUB) films, in chronic intestinal pseudo-obstruction, 202, 204f
KUB. See Kidney, ureter, and bladder (KUB) films.

L

Lactase (LactAid; Lactase), for lactose intolerance, 149-150
Lactase deficiency
    congenital, 146-147
    primary, 147, 147t
    secondary (acquired), 147

D-Lactic acidosis, in small bowel bacterial overgrowth, 219
Lactobacillus johnsonii La1, for Helicobacter pylori infection, 107
Lactobacillus paracasei ST11, for Helicobacter pylori infection, 107
Lactose breath test, 148-149, 148f, 149f
Lactose intolerance, 146-150
    case approach for, 150
    case presentation of, 146
    in celiac disease, 27
    description of, 146
    diagnostic testing for, 148-149
    differential diagnosis of, 148, 148t
    epidemiology of, 146-147, 147t
    pathophysiology of, 147-148
    treatment of, 149-150
Ladd procedure, for volvulus, 154, 156
Lamivudine, for viral hepatitis, 291t, 295-296
Lansoprazole (Prevacid), for gastroesophageal reflux disease, 83t, 85
Laparoscopic therapy, for achalasia, 16-17
Large foreign body ingestions, diagnostic testing and management for, 68
Laryngospasm, gastroesophageal reflux disease and, 75
Laser photocoagulation, for gastrointestinal bleeding, 94
Laxatives, 32, 37t
Lead
    ingestion of, diagnostic testing and management for, 69
    serum level of, in constipation, 33t
Leiomyoma(s), esophageal, achalasia versus, 14
Length, measurement of, 49
LES. See Lower esophageal sphincter (LES).
LFTs. See Liver function tests (LFTs).
Lifestyle management, for gastroesophageal reflux disease, 82
Linear growth, measurement of, 49
Listeria infection(s), inflammatory bowel disease and, 132
Liver biopsy
    in $α_1$-AT deficiency, 235, 235f
    in congenital hepatic fibrosis, 258t
    in jaundice, 281
    in Wilson disease, 301
Liver disease
    cystic fibrosis and, 316
    end-stage, neonatal, 262, 263t
    metabolic. See Metabolic liver disease.
    in Wilson disease, 300t, 300
Liver failure, indolent, metabolic causes of, 270, 271t
Liver function tests (LFTs)
    in congenital hepatic fibrosis, 258t
    in jaundice, 280
Liver transplantation (LT)
    for Alagille syndrome, 230
    for $α_1$-AT deficiency, 235
    for hemochromatosis, 264
    for Wilson disease, 303
Long foreign body ingestion(s), diagnostic testing and management for, 68
Lower esophageal sphincter (LES), gastroesophageal reflux disease and, 75-76
LT. See Liver transplantation (LT).
Lymphoma(s), 9

M

Magnet ingestion(s), diagnostic testing and management for, 69, 69f
Magnetic resonance cholangiography, in congenital hepatic fibrosis, 258t
    of abdominal masses, 7
    in cholelithiasis, 247, 248t
    in pancreatitis, 325, 326t
Magnetic resonance imaging (MRI)
    of abdominal masses, 6, 7
    in achalasia, 14
    in constipation, 33t

Malnourishment, failure to thrive and. *See* Failure to thrive.
Malnutrition, in small bowel bacterial overgrowth, 218-219
Malrotation. *See* Intestinal malrotation.
Manometry
 anorectal
  in chronic intestinal pseudo-obstruction, 204
  in constipation, 33t
 antroduodenal, in chronic intestinal pseudo-obstruction, 202, 204, 205f
 colonic
  in chronic intestinal pseudo-obstruction, 204, 206f
  in constipation, 33t
 esophageal
  in achalasia, 15, 17
  in chronic intestinal pseudo-obstruction, 202
 sphincter of Oddi, in chronic intestinal pseudo-obstruction, 204
Marshall, Barry, 98
MCAD deficiency. *See* Medium-chain acyl-CoA dehydrogenase (MCAD) deficiency.
MD. *See* Meckel's diverticulum (MD).
MDR3. *See* Multidrug resistant protein 3 deficiency (MDR3).
Measles, inflammatory bowel disease and, 132
Meat impactions, 65
Meckel, Johann, 158
Meckel-Gruber syndrome, 257t
Meckel's diverticulum (MD), 158-161
 case approach for, 160, 161f
 case presentation of, 158
 clinical features of, 159
 description of, 158
 diagnostic testing for, 159-160, 160t
 differential diagnosis of, 159, 159t
 epidemiology of, 158-159
 malrotation with, 152
 pathophysiology of, 159
 treatment of, 160
Meckel's scan, 159-160, 160t
Meconium ileus (MI), 116
 cystic fibrosis and, 316-317, 318t
Meconium ileus equivalent, cystic fibrosis and, 317-318
Meconium plug syndrome, 116
Medium-chain acyl-CoA dehydrogenase (MCAD) deficiency, 271
Medulloblastoma(s), in Turcot's syndrome, 197
Megacolon, in Hirschsprung's disease, 114
Melena, 89
MEN. *See* Multiple endocrine neoplasia (MEN).
Mepolizumab (anti-IL-5), for eosinophilic esophagitis, 45-46
6-Mercaptopurine (6-MP; Purinethol)
 for inflammatory bowel disease, 139-140
 for ulcerative colitis, 138t
Mesalamine (Asacol; Pentasa; Rowasa)
 for inflammatory bowel disease, 139
 for ulcerative colitis, 138t
Mesalazine, for inflammatory bowel disease, 139
Mesoblastic nephromas, 10
Metabolic disorders, 229t
Metabolic liver disease, 267-275
 case approach for, 274
 case presentation of, 267
 description of, 267
 diagnostic testing for, 272-273, 272t, 273t
 differential diagnosis of, 270-272, 271t
 epidemiology of, 268
 pathophysiology of, 268-270
 treatment of, 274
Metabolic screen, in chronic intestinal pseudo-obstruction, 204, 207f
Methane, measurement of, in lactose intolerance, 149
Methane breath test, in small bowel bacterial overgrowth, 220
Methotrexate, for inflammatory bowel disease, 139
Methylprednisolone, for eosinophilic esophagitis, 45
Metoclopramide (Reglan)
 for chronic intestinal pseudo-obstruction, 207
 for gastroesophageal reflux disease, 83t, 84

Metronidazole (Flagyl)
 for Crohn's disease, 138t
 for *Helicobacter pylori* infection, 107-108
 for infectious diarrhea, 129t
 for inflammatory bowel disease, 139
MI. *See* Meconium ileus (MI).
MIBG scans, for abdominal masses, 11, 11f
Microsporidia infection(s), 183t
Midparental height (MPH), 54
Mid-upper arm circumference, measurement of, 49, 52
MII. *See* Multichannel intraluminal impedance (MII).
Milk protein allergy, 116
Milk scans, in gastroesophageal reflux disease, 78, 80t
Mitochondrial cytopathy, 263t
6-MP. *See* 6-Mercaptopurine (6-MP; Purinethol).
MPH. *See* Midparental height (MPH).
MRCP. *See* Magnetic resonance cholangiopancreatography (MRCP).
MRI. *See* Magnetic resonance imaging (MRI).
Multichannel intraluminal impedance (MII), in gastroesophageal reflux disease, 80t, 81
Multidrug resistant protein 3 deficiency (MDR3), jaundice and, 279
Multiple endocrine neoplasia (MEN), type 2, Hirschsprung's disease and, 114-115
Murmurs, in Alagille syndrome, 230
Mycophenolate mofetil, for autoimmune hepatitis, 240

N

NASH. *See* Nonalcoholic steatohepatitis (NASH).
Nasogastric irrigation, for gastrointestinal bleeding, 89-90
Necator americanus infection(s), 179
Necrotizing enterocolitis, 163-168
 case approach for, 166, 168
 case presentation of, 163-164
 complications of, 165
 description of, 163
 diagnostic testing for, 165, 166f, 167f, 167t
 differential diagnosis of, 165
 epidemiology of, 164
 pathophysiology of, 164-165
 staging criteria for, 165, 167t
 treatment of, 165-166
Nematode infection(s), 176-179, 177f, 178f, 184t-185t
Neonatal growth charts, 52
Nephroma(s), mesoblastic, 10
Nephronolithiasis, in congenital hepatic fibrosis, 256
Neural crest migration disorders, Hirschsprung's disease and, 114-115
Neuroblastoma(s), 10, 12
Neuropsychiatric manifestations, in Wilson disease, 300t, 300, 303
Neutralization, contraindication to, in caustic ingestions, 21
Newborns. *See also specific conditions.*
 abdominal masses in, 5t
 conjugated hyperbilirubinemia in, 228
 hemochromatosis in, 271
 hepatitis in, 229t
 liver failure in, 262, 263t
 screening of, by state, 273, 273t
Nexium (esomeprazole), for gastroesophageal reflux disease, 83t
Nifedipine, for achalasia, 16
Nissen fundoplication, for gastroesophageal reflux disease, 84-85, 84t
Nitazoxamine, for infectious diarrhea, 129t
Nitric acid synthase (NOS), as dysmotility marker, 201-202
Nizatidine (Axid), for gastroesophageal reflux disease, 83t
Nonalcoholic steatohepatitis (NASH), Wilson disease *vs.*, 300

Nonoperative reduction, for intussusception, 143-144
NOS. *See* Nitric acid synthase (NOS).
NPHP1-5 gene, 256
Nuclear medicine. *See* Scintigraphic studies; *specific studies.*
Nutritional status, anthropometric measurements of, 49, 52-54, 52t, 53t
Nutritional therapy
 for Alagille syndrome, 230, 231t
 for caustic ingestions, 21
 for celiac disease, 26-27, 26t-28t
 for chronic intestinal pseudo-obstruction, 205-206
 for constipation, 32
 for cystic fibrosis, 319
 for eosinophilic esophagitis, 44-45
 for failure to thrive, 55, 61-62
 for gastroesophageal reflux disease, 82
 for inflammatory bowel disease, 135, 138
 for irritable bowel syndrome, 39
 for jaundice, 281-282
 for short bowel syndrome, 213, 214f
 for small bowel bacterial overgrowth, 221

O

Obesity, cholelithiasis and, 244
Occult blood tests, 88
Octreotide
 for chronic intestinal pseudo-obstruction, 207
 for gastrointestinal bleeding, 92
Omeprazole (Prilosec)
 for gastroesophageal reflux disease, 83t
 for *Helicobacter pylori* infection, 107
Ondansetron, for chronic intestinal pseudo-obstruction, 207
Ondine's curse, Hirschsprung's disease and, 114
Ophthalmologic manifestations
 in inflammatory bowel disease, 133
 in Wilson disease, 300t
Oral rehydration therapy, for infectious diarrhea, 126-127, 128t
Orogastric intubation, for necrotizing enterocolitis, 165-166
Orthopedic manifestations, in Wilson disease, 300t
Ova and parasites test, in infectious diarrhea, 127t
Ovarian neoplasm(s), 10-11

P

Pancreas
 agenesis of, pathophysiology and epidemiology of, 308-309, 310t, 311
 annular
  pathophysiology and epidemiology of, 309, 310t, 311
  treatment of, 312
 congenital anomalies of, 307-312. *See also specific anomalies.*
  case approach for, 312
  case presentation of, 307-308
  description of, 307, 308t
  diagnostic testing for, 310-311, 310t, 311f
  differential diagnosis of, 310, 310t
  pancreatic development and, 308, 308f
  pathophysiology and epidemiology of of, 308-309
  treatment of, 311-312
 heterotopic
  diagnosis and treatment of, 310t
  pathophysiology and epidemiology of, 309, 311
  treatment of, 312
Pancreas divisum
 pathophysiology and epidemiology of, 309, 310t, 311, 311f
 treatment of, 311
Pancreatic carcinoma(s), 10

Pancreatic cyst(s), pathophysiology and epidemiology of, 309, 310t
Pancreatic dysplasia, pathophysiology and epidemiology of, 308-309, 310t, 311
Pancreatic enzyme supplementation
 for pancreatitis, 327
 for Shwachman-Diamond syndrome, 333
Pancreatic hypoplasia, pathophysiology and epidemiology of, 308-309, 310t, 311
Pancreatic insufficiency (PI), cystic fibrosis and, 315-316, 316t, 317t
Pancreatic neoplasm(s), 10
Pancreatic pseudocyst(s), 9
 in pancreatitis, 327
Pancreatitis, 312, 322-328
 acute
  complications of, 327
  diagnostic testing for, 325, 325f, 326f
  etiology of, 324, 324t
  severity and grading systems for, 326
  treatment of, 326-327
 case approach for, 327-328
 case presentation of, 322
 chronic
  diagnostic testing for, 325-326
  etiology of, 324, 325t
  treatment of, 327
 description of, 322
 epidemiology of, 322-323, 323t
 familial, 324
 genetic testing for, 326
 pathophysiology of, 323-324
Pantoprazole (Protonix), for gastroesophageal reflux disease, 83t
Papain, for foreign body dissolution, 71
Papillary-cystic epithelial neoplasms, pancreatic, 10
Paraesophageal hernia, following Nissen fundoplication, 84t
Parasitic infection(s), 170-181
 amebic, 172-176, 173f-175f
 blood fluke, 179-181, 180f
 case approach for, 181
 case presentation of, 170
 cestode, 183t-184t
 description of, 170
 epidemiology of, 170-171
 nematode, 176-179, 177f, 178f, 184t-185t
 protozoan, 171-172, 172f, 173f, 182t-183t
Paromomycin, for infectious diarrhea, 129t
Paroxetine, for irritable bowel syndrome, 39
Parvovirus B19 infection(s), neonatal liver failure and, 263t
Peginterferon, for viral hepatitis, 291, 291t
D-Penicillamine, for Wilson disease, 302-303
Pentasa (mesalamine)
 for inflammatory bowel disease, 139
 for ulcerative colitis, 138t
Pepcid (famotidine), for gastroesophageal reflux disease, 83t
Peptic ulcer(s), Helicobacter pylori infection and. See Helicobacter pylori infection(s).
Perianal anomalies, 187-191
 case approach for, 190-191
 case presentation of, 187
 definitions of, 188
 description of, 187
 diagnostic testing for, 189
 differential diagnosis of, 188-189, 189t
 epidemiology of, 187
 pathophysiology of, 188
 treatment of, 189-190
Perirectal abscess(es), 187, 189t
Perirectal infection(s), 187
Peutz-Jeghers syndrome (PJS), 193t, 196-197, 196f, 196t
Peyer's patches, intussusception and, 142
PFIC. See Progressive familial intrahepatic cholestasis (PFIC).
pH monitoring
 esophageal
  in eosinophilic esophagitis, 44
  in gastroesophageal reflux disease, 79-80, 80t

pH monitoring (Continued)
 wireless, in gastroesophageal reflux disease, 80-81, 80t
Pharmacologic therapy. See Drug therapy; specific drugs.
Phosphomannose isomerase deficiency, 256
Photocoagulation, laser, for gastrointestinal bleeding, 94
Phytobezoars, diagnostic testing and management for, 70-71
PI. See Pancreatic insufficiency (PI).
Pigment gallstones, 244, 244t, 245
Pilonidal abscess(es), 187, 189t
PJS. See Peutz-Jeghers syndrome (PJS).
Plain films
 of abdominal masses, 5
 in cholelithiasis, 246
 in constipation, 33t
 in food impactions, 69-70
 in gastrointestinal bleeding, 90
 in malrotation, 153-154
 in Meckel's diverticulum, 159
 in pancreatitis, 326
Pneumatic dilatation, for achalasia, 16
Polycystic liver disease, isolated, 256
Polyp(s), 192-198
 case presentation of, 192
 classification and histology of, 192-193, 194f
 clinical presentation of, 192, 193t
 colonic, removal of, 94-95, 94f, 95f
 description of, 192, 193t
 in familial adenomatous polyposis, 193t, 196t, 197-198, 197f, 198f
 genetic screening and, 198
 hamartomatous, 193-197
  in Bannayan-Riley-Ruvalcaba syndrome, 193t, 195-196, 196t
  in Cowden's syndrome, 193t, 195-196, 196t
  juvenile, 193-194, 194f
  in juvenile polyposis syndrome, 193t, 194-195, 195f, 196t
  in Peutz-Jeghers syndrome, 193t, 196-197, 196f, 196t
 neoplasia and, 194, 195
Polypectomy snares, for foreign body removal, 68
Ponderal growth, measurement of, 49
Positioning therapy, for gastroesophageal reflux disease, 82
Potassium hydroxide, in batteries, 67
PPIs. See Proton pump inhibitors (PPIs).
Prednisolone, for inflammatory bowel disease, 139
Prednisone, for autoimmune hepatitis, 239, 240t
Pregnancy, 11
Premature infants
 feeding, 164-165
 necrotizing enterocolitis in. See Necrotizing enterocolitis.
Prenatal history, failure to thrive and, 56
Prevacid (lansoprazole), for gastroesophageal reflux disease, 83t, 85
Prilosec (omeprazole)
 for gastroesophageal reflux disease, 83t
 for Helicobacter pylori infection, 107
Primary sclerosing cholangitis (PSC), 285-288
 case approach for, 288
 case presentation of, 285
 description of, 285
 diagnostic testing for, 286, 287t
 differential diagnosis of, 287t
 epidemiology of, 285-286, 286t
 overlap with autoimmune hepatitis, 248
 pathophysiology of, 286
 treatment of, 287-288
PRKCSH gene, 256
Probiotics, for small bowel bacterial overgrowth, 221
Progressive familial intrahepatic cholestasis (PFIC), jaundice and, 279
Prokinetics
 for chronic intestinal pseudo-obstruction, 206-207
 for gastroesophageal reflux disease, 83t, 84

Propulsid (cisapride), for gastroesophageal reflux disease, 83t, 84
Protease inhibitor typing, in α_1-AT deficiency, 234-235
Proton pump inhibitors (PPIs)
 for eosinophilic esophagitis, 45
 for gastroesophageal reflux disease, 77, 83, 83t
 for Helicobacter pylori infection, 107
Protonix (pantoprazole), for gastroesophageal reflux disease, 83t
Protozoan infection(s), 171-172, 172f, 173f, 182t-183t
PSC. See Primary sclerosing cholangitis (PSC).
Pseudocyst(s), pancreatic, 9
 in pancreatitis, 327
PTEN gene
 Bannayan-Riley-Ruvalcaba syndrome and, 196
 Cowden's syndrome and, 196
Public health, infectious diarrhea and, 127-128
Pulmonary stenosis, in Alagille syndrome, 230
Purinethol (6-mercaptopurine)
 for inflammatory bowel disease, 139-140
 for ulcerative colitis, 138t
Pyloric stenosis, 8
Pyridoxine, for Wilson disease, 303

R

Rabeprazole (Aciphex), for gastroesophageal reflux disease, 83t
Radionuclide tests. See Scintigraphic studies.
Radiopaque marker transit studies, in constipation, 33t
Ranitidine (Zantac), for gastroesophageal reflux disease, 83t, 85
Rectal abscess(es), 190
Rectal biopsy
 in constipation, 33t
 in Hirschsprung's disease, 116-118, 117f
Rectal duplication cysts, 116
Rectal fistulas, 190
Rectal prolapse, 187, 189t
 cystic fibrosis and, 318
Rectal strictures, in Hirschsprung's disease, 119
Reducing sugars, measurement of, in lactose intolerance, 149
Reglan (metoclopramide)
 for chronic intestinal pseudo-obstruction, 207
 for gastroesophageal reflux disease, 83t, 84
Regurgitation
 in achalasia, 14
 in gastroesophageal reflux disease, 75
Remicade (infliximab)
 for inflammatory bowel disease, 140
 for ulcerative colitis, 138t
Renal anomalies, in Alagille syndrome, 229
Renal manifestations, in Wilson disease, 300t
Renal neoplasm(s), 10
Ribavirin, for viral hepatitis, 291t
Rotavirus enzyme immunoassay, in infectious diarrhea, 127t
Rotavirus infection(s), diarrhea due to, 124
Roth Net retrieval device, for foreign body removal, 68
Round worms, 176-179, 177f, 178f, 184t-185t
Rowasa (mesalamine)
 for inflammatory bowel disease, 139
 for ulcerative colitis, 138t
Rozycki syndrome, 15
Rubella, neonatal liver failure and, 263t
Rumination syndrome, achalasia versus, 14

S

Sacrococcygeal teratoma(s), 10
Salmonella infection, diarrhea due to, treatment of, 129t
Sandifer's syndrome, 75

Sarcoma(s), 9
  hepatic, embryonal, 9
SBBO. See Small bowel bacterial overgrowth (SBBO).
SBDS gene, 331
SBS. See Short bowel syndrome (SBS).
Schistosoma infection(s), 179-181, 180f
Scintigraphic studies
  of abdominal masses, 7
  in achalasia, 15
  in cholelithiasis, 247, 248t
  in gastroesophageal reflux disease, 78, 80t
  in gastrointestinal bleeding, 90-91
  in jaundice, 281
  in Meckel's diverticulum, 159-160, 160t
SDS. See Shwachman-Diamond syndrome (SDS).
SEC63 gene, 256
Secretin-pancreozymin test, in pancreatitis, 326
Sertoli-Leydig tumor(s), 11
Serum thyroxine, in constipation, 33t
Sharp foreign body ingestion(s), diagnostic testing and management for, 67-68, 68f
Shigella infection(s)
  diarrhea due to, treatment of, 129t
  S. dysenteriae infection(s), diarrhea due to, 124
Short bowel syndrome (SBS), 211-215
  case approach for, 215
  case presentation of, 211
  description of, 211
  diagnostic testing for, 213, 213f
  epidemiology of, 211, 212f
  pathophysiology of, 211-212, 212f
  treatment of, 213-215
    of complications, 213-214, 214f
    nutritional, 213, 214f
    surgical, 214-215
Short-segment Hirschsprung's disease, treatment of, 119
Shwachman-Diamond syndrome (SDS), 329-334
  case approach for, 334
  case presentation of, 329, 330f, 331f
  description of, 329
  diagnostic testing for, 333, 333t
  differential diagnosis of, 331-333, 332f, 332t, 333f
  epidemiology of, 329, 331
  pathophysiology of, 331, 332t
  treatment of, 333
Skeletal system, cross-sectional evaluation of, in Shwachman-Diamond syndrome, 332
Skin manifestations, in inflammatory bowel disease, 133
Small bowel bacterial overgrowth (SBBO), 217-222
  case approach for, 221-222, 222f
  case presentation of, 217
  cystic fibrosis and, 318-319
  description of, 217
  diagnostic testing for, 219-220, 220t
  epidemiology of, 217-218, 218t
  pathophysiology of, 218-219
  in short bowel syndrome, treatment of, 214
  treatment of, 206, 220-221
    dietary, 221
    medical, 220-221
    surgical, 221
Small left colon syndrome, 116
Small-bowel obstruction, following Nissen fundoplication, 84t
Smith-Lemli-Opitz syndrome, Hirschsprung's disease and, 115
Soave-Boley operation, for Hirschsprung's disease, 118, 118f
Socioeconomic stressors, failure to thrive and, 61
Sodium hydroxide, in batteries, 67
Sphincter of Oddi manometry, in chronic intestinal pseudo-obstruction, 204
Splenomegaly, in Alagille syndrome, 228
Step-down approach, for gastroesophageal reflux disease, 84
Step-up approach, for gastroesophageal reflux disease, 84
Steroids, for jaundice, 282-283

Stool antigen test, for *Helicobacter pylori* infection, 102-103
Stool culture, in infectious diarrhea, 127t
Stool enzyme immunoassay, in infectious diarrhea, 127t
Stool guaiac test, in infectious diarrhea, 127t
Stool PCR, in infectious diarrhea, 127t
Stool pH, in lactose intolerance, 149
Straight pins, ingested, 68
Streptococcus infection(s), inflammatory bowel disease and, 132
Stricture(s)
  in primary sclerosing cholangitis, treatment of, 288
  in short bowel syndrome, 215
Strongyloides stercoralis infection(s), 176
Suction rectal biopsy, in Hirschsprung's disease, 117-118, 117f
Sulfasalazine, for inflammatory bowel disease, 139
Surgical therapy
  for achalasia, 16-17
  for Alagille syndrome, 230
  for anorectal anomalies, 189-190
  for caustic ingestions, 21, 21t
  for chronic intestinal pseudo-obstruction, 207, 208-209
  for familial adenomatous polyposis, 197-198
  for gastroesophageal reflux disease, 84-85, 84t
  for gastrointestinal bleeding, 95
  for gastrointestinal bleeding diagnosis, 92
  for hemochromatosis, 264
  for Hirschsprung's disease, 118-119, 118f
  for inflammatory bowel disease, 140
  for Meckel's diverticulum, 160
  for short bowel syndrome, 214-215
  for small bowel bacterial overgrowth, 221
  for trichobezoar removal, 71
  for volvulus, 154, 156
Sweat test
  in cystic fibrosis, 317t
  for pancreatic anomalies, 310
Swenson operation, for Hirschsprung's disease, 118, 118f
Systemic diseases, pancreatitis and, 324

T

Taenia saginata infection(s), 183t
Taenia solium infection(s), 184t
Tagamet (cimetidine)
  for gastroesophageal reflux disease, 83t
  in Meckel's diverticulum, 160
Tagged white blood cell scans, of abdominal masses, 7
Tapeworms, 183t-184t
Tegaserod
  for chronic intestinal pseudo-obstruction, 207
  for irritable bowel syndrome, 39
Teratoma(s), sacrococcygeal, 10
Tetracycline, for *Helicobacter pylori* infection, 107
Thermal electrocoagulation, for gastrointestinal bleeding, 93
Thrombin injections, for gastrointestinal bleeding, 92-93
Thromboembolic disease, in inflammatory bowel disease, 134
Thyroid-stimulating hormone, in constipation, 33t
TMP-SMX. See Trimethoprim-sulfamethoxazole (TMP-SMX).
Total colonic aganglionosis, treatment of, 119
Toxic disorders, 229t
Travel history, failure to thrive and, 60
Trichinella spiralis infection(s), 185t
Trichobezoars, diagnostic testing and management for, 70, 71f
Trichuris trichuria infection(s), 178, 178f
Tricyclic antidepressants, for irritable bowel syndrome, 39
Trientine, for Wilson disease, 302, 303

Trimethoprim-sulfamethoxazole (TMP-SMX), for infectious diarrhea, 129t
Triple-A syndrome, 15
Trisomy 21, Hirschsprung's disease and, 114
Tropheryma whippelii infection(s), 171
Trypsin, autodestruct mechanism of, pancreatitis and, 323-324
Trypsinogen, pancreatitis and, 323, 324
TT virus (TTV), *Helicobacter pylori* infection and, 99-100
Tubo-ovarian abscess(es), 9
Turcot's syndrome, 197
Tyrosinemia, 263t
  epidemiology of, 268
  pathophysiology of, 268-269, 268f
  treatment of, 274

U

UBT. See Urea breath test (UBT).
UDCA. See Ursodeoxycholic acid (UDCA).
UGI studies. See Upper gastrointestinal (UGI) studies.
Ulcerative colitis. See also Inflammatory bowel disease (IBD).
  clinical features of, 132-133
Ultra-short-segment Hirschsprung's disease, treatment of, 119
Ultrasound
  of abdominal masses, 5-6
  in chronic intestinal pseudo-obstruction, 202
  in congenital hepatic fibrosis, 258t
  in gastrointestinal bleeding, 91
  in intussusception, 143, 143f
  in jaundice, 281
  in pancreatitis, 325, 325f
  transabdominal
    in cholelithiasis, 246, 247f, 248t
    in pancreatitis, 326
Umbilical hernias, incarcerated, 8
Undernutrition, failure to thrive and. See Failure to thrive.
Upper gastrointestinal (UGI) studies
  of abdominal masses, 7
  in achalasia, 14
  in malrotation, 154, 155f
  in Meckel's diverticulum, 159
Urachal remnant, 9
Urea breath test (UBT), for *Helicobacter pylori* infection, 100-101, 102
Urecholine (bethanechol), for gastroesophageal reflux disease, 83t, 84
Urinary retention, 11
Urine antibody test, for *Helicobacter pylori* infection, 103
Urine tests
  in jaundice, 280
  in small bowel bacterial overgrowth, 220t
Urologic manifestations, in inflammatory bowel disease, 134
Ursodeoxycholic acid (UDCA)
  for cholelithiasis, 250
  for jaundice, 282
  for primary sclerosing cholangitis, 287
Ursodiol, for hepatic fibrosis, 316

V

Vancomycin, for infectious diarrhea, 129t
Varices, esophageal
  bleeding, therapy for, 93-94, 93t, 94f
  in congenital hepatic fibrosis, 258
Vasoactive intestinal peptide-secreting tumors, 10
Vasopressin, for gastrointestinal bleeding, 92
Vibrio cholerae infection(s), diarrhea due to, 124
Video capsule endoscopy, in gastrointestinal bleeding, 91

VIPoma(s), 10
Vitamin A, for infectious diarrhea, 127
Vitamin C, with *Helicobacter pylori* infection, 105
Vitamin deficiencies, in inflammatory bowel disease, 138
Vitamin supplementation, for Shwachman-Diamond syndrome, 333
Volvulus, 116, 152-157
    case approach for, 156
    case presentation of, 152
    description of, 152
    diagnostic testing for, 153-154, 155f
    differential diagnosis of, 153, 154t
    epidemiology of, 152
    pathophysiology of, 153, 153f
    treatment of, 154, 156
Vomiting
    of blood, 88-89
    contraindication to, in caustic ingestions, 21
    differential diagnosis of, 153, 154t
    in gastroesophageal reflux disease, 75

W

Waardenburg-Shah syndrome, Hirschsprung's disease and, 114
Warren, Robert, 98
Weight, measurement of, 49
Weight velocity, tracking, 53, 53t
Western blot test, for *Helicobacter pylori* infection, 101
Whipple's disease, 171
Whipworms, 178, 178f
Wilms' tumor(s), 10
Wilson, Kinnear, 298
Wilson disease, 271, 298-304
    asymptomatic relatives and, 301-302
    case approach for, 303
    case presentation of, 298-299
    description of, 298, 300t
    diagnostic testing for, 300-302, 301f
    differential diagnosis of, 300
    epidemiology of, 299
    genetic testing in, 302
Wilson disease (*Continued*)
    pathophysiology of, 299-300
    treatment of, 298, 302-303, 302f
Wireless pH monitoring, in gastroesophageal reflux disease, 80-81, 80t
Wolman's disease, 271

Y

Yersinia enterocolitica infection(s), diarrhea due to, treatment of, 129t

Z

Zantac (ranitidine), for gastroesophageal reflux disease, 83t, 85
Zellweger syndrome, 263t
Zinc supplementation, for infectious diarrhea, 127
Zinc therapy, for Wilson disease, 303